MEDICAL RADIOLOGY

Diagnostic Imaging and Radiation Oncology

Radiology of the Lower Urinary Tract

With Contributions by
E.S. Amis · W. Anzböck · L.R. Bigongiari · K.S. Cho · E.J. Doganiero
G.W. Friedland · P.F. Fritzsche · W. Hruby · B. Hsu · W. Krampla · E.K. Lang
H.M. Levy · R.F. Mattrey · R.W. McCallum · R.M. Morse · D.S. Moss
H. Mosser · J. Ortenberg · J.A. Parker · I. Perkash · J.M. Pisco · G.L. Popky
M.I. Resnick · L.M. Sanders · G.M. Segall · D.B. Spring · M. Urban
J.C. Winters · H. Zarnow

Edited by

Erich K. Lang

Foreword by

Martin W. Donner and Friedrich H.W. Heuck

With 293 Figures and 14 Tables

Springer-Verlag
Berlin Heidelberg New York London Paris
Tokyo Hong Kong Barcelona Budapest

ERICH K. LANG, M.D.
Professor and Chairman

Department of Radiology, School of Medicine
Louisiana State University, Medical Center
1542 Tulane Avenue, New Orleans, LA 70122-2822, USA

MEDICAL RADIOLOGY · Diagnostic Imaging and Radiation Oncology

Continuation of
Handbuch der medizinischen Radiologie
Encyclopedia of Medical Radiology

ISBN 3-540-53720-1 Springer-Verlag Berlin Heidelberg New York
ISBN 3-387-53720-1 Springer-Verlag New York Berlin Heidelberg

Library of Congress Cataloging-in-Publication Data
Radiology of the lower urinary tract/with contributions by E.S. Amis . . .[et al.]; edited by Erich K. Lang; foreword by Martin W. Donner and Friedrich H.W. Heuck. p. cm. – (Medical radiology)
Includes index.
ISBN 3–540–53720–1 (alk. paper) – ISBN 0–387–53720–1 (alk. paper)
1. Urinary organs-Imaging. I. Amis, E. Stephen. II. Lang, Erich K. (Erich Karl), 1929– . III. Series. [DNLM: 1. Urography. 2. Urologic Diseases-radiography. 3. Bladder-radiography. 4. Genitalia, Male-radiography. WJ 141 R128 1994] RC874.R33 1994 616.6′07572 – dc 20 DNLM/DLC
93-49790

Typesetting: Best-set Typesetter Ltd., Hong Kong
SPIN: 10008929 21/3130-543210 – Printed on acid-free paper

Foreword

Following the favorable reception accorded *Radiology of the Upper Urinary Tract* (edited by E.K. Lang), a complementary volume on the lower urinary tract was naturally demanded, serving to complete the coverage of current radiologic diagnosis of the urinary tract.

The ureter, bladder, and urethra are considered in separate chapters that appraise the value of the various diagnostic radiologic methods in respect of the disease processes and for differential diagnosis.

Particular emphasis is placed on the radiologic findings when the efferent urinary tract is of abnormal form. In the chapter on functional tests of the urinary tract and analysis of excretory disorders, the most recent knowledge from the field of urodynamics is presented. The pathophysiology of vesicoureteral reflux also receives due consideration, and special attention is drawn to the well-structured chapter on radiologic diagnosis of the ureter following surgical procedures, for the important purpose of controlling urinary flow function.

The application of the new radiologic methods for the detection and differential diagnosis of diseases of the male reproductive organs is discussed extensively and critically. Indirect disorders of the urinary tract due to prostatic disease are also considered.

The extensive literature citations include important communications from study groups at European centers. Moreover, against the current trend, important older publications are cited that are fundamental to an understanding of pathomorphologic diagnosis. This serves to prevent an unjustifiable, excessively positive evaluation of the newer investigative methods; such an evaluation often leads proven methods to be neglected, though their use is essential. A danger exists that some pathologic findings, such as discreet alterations of the mucous membrane of the urinary tract, which can only be recognized when diagnostic methods offer sufficient spatial resolution, will no longer be detected and consequently no longer be sought.

The present volume offers comprehensive coverage of the possible applications of diagnostic radiology of the lower urinary tract and should prove of value in daily clinical routine.

M.W. Donner(†), Baltimore

F.H.W. Heuck, Stuttgart

Preface

Advances in diagnostic and interventional radiology, endourology, and clinical urology are occurring at an unprecedentedly rapid rate, often causing wholesale changes in traditional concepts of urologic diagnosis. To meet the formidable challenge of obsolescence, we elected to publish our volumes on radiology of the urinary tract at different dates. This approach, as well as the use of a large group of internationally known experts in the field of uroradiology to write the different chapters, has allowed us to reduce significantly the interim between writing of chapters and the final publication in book form. The second volume of this series, *Radiology of the Lower Urinary Tract*, benefits from this approach and includes discussions of the newest imaging modalities and the latest interventional uroradiologic and endourologic procedures, as well as extensive and up-to-date references. The text is written to satisfy the needs of the practicing radiologist and urologist but also to offer up-to-date information and references to the researcher. The text is embellished with 432 carefully selected and representative illustrations.

Interventional uroradiology has become an important nonsurgical alternative for patient management. Interventional uroradiologic techniques are presented in minute detail to allow the reader not only to establish their value in treatment or diagnosis of a given condition, but also hopefully to serve as a source guiding the performance of these interventions.

Radiology of the Lower Urinary Tract is divided into 19 chapters. In each chapter the pertinent clinical, laboratory, and pathologic findings of the disease entities are presented and the contributions of diagnostic and interventional uroradiologic techniques elucidated. Detailed discussions of embryology, anatomy, and pathophysiology are added to facilitate understanding of the disease process and anticipated complications, and form the rationale for interventions.

The first five chapters deal with conditions of the ureter, two chapters with disease of the bladder, and one chapter with vesicoureteral reflux. This last chapter discusses the concept held by the practicing urologist and emphasizes data needed for treatment of such patients.

The following eight chapters deal with anatomy, physiology, and diagnosis of diseases of the prostate. A comprehensive picture from clinical screening examinations for prostatic neoplasms, to detailed diagnostic assessment by the most advanced imaging as well as interventional techniques is assembled. The presentation is backed by an extensive and up-to-date bibliography.

One chapter is devoted to neurogenic disease afflicting the bladder and physiology of incontinence. The pathophysiology of these conditions is discussed and their diagnosis by imaging techniques and urodynamic studies presented.

The chapter on the testis and scrotum brings to the attention of the reader the most recent diagnostic advances in magnetic resonance, ultrasound, as well as Doppler color ultrasound imaging techniques for assessment of this system.

A chapter on the urethra reviews the complex normal anatomy and then presents diagnostic techniques for identification of disease and injury of this organ.

A separate chapter deals with diagnosis of diseases of the seminal vesicles by today's imaging techniques. Once again, an appropriate introduction into the embryology and anatomy of this organ system facilitates understanding of the pathophysiology.

Although some information has been duplicated in various chapters, this approach was introduced to: (1) make information more readily available to the reader, and (2) present a different point of view with different emphasis. Idiosyncrasies of individual authors and their points of view have been respected and maintained.

It is hoped by the contributors and the editor that this work will be accepted as the standard working and reference text of radiology of the lower urinary tract.

Erich K. Lang, New Orleans

Contents

1 Ureteral Neoplasms

JANET A. PARKER, ENRICO J. DOGANIERO, and GEORGE L. POPKY

CONTENTS

1.1 Introduction

Primary neoplasms of the ureter are uncommon; they account for less than 1% of urinary tract tumors and are found in 1 in 11000 autopsies (LEDER and DUNNICK 1990; MURPHY 1989). Fewer than 3000 cases have appeared in the literature since the first authenticated case was reported in 1878 (POLLACK 1990).

Ureteral cancer is more common in males, with a male/female ratio of 3:1 (ZORETIC and GONZALES 1983). It is rarely seen prior to the fifth decade of life; the mean age of patients with ureteral carcinoma is 63 years (WITTERS et al. 1987).

The distal third of the ureter is involved in 50%–70% of cases, the middle third in 15%–25%, and the upper third in 10%–12% (SCOTT and McDONALD 1970).

A propensity for multicentricity is an important feature of urothelial carcinomas in general. Upper urinary tract tumors are multicentric in 22%–44% of cases; 12% of patients with ureteral cancer have multiple sites involved at the time of diagnosis, and 4% present with bilateral ureteral involvement (MILLS and VAUGHAN 1983). Synchronous or metachronous bladder cancer is seen in 30%–50% of cases (ZORETIC and GONZALES 1983). The detection of any urothelial neoplasm necessitates careful and repeated evaluation of the entire urinary tract.

JANET A. PARKER, M.D., Professor of Radiology; ENRICO J. DOGANIERO, D.O., Instructor with Radiology; GEORGE L. POPKY, M.D., Professor and Chairman; Department of Radiological Sciences, PCOM, Graduate Health System, City Avenue Hospital, 4150 City Avenue, Philadelphia, PA 19131, USA

1.2 Pathology

The overwhelming majority of primary ureteral neoplasms are urothelial, and well over 90% of these are transitional cell tumors. At least 60% of these are papillary, generally well differentiated, noninvasive, low-grade tumors. Nonpapillary transitional cell carcinomas may present as flat, nodular, or ulcerated lesions. They tend to invade and metastasize early (LEDER and DUNNICK 1990; BENNINGTON and BECKWITH 1975; SKINNER and LEISKOVSK 1988).

Squamous cell carcinomas and adenocarcinomas represent about 5% and 2% of ureteral carcinomas respectively (BATATA et al. 1975). They are rare lesions, usually associated with chronic irritation, inflammation, and/or ureteral stones. They are rapidly invasive and have a uniformly poor prognosis (MURPHY 1989).

A variety of rare neoplasms and nonneoplastic tumorous conditions, including leiomyoma, neurofibroma, hemangioma, leiomyosarcoma, mixed mesodermal tumor, amyloid, endometriosis, cholesteatoma, inverted papilloma, spindle cell carcinoma, signet ring adenocarcinoma, and undifferentiated carcinoma have been reported in the ureter (MURPHY 1989; DELAHUNT et al. 1992; KINI et al. 1991).

Endometriosis of the ureter, while rare, may cause progressive ureteral obstruction with loss of renal function in 25%–43% of cases (PATEL et al. 1992; RYAN and BOOTH 1992).

The most common benign mesodermal ureteral tumor is the fibroepithelial polyp, found in the proximal ureter and almost always solitary. Usually seen in adults, fibroepithelial polyps may also be seen in children, in whom they are a rare cause of ureteral obstruction. Boys are affected in about 81% of cases, and the left ureter is involved in 70%. Appropriate treatment is local excision. The prognosis is excellent (GALIFER et al. 1988; LIDDELL et al. 1991; DEBRUNGNE et al. 1980).

Metastatic disease involving the ureter, except by direct extension, is rare. It can occur by urinary, hematogenous, lymphatic, and direct routes. The ureter can be involved by metastases from downstream seeding from a primary renal or renal pelvis tumor, or by upstream seeding from a bladder neoplasm. Tumors of the bladder and renal pelvis may also involve the ureters through direct intraureteral extension. Metastatic lesions by hematogenous and lymphatic routes can occur from almost any primary site. Seeding of neoplasms from the gonadal vein to the ureteric vein and implantation in the ureter is observed with neoplasms of the female pelvic organs. Particularly on the left side, seeding and tumor implantation may be observed all the way to the level of the renal pelvis since the gonadal vein ends in the left renal vein (FRIEDENBERG et al. 1976). The maligancies metastasizing to the ureter most commonly are cancers of the breast, stomach, and colon and melanoma (GELISTER et al. 1992). Direct extension from pelvic or retroperitoneal malignancies to the ureter is more common and is most frequently due to extension from carcinoma of the cervix. Malignancies primary in the rectosigmoid, prostate, or pancreas and lymphomas may also involve the ureter extrinsically. Ureteral stenosis is the characteristic finding in these lesions. CT scans demonstrate a thickened regular ureteral wall at the level of the narrowing. Early recognition and appropriate treatment for relief of obstruction may prolong survival in these patients (POLLACK 1990; GELISTER et al. 1992; PUECH et al. 1987; AMBOS et al. 1979).

Metastatic disease is more common in ureteral than in bladder cancers, occurring in more than 10% of patients. This is attributed to the extensive lymphatic and vascular system in the thin wall of the ureter. When metastases from primary ureteral cancer are present, they involve the retroperitoneal nodes in 34% of cases, distant nodes in 17%, the liver in 17%, lumbar or sacral vertebrae in 15%, lungs or kidneys in about 10%, and adrenals, brain, pancreas, and skin less frequently (POLLACK 1990; SCOTT and McDONALD 1970).

Table 1.1. TNM staging system

Primary tumor (T)	
TX	Primary tumor cannot be assessed
T0	No evidence of primary tumor
Tis	Carcinoma in situ
Ta	Papillary nonivasive carcinoma
T1	Tumor invades subepithelial connective tissue
T2	Tumor invades muscularis
T3	Tumor invades beyond muscularis into periureteric or peripelvic fat or renal parenchyma
T4	Tumor invades adjacent organs or through the kidney into perinephric fat
Regional lymph nodes (N)	
NX	Regional lymph nodes cannot be assessed
N0	No regional lymph node metastasis
N1	Metastasis in a single lymph node, 2 cm or less in greatest dimension
N2	Metastasis in a single lymph node, more than 2 cm but not more than 5 cm in greatest dimension, or multiple lymph nodes, none more than 5 cm in greatest dimension
N3	Metastasis in a lymph node more than 5 cm in greatest dimension
Distant metastasis (M)	
MX	Presence of distant metastasis cannot be assessed
M0	No distant metastasis
M1	Distant metastasis

Table 1.2. Stage grouping (TNM system)

Stage	0	Tis	N0	M0
		Ta	N0	M0
Stage I	A	T1	N0	M0
Stage II	B	T2	N0	M0
Stage III	C	T3	N0	M0
Stage IV	D	T4	N0	M0
		Any T	N1, N2, N3	M0
		Any T	Any N	MI

1.3 Staging and Grading

In 1971, GRABSTALD et al. first suggested a staging system for renal pelvic tumors based on histology and extent of tumor; this has remained the basis for staging urinary tract cancers. The American Joint Committee on Cancer first published a TNM staging system and a grading system for carcinomas of the renal pelvis and ureter in 1988 (Tables 1.1, 1.2) (BEAHRS 1988). This system requires that clinical assessment of the primary tumor include radiographic imaging, endoscopic evaluation, and ureteroscopy when applicable. Clinical evaluation for metastases includes radiographic, radioisotopic, and laboratory studies. For pathologic staging histologic confirmation of extent of disease is required (Table 1.3).

Table 1.3. Histopathologic grading, according to the American Joint Committee on Cancer. (Modified from BEAHRS 1988)

GX	Grade cannot be assessed
G1	Well differentiated
G2	Moderately well differentiated
G3	Poorly differentiated
G4	Undifferentiated

Table 1.4. Correlation between 5-year survival rates and pathologic stage

Pathologic stage			5-year survival
0		T0	100%
I	A	T1	80%
II	B	T2	50%
III	C	T3	33%
IV	D	T4	0%–10%

1.4 Prognosis

The prognosis for patients with ureteral neoplasms is dependent on histologic type, grade, and stage of the tumor. Nontransitional cell carcinomas (squamous cell, adeno carcinoma, undifferentiated) have a uniformly poor prognosis. Even those of low histologic grade invade and metastasize early (HENEY et al. 1981).

The papillary transitional cell carcinomas that are well differentiated and noninvasive have an excellent prognosis. The nonpapillary lesions that are high grade, high stage have a poor prognosis. Five-year survival figures (MURPHY 1989; POLLACK 1990; ZORETIC and GONZALES 1983; BATATA et al. 1975; BADALAMENT et al. 1990; YOSHINO et al. 1990; STROBEL et al. 1984) show a high correlation of survival with stage (Table 1.4).

Histologic grade is also of prognostic significance. HUBEN et al. (1988) report a median survival of 67 months in 25 patients with grade I and II cancers, compared to 14 months in 29 patients whose cancers were grade III and IV ($P = 0.0004$).

The prognostic value of DNA ploidy in upper urinary tract transitional cell carcinomas remains uncertain. BADALAMENT et al. (1990) reported that in their univariate analysis, DNA ploidy was the only significant predictor of disease-free survival ($P = 0.04$). Patients with aneuploid tumors had a disease-free median survival of 19 months versus 59 months for those with diploid tumors. Tumor stage, however, was the only significant factor associated with overall survival in univariate and multivariate analysis ($P = 0.02$ and 0.005 respectively). In patients with high-grade, high-stage tumors DNA ploidy does not provide additional prognostic information. However, the presence of DNA aneuploidy in low-grade, low-stage tumors may identify a set of patients at increased risk of death from upper urinary tract cancers.

1.5 Etiology

The exact etiology of urothelial cancers is not known. Many environmental carcinogens have been implicated in this malignancy. Chronic exposure to *ortho*-aminophenol compounds contained in aniline dyes used in textile, plastic, and printing industries is known to be associated with uroepithelial tumors. N-Hydroxylation of these compounds by enzymes in the urine results in the production of carcinogenic compounds (SKINNER and LEISKOVSK 1988; ROBBINS and COTRAN 1988).

Cigarette, pipe, and cigar smoking increases the risk of transitional cell carcinoma. A proposed mechanism is interference with tryptophan metabolism resulting in increased excretion of metabolites of tryptophan that have structural similarities to the *ortho*-aminophenol compounds. In their population-based case control study, Ross et al. (1989) identified cigarette smoking as the major risk factor for cancers of the renal pelvis and ureter, with smokers having a relative risk of 4.5 compared to nonsmokers ($P = 0.0001$).

The statistical association between abuse of phenacetin-containing analgesics and upper urinary tract carcinoma is convincing. The major metabolite of phenacetin is N-acetyl *para*-aminophenol, which resembles other known urothelial carcinogens (JOHANSSON et al. 1974).

Papillary transitional cell tumors of the ureters occur more frequently in Balkan countries than in any other area of the world. In 1968 PETKOVIĆ reported an increased incidence of upper urinary tract tumors in populations at risk for Balkan endemic nephropathy (BEN). Upper urinary tract tumors are 100 times more frequent in areas where BEN is endemic than in nonendemic areas. BEN is a chronic tubulointerstitial kidney disease restricted to well-defined geographic areas along tributaries of the Danube in Yugoslavia, Bulgaria, and Romania. BEN is more common in women than in men, accounting for the sex distribution of upper urinary tract tumors in endemic areas, where the male to female ratio is 1.7 to 1, compared to large cities where BEN is not present and where the male to female ratio is 5.2 to 1. A common etiology for both the nephropathogenic and carcinogenic processes has been suggested. Both genetic and environmental factors are thought to be operative (PETRONIC et al. 1991; CUKURANAVIC et al. 1991). Ochratoxin A may play a role. It is ubiquitous in regions where BEN is common and has been demonstrated to damage the renal cortex and induce renal parenchymal carcinomas in experimental animals (BACH 1991).

The association of urothelial tumors with cyclophosphamide administration has been documented since 1971 (BRENNER and SCHELLHAMMER 1987). The first case of ureteral cancer following cyclophosphamide therapy was reported in 1982 (SHETTY and TABACOCHALI 1987). Neoplasms have been observed only after prolonged exposure to cyclophosphamide and a minimum dose of 90 g. There is usually a long latency between exposure and urothelial neoplasia. The ureteral cancers associated with cyclophosphamide therapy tend to be high grade and extremely aggressive (BENNINGTON and BECKWITH 1975).

Patients with bladder carcinoma and associated vesicoureteral reflux have approximately a 15-fold greater risk of upper urinary tract cancer than those without vesicoureteral reflux (DAS 1985).

An increased index of suspicion and close surveillance for ureteral cancer is required in patients at increased risk, including patients with a history of exposure to environmental carcinogens, heavy smoking, analgesic (phenacetin) abuse, cyclophosphamide therapy, BEN, bladder cancer with associated vesicoureteral reflux, or any urothelial neoplasm.

1.6 Clinical Presentation

Approximately 20% of the patients with ureteral neoplasms will be asymptomatic (ZORETIC and GONZALES 1983; GHUZI et al. 1979). Hematuria, either gross or microscopic, is a presenting symptom in 50%–75% of cases (SCOTT and MCDONALD 1970). Flank pain is present in 25%–30% (LEDER and DONNICK 1990; GHUZI et al. 1979).

A palpable mass due to a hydronephrotic kidney will be found in up to 30%. Frequency and dysuria are less common presenting symptoms. Despite its infrequency, ureteral neoplasm should be a diagnostic consideration in patients who present with otherwise unexplained hematuria and/or flank pain (BADALAMENT et al. 1990).

1.7 Diagnostic Procedures

Radiologic evaluation is critical for the detection, clinical staging, and follow-up evaluation of patients with ureteral neoplasms.

Plain films of the chest and abdomen are useful for detection of ureteral stones, an enlarged kidney due to hydronephrosis, or evidence of pulmonary or osseous metastatic disease.

Excretory urography is a primary tool in establishing the diagnosis of ureteral neoplasm(s). It will demonstrate a nonfunctioning kidney in 25%–50% of patients and hydronephrosis with or without hydroureter in 25%–35%. One or more ureteral defects will be evident with or without hydronephrosis in up to 25% of cases (LEDER and DUNNICK 1990; POLLACK 1990; WITTERS et al. 1987; GHUZI et al. 1979). The surface of a ureteral defect due to transitional cell carcinoma may be smooth, irregular, or stippled. The "stipple sign" results from the trapping of contrast in the interstices of a papillary tumor (POLLACK 1990).

If the kidney is not functional because of prolonged obstruction, excretory urography will not be diagnostic. Retrograde or antegrade ureterography will be necessary.

Retrograde ureterography has a diagnostic accuracy of between 70% and 90% in the diagnosis of ureteral tumors. It is presently the most useful diagnostic procedure for the study of intraluminal ureteral lesions (LEDER and DUNNICK 1990). The significant finding on retrograde ureterography is the presence of single or multiple filling defects. These may have a wide range of radiologic presentations. The classic papillary tumor with a long stalk is quite mobile and may demonstrate the "flip-flop" phenomenon (SWANSON and ZINCKE 1983). Unique to mobile ureteral carcinomas is the so-called goblet sign. This is the "champagne glass"-shaped dilatation of the ureter below the tumor. It is caused, in part, by repeated prolapse of the tumor during ureteral peristalsis. It may result in Bergman's sign – coiling of the ureteral catheter in the dilated ureter below the tumor.

Fig. 1.2. A retrograde ureterogram demonstrates the classical "champagne glass" configuration of the right mid ureter indicative of relatively low-grade papillary transitional cell carcinoma. (Courtesy of E.K. LANG, M.D.) ▷

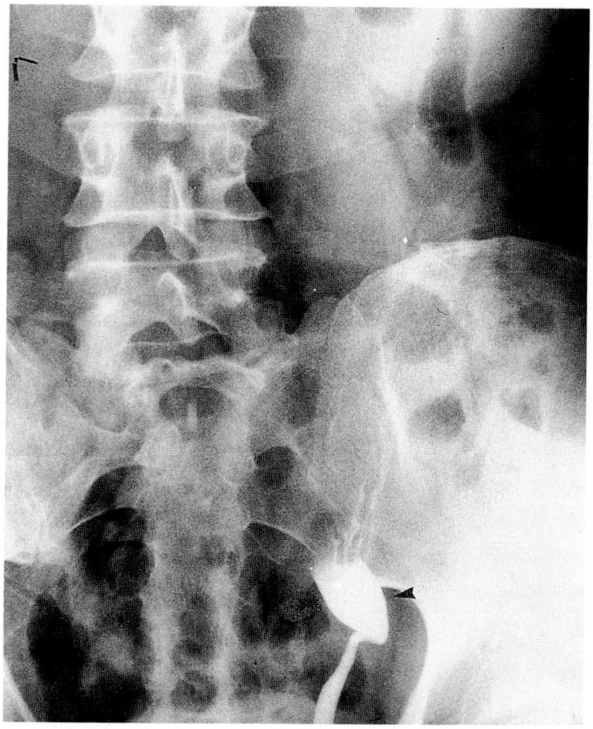

Fig. 1.1. A retrograde ureterogram demonstrates dilatation of the segment of the ureter distal to an obstruction (*arrows*). This "champagne glass" configuration is characteristic for a low-grade papillary transitional cell carcinoma. (Courtesy of E.K. LANG, M.D.)

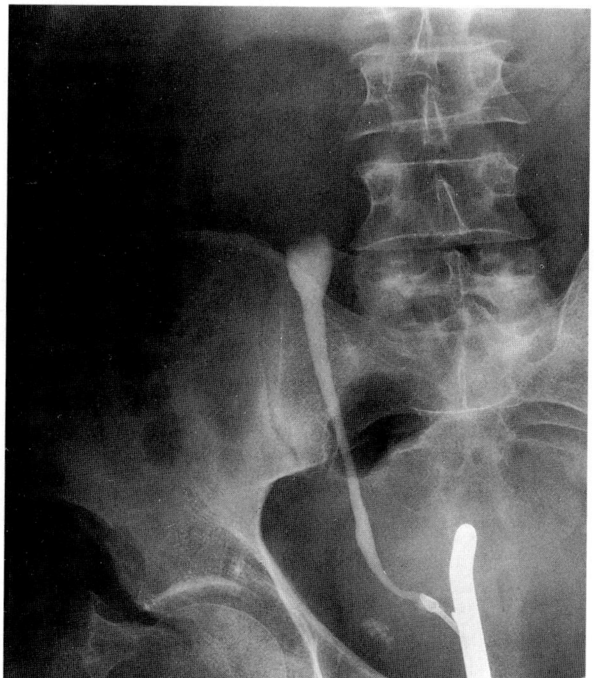

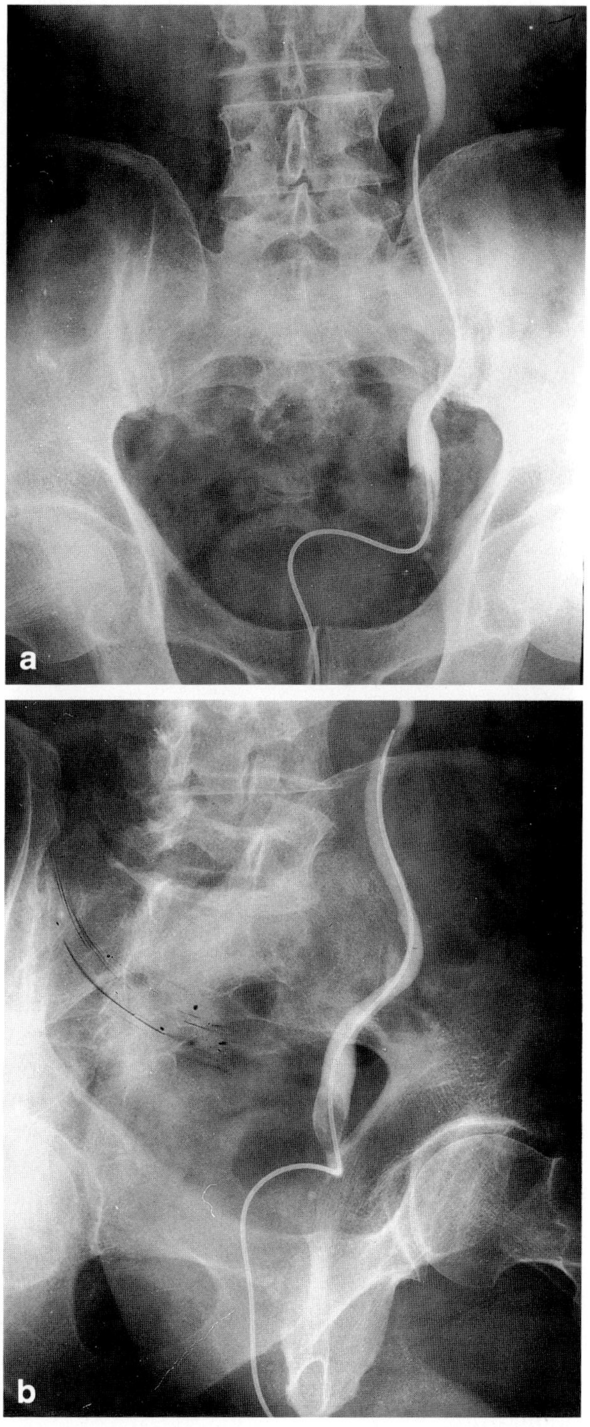

Fig. 1.3 a,b. A ureteral catheter has been advanced above a 1.5 × 1 cm papillary tumor in the distal left ureter. The ureter above the mass is likewise dilated. The ease of passing a catheter in a retrograde fashion above the lesion indicates that the tumor has gradually dilated the ureter and there is no fixation of the wall of the ureter. Note the lace-like pattern indicating slight nodularity of the papillary tumor projecting into the lumen of the ureter. (Courtesy of E.K. LANG, M.D.)

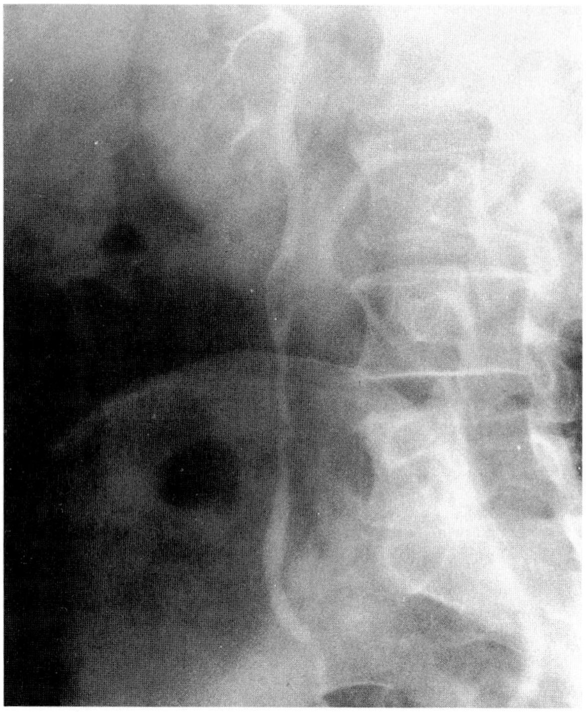

Fig. 1.4. The intravenous urogram demonstrates an approximately 2 × 1 cm oval defect in the mid-right ureter. Note some dilatation of the ureter above and below the lesion, but unabated passage of contrast medium-laden urine in the gutters around the tumor. The normal appearance of the calyces attests atest to the nonobstructive nature of the lesions. (Courtesy of E.K. LANG, M.D.)

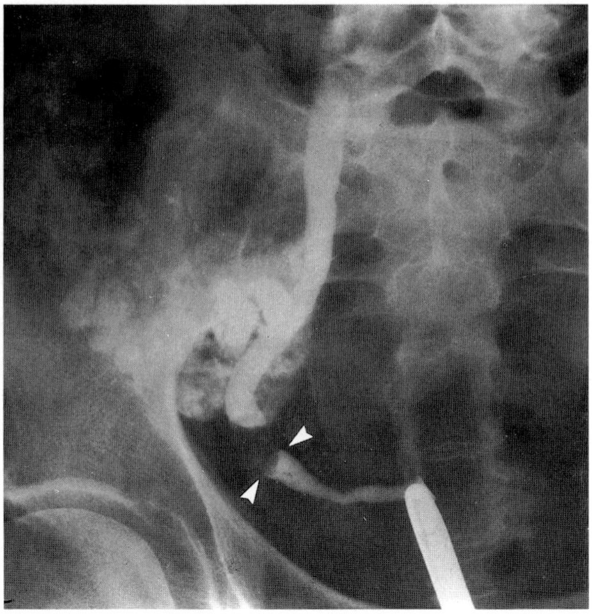

Fig. 1.5. A mass is demonstrated in the distal right ureter on a retrograde ureterogram. Note "a shoulder effect" (*arrows*) as well as dilatation of the entire ureter above the lesion. This indicates some degree of obstruction and also early infiltration of the wall of the ureter resulting in "tumor shoulder". (Courtesy of E.K. LANG, M.D.)

Nonpapillary tumors generally present as fixed or ovoid filling defects which may show evidence of ulceration. Sometimes the tumor may mimic an inflammatory stricture (POLLACK 1990). It is very important to obtain cytologic or biopsy specimens during the procedure. Diverse findings on retrograde ureterograms are presented in Figs. 1.1–1.10.

Retrograde ureterography is not always satisfactory. Often it cannot demonstrate the superior surface of a ureteral tumor or detect the presence of lesions in the renal pelvis or ureter above the obstructing mass. It may be technically difficult and should always be performed with fluoroscopic monitoring.

Antegrade pyeloureterography permits visualization of the superior surface of a ureteral tumor and identification of abnormality above it. It is, however, a somewhat more invasive procedure, and more likely than the retrograde approach to be technically unsatisfactory.

The presence of one or more ureteral filling defects on excretory urography or retrograde or

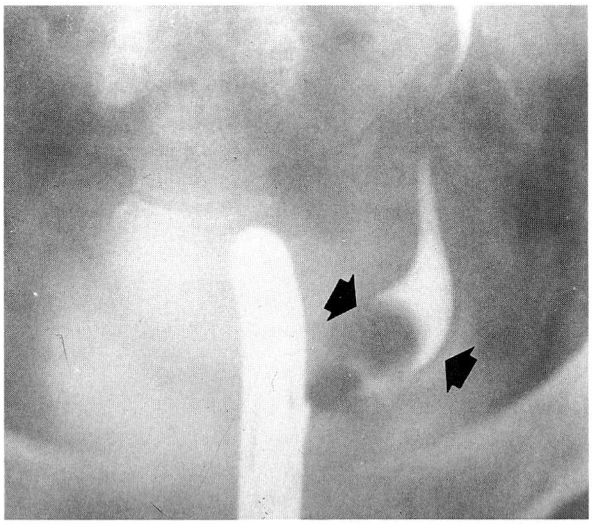

Fig. 1.6. A mass is demonstrated in the intramural segment of the left ureter (*arrows*). This represented one of several papillary transitional cell tumors in the left ureter and kidney pelvis. (Courtesy of E.K. LANG, M.D.)

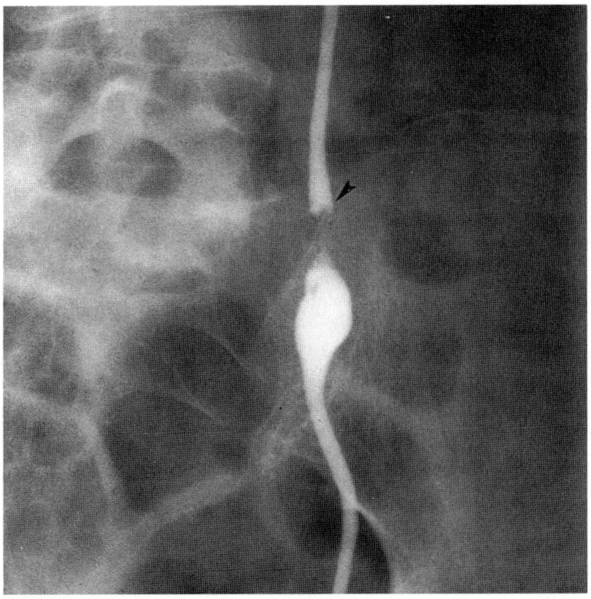

Fig. 1.7. An "applecore deformity" of a 1.5-cm segment of the left ureter is shown below the lesion; the ureter is dilated, and the upper edge of the lesion shows several nodular irregularities (*arrowtip*). This appearance suggests a low-grade transitional cell papillary tumor that has degenerated into an undifferentiated transitional cell tumor which is now invading the wall of the ureter. Histologic examination of the specimen revealed grade 1 through grade 4 tumor elements. (Courtesy of E.K. LANG, M.D.)

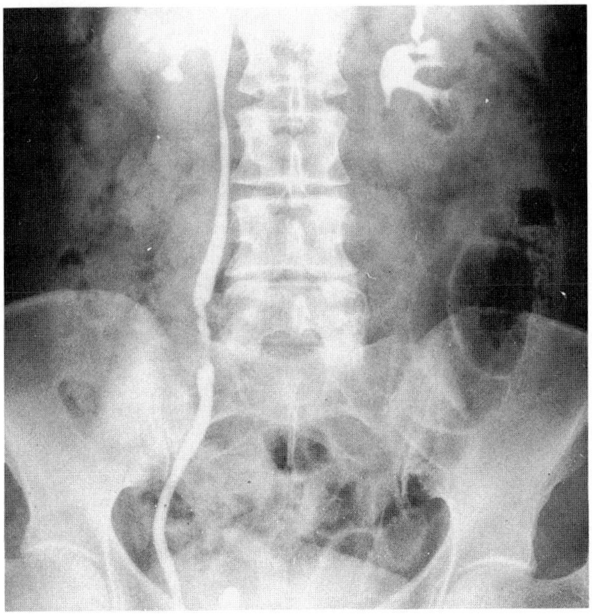

Fig. 1.8. A retrograde ureterogram demonstrates a 3-cm stenotic lesion with a corkscrew appearance involving the right mid ureter. The appearance is characteristic for an undifferentiated transitional cell carcinoma invading the wall of the ureter. (Courtesy of E.K. LANG, M.D.)

antegrade studies is not diagnostic of ureteral neoplasm. Ureteral filling defects are nonspecific and are seen with a number of benign and malignant processes. The differential diagnosis of solitary ureteral defects, in addition to neoplasm, includes stone, blood clot, vascular imprint, ureteral kink, sloughed papilla, fungus ball, cholesteatoma, malacoplakia, amyloidosis, and congenital cyst or web. Most of these lesions can also cause multiple or diffuse ureteral filling defects (FEIN and MCCLENNON 1986; WILLIAMSON et al. 1986).

Ultrasonographic techniques will not demonstrate ureteral tumors because of overlying bone and gas-filled bowel. Ultrasonography can be useful, however, in demonstrating hydronephrosis (GHUZI et al. 1979).

Computed tomography (CT) is more useful for staging than for detecting ureteral neoplasms. It

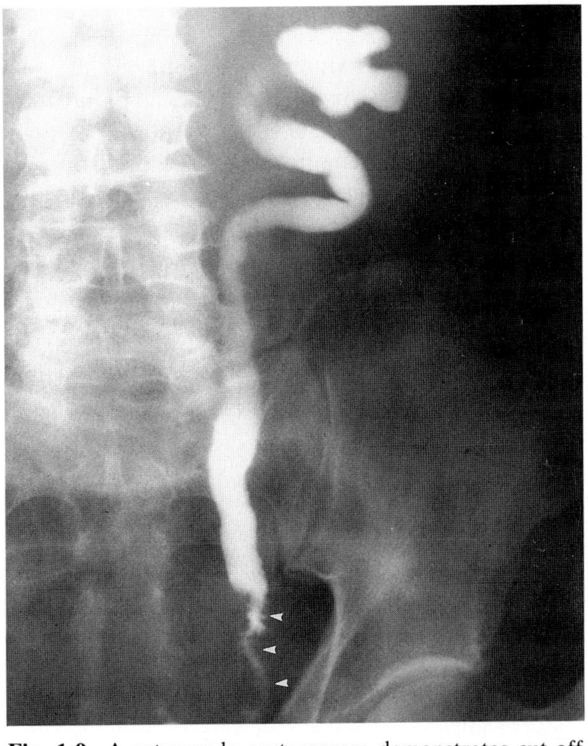

Fig. 1.9. A retrograde ureterogram demonstrates cut-off in the distal left ureter with a resulting "champagne glass" deformity. Above that the ureter is narrowed over a 6-cm segment with a feathery and serated appearance (*white arrowheads*). The former manifestation suggests a relatively low-grade papillary transitional cell carcinoma, the latter an infiltrating transitional cell carcinoma with resultant lymphatic obstruction. The resected specimen demonstrated lymphectasia and an infiltrating transitional cell carcinoma with papillary elements and histologic grade 1 through 3. (Courtesy of E.K. LANG, M.D.)

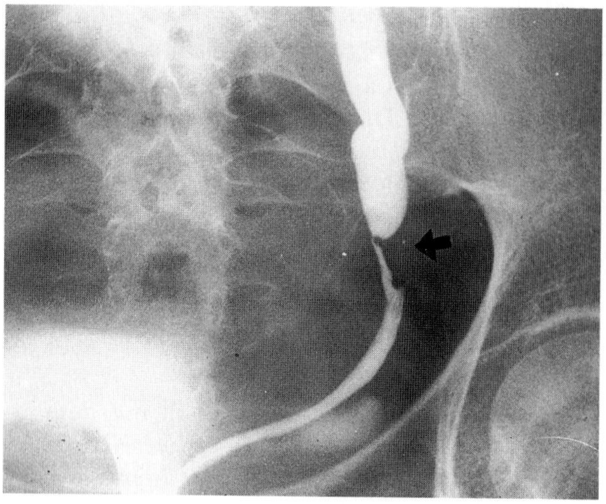

Fig. 1.10. A retrograde ureterogram demonstrates a stenotic lesion in the left ureter with dilatation of the ureter above. Two nodular masses protrude into the stenotic lesion, representing prominent tumor growth from a basically infiltrative grade 3 transitional cell carcinoma. (Courtesy of E.K. LANG, M.D.)

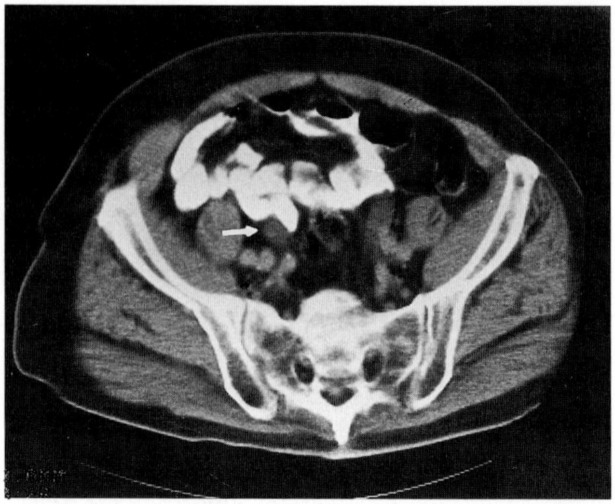

Fig. 1.11. A computed tomogram through the pelvis demonstrates a right ureter with faint staining of the thickened wall (*white arrows*). Several staining 1-cm nodes did not harbor transitional cell carcinoma. (Courtesy of E.K. LANG, M.D.)

can, however, be valuable in identifying the primary tumor in an obstructed ureter. The ureteral tumor will appear as a soft tissue mass greater in density than the urine in the dilated ureter above it. The primary may also appear as a thickening of the ureteral wall (Figs. 1.11, 1.12).

It is important to obtain a precontrast study to avoid nonvisualization of the ureteral tumor because of volume averaging (KENNEY and STANLEY 1987). The ability of CT to demonstrate direct tumor extension through the ureteral wall is important since this is a sensitive indicator of high-stage disease. In the absence of this finding, however, CT is of limited value (BADALAMENT et al. 1992).

Results must be viewed with caution, particularly when precise preoperative clinical staging is essential (McCOY et al. 1991). CT and MRI have been found to be effective in the assessment of contiguous extension of the tumor into the periureteral fat (MILESTON et al. 1990; WINALSKI et al. 1990).

Angiography is generally not needed for detection of ureteral tumors. If it is performed, the ureteral neoplasm is seen as a hypovascular mass. Arterial encasement and neovascularity may be demonstrated in the region of the tumor (LEDER and DUNNICK 1990; POLLACK 1990).

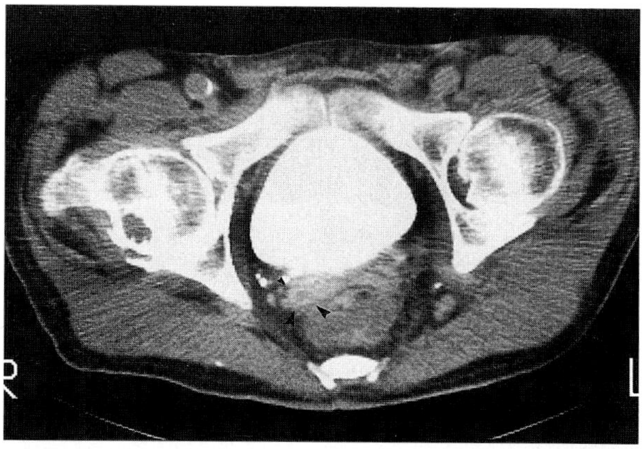

Fig. 1.12. Following administration of intravenous contrast medium a computed tomogram in the true pelvis demonstrates the thickened and staining wall of the right ureter (*arrowheads*). The low-density center represents nonopaque urine due to total obstruction of the ureter by a neoplasm extending from the parametrial segment into the intramural segment of the right ureter. An edematous appearance of the right parametrium is noted; however, histologically there was no extension of the ureteric neoplasm. (Courtesy of E.K. LANG, M.D.)

1.8 Treatment

The primary treatment of ureteral carcinoma is surgical, but there is considerable controversy regarding the best surgical procedure. Classic radical treatment consists of nephroureterctomy with removal of a bladder cuff (LEDER and

Dunnick 1990). This procedure continues to be advocated by many who cite the frequency of clinically unrecognized multiple ipsilateral tumor involvement discovered only on histologic examination of the entire ureter (Hatch et al. 1988). In addition, recurrence rates of 20%–43% have been reported with lesser procedures, with the majority of recurrences being of increased grade and/or stage (Charbit et al. 1991). However, nephroureterectomy is contraindicated in patients who have only one kidney, have bilateral synchronous ureteral tumors, have poor renal function, are poor risks for surgery, or have evidence of nodal or hematogenous metastatic disease (Pollack 1990; Zoretic and Gonzales 1983; Witters et al. 1987). More conservative therapeutic options are available for the majority of patients with ureteral neoplasms. Segmental resection is the major alternative to nephroureterectomy. It appears to be effective in those patients who have a single tumor of low histologic grade and early stage involving the distal third of the ureter. Witters et al. (1987) reported survivals of 80% in patients undergoing segmental resection compared with 64% in patients undergoing complete nephroureterectomy with bladder cuff excision.

Accurate pretreatment assessment is essential to define those groups of patients whose cancers may be amenable to local resection, those who would benefit from nephroureterectomy with removal of a bladder cuff, and those who, because of metastatic disease, will not be cured by either local resection or radical surgery.

Technological advances of the past decade have enabled urologists to utilize endourologic techniques for diagnosis and treatment of ureteral neoplasms. Blute et al. (1989) report a diagnostic accuracy of 90% (19 of 21) and a control rate of 85% (11 of 13) following endourologic procedures. They recommend that conservative endourologic techniques be considered for the management of selected cases. Endoscopic intervention may be of particular importance in older patients whose tolerance of nephroureterectomy is poor (Moldwin et al. 1990). Because patient numbers are few and follow-up has been limited, the long-term effectiveness of endourologic treatment has not yet been documented. Ideally, only patients who have small, single, low-grade, papillary tumors confined to the mucosa and negative random biopsies of contiguous mucosa are suitable candidates (Carson 1991).

Recent improvements in laser technology including small-caliber quartz fibers for the neodymium yttrium aluminum garnet (Nd:YAG) laser have made endoscopic laser treatment feasible. Tumor destruction can be accomplished with the Nd:YAG laser placed through a flexible ureteroscope. Following adequate treatment a double-J ureteral stent must be placed and remain in position for a time adequate to permit ureteral healing. Ureteroscopic and radiographic follow-up of these patients must be carried out to identify recurrence or development of new lesions (Carson 1991; Grossman et al. 1992).

The role of adjuvant radiation therapy in the management of ureteral neoplasms is not clear. In their recent review of radiation therapy in locally advanced transitional cell carcinomas of the renal pelvis or ureter following curative resection, Cozad et al. (1992) report actuarial 5-year local control rates of 88% in patients who received adjuvant radiation therapy and 34% in those who did not. Local failure occurred in 9 of the 17 who did not receive radiation and one of the nine who did ($P = 0.07$). Brookland and Richter (1985) report similar results in a series of 95 patients, 23 of whom had high-grade and/or high-stage lesions. Eleven received postoperative radiation therapy. None of the radiated patients failed with local disease only. One had both local and distant recurrence. In the nonirradiated group of 12, five patients had local failure and there were twice the number of failures overall.

Adjuvant radiation therapy markedly reduces the risk of local failure but has no impact on distant disease, which occurs in approximately 50% of patients with high-stage, high-grade tumors. Effective adjuvant therapy will require effective systemic therapy in addition to adjuvant local radiation.

Combination chemotherapy, primarily CMV (cisplatin, methotrexate, vinblastine) regimens were initially evaluated in the early 1980s. Complete response rates of 20%–30% and combined complete and partial response rates of 50%–60% were reported (Yagoda 1985). A more recent report of CMV chemotherapy for advanced transitional cell carcinoma by Jeffrey and Meade (1992) confirms a complete response rate of 28%. The median survival of complete responders was 13 months compared to 7 months for the entire group and 3 months for untreated patients. Toxicity was significant. Tannock et al. (1989) reported the Princess Margaret Hospital experience with MVAC (methotrexate, vinblastine, doxorubicin, cisplatin) chemotherapy in the treatment of locally extensive metastatic transitional cell carcinoma. Four of the 30 patients with measurable disease were complete responders. The toxicity of the regimen was severe. They concluded that despite the fact that an occasional patient may benefit from presently available chemotherapy, it is clear that less toxic, more effective agents are needed. Nevertheless, mitomycin C does appear to be effective in preventing recurrence of urothelial tumors after resection of the primary (EASTHAN and HUFFMAN 1993).

Appropriate primary and adjuvant therapy for ureteral neoplasms remains controversial.

References

Ambos MA, Bosniak MA, Megbow AJ (1979) Ureteral involvement by metastatic disease. Urol Radiol: 103–112

Bach PH (1991) A molecular basis for target cell toxicity and upper urothelial carcinoma in analogesic abusers and patients with Balkan endemic nephropathy. In: Castegnaro M, Plestina R, Dirheimer G, Chernozemsky IN, Bartsch H (eds) Mycotoxins, endemic nephropathy and urinary tract tumors. IARC 115:215–227

Badalament RA, O'Toole RV, Kenworthy P et al. (1990) Prognostic factors in patients with primary transitional cell carcinoma of the upper urinary tract. J Urol 144: 859–863

Badalament RA, Bennett WF, Bova JG, Kenworthy PR, Wise HA II, Smith S, Perez J (1992) Computed tomography of primary transitional cell carcinoma of upper urinary tracts. Urology 40:71–76

Batata MA, Whitmore WF, Hilaris BS, Tokita N, Grabstald H (1975) Primary carcinoma of the ureter: a prognostic study. Cancer 35:1626–1632

Beahrs O (1988) Renal pelvis and ureter. Manual for staging of cancer. American Joint Committee on Cancer, 3rd edn, pp 205–207

Bennington JL, Beckwith JB (1975) Tumors of the kidney, renal pelvis and ureter. Armed Forces Institute of Pathology, Washington, DC

Blute ML, Segura JW, Patterson DE, Benson RC Jr, Zincke H (1989) Impact of endourology on diagnosis and management of upper urinary tract urothelial cancer. J Urol 141:1298–1301

Brenner DW, Schellhammer PF (1987) Upper tract urothelial malignancy after cyclophosphamide therapy. J Urol 137:1226–1227

Brookland PK, Richter MP (1985) The postoperative irradiation of transitional cell carcinoma of the renal pelvis and ureter. J Urol 133:952–955

Carson CC III (1991) Endoscopic treatment of upper and lower urinary tract lesions using lasers. Semin Urol 9:185–191

Charbit L, Gendreau M, Mees, Cukier J (1991) Tumors of the upper urinary tract: 10 years of experience. J Urol 146:1243–1246

Cozad SC, Smalley SR, Austenfeld M, Noble M, Jennings S, Reymond R (1992) Adjuvant radiotherapy in high stage transitional cell carcinoma of the renal pelvis and ureter. Int J Radiat Oncol Biol Phys 24:743–745

Cukuranavic R, Ignjatovic M, Stefanovic V (1991) Urinary tract tumors and Balkan nephropathy in the South Morava river basin. Kidney Int 40 [Suppl 34]:S80–83

Das S (1985) Upper urinary tract transitional cell carcinoma in patients with bladder carcinoma and vesicoureteral reflux. J Urol 133:468–471

Debrungne FMJ, Niodner WA, Daenekindt AA (1980) Fibroepithelial polyp of the ureter. Urology 16:355–359

Delahunt B, Nacey JN, Meffan PJ, Clark MG (1992) Signet ring cell adenocarcinoma of the ureter. Br J Urol 69:555–556

Easthan JA, Huffman JL (1993) Technique of mitomycin C instillation in the treatment of upper urinary tract urothelial tumors. J Urol 150:324–325

Fein AB, MuClennon BL (1986) Solitary filling defects of the ureter. Semin Roentgenol 21:201–213

Friedenberg RN, Becker JA, Elkin M, Lang EK (1976) ACR self evaluation program, genital urinary tract, 10. ACR, Chicago, TP 201–210

Galifer RB, Aubert D, Couture A, Veyrac C, Barneon C, Kotter R (1988) Fibrous epithelial polyps of the pyeloureteral junction in children. Chir Pediatr 29: 318–324

Gelister JSK, Falzon M, Crawford R, Chapple CR, Hendry WF (1992) Urinary tract metastases from renal carcinoma. Br J Urol 69:250–252

Ghuzi MR, Morales PA, Al-Askari S (1979) Primary carcinoma of ureter. Urology 14:18–21

Grabstald H, Whitmore WF, Melamed MR (1971) Renal pelvic tumors. JAMA 218:845–854

Grossman HB, Schwartz SL, Konnak JW (1992) Ureteroscopic treatment of urothelial carcinoma of the ureter and renal pelvis. J Urol 148:275–277

Hatch TR, Hefty TR, Barry JM (1988) Time-related recurrence rates in patients with upper tract transitional cell carcinoma. J Urol 140:40–41

Heney NM, Nocks BN, Daly J, Blitzer PH, Parkhurst EC (1981) Prognostic factors in carcinoma of the ureter. J Urol 125:632–636

Huben RP, Mounzer AM, Murphy GP (1988) Tumor and stage as prognostic variables in upper tract urothelial tumors. Cancer 62:2016–2019

Jeffery GM, Mead GM (1992) CMV chemotherapy for advanced transitional cell carcinoma. Br J Cancer 66: 542–546

Johansson S, Angervall L, Bengtsson U, Wahlqvist L (1974) Uroepithelial tumors of the renal pelvis associated with abuse of phenacetin containing analgesics. Cancer 33:743–753

Kenney PJ, Stanley RJ (1987) Computed tomography of ureteral tumors. J Comput Assist Tomogr 11:102–107

Kini U, Shariff S, Thomas J (1991) Mixed mesodermal tumours of the ureter. J Surg Oncol 46:208–210

Leder RA, Dunnick NR (1990) Transitional cell carcinoma of the pelvicalices and ureter. AJR 155:713–722

Liddell RM, Weinberger E, Schofield DE, Pelman RS (1991) Fibroepithelial polyp of the ureter in a child. AJR 157:1273–1274

McCoy JG, Honda H, Reznicek M, Williams RD (1991) Computerized tomography for detection and staging of localized and pathologically defined upper tract urothelial tumors. J Urol 146:1500–1503

Mileston B, Friedman AC, Seidmon EJ et al. (1990) Staging of ureteral transitional cell carcinoma by CT and MRI. Urology 36:346–349

Mills C, Vaughan EO Jr (1983) Carcinoma of the ureter: natural history, management and 5 year survival. J Urol 129:275–283

Moldwin RM, Orihuela E, Smith AD (1990) Conservative management for transitional cell carcinoma of the upper urinary tract. Clin Geriatr Med 6:163–171

Murphy W (1989) Urologic pathology. W.B. Saunders, Philadelphia, pp 128–131

Patel U, Thorpe P, Ramsay JWA, Shepherd JH, Kirby RS, Hendry WF (1992) Endometriosis of the ureter. Br J Urol 69:495–498

Petronic VJ, Bukurov NS, Djokic MR et al. (1991) Balkan endemic nephropathy and papillary transitional tumors of the renal pelvis and ureters. Kidney Int 40 [Suppl 34]:S77–79

Pollack HM (1990) Clinical urography. W.B. Saunders, Philadelphia, pp 1324–1353

Puech JL, Song MY, Joffre F, Rousseau H, Trocard J, Plante P (1987) Ureteral metastases: computed tomographic findings. Eur J Radiol 2:103–106

Robbins SL, Cotran RS (1988) Pathologic disease, 4th edn. W.B. Saunders, Philadelphia, pp 1083–1098

Ross RK, Paganini-Hill A, Landolph J, Gerkins V, Henderson BE (1989) Analgesics, cigarette smoking and other risk factors for cancer of the renal pelvis and ureter. Cancer Res 49:1045–1048

Ryan JF, Booth CM (1992) Endometriosis of the ureter. Br J Urol 69:430–431

Scott WW, McDonald DF (1970) Tumors of the ureter. In: Campbell, MF, Harrison JH (eds) Urology. W.B. Saunders, Philadelphia

Shetty SD, Tabacochali MA (1987) Cyclophosphamide and ureteric carcinoma. Br J Urol 60:274

Skinner DG, Leiskovsk G (1988) Diagnosis and management of genitourinary cancer. W.B. Saunders, Philadelphia, pp 323–336

Strobel SL, Jasper WS, Gogate SA, Sharma HM (1984) Primary carcinoma of the renal pelvis and ureter. Evaluation of clinical and pathologic features. Arch Pathol Lab Med 108:697–700

Swanson SK, Zincke H (1983) "Flip-flop" phenomenon on retrograde ureterography establishes the diagnosis of ureteral tumor. Urology 21:542–543

Tannock I, Gospodarowicz M, Connolly J, Jewett M (1989) M-VAC (methotrexate, vinblastine, doxorubicin and cisplatin) chemotherapy for transitional cell carcinoma: The Princess Margaret Hospital experience. J Urol 142:289–292

Williamson B Jr, Hartman GW, Hattery RR (1986) Multiple and diffuse ureteral filling defects. Semin Roentgenol 21:214–223

Winalski CS, Lipman JC, Tumeh SS (1990) Ureteral neoplasms. Radiographics 10:271–282.

Witters S, Vereecken RL, Baert L, VanDamme B (1987) Primary neoplasms of the ureter: a review of twenty-eight cases. Eur Urol 13:256–258

Yagoda A (1985) Progress in treatment of advanced urothelial tract tumors. J Clin Oncol 3:1448–1450

Yoshino S, Takahashit, Tach, Bana Y, Kokuhom, Yamauchit (1990) A clinical study on transitional cell carcinoma of the renal pelvis and ureter. Acta Urol Jpn 36:541–547

Zoretic S, Gonzales J (1983) Primary carcinoma of ureters. Urology 21:354–356

2 Traumatic Lesions of the Ureter

ERICH K. LANG

CONTENTS

2.1 Introduction

The protected location of the ureter makes injury rather uncommon. Although the incidence of surgically induced injuries to the urinary tract is low, iatrogenic trauma is the leading cause of ureteral injuries (Table 2.1) (BRUBACKER and WILBANKS 1991; DOWLING et al. 1986; BRIGHT and PETERS 1977). The majority of iatrogenic ureteral injuries occur during gynecologic surgery, with more than half occurring during simple hysterectomy for benign disease (BRUBACKER and WILBANKS 1991; ZINMAN et al. 1978). Urinary tract surgery is responsible for about 30% of the injuries; abdominal surgical procedures such as abdominal perineal resection, pelvic tumor surgery, lyses of adhesions, aortic bypass surgery, and orthopedic and neurosurgical procedures account for the remaining relatively small group of ureteral injuries. Penetrating and blunt trauma are responsible for a small number of ureteral injuries but pose major management problems because there are often associated injuries to other structures (GUERRIERO 1989).

2.2 Iatrogenic Injury

Injury to the ureter during gynecologic surgery may result in anatomic or functional lesions such

ERICH K. LANG, M.D., Professor and Chairman, Department of Radiology, School of Medicine, Louisiana State University, Medical Center, 1542 Tulane Avenue, New Orleans, LA 70112-2822, USA

Table 2.1. Etiologies of ureteral injuries

I. Iatrogenic injuries
- A. Gynecologic and obstetric interventions
  1. Vaginal hysterectomy
  2. Sentinel hysterectomy
  3. Wertheim radical hysterectomy
  4. Salpingo-ovariectomy
  5. Ovariectomy
  6. Myomectomy
  7. Colpocleisis
  8. Marshall-Marchettie suspension
  9. Cystocele repair
  10. Vesicovaginal fistula repair
  11. Fimbriolysis – laparoscopic
  12. Fimbrioplasty – laparoscopic
  13. Lysis of periovarian adhesions – laparoscopic
  14. Cesarean section
  15. Forceps delivery
  16. D and C
- B. Urologic surgery
  1. Ureterolithotomy
  2. Segmental bladder resection
  3. Diverticulectomy of the bladder
  4. Radical prostatectomy
  5. Dismembered pyeloplasty
  6. YV pyeloplasty
  7. Enterovesical fistula repair
  8. Transureteral ureterostomy
  9. Ureteroneocystostomy
- C. Other surgical procedures
  1. Colon surgery
  2. Duodenal surgery
  3. Pancreatic surgery
  4. Aortic aneurysm repair
  5. Aortoiliac or aortobifemoral bypass graft
  6. Laminectomy
  7. Salpingectomy
  8. Laser surgery
  9 Retroperitoneal node dissection
  10. Percutaneous diskectomy
- D. Endoscopic procedures
  1. Ureteroscopy
  2. Stone basketing
  3. Retrograde pyelography
  4. Transurethral resection of the prostate (TURP)
  5. TURP – bladder tumor
  6. Antegrade percutaneous occlusion of ureter
- E. Radiation injuries
  1. External radiation therapy
  2. Interstitial implant therapy

II. External trauma
- A. Penetrating injuries
- B. Blunt injuries

as detrusor overactivity, postvoid dribbling, or urinary retention (BRUBACKER and WILBANKS 1991). The latter functional disorders probably reflect injury to neural transmitters and pathways (FARGHALY et al. 1986; PARYS et al. 1989; LANGER et al. 1989; VERVEST et al. 1988, 1989).

The incidence of ureteral injury in patients undergoing major gynecologic procedures has been reported to be in the range 0.5%–2.2% (ST. LEZIN and STOLLER 1991; MANN et al. 1988). However, Wertheim radical hysterectomy, or one of its modifications, has been reported to entail an incidence of injury from 10% to 30% (HOE et al. 1992). Abdominal hysterectomy accounts for 38% of all iatrogenic injuries to the ureter. Preoperative radiation therapy is an added risk factor that is prone to increase in particular the incidence of ureteral fistulas (ST. LEZIN and STOLLER 1991; LARSON et al. 1987; RISS et al. 1988; UNDERWOOD et al. 1979). Ureteral dissection and difficult mobilization may result in laceration and devascularization. Devitalization of the ureter may lead first to ischemic ureteral strictures and ultimately to fistulization (BRUNSCHWIG 1960; PIVER et al. 1974; GREEN et al. 1962; GAL and BUCHSBAUM 1983).

The important anatomic relationships of the ureter to blood vessels are as follows: The left ureter crosses anteriorly to the left colic and inferior mesenteric vessels, while the right ureter passes posterior to the right colic and ileocolic vessels in the root of the mesentery. Before entering the pelvis, the ureter passes under the gonadal vessels and then crosses the iliac vessels. The male ureter runs anterior to the obturator nerve and vessels. The female ureter courses posterior to the infundibulopelvic ligament, which contains the ovarian vessels. It is then anterior to the superior vesical and uterine arteries. The ureter then lies in the base of the broad ligament 2 cm lateral to the cervix. At this point the ureter is again crossed by the uterine artery.

There continues to be debate over the precise arterial supply to the ureter. The abdominal component of the ureter is regularly supplied by a branch directly from the abdominal aorta or by branches from the renal or ovarian artery. The mid portion receives supply from branches of the common or internal iliac arteries. The pelvic portion is supplied by the superior and inferior vesical arteries as well as by branches from uterine, internal pudendal, and mid rectal arteries. The upper and mid segments of the ureter have their vascular supply along the medial side, whereas the pelvic ureter receives its vascular supply from the lateral side (BRUBAKER and WILBANKS 1991). Maintenance of the ureteral attachment to the medial leaf of the pelvic peritoneum is important to preserve its longitudinal supply (BRUBAKER and WILBANKS 1991). Preservation of the superior vesical artery, when ligating the uterine artery and before transecting the cardinal ligament, is an important measure to prevent ischemic ureteral stricture (SMITH 1975; PIVER et al. 1974).

Table 2.2. Types of surgical ureteral injuries. (Adapted from ST. LEZIN and STOLLER 1991)

Open surgery
Transaction
Suture ligation
Crush injury
Devascularization
Cicatricial fibrotic stricture
Cautery thermal injury
Endourologic surgery
Perforation
Avulsion
Mucosal false passage
Ischemic necrosis
Stricture formation
Intussusception

Risk factors of ureteral injury during abdominal and pelvic operations include endometriosis, retroperitoneal fibrosis, pelvic inflammatory disease, diverticulitis, and neoplastic disease (ST. LEZIN and STOLLER 1991). Depending on the route of surgical approach, different injury patterns may be anticipated. An abdominal route of surgery predisposes to injury of the ureter (a) at the level of the infundibulo-pelvic ligament, (b) in the region of crossing of the uterine vessels, (c) during suture closure at the cervicovaginal angle, or (d) during pelvic reperitonealization (particularly in its course in the broad ligament). Conversely, a vaginal surgical approach puts the ureter at risk at the point of clamping to control hemorrhage or at the point of prolapse of the ureter (BRUBAKER and WILBANKS 1991).

Open surgery places the ureter at risk of transection, suture ligation, crush injury, cautery thermal injury, devascularization with attendant ischemic necrosis and cicatricial fibrotic strictures (ST. LEZIN and STOLLER 1991). Ligation and strictures are by far the most common injuries; however, ureterovaginal fistula formation has been described with an incidence as high as 28% (SCHWIMMER 1974).

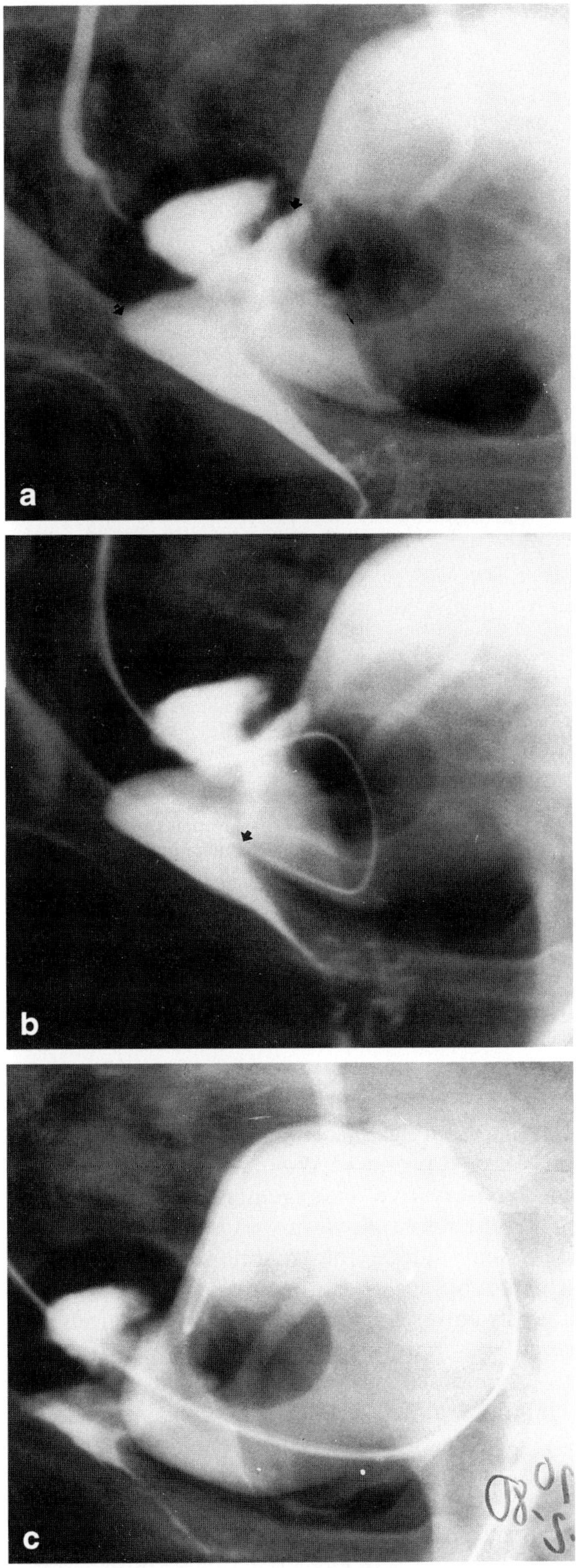

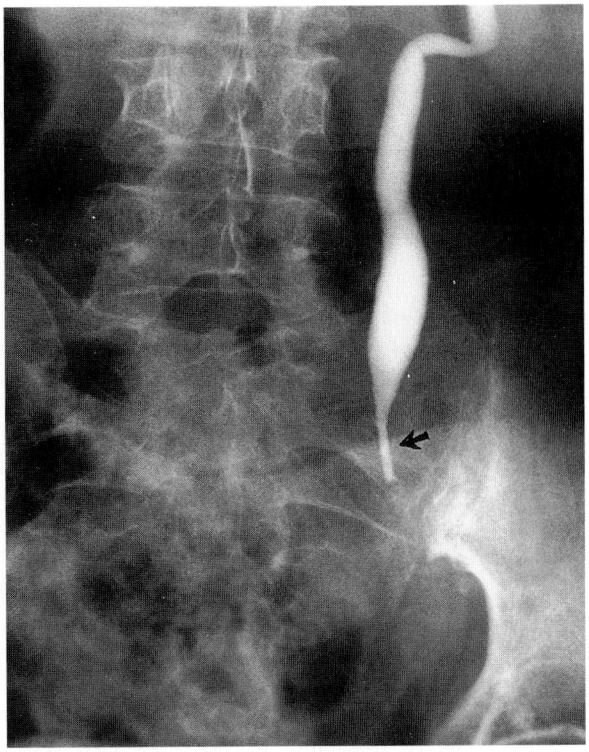

Fig. 2.2. An antegrade ureterogram demonstrates pipestem narrowing and complete obstruction of the left ureter at the level of S1. This is attributable to devascularization and radiation fibrosis due to overdosing by external beam irradiation and brachytherapy

◁

Fig. 2.1. **a** An antegrade ureterogram demonstrates communication between the right ureter and the vagina, which is densely opacified. During vaginal hysterectomy, a segment of the ureter was resected and the free end of the ureter fixed by sutures when closing the vaginal cuff. **b** An attempt to pass a guidewire into the bladder demonstrates the preferential passage into the vagina due to suture fixation of the ureter (LANG 1988). **c** After freeing the ureter by cutting the suture with a knife mounted on the guidewire, the bladder is re-entered using a transseptal guidewire, and a stent is placed from the renal pelvis to the bladder. (LANG 1988)

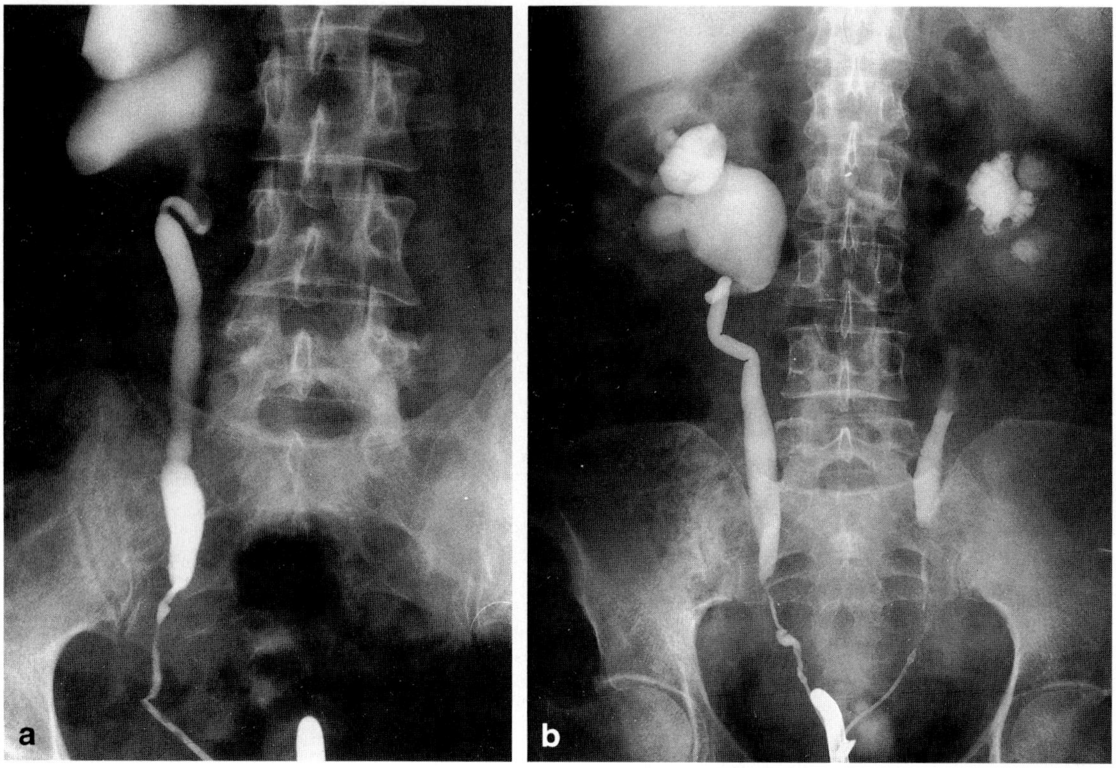

Fig. 2.3. **a** A retrograde ureterogram demonstrates classical stricture formation in the parametrial segment of the right ureter. Tilt of the brachytherapy applicator resulted in overdose to this segment of the ureter. **b** Note the medial path of both pelvic ureters, indicating prior radical pelvic surgery. The strictures of the pelvic segments of the ureter are caused by devascularization and fibrosis secondary to stripping of the lymphatics of the ureter during Wertheim hysterectomy and by radiation therapy

Vaginal hysterectomy is a not uncommon cause of ureteral disruption due to inadvertent resection of a segment of the ureter in the parametrium (Fig. 2.1a,b). Crush injury to the ureter by clamps, while dissecting along the uterus, is another common cause of late formation of strictures.

Because of the relative resistance to the effect of radiation, most ureteral strictures seen in association with radiation therapy are attributable to the desmoplastic effect accompanying the destruction of malignant disease or recurrent tumor (UNDERWOOD et al. 1977). However, injury as a consequence of excessive radiation by external beam and interstitial therapy can also cause ischemic strictures (ST. MARTIN et al. 1953; LANG et al. 1973). Involvement of the parametrium by the neoplasm may fix the ureter and cause tilt of the brachytherapy applicators. Thereby, the ureter on the involved side may be exposed to an excessive dose rate while an inadequate dose is delivered to the contralateral side. This sets the stage for ischemic changes of the ureter resulting in late stenosis of the ipsilateral ureter and obstruction of the contralateral ureter by uncontrolled neoplasm (Figs. 2.2, 2.3).

Inadvertent ligation of the ureter by silk or other nonabsorbable suture material will usually mandate surgical correction. Chromic catgut sutures are prone to dissolution in 2–3 weeks, and conservative management by temporizing percutaneous nephrostomy and/or placement of a stent may suffice for treatment of ureters obstructed by such suture entrapment. However, late strictures may result from the attendant vascular compromise. Once again, such strictures are sometimes successfully handled by balloon dilatation, while on other occasions endoureterotomy and stenting may be necessary to correct them (EISENKOP et al. 1982) (Figs. 2.4, 2.5). Salpingo-ovariectomy is another procedure that may cause ureteral injury.

Cesarian section has a low rate of injury to the ureter in the range of 0.1%–1% (ST. LEZIN and STOLLER 1991; EISENKOP et al. 1982). Avulsion

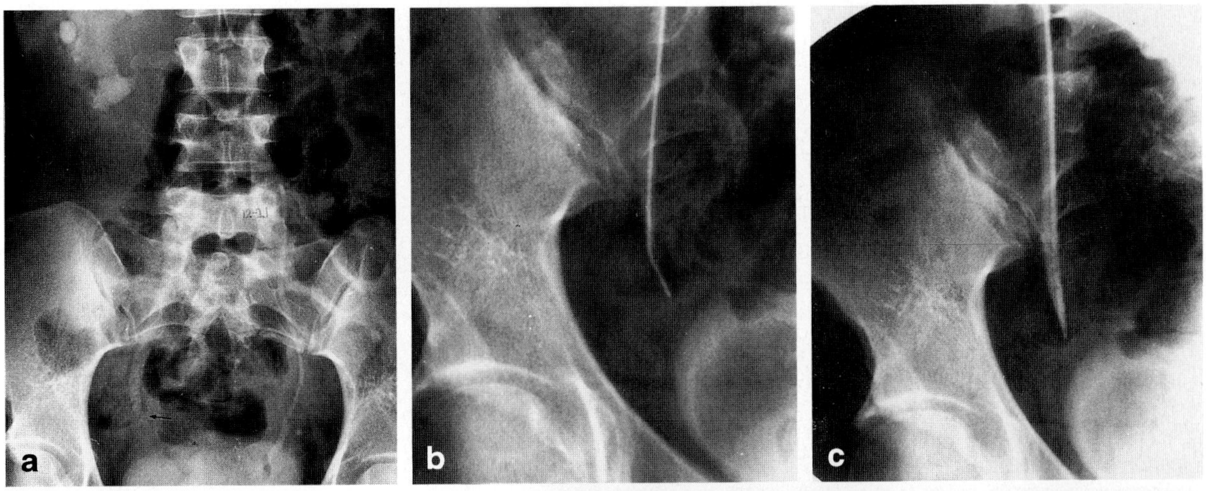

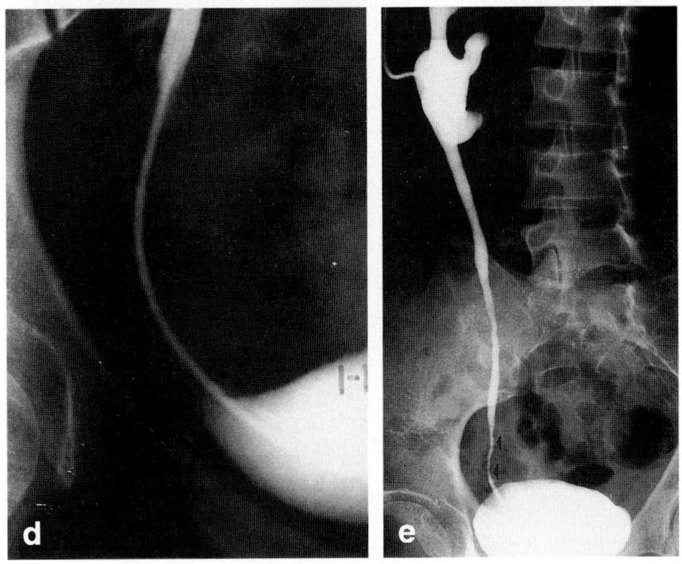

Fig. 2.4. **a** An intravenous urogram demonstrates moderate hydronephrosis of the right kidney and collumination of the right ureter to about its point of entry into the parametrial segment (*arrow*). **b** Percutaneous nephrostomy has been performed. A guidewire has been advanced to and is probing the obstruction caused by sutures inappropriately placed during pelvic surgery days earlier. **c** A stiff Amplatz guidewire is forced through the area of obstruction. **d** A stent is placed across the site of obstruction and retained for 4 weeks. **e** A follow-up antegrade pyelogram demonstrates only minimal changes in the parametrial segment of the right ureter attributable to residual mucosal edema. In this case, a late stricture did not develop; the patient, however, was carefully followed with radionuclide urography to monitor right renal function. (LANG 1986)

of the ureter at the ureterovesical junction has been reported as a complication of high forceps delivery (Fig. 2.6).

The elevation of laparoscopy from a diagnostic to a combined diagnostic and therapeutic procedure has been accompanied by an increasing incidence of ureteral injury (GRAINGER et al. 1990; GOMEL and JAMES 1991; STENGEL et al. 1974). Laparoscopic fulguration and electrocoagulation in the treatment of endometriosis are a common cause of ureteral injury (Fig. 2.7). The electrical current may damage the vascular supply to the coagulated tissue beyond the extent of the apparent lesion, leading to delayed tissue necrosis (GRAINGER et al. 1990; SCHWIMMER 1974). Similarly, the ureter may be injured by cautery during application of current for the purpose of sterilization. This type of injury is usually recognized promptly. Within 48–72 h, patients present with fever, abdominal pain, peritonitis, and leukocytosis (GRAINGER et al. 1990). Fistulization between the ureter and fallopian tube can result if coagulation is set in the isthmic segment of the tube and in proximity to the ureter (Fig. 2.8). Electrocoagulation at the utero-sacral ligament is one other potential cause of ureteral injury (GOMEL and JAMES 1991).

Abdominal peritoneal resection is the most common open surgery associated with ureteral injuries; it accounts for up to 9% of all ureteral injuries (ST. LEZIN and STOLLER 1991; NUMAN et al. 1991; DALY and HIGGINS 1988; BRIGHT and PETERS 1977). The incidence of ureteral injury during abdominal peritoneal resection ranges from 0.3% to 5.7% (ZINMAN et al. 1978; HOGHES et al. 1984; ANDERSSON and BERGDAHL 1976). The

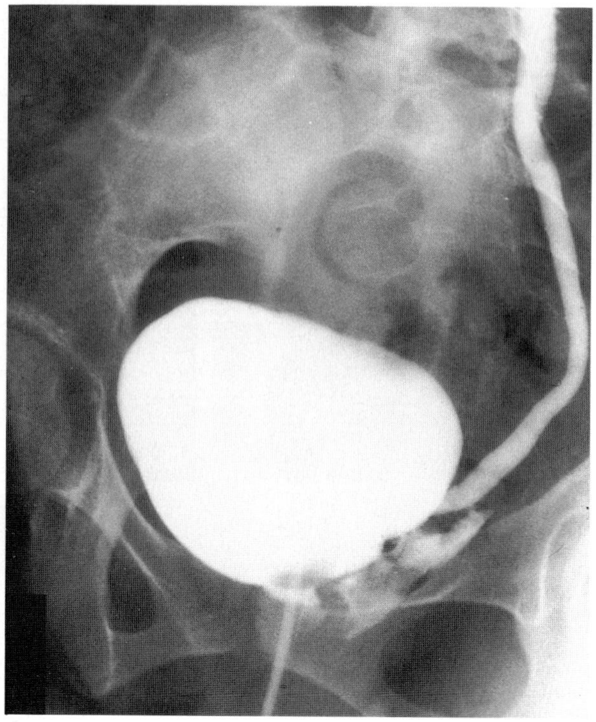

Fig. 2.6. An antegrade ureterogram demonstrates extravasation of contrast medium into the perivesical space. Filling from a prior cystogram demonstrates irregularity of the left posterolateral bladder wall and the left trigone area. The ureter had been avulsed during a high forceps rotation; likewise, there had been a tear of the trigone area of the bladder with a substantial hematoma in the abutting perivesical space

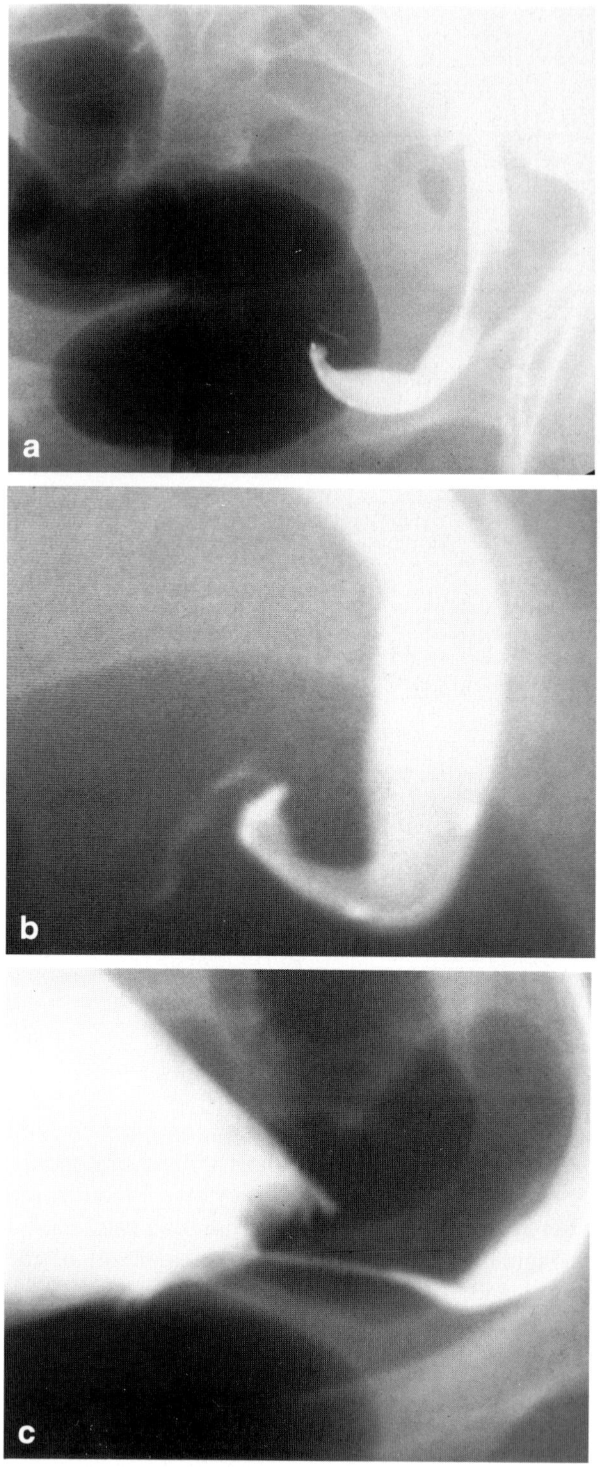

◁

Fig. 2.5. **a** An antegrade ureterogram demonstrates complete obstruction of the left ureter by sutures inappropriately placed during a Marshall-Marchettie bladder suspension and urethropexy procedure. **b** A sheath has been advanced to the site of obstruction and a guidewire with a small knife blade advanced through the sheath to make a longitudinal cut through the ureter and suture and thus free the ureter. **c** Finally, a guidewire has been advanced into the bladder and a stent placed in position. Uroepithelium will readily cover the defect. This procedure obviates the risk of late stricture formation that accompanies compromise of vascular supply to this segment of the ureter

left ureter is most likely to be injured due to its proximity to the mesosigmoid (Andersson and Bergdahl 1976) (Fig. 2.9).

The increased popularity of retrograde and antegrade ureteroscopy has been accompanied by a rise in iatrogenic injuries of the ureter, particularly attendant to the use of ridged endoscopes (Fig. 2.10). It is, however, hoped that with the availability of smaller caliber ridged endoscopes, dependable flexible ureteroscopes, and newer devices for intraureteral lithotripsy, the safety margin for these procedures will widen (Huffman

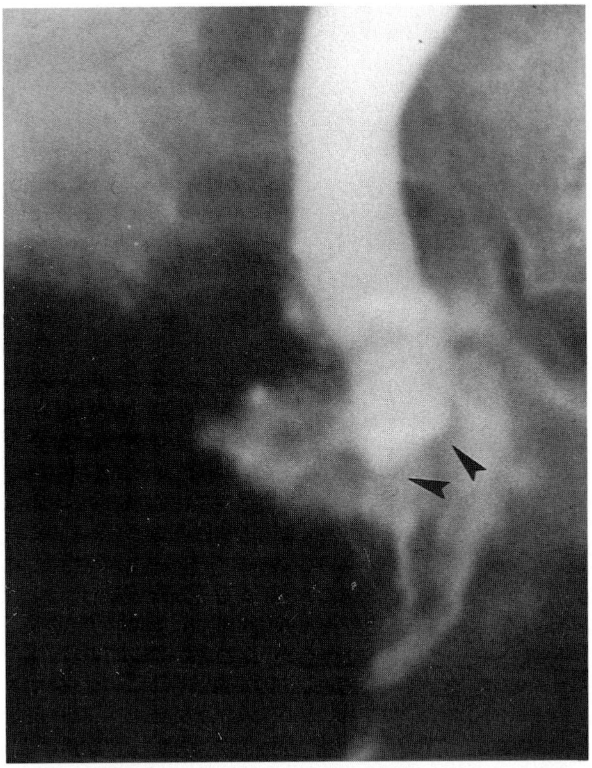

Fig. 2.7. Following fulguration of endometrial implants, there is evidence of necrosis at the wall of the ureter and extravasation of contrast medium into periureteral tissues (*arrowheads*)

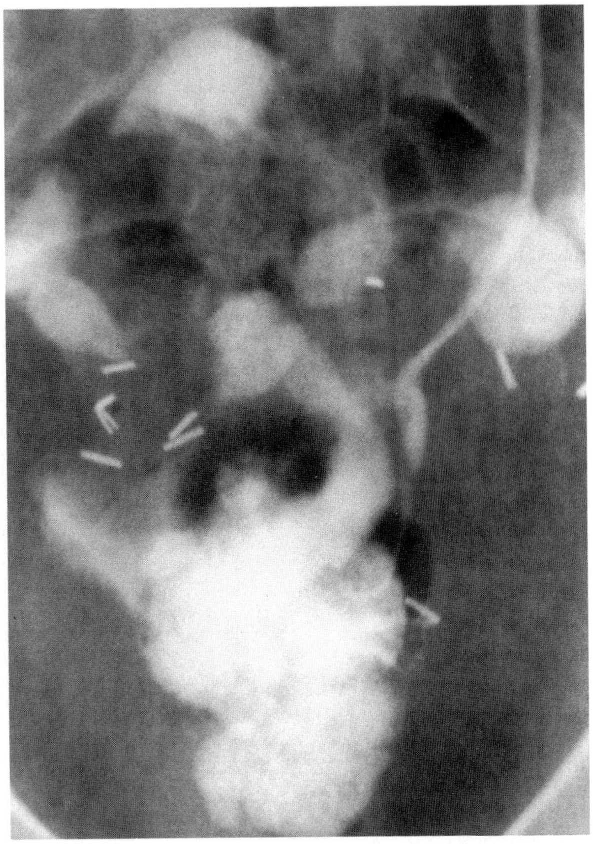

△

Fig. 2.9. An antegrade left ureterogram demonstrates medial deviation of the left ureter, near or complete obstruction of the ureter, and opacification of ileal loops as well as of packing material in the rectal fossa. Injury to the ureter occurred during abdominal perineal resection

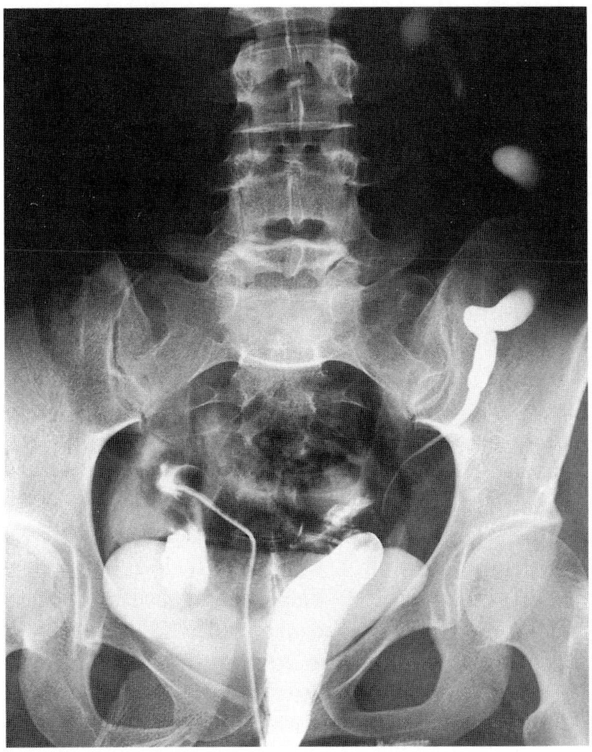

◁

Fig. 2.8. Following laparoscopic cautery of the fallopian tubes for the purpose of sterilization, a ureteral fallopian tube fistula results. A hysterosalpingogram of the left moiety of a subseptated uterus shows filling of the left ureter and finally also of the bladder

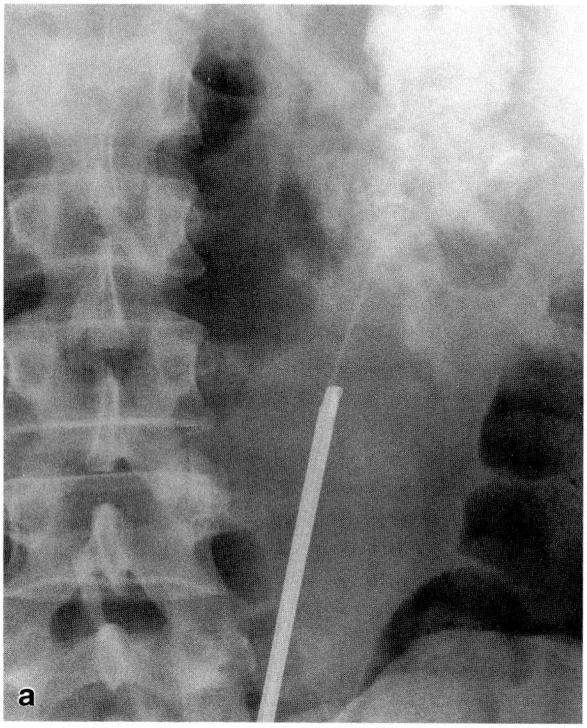

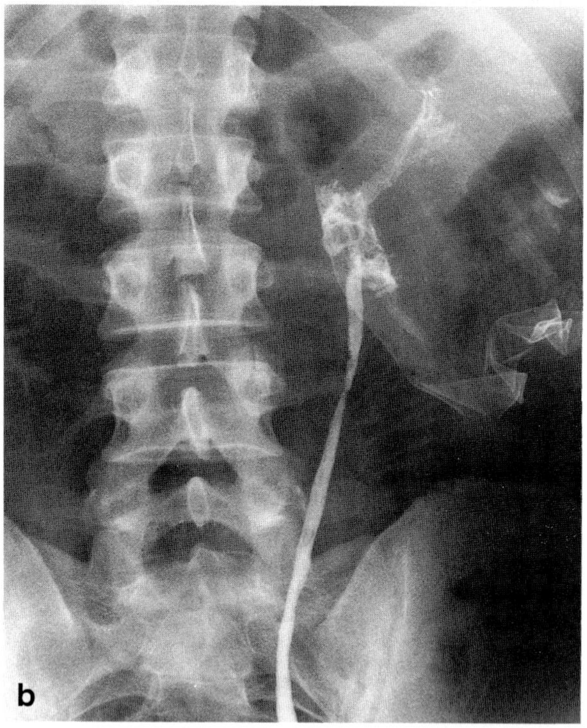

Fig. 2.10. **a** A ridged ureteroscope has been advanced in a retrograde fashion. A guidewire with channel is advanced into what was presumed to be the left renal pelvis. Injection through the guidewire channel reveals extravasation into peripelvic tissues. **b** A subsequent retrograde ureterogram demonstrates the site of perforation of the left ureter near the ureteropelvic junction

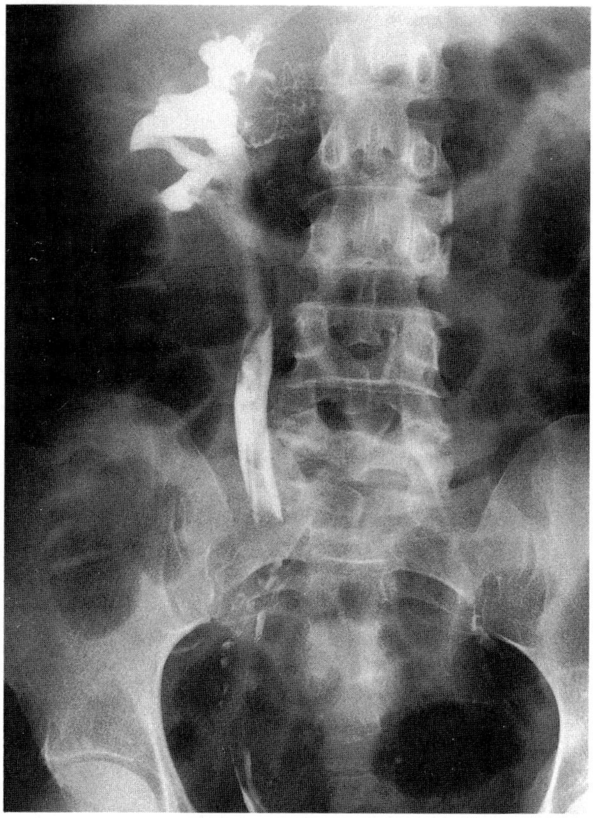

Fig. 2.11. Retrograde passage of a ureteral catheter over a preinserted guidewire has resulted in a partial thickness injury to the ureteral wall. Note the negative shadow cast by the ureter enveloped by a mantle of contrast medium, injected in an area of dissection in the muscularis of the ureter but curtailed by the adventitia

1989). However, even with improved instrumentation, operator error, whether in judgement or technique, can lead to disastrous complications. It is, therefore, incumbent upon the endoscopist to be familiar with the types of injury that may occur as well as the appropriate means for diagnosing such injuries and their treatment.

Injuries such as perforation, false passage, and avulsion are commonly recognized acutely and appropriate intervention is instituted (HUFFMAN 1989; BENJAMIN et al. 1987; BIESTER and GILLENWATER 1986; KRAMOLOWSKY 1987; SOSA and HUFFMAN 1988; STACKL and MARBERGER 1986; SCHULTZ et al. 1987; WEINBERG et al. 1987; CORRIERE 1987). Avulsion of the ureter is without doubt the most severe complication. False passage with a partial thickness injury to the ureteral wall, which does not extend through the adventitia, is perhaps the least consequential injury (Fig. 2.11). HUFFMAN (1989) reviewed 1696 ureteroscopic procedures reported in 15 series and computed a rate of

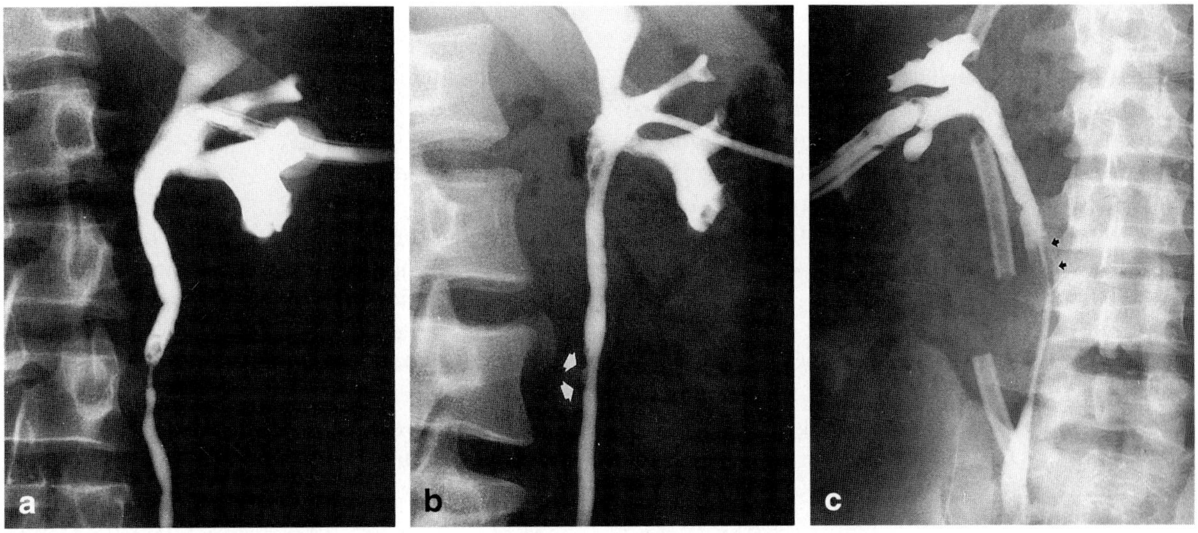

Fig. 2.12. **a** An antegrade ureterogram demonstrates a stricture in the left ureter and several small calculi immediately above the stricture. **b** A follow-up antegrade pyelogram demonstrates satisfactory dilatation of the stricture by prior transluminal balloon dilatation, but also extrusion of a calculus through the wall of the ureter (*white arrows*). **c** While basketing a calculus with a rigid ureteroscope, a submucosal false passage has been created. The antegrade ureterogram demonstrates the compromised true lumen of the ureter enveloped by a thick mantle of submucosal to subadventitial hematoma in the area of dissection (*arrows*)

injury of 9%, 1.6% of which necessitated surgical intervention.

Iatrogenic injury to some degree varies according to the site. The intramural and juxtavesical ureter has more muscular support than the proximal ureter or pelvic segment. Moreover, the number of mucosal cells is substantially greater in the lower ureter. Thus, there is less likelihood of complete perforation in the intramural tunnel or distal ureter than in the proximal ureter or pelvis. False passage, however, is common in the distal ureter.

Flexible instruments in general are less likely to cause traumatic injury than ridged instruments. The contiguous blood supply to the ureteral mucosa increases the probability of significant complications attendant upon submucosal dissection by instrument. Minor endoscopic injury can, therefore, lead to devascularization, necrosis, and later stricture formation. Thermal injury secondary to intraureteral lithotripsy is likewise prone to cause secondary strictures. Ultrasonic lithotripsy and laser lithotripsy can cause thermal injury to the ureteral wall and secondary strictures (Dretler et al. 1987; Green and Lytton 1985; Huffman 1988). Electrohydrolic lithotripsy entails the greatest temperature increase and accordingly is associated with the highest incidence of ureteral injury. The advent of balloon dilatation, replacing the use of metal bougies, has decreased the frequency of perforation at the intramural tunnel (Huffman 1988).

Avulsion of the distal ureter can be treated by ureteral reimplantation, sometimes in combination with a psoas hitch or Boari flap (Huffman 1989). Avulsion in the middle or proximal ureter, however, usually calls for bowel interposition or autotransplantation. Most other endoscopic injuries of the ureter can be handled by conservative management, i.e., placement of a stent.

Overzealous use of ureteroscopy is perhaps the most common cause of ureteral injury. The sobering message regarding the potential complications of ureteroscopy should lead to careful patient selection and practice of prevention of such injuries rather than to denigration of this technique, which offers unique advantages. Fluoroscopy, in particular, is a sine qua non for the safe performance of this procedure.

In addition to injury of the ureter by the ridged tip of an ultrasonic lithotriptor, extrusion of calculi into the perinephric or periureteral tissues is a distinct risk accompanying this procedure (Moretti et al. 1991) (Fig. 2.12a,b). In general, these patients can be managed conservatively, although secondary strictures may develop. It is, however, questionable whether these strictures are caused by the extruded calculus or are secondary to an electrical injury as a result of the electrohydrolic lithopaxy (BRANNEN et al. 1985; LEE et al. 1987; VERSTANDIG et al. 1986).

Extruded struvite fragments must be considered a more serious risk, since not infrequently they lead to perinephric abscess formation (LANG 1987a). Stenting of the injured ureter and treatment with antibiotics will generally suffice in the management of calculi extruded during ureteroscopic manipulation.

Stone basketing can lead to denudation of the ureteral mucosa, submucosal false passages, and even avulsion of the distal ureter. Management is akin to similar injuries resulting from ureteroscopy (Fig. 2.12c).

Ureteral obstruction may occur at the aorto-iliac and aorto-bifemoral anastomosis site as a complication of arterial bypass surgery. BLASCO and SALADIE (1991) found a 20% incidence of asymptomatic hydronephrosis after aortovascular bypass surgery; symptomatic hydronephrosis occurred in only 2%.

Urologic complications associated with vascular reconstruction are often related to anatomic abnormalities secondary to vascular disease (SPIRNAK et al. 1989; FRY et al. 1983). Retroperitoneal fibrosis caused by bypass graft surgery is a real risk factor for the involved ureter (BROCK and SOLOWAY 1980; MEGIBOW et al. 1979–1980). Edema of the ureter following transection of its lymphatics during freeing from the retroperitoneal bed and fibrosis engendered by blood and serum enveloping denuded adventitia are the pathophysiologic bases for stricture formation and hyalinization of fibrous tissue simulating retroperitoneal fibrosis. However, 90% of ureteral obstruction following aortic graft insertion is transient and will resolve within 3 months (GOLDENBERG et al. 1988).

If a ureter is compressed by the bypass graft placed anterior to the ureter, the recommended corrective procedure is to divide the graft and reposition the ureter anterior to the graft rather than to divide the ureter (SPIRNAK et al. 1989; FRY et al. 1983). SPIRNAK et al., in eight patients, reported no graft complications if the diagnosis of ureteral injury was established promptly and primary repair of the ureter instituted. Lack of such complications is probably attributable to the presence of sterile urine as well as the prophylactic use of broad-spectrum antibiotics. Mid ureteral injuries are best managed by watertight uretero-ureterostomy, sealing with omentum, and placement of a double J stent. Distal ureteral injuries should be handled by ureteroneocystostomy, possibly in combination with a psoas hitch.

2.3 External Trauma

Ureteral and renal pelvic injuries secondary to external trauma are relatively uncommon, accounting for less than 1% of all urologic trauma (PRESTI et al. 1989). Penetrating trauma is a more frequent cause than blunt trauma. There is a frequent association with injury to the small bowel, stomach, pancreas, liver, spleen and major blood vessels (CASS and CASS 1983; CASS 1983; BRIGHT and PETERS 1977). Immediate recognition of ureteral injury is important (MCGINTY and MENDEZ 1977). MCGINTY and MENDEZ (1977) reported a 32% incidence of nephrectomy in cases of delayed recognition of ureteral injury. Unfortunately, both intravenous urography (IVU) and initial urine analysis may be unreliable indicators of ureteral injury (PRESTI et al. 1989). PRESTI et al. (1989) noted absence of hematuria in 5 of 16 patients with ureteral and renal pelvic injuries as well as normal or nondiagnostic intravenous urograms in 8 of 11 such patients. In fact, as regards hematuria a false-negative rate of up to 40% has been reported in patients with proven injury to the ureter (LANG 1981).

The management of associated injuries requires early and immediate attention. Adequate urinary diversion can usually be achieved by internal double J ureteral stenting, thus deferring reconstruction of the urinary tract (PRESTI et al. 1989; CASS and CASS 1983; CASS 1983; BRIGHT and PETERS 1977).

Projectile injury can either sever the ureter or cause secondary damage from the transmitted shock wave (HOLDEN et al. 1976; STUTZMAN 1977; ROHNER 1971; SPIRNAK et al. 1985; LANG 1981; FISHER et al. 1972; CASS 1984; EICKENBERT and AMIN 1976; FACKLER et al. 1986; LIROFF et al. 1977) (Figs. 2.13–2.16). Despite the fact that only 48 cases of gunshot injury to the ureter were reported in World War II, the recent literature indicates an increase in civilian gunshot injuries to the ureter (FISHER et al. 1972; KHASHU et al. 1975). Associated injuries to intraabdominal organs are present in virtually all cases (LANG 1981). However, the extent of these other organ injuries, including perforations of the bowel, should not preclude primary repair of the ureteral injury.

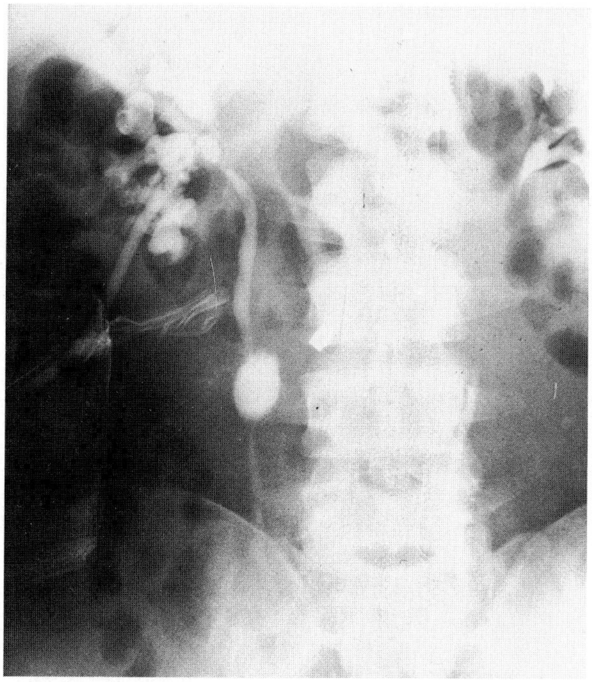

Fig. 2.13. An antegrade pyelogram demonstrates extravasation of contrast medium-laden urine into a urinoma from an incomplete tear of the mid portion of the right ureter

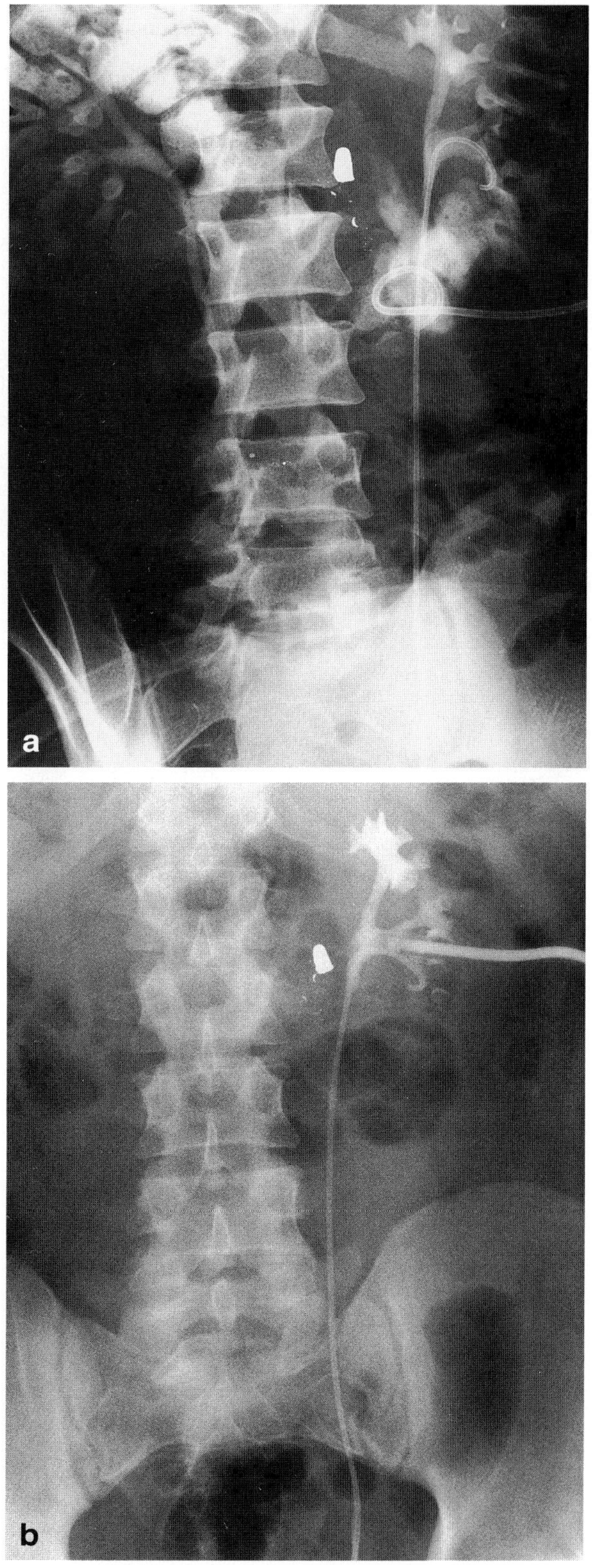

▷

Fig. 2.14. **a** Extravasation of contrast medium-laden urine is demonstrated from the left upper ureter, which has been partially severed by a projectile. A stent is seen in position from the left renal pelvis to the bladder. The urinoma is drained by a percutaneous drainage catheter. **b** A follow-up study no longer shows extravasation at the site of partial severance of the ureter. Drainage appears to be via the stent into the bladder; the defect has probably been covered by uroepithelium

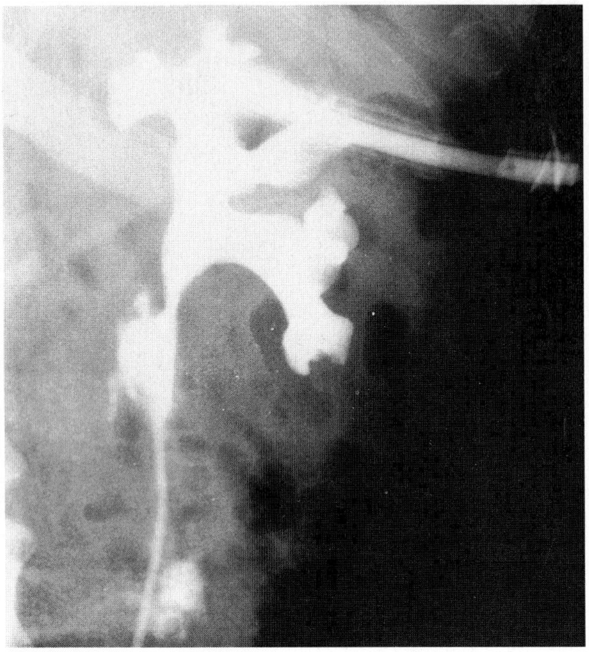

Fig. 2.15. A follow-up antegrade pyelogram, some 6 weeks after placement of a stent following acute projectile injury to the retroperitoneum and peritoneal organs, demonstrates extravasation at two sites. This is felt to be caused by late necrosis attendant upon the effect of a shockwave generated by the passing high velocity projectile and causing thrombosis of small vessels supplying the ureter

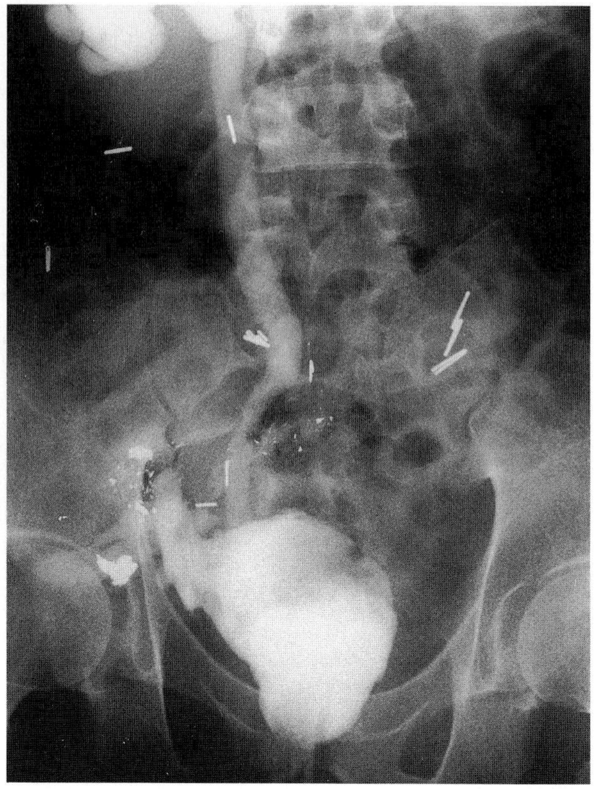

Fig. 2.16. An intravenous urogram demonstrates extravasation in the right half of the true pelvis. The ureter, severed by a projectile, has been reimplanted in the bladder; however, the ureteroneocystostomy broke down owing to devascularization of the ureter caused by the shockwave produced by the passing high velocity projectile

All patients with gunshot or other penetrating injuries located in the vicinity of the urinary tract should routinely undergo imaging studies to rule out urinary tract injuries regardless of findings from other studies, including urinanalysis (LANG 1981). Ureteral injury should be suspected if a retroperitoneal hematoma or fluid collection is present (Figs. 2.13, 2.14a). Injury to the bladder should provoke a high index of suspicion of associated ureteral injury. Passage of a projectile in the vicinity of the ureter may present with delayed manifestations. Damage from the transmitted shock wave can cause thrombosis of small blood vessels resulting in ureteral ischemia; stricture formation or fistulization may be the consequence (ROHNER 1971) (Figs. 2.15, 2.16). Simultaneous injury to the pancreas can liberate digestive enzymes, which greatly fosters fistulization (SEILER et al. 1991) (Fig. 2.17).

Blunt trauma is a rare cause of injury to the ureter; however, ureteral avulsion can be the consequence of acute acceleration/deceleration trauma (CAMPBELL et al. 1993; SEILER et al. 1991; WALLIJN et al. 1975; PALMER and DRAGO 1981; BEAMUD-GOMEZ et al. 1986; LIVNE and GONZALES 1985; REZNICHEK et al. 1973). Hyperextension following sudden acceleration or deceleration sets the stage for this injury (PALMER and DRAGO 1981). The injury mechanism is the result of two successive events: first, the ureter tenses like a bowstring and thereafter it is lashed against the transverse process of the lumbar vertebrae attendant to the sudden motion of the collecting system (PALMER and DRAGO 1981; LABERGE et al. 1979). Hematuria, microscopic or gross, is present in only about 66% of the patients (PALMER and DRAGO 1981). Again, injury to other organ systems often requires more immediate attention.

Contrast-enhanced computed tomography (CT) scans, and particularly delayed CT scans demonstrating small irregular collections of contrast medium medial to the kidney, offer the most

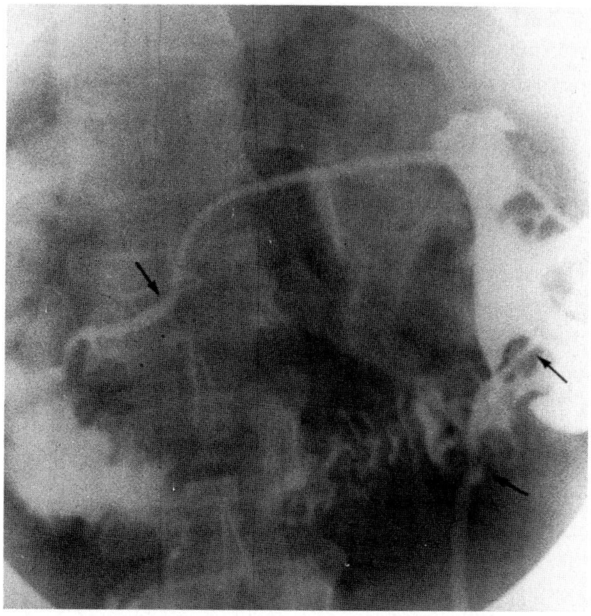

Fig. 2.17. Note the presence of a ureteral pancreatic fistula (*arrows*) resulting in opacification of the pancreatic duct and the duodenum by contrast medium-laden urine. (LANG 1981)

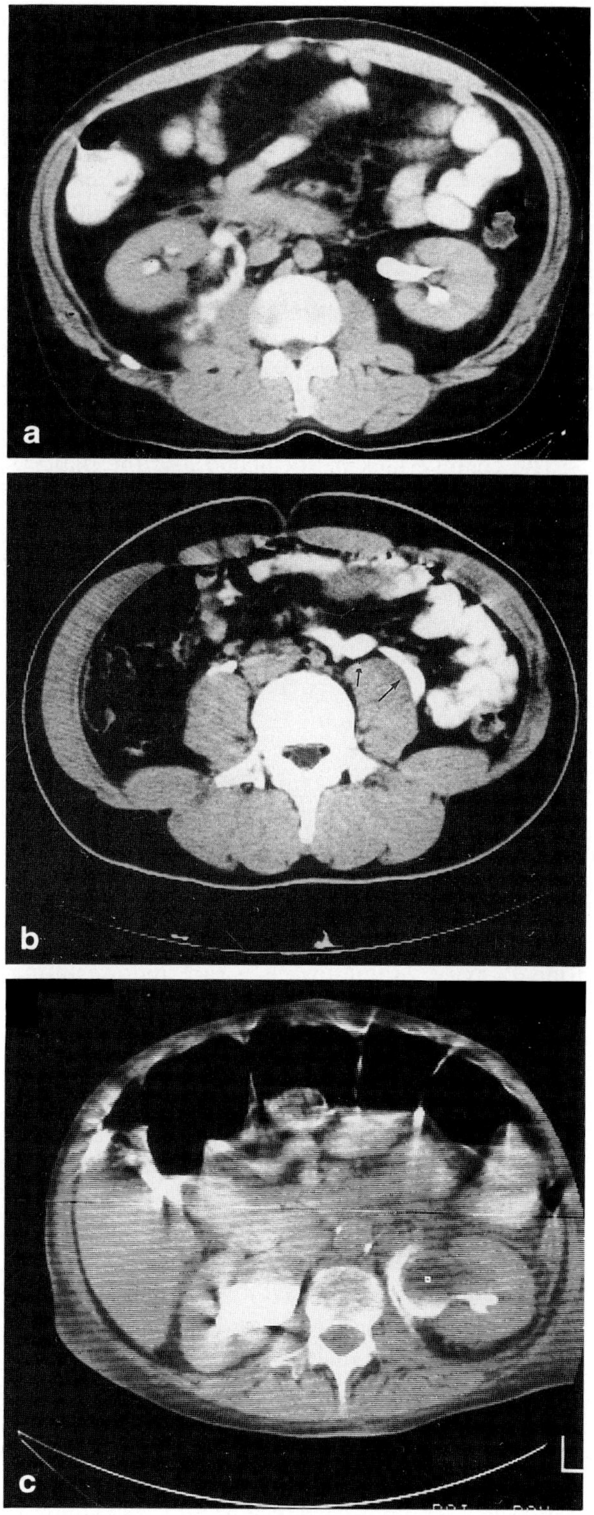

▷

Fig. 2.18. **a** A CT scan demonstrates extravasation from a dehiscence at the ureteropelvic junction and puddling of contrast medium medial to the kidney. **b** A CT scan demonstrates a ureterobilial fistula on the left side (*arrows*). **c** Extravasation in the peripelvic space is appreciated on a post-enhancement CT scan. The pelvis itself is devoid of opacified urine. This appearance is characteristic for opacification via peripelvic lymphatics in patients with obstruction of the ureter

consistent imaging findings suggesting traumatic avulsion (TEMPLETON et al. 1988) (Fig. 2.18). Lack of visualization of the afflicted ureter on sequential slices and demonstration of the aforementioned type of extravasation are considered telltale indications of avulsion of the ureter at the ureteropelvic junction. Initially, undetected avulsion of the ureteropelvic junction may present with pleural effusion and an elevated creatinine level in the effusion (SELIER et al. 1991). It is postulated that the urine reaches the pleural space by increased lymphatic drainage (CORRIERE et al. 1968).

Ideally, traumatic ureteropelvic disruption is diagnosed prior to extensive local reaction, and reconstruction should be possible by pyeloplasty or ureterocalicostomy (LYTTON and SCHIFF 1981). Alternatively, autotransplantation of the kidney may be utilized. Ileal interposition may be the procedure of choice after severe scarring has occurred (LYTTON and SCHIFF 1981; CASALE et al. 1985).

2.4 Presenting Symptoms

Recognition of iatrogenic ureteral injury is often delayed by 7–10 days (DOWLING et al. 1986; WALLIJN et al. 1975; PALMER and DRAGO 1981; FLYNN et al. 1979). DOWLING et al. (1986) reported immediate diagnosis of ureteral injury at the time of surgery in only 4 of 27 patients. The time-honored technique of verifying ureteral integrity and patency after pelvic or abdominal surgery in proximity to the ureter utilizes intravenous injections of 5 ml indigo carmine. Ejaculation of dye from both ureteral orifices should be observed.

The relative lack of specificity and the paucity of symptoms explain the frequent delay in diagnosis (BOYD 1987). Symptoms range from total absence of any discernible manifestations to a severe symptom complex with febrile reaction and marked biochemical alterations (DOWLING et al. 1986; ST. MARTIN et al. 1953; FLYNN et al. 1979). Postoperative anuria is a severe symptom that should prompt urgent evaluation of ureteral patency (BRUBAKER and WILBANKS 1991). Unilateral ureteral ligation, again, may be silent or may produce prompt flank pain. Partial or complete transactions may cause fever, pain, retroperitoneal urinoma formation, ileus, and abdominal distention (BARANYAI 1987). The serum creatinine should rise as urine is reabsorbed from the peritoneal cavity. Hematuria is a rare manifestation and, if present, tends to be microscopic and transient (PALMER and DRAGO 1981).

Urinary leakage, other than from the urethra, should lead to a search for a fistula. In general, urinary leakage becomes manifest only after a delay of 7–10 days (UNDERWOOD et al. 1977; WALLIJN et al. 1975). The diagnosis can be aided by analysis of drainage fluid for urea nitrogen and creatinine (GUERRIERO 1989). A ureterovaginal fistula may be recognized by various dye and radiologic tests (BRUBAKER and WILBANKS 1991). Dye testing should include testing with Congo red in the bladder through a urethral catheter. Intravenous blue dye (indigo carmine) should also be given. A tampon is placed in the vagina. The presence of red dye alone suggests a vesicovaginal fistula, whereas the presence of blue dye suggests a uretero-vaginal fistula. If both dyes are seen, multiple fistulae are present.

Ureteral fistulae may also occur in other locations, e.g., ureteroenteric or ureterocutaneous fistulae (Fig. 2.18b).

Intraoperative recognition of vascular injury to the ureter is based on discoloration, lack of peristalsis, and absence of ureteral bleeding from cut surfaces of the ureter.

2.5 Diagnostic Imaging Studies

Diagnostic imaging studies are performed to ascertain the presence and identify the site and nature of injury to the ureter or ureteropelvic junction as well as to other parenchymal or retroperitoneal organs. Plain radiographs are useful to identify skeletal injuries and foreign bodies.

Intravenous urography remains a key examination for assessment of ureteral injury. However, its sensitivity for identifying extravasation of urine and, therefore, potential ureteral injury has been reported to be as low as 27% (PRESTI et al. 1989). The status of kidney function and the magnitude of extravasation influence the ability to demonstrate such a leak. Intravenous urograms obtained in the immediate postoperative period are often of suboptimal quality and the yield for identifying ureteral injury may, therefore, be low (LARSON et al. 1987). Conversely, high dose infusion pyelograms obtained in clearly symptomatic patients tend to have a higher yield.

Hydronephrosis is the most common urographic manifestation of ureteral injury, being present in more than 90% of such patients. (FLYNN et al. 1979). However, some dilatation of the ureter and collecting system is a common transient postoperative manifestation in patients who have had pelvic, retroperitoneal, or gynecologic surgery (GAL and BUCHSBAUM 1983; LARSON et al. 1987; BUCHSBAUM 1986). A sustained and dense nephrogram and delayed appearance of contrast medium in the collecting system in association with progressive hydronephrosis are other manifestations of ureteral trauma (BUCHSBAUM 1986; MALLIK 1960).

Avulsion of the ureter and/or dehiscence at the ureteropelvic junction often show a normal intrarenal collecting system and prompt excretion of contrast medium. Extravasation of contrast medium-laden urine medial to the renal pelvis and ureter is the diagnostic finding (BEAMUD-GOMEZ et al. 1986; KENNEY et al. 1987). However, this appearance is closely mimicked by opacification of peripelvic lymphatics in patients with obstruction secondary to calculus or neoplasm (LANG 1983) (Fig. 2.18c).

Urographic demonstration of ureteral fistulae is successful in only 25% of patients. Extravasation of opacified urine into urinomas, however, is recognized at a much higher rate (DOWLING et al. 1986; SCHULTZ et al. 1987; HOLDEN et al. 1976).

Retrograde and/or antegrade ureterograms are the gold standard for affirming the presence of ureteral injury and defining its magnitude and characteristics, e.g., associated fistulas and urinomas. Retrograde ureterography has been proposed as the modality for ascertaining continuity or dehiscence of the ureter in patients examined with a delay of 36h or greater (LANG 1983). Forceful antegrade or retrograde injections are better able to demonstrate small ureteral perforations that may be temporarily sealed by edema or clot and fail to visualize on intravenous urograms.

Computed tomography is capable of identifying even minimal extravasation of contrast medium-laden urine because of its high sensitivity to minor differences in attenuation coefficients. This high sensitivity makes possible differentiation of liquefying hematomas from urinomas. Contrast-enhanced and delayed CT scans are the method of choice for assessing ureteral avulsion or traumatic dehiscence of the ureteropelvic junction (KENNEY et al. 1987). Other characteristic findings heralding this complication are a negative defect within a pool of extravasated opacified urine and lack of opacification of the afflicted ureter on any of the sequential slices through the lower abdomen and pelvis (KENNEY et al. 1987) (Fig. 2.19).

In addition, CT and dynamic CT are the procedures of choice to assess tissue viability of parenchymal organs (LANG 1983). Delayed, heterogeneous, decreased, or absent enhancement indicates reduced or absent capillary perfusion of the afflicted tissues. Moreover, the ability of CT to detect minute amounts of free air provides a highly sensitive parameter for diagnosis of injury to hollow viscera (FEDERLE et al. 1984).

Radionuclide studies are, likewise, highly sensitive for detection of minute extravasation (MCCONNELL et al. 1981; DELANGE et al. 1982). In general, the diagnosis is easiest on delayed scintiscans showing accumulation of the radioactive tracer material in an abnormal location. Moreover, radionuclide studies may also confirm obstruction.

Dynamic gadolinium diethylenetriamine pentaacetic acid (DTPA)-enhanced MRI may differentiate acute from chronic ureteral obstruction and a dilated nonobstructed from an obstructed renal unit (SEMELKA et al. 1990).

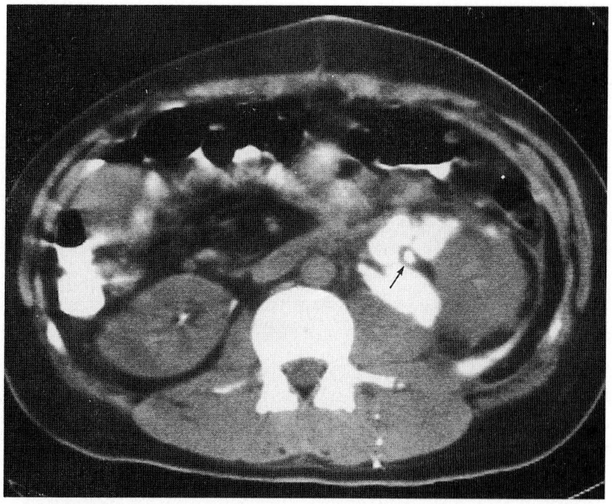

Fig. 2.19. A CT scan demonstrates extravasation of contrast medium medial to the kidney. There is evidence of opacification of the ureter (*arrow*), indicating that only a partial dehiscence exists

Uretero–arterial or ureterovenous fistulas occur most commonly as a consequence of erosion caused by an indwelling ureteral stent (BHARGAVA and YUSEF 1987; SMITH 1984; WHEATLEY et al. 1981; NELSON and FRIED 1981; TOOLIN et al. 1984; ADAMS 1984; KAR et al. 1984). Stone disease, pelvic surgery, and instrumentation with ridged ureteroscopes or basketing of calculi likewise may cause ureterocaval, ureterovenous, and uretero–arterial fistulas. Arteriography or phlebography is the procedure of choice to document uretero-vascular communications (TOOLIN et al. 1984).

2.6 Treatment

Treatment of surgical ureteral injuries is governed by the site and length of the damaged segment. The choice of repair is also influenced by underlying factors such as uncontrolled cancer, infection, retroperitoneal fibrosis, devascularization attendant upon prior radiation therapy, or presence of a vascular graft (ST. LEZIN and STOLLER 1991; TARKINGTON et al. 1991). Whenever possible, immediate reconstruction of ureteral continuity should be attempted (TARKINGTON et al. 1991).

Injuries recognized during open surgery are best repaired immediately. Areas of questionable viability should be debrided to avoid late necrosis

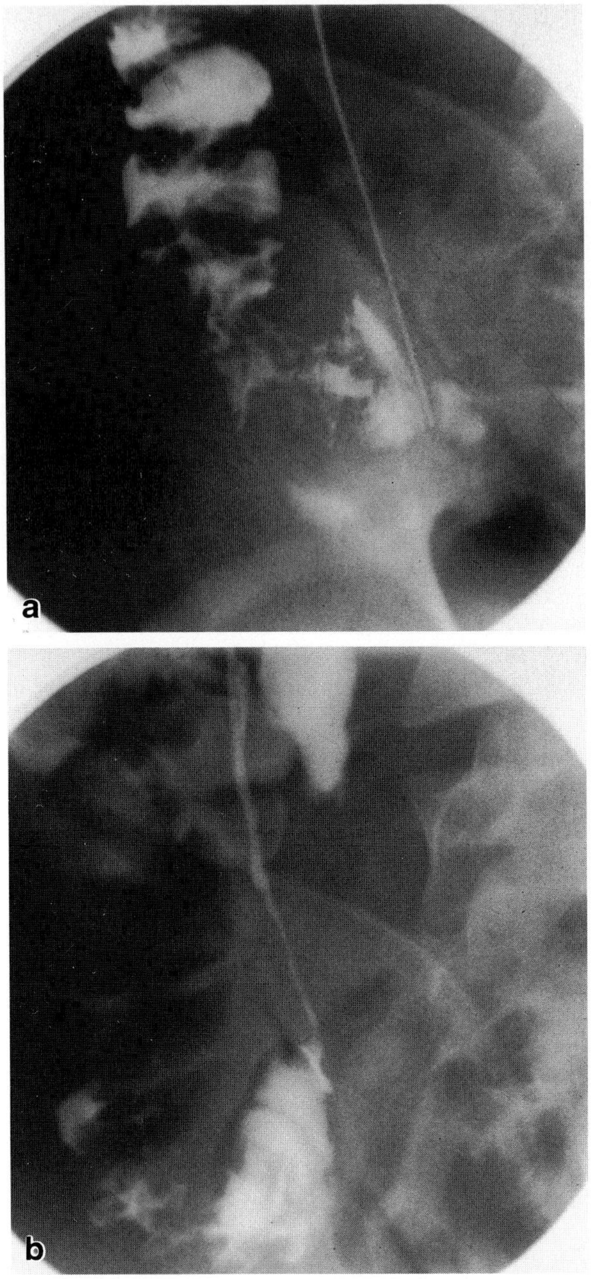

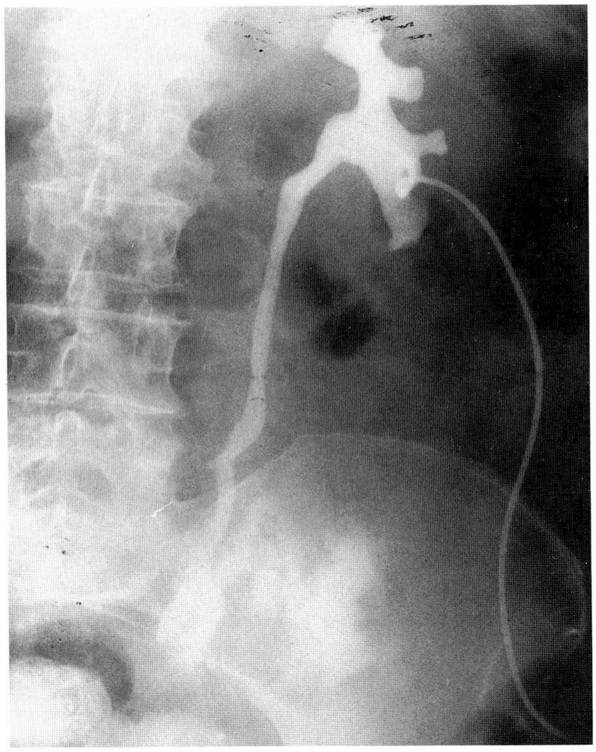

Fig. 2.21. An antegrade pyelogram demonstrates extravasation at the level of the uretero-ileostomy. The anastomosis must be taken down and a new one performed to viable components of the ileal loop

◁

Fig. 2.20. **a** A catheter has been advanced through a right nephrostomy tube and the right ureter into the appendix. The injection phase demonstrates opacification of the right colon. **b** An antegrade ureterogram demonstrates continued drainage from the right ureter through the appendix into the cecum. The lower anastomosis of the ureter was improperly performed to the appendix, thus causing a ureteral – appendiceal fistula

of nonviable ureter with formation of delayed fistulas, urinomas, and strictures (St. Lezin and Stoller 1991). Whenever possible, the repair site is isolated from infection or cancer. In the case of associated vascular injury or presence of a graft, interposition of the omentum between the ureteral repair site and the injured vessel will assure blood supply to the ureter and help prevent contamination of the artery (Guerriero 1989).

Injuries resulting from ligation and crushing of the ureter with a clamp often can be handled by removal of the inappropriately placed suture or clamp and ureteral stenting, if the ureter appears to be viable after removal of the compression (Brubaker and Wilbanks 1991; Tarkington et al. 1991; Daly and Higgins 1988; Lang 1988). Debridement of the involved segment is necessary if viability is uncertain. Ureteral reanastomosis or ureteroneocystomy after resection of the involved segment of the ureter is then the recommended procedure (St. Lezin and Stoller 1991; Zinman et al. 1978).

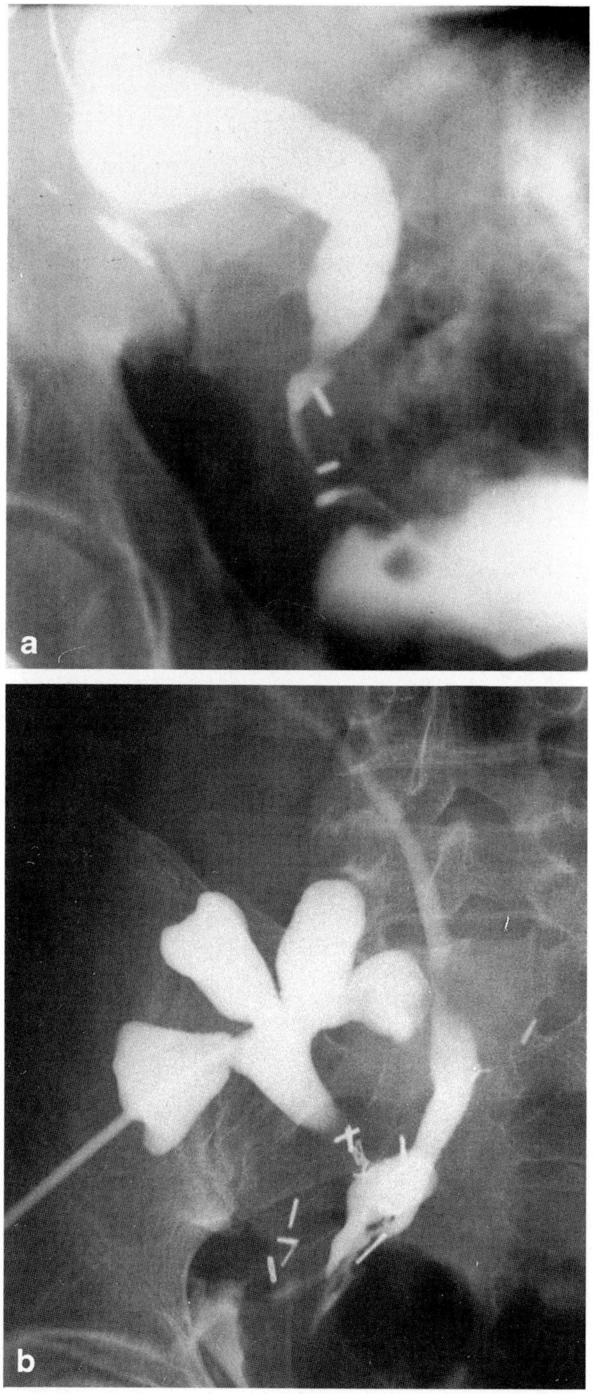

Fig. 2.22. **a** An antegrade pyelogram of a transplanted kidney demonstrates stenosis at the ureteroneocystostomy site as well as multiple studded defects suggesting small urinomas secondary to leakage from the partially dehiscent reimplantation site. **b** Anastomosis of the native ureter to the transplant renal pelvis to bypass the strictured cadaver transplant ureter

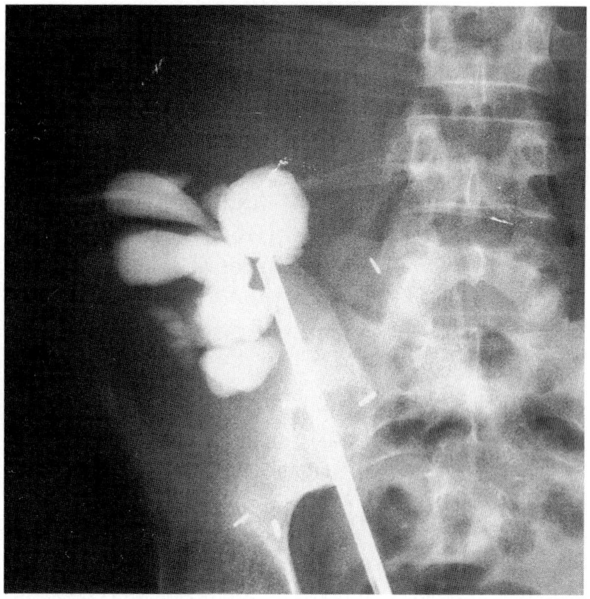

Fig. 2.23. A rigid ureteroscope has been advanced through the native ureter to perform a percutaneous ureterocalicostomy with the intent of bypassing the totally obstructed cadaver transplant ureter

For repair of ureteral injury involving the distal ureter, a common site of injury sustained during gynecologic procedures, antireflux ureteroneocystostomy is the simplest and most effective method of surgical correction. Percutaneous ureteroneocystostomy is an excellent alternative, particularly in the repair of ureteral dehiscence attendant upon vaginal hysterectomy (LANG 1988) (Fig. 2.1c). If a long segment defect needs to be bridged, the psoas hitch or Boari bladder flap procedure is advocated (BOXER et al. 1978; WILLIAMS and PORTER 1966; KONIGSBERG et al. 1975).

For correction of extensive injuries in the mid ureter, transuretero-ureterostomy should be considered (ST. LEZIN and STOLLER 1991; HENDREN and HENSLE 1980; HODGES et al. 1980).

For injuries in the proximal ureter, uretero-ureterostomy will usually suffice (ST. LEZIN and STOLLER 1991). Autotransplantation or intestinal interposition is an alternative procedure if a long defect in the proximal ureter needs to be bridged (SEILER et al. 1991; BODIE et al. 1986; BOXER et al. 1979). Occasionally, the appendix provides an opportune pedicle graft which can be interposed to bridge long defects of the right upper ureter (KOMATZ and ITOH 1990) (Fig. 2.20). Dehiscence or breakdown of ureteroenteric anastomoses generally mandates surgical revision (Fig. 2.21). Dehiscence or obstruction at the ureteroneocystostomy site of transplant kidneys is best treated by ureteropyelotomy or ureterocalicostomy using the native ureter, if retained (Figs. 2.22, 2.23). However, recent advances in interventional radiologic and endourologic techniques have vastly increased conservative management, particularly of the partially dehiscent ureter (FLYNN et al. 1979; HODGES et al. 1980; BHATTACHARYA et al. 1986; LANG 1987b; HUFFMAN et al. 1983).

References

Adams PS Jr (1984) Iliac artery-ureteral fistula developing after dilatation and stent placement. Radiology 153: 647–648

Andersson A, Bergdahl L (1976) Urologic complications following abdominoperineal resection of the rectum. Arch Surg 111:969

Baranyai E (1987) Injuries of ureteral lower segment and the bladder during surgery. Acta Chir Hung 28: 149–154

Beamud-Gomez A, Martinez-Verduch M, Estornell-Moragues F et al. (1986) Rupture of ureteropelvic junction nonpenetrating trauma. J Pediatr Surg 21: 702–705

Benjamin JC, Donaldson PJ, Hill JT (1987) Ureteric perforation after ureteroscopy: conservative management. Urology 29:623–624

Bhargava A, Yusef R (1987) Ureterovenous fistula: an unusual complication of ureteric catheterization. Br J Urol 60:373

Bhattacharya S, Overton S, Yang R, Raz S (1986) Repair of upper ureteric obstruction with Boari flap and psoas hitch. Urology 27:451–453

Biester R, Gillenwater JY (1986) Complications following ureterscopy. J Urol 136:382

Blasco F-J, Saladie J-M (1991) Ureteral obstruction and ureteral fistulas after aortofemoral or aortoiliac bypass surgery. J Urol 145:237–240

Bodie B, Novick AC, Rose M, Straffon RA (1986) Long-term results with renal autotransplantation for ureteral replacement. J Urol 136:1187–1191

Boxer RJ, Johnson SF, Ehrlich RM (1978) Ureteral substitution. Urology 12:269

Boxer RJ, Fritzsche P, Skinner DG et al. (1979) Replacement of the ureter by small intestine: clinical application and results of the ileal ureter in 89 patients. J Urol 121:728–732

Boyd ME (1987) Care of the ureter in pelvic surgery. Can J Surg 20:234–236

Brannen GE, Bush WH, Correa RJ, Gibbons RP, Elder JJ (1985) Kidney stone removal, percutaneous versus surgical lithotomy. J Urol 133:6

Bright TC III, Peters PC (1977) Ureteral injury secondary to operative procedures. Urology 9:22–26

Bright TC III, Peters PC (1977) Ureteral injuries due to external violence. 10 years' experience with 59 cases. J Trauma 17:616–620

Brock J, Soloway MS (1980) Retroperitoneal fibrosis and aortic aneurysm. Urology 15:14–16

Brubaker LT, Wilbanks GD (1991) Urinary tract injuries in pelvic surgery. Surg Clin North Am 71:963–976

Brunschwig A (1960) Surgical treatment of stage I cancer of the cervix. Cancer 13:34–36

Buchsbaum HJ (1986) The urinary tract and radical hysterectomy. In: Buchsbaum HJ, Schmidt JD (eds) Gynecologic and obstetric urology, 2nd edn. W.B. Saunders, Philadelphia, pp 151–167

Calame RJ, Nelson JH Jr (1967) Ureterovaginal fistula as a complication of radical pelvic surgery. Arch Surg 94:876–880

Campbell EW Jr, Filderman PS, Jacobs SC (1992) Ureteral injury due to blunt and penetrating trauma. Urol 40: 216–220

Casale AJ, Colodny AH, Bauer SB, Retik RB (1986) The use of bowel interposed between proximal and distal ureter in urinary tract reconstruction. J Urol 134: 737–740

Cass AS (1983) Blunt renal pelvic and ureteral injury in multiple-injured patients. Urology 22:268–270

Cass AS (1984) Ureteral contusion with gunshot wounds. J Trauma 24:59–60

Cass AS, Cass BP (1983) Immediate surgical management of severe renal injuries in multiple-injured patients. Urology 21:140–145

Corriere JN (1987) Ureteral injuries. In: Gillenwater JY, Grayhack JT, Howards SS, Duckett JW (eds) Adult and pediatric urology. Year Book Medical, Chicago, p 436

Corriere JN Jr, Miller WT, Murphy JJ (1968) Hydronephrosis as a cause of pleural effusion. Radiology 90:79

Daly JW, Higgins KA (1988) Injury to the ureter during gynecologic surgical procedures. Surg Gynecol Obstet 167:19–25

DeLange EE, Paurvels EKJ, Lobatto S et al. (1982) Scintigraphic detection of urinary leakage after kidney transplantation. Eur J Nucl Med 7:55–57

Dowling RA, Corriere GN Jr, Sandler CM (1986) Iatrogenic ureteral injury. J Urol 135:912–915

Dretler SP, Watson G, Parrish JA (1987) Pulsed dye laser fragmentation of ureteral calculi: initial clinical experience. J Urol 137:386

Eickenbert HU, Amin M (1976) Gunshot wounds to the ureter. J Trauma 16:562–565

Eisenkop SM, Richman R, Platt LD, Paul RH (1982) Urinary tract injury during Caesarean section. Obstet Gynecol 60:591–596

Fackler JL, Bellamy FR, Malinowski JA (1986) Wounding mechanism of projectiles striking at more than 1.5 km/sec. J Trauma 26:250–254

Farghaly SA, Hindmarsh JR, Worth PHL (1986) Post-hysterectomy urethral dysfunction: evaluation and management. Br J Urol 58:299–308

Federle MP, Chun G, Jeffery RB Jr, Rayor R (1984) Computed tomographic findings in bowel infarction. AJR 142:91–95

Fisher S, Young DA, Malin JM et al. (1972) Ureteral gunshot wounds. J Urol 108:238

Flynn JT, Tiptaft RC, Woodhouse CRJ et al. (1979) The early aggressive repair of iatrogenic ureteric injuries. Br J Urol 51:454–457

Fry DE, Milholen L, Harbrecht PJ (1983) Iatrogenic ureter injury: options in management. Arch Surg 118:454–458

Gal D, Buchsbaum HJ (1983) A cinefluoroscopic study of ureteral function following radical hysterectomy. Obstet Gynecol 61:82–86

Goldenberg SL, Gordon PB, Cooperberg PL, McLoughlin MG (1988) Early hydronephrosis following aortic bifur-

cation graft surgery: a prospective study. J Urol 140: 1367–1372
Gomel V, James C (1991) Intraoperative management of ureteral injury during operative laparoscopy. Fertil Steril 55:416–419
Grainger DA, Sodersrom RM, Schiff SF et al. (1990) Ureteral injuries at laparoscopy: insights into diagnosis, management and prevention. Obstet Gynecol 75:839–843
Green DF, Lytton B (1985) Early experience with electrohydraulic lithotripsy of ureteral calculi using direct vision ureteroscopy. J Urol 133:767–769
Green TH, Meigs JV, Ulfelder H, Curtin RR (1962) Urologic complications of radical Wertheim hysterectomy: incidence, etiology, management, and prevention. Obstet Gynecol 20:293–312
Guerriero WG (1989) Ureteral injury. Urol Clin North Am 16:237–248
Hendren WH, Hensle TW (1980) Transureteroureterostomy: experience with 75 cases. J Urol 123:826–831
Hodges CV, Barry JM, Fuchs EF et al. (1980) Transureteroureterostomy: 25-year experience with 100 patients. J Urol 123:834–839
Hoe JWM, Tan EC, Tung KH et al. (1992) Percutaneous dilatation of benign ureteric strictures following radical hysterectomy. Eur Radiol 2:62–68
Holden S, Hicks CC, O'Brien DP III et al. (1976) Gunshot wounds of the ureter: a 15 year review of 63 consecutive cases. J Urol 116:562–564
Huffman JL (1988) Approach to upper tract calculi. In: Huffman JL, Bagley DM, Lyon ES (eds) Ureteroscopy. W.B. Saunders, Philadelphia, p 85
Huffman JL (1989) Ureteroscopic injuries to the upper urinary tract. Urol Clin North Am 16:249–254
Huffman JL, Bagley DH, Lyon ES (1983) Extending cystoscopic technique into the ureter and renal pelvis: experience with ureteroscopy and pyeloscopy. JAMA 250:2002–2005
Hughes ESR, McDermott FT, Polglase AL, Johnson WR (1984) Ureteric damage in surgery for cancer of the large bowel. Dis Colon Rectum 27:293–297
Kar A, Angwafo FF, Jhunjhunwala JS (1984) Uretero-arterial and uretero-sigmoid fistula associated with polyethylene indwelling ureteral stent. 132:755–757
Kenney PJ, Panicek DM, Witanowski LS (1987) Computed tomography of ureteral disruption. J Comput Assist Tomogr 11:480–484
Khashu BL, Seery WH, Smulewicz JJ et al. (1975) Gunshot injuries to ureter. Urology 6:182
Komatz Y, Itoh H (1990) A case of ureteral injury repaired with appendix. J Urol 144:132–133
Konigsberg H, Blunt KJ, Muecke ED (1975) Use of Boari flap in lower ureteral injuries. Urology 5:751–755
Kramolowsky EV (1987) Ureteral perforation during ureteroscopy. J Urol 138:36–38
Laberge I, Homsy YL, Dadour G, Beland G (1979) Avulsion of the ureter by blunt trauma. Urology 13:172–178
Lang EK (1981) Diagnosis and management of ureteral fistulas by percutaneous nephrostomy and antegrade stent catheter. Radiology 138:311–317
Lang EK (1983) Assessment of renal trauma by dynamic computed tomography. Radiographics 3:566–584
Lang EK (1985) Antigrade ureteral stenting for dehiscence, strictures and fistulae. AJR 143:795–801
Lang EK (1986) Transluminal dilatation of ureteropelvic junction strictures, ureteral strictures and strictures at uretero-neocystostomy sites. Rad Clin NA 24:601–613
Lang EK (1987a) Percutaneous nephrolithotomy and lithotripsy: a multi-institutional survey of complications. Radiology 162:25–30
Lange EK (1987b) Nonsurgical treatment of ureteral fistulas. Semin Int Radiol 4:53–69
Lange EK (1988) Percutaneous ureterocystostomy and ureteroneocystostomy. AJR 150:1065–1068
Lang EK, Wood M, Brown R et al. (1973) Complications in the urinary tract related to treatment of carcinoma of the cervix. South Med J 66:228–236
Langer R, Neuman M, Ron-EL R et al. (1989) The effect of total abdominal hysterectomy on bladder function in asymptomatic women. Obstet Gynecol 74:205–211
Larson DM, Malone JR Jr, Copeland LJ et al. (1987) Ureteral assessment after radical hysterectomy. Obstet Gynecol 69:612–616
Lee WJ, Smith AD, Cubelli V et al. (1987) Complications of percutaneous nephrolithotomy. AJR 148:177
Liroff SA, Pontes JES, Pierce JM Jr (1977) Gunshot wounds of the ureter: 5 years of experience. J Urol 118:551–553
Livne M, Gonzales ET Jr (1985) Genitourinary trauma in children. Urol Clin North Am 12:53–65
Lytton B, Schiff M (1981) Interposition of an ileal segment for repair of ureteral injuries. J Urol 125:739–743
Mallik MKB (1960) A study of the ureters following Wertheim's hysterectomy. J Obstet Gynaecol Br Emp 67:556–560
Mann WJ, Arato M, Patsner B, Stone ML (1988) Ureteral injuries in an obstetrics and gynecologic training program: etiology and management. Surg Gynecol Obstet 72:82–87
McConnell BJ, McConnell RW, Guiberteau MJ (1981) Radionuclide imaging in blunt trauma. Radiol Clin North Am 19:37–51
McGinty DM, Mendez R (1977) Traumatic ureteral injuries with delayed recognition. Urology 10:115–117
Megibow AJ, Ambos MA, Bosniak MA (1979–1980) Computed tomographic diagnosis of ureteral obstruction secondary to aneurysmal disease. Urol Radiol 1:211–215
Moretti KL, Miller RA, Kellett MJ, Wickham JE (1991) Extrusion of calculi from upper urinary tract into perinephric and periureteric tissues during endourologic stone surgery. Urology 28:447–449
Nelson HN, Fried FA (1981) Iliac artery-ureteral fistula associated with Gibbons catheter, case report and review of literature. J Urol 125:878–880
Novak F (1969) The prevention of uretero-vaginal fistulas after Wertheim operation. Int J Gynaecol Obstet 7: 301
Numan M, Eidelman A, Langer R et al. (1991) Iatrogenic injuries to the ureter during gynecologic and obstetric operations. Surg Gynecol Obstet 173:268–272
Palmer JM, Drago JR (1981) Ureteral avulsion from nonpenetrating trauma. J Urol 125:108–111
Parsons L, Cesare P, Friedell GH (1959) Primary surgical treatment of invasive cancer of the cervix. Surg Gynecol Obstet 109:279–286
Parys BT, Haylen BT, Hutton JL et al. (1989) The effects of simple hysterectomy on vesicourethral function. Br J Urol 64:594–601
Peterson NE, Schulze KA (1987) Selective diagnostic uroradiography for trauma. J Urol 137:449–451
Piver MS, Rutledge F, Smith JP (1974) Five classes of extended hysterectomy for women with cervical cancer. Obstet Gynecol 44:265–272

Presti JC Jr, Carroll PR, McAninch JW (1989) Ureteral and renal pelvic injuries from external trauma: diagnosis and management. J Trauma 129:370–374
Rabinowitz JG, Keller RJ, Wolf BS (1966) Benign peripelvic extravasation associated with renal colic. Radiology 86:220–226
Reznichek RC, Brosman SA, Rhodes DB (1973) Ureteral avulsion from blunt trauma. J Urol 109:812–816
Riss P, Koelbl H, Neunteufel W, Janisch H (1988) Wertheim radical hysterectomy 1921–1986: changes in urologic complications. Gynecol Obstet 241:249
Rohner TJ Jr (1971) Delayed ureteral fistula from high velocity missiles: report of 3 cases. J Urol 105:63–64
Schultz A, Kristensen JK, Bilde T, Eldrup J (1986) Ureteroscopy: results and complications. J Urol 137:865–866
Schwimmer WB (1974) Electrosurgical burn injuries during laparoscopic sterilization: treatment and prevention. Obstet Gynecol 44:526–530
Seiler RK, Filmer RB, Reitelman C (1991) Traumatic disruption of the ureteropelvic junction managed by ileal interposition. J Urol 146:392–395
Sekiba K (1985) Radical hysterectomy for cancer of the uterine cervix. Semin Surg Oncol 1:95–104
Semelka RC, Hricak H, Tomei E (1990) Obstructive nephropathy: evaluation with dynamic Gd-DTPA-enhanced MR imaging. Radiology 175:797–803
Smith AM (1975) Injuries of the pelvic ureter. Surg Gynecol Obstet 140:761–764
Smith RB (1984) Ureteral common iliac artery fistula: a complication of internal double-J ureteral stent. J Urol 132:113
Sosa RE, Huffman JL (1988) Complications of ureteroscopy. In: Fullman JL, Bagley DH, Lyon ES (eds) Ureteroscopy. W.B. Saunders, Philadelphia, p 157
Spirnak JP, Persky L, Resnick MI (1985) The management of civilian ureteral gunshot wounds: a review of 8 patients. J Urol 134:733–736
Spirnak JP, Hampel N, Resnick MI (1989) Ureteral injuries complicating vascular surgery: Is repair indicated? J Urol 141:13–14
St. Lezin MA, Stoller ML (1991) Surgical ureteral injuries. Urology 38:497–506
St. Martin EC, Trichel BE, Campbell JH, Locke CM (1953) Ureteral injuries in gynecologic surgery. J Urol 70:51–57
Stackl W, Marberger M (1986) Complications of ureteroscopy. J Urol 136:386
Stengel JN, Felderman ES, Zamora D (1974) Ureteral injury. Complication of laparoscopic sterilization. Urology 4:341–342
Stutzman RE (1977) Ballistics and the management of ureteral injuries from high velocity missiles. J Urol 118:947–949
Symmonds RE (1976) Ureteral injuries associated with gynecologic surgery: Preventative management. Clin Obstet Gynecol 19:623–628
Tarkington MA, Dejter SW Jr, Bresette JF (1991) Early surgical management of extensive gynecologic ureteral injuries. Surgery 173:17–21
Templeton PA, Mirvis SE, Whitley NO (1988) Traumatic avulsion of the ureter: computed tomography correlation. J Comput Tomogr 12:159
Toolin E, Pollack HM, McLean TK et al. (1984) Ureteral-arterial fistula, case report. J Urol 132:553–554
Underwood PB Jr, Lutz MH, Smoak DL (1977) Ureteral injury following irradiation therapy for carcinoma of the cervix. Obstet Gynecol 49:663
Underwood PB Jr, Wilson WC, Kreutner A et al. (1979) Radical hysterectomy: a critical review of twenty-two years' experience. Am J Obstet Gynecol 134:889
Verstandig AG, Banner MP, Van arsdalen KN, Pollack HM (1986) Upper urinary tract calculi, extrusion into perinephric and periureteric tissues during percutaneous management. Radiology 158:215–218
Verest HAM, deJonge MK, Verest TMJS et al. (1988) Micturition symptoms and urinary incontinence after non-radical hysterectomy. Acta Obstet Gynaecol Scand 67:141–147
Verest HAM, van Venrooij GEPM, Barents JW et al. (1989) Non-radical hysterectomy and the function of the lower urinary tract. Acta Obstet Gynecol Scand 68:231–237
Wallijn E, DeSy W, Fonteyne E (1975) Blunt ureteral trauma with perineal urine fistulization: review of the literature. J Urol 114:942–945
Weinberg JJ, Ansong K, Smith AD (1987) Complications of ureteroscopy in relation to experience: report of survey and author expericence. J Urol 137:384–385
Wheatley JK, Ansley JD, Smith RB et al. (1981) Uretero-arterial fistula. Urology 18:498–502
Williams JL, Porter RW (1966) The Boari bladder flap in lower ureteric injuries. Br J Urol 38:528–553
Witters S, Cornelissen M, Vereecken R (1986) Iatrogenic ureteral injury: aggressive or conservative treatment? Am J Obstet Gynecol 155:582
Zinman LM, Libertino JA, Roth RA (1978) Management of operative ureteral injury. Urology 12:290–293

3 Ureteral Strictures

ERICH K. LANG and PEGGY F. FRITZSCHE

CONTENTS

3.1 Introduction

Catheter dilatation of ureteral strictures was reported as early as 1890 (MURPHY 1972). The procedure, however, did not become widely used because of numerous complications. Today, surgical techniques such as end-to-end anastomosis after resection of the stricture, transureterostomies, and augmentation or interposition procedures compete with percutaneous management of ureteral strictures (BANNER et al. 1983; DEWEERD et al. 1969; LANG and GLORIOSO 1988). Percutaneous management of ureteral strictures is a natural evolution of the percutaneous nephrostomy and angiographic techniques for dilatation of vascular stenosis (DIXON et al. 1982; GRUNTZIG and HOPFF 1974; KADIR et al. 1982). Continued improvements in guidewires and catheter equipment have improved both the efficacy and the safety of dilatation technique.

Since 1977, multiple reports have suggested that the benign ureteral strictures can be successfully treated with a combination of balloon catheters, tapered dilating catheters, and temporary ureteral stents (BANNER et al. 1983; BARBARIC et al. 1977; BIGONGIARI et al. 1979; JOHNSON et al. 1987; LANG 1984a, 1986, 1987; MARTIN et al. 1982; WITHERINGTON and SHELOR 1980; KAPLAN et al. 1982; LIEBERMAN et al. 1982; LIST et al. 1983). The percutaneous transluminal dilatation procedure spares the patient the cost and risk of an extensive surgical procedure, and for many types of strictures offers the patient a potentially equally effective and perhaps safer approach. Such management is particularly attractive since many of these injuries arise as a complication of previous surgery and reoperation for repair is more difficult.

However, most recent data indicate the need for stratification of patients according to underlying etiology of such strictures, demographic criteria, and particularly estimation of viability, i.e., vascular supply to the stricture and adjacent ureter (LANG and THOMAS 1992). While the results of balloon dilatation of short strictures of the ureter with apparently intact vascular supply and without underlying malignant etiology are most acceptable (in the 50%–80% cure range), surgical procedures such as endopyelotomy or endoureterotomy offer better results for strictures at the ureteropelvic junction or long strictures of the ureter (see Sect. 3.3).

The more complex surgical procedures such as transverse ureteroureterostomy or interposition procedures are generally reserved for the management of strictures refractory to the less invasive techniques or those occurring in patients with underlying neoplastic disease and, often, prior surgical or radiotherapeutic interventions. However, even patients with strictures caused by recurrent neoplastic disease are sometimes efficaciously managed by transluminal dilatation and placement of permanent indwelling stents (LUGMAYR and PAUER 1992; CORNŬD et al. 1991). While most strictures in the past were secondary to open surgery or trauma, the increase in ureteral manipulation has introduced a new source of ureteral injuries. Fortunately, strictures resulting from such injuries are usually amenable to percutaneous management. Today most benign ureteral strictures deserve at least an attempt at transluminal dilatation.

ERICH K. LANG, M.D., Professor and Chairman, Department of Radiology, School of Medicine, Louisiana State University, Medical Center, 1542 Tulane Avenue, New Orleans, LA 70112-2822, USA

PEGGY F. FRITZSCHE, M.D., Professor of Radiology, Loma Linda University, Medical Center, Schuman Pavilion, Room 2605 East, 11234 Anderson Street, Loma Linda, CA 92354, USA

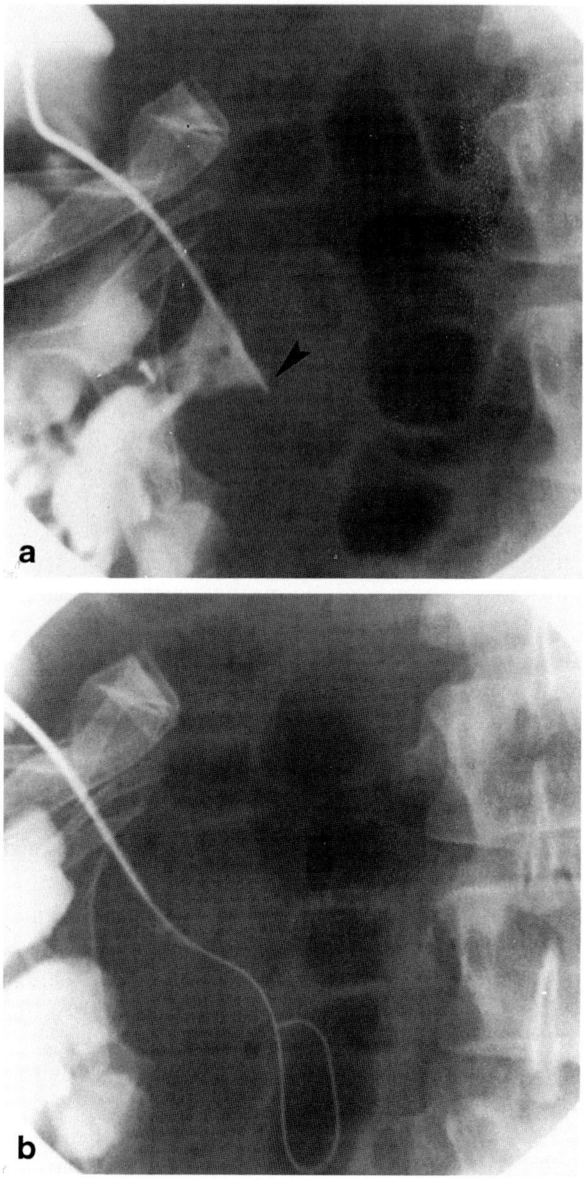

Fig. 3.1. **a** The posterior superior calyx of the right kidney has been accessed to offer a straight pathway to the ureteral pelvic junction in this patient with an apparent obstruction following a dismembered pyeloplasty. A Headhunter catheter has been introduced and the tip has engaged the ureteropelvic junction (*arrowhead*). **b** A guidewire has been advanced through the stricture into the upper right ureter. Bougie dilatation of the stricture is now carried out with tapered, progressively larger straight Teflon catheters. (LANG 1986)

3.2 Technique of Transluminal Dilatation

An optimal approach for transluminal dilatation is selected on the basis of etiologic, morphologic, and topographic information about the stricture (LANG 1984, 1987; LANG and GLORIOSO 1988). Strictures of the lower and pelvic ureter are often approached most easily via a retrograde pathway. Conversely, most strictures of the ureteropelvic junction, upper ureter, and midureter and those occurring at ureteral ileal anastomoses or involving the ureters of transplanted kidneys are most easily accessible via an antegrade approach.

Dilatation is usually performed 2–3 days after a percutaneous nephrostomy to allow for tract maturation. Entry into the collecting system via an interpolar calyx is recommended for antegrade transluminal dilatation of all strictures except those at the ureteropelvic junction and those occurring in transplant kidneys (BECKMANN and ROTH 1987). In the latter cases, entry via the superior calyceal group is ideal because of the direct path to the area of interest (Fig. 3.1).

For optimal guidewire and catheter selection, antegrade urography is suggested to outline the anatomy. Often, the orifice of the stricture is eccentric to the dilated segment of the ureter. The best combination for crossing a stricture is a slightly curved catheter with a floppy tip straight guidewire. Rotation of the catheter while simultaneous gently probing with the guidewire facilitates engagement of the eccentric opening of the stricture (Fig. 3.2a). The stricture can be studied in detail by injection of contrast medium through the catheter. A forceful injection of dilute contrast medium through the catheter engaged in the stricture can also hydrodilate such strictures (LANG 1987; LANG and GLORIOSO 1988) (Fig. 3.2b). Once the stricture is engaged, a floppy tip guidewire can be advanced into either the bladder or the ileal conduit (Fig. 4.2c). The Torumo guidewire (glidewire, Medi-tech, Watertown, Mass.) is useful in crossing severe stenosis.

After the guidewire has crossed the stricture, the slightly curved tip catheter is removed and a straight Teflon catheter or Lieberman sheath system (Cook, Bloomington, Ind.) is inserted. After the Lieberman sheath (8.5 F) has been advanced through the stricture, the inner tapered catheter (6.5 F) is removed and a rigid wire is inserted. The Lunderquist "coat hanger" wire (Cook) or Amplatz super stiff wire (Medi-tech) facilitates advancement and seating of the balloon

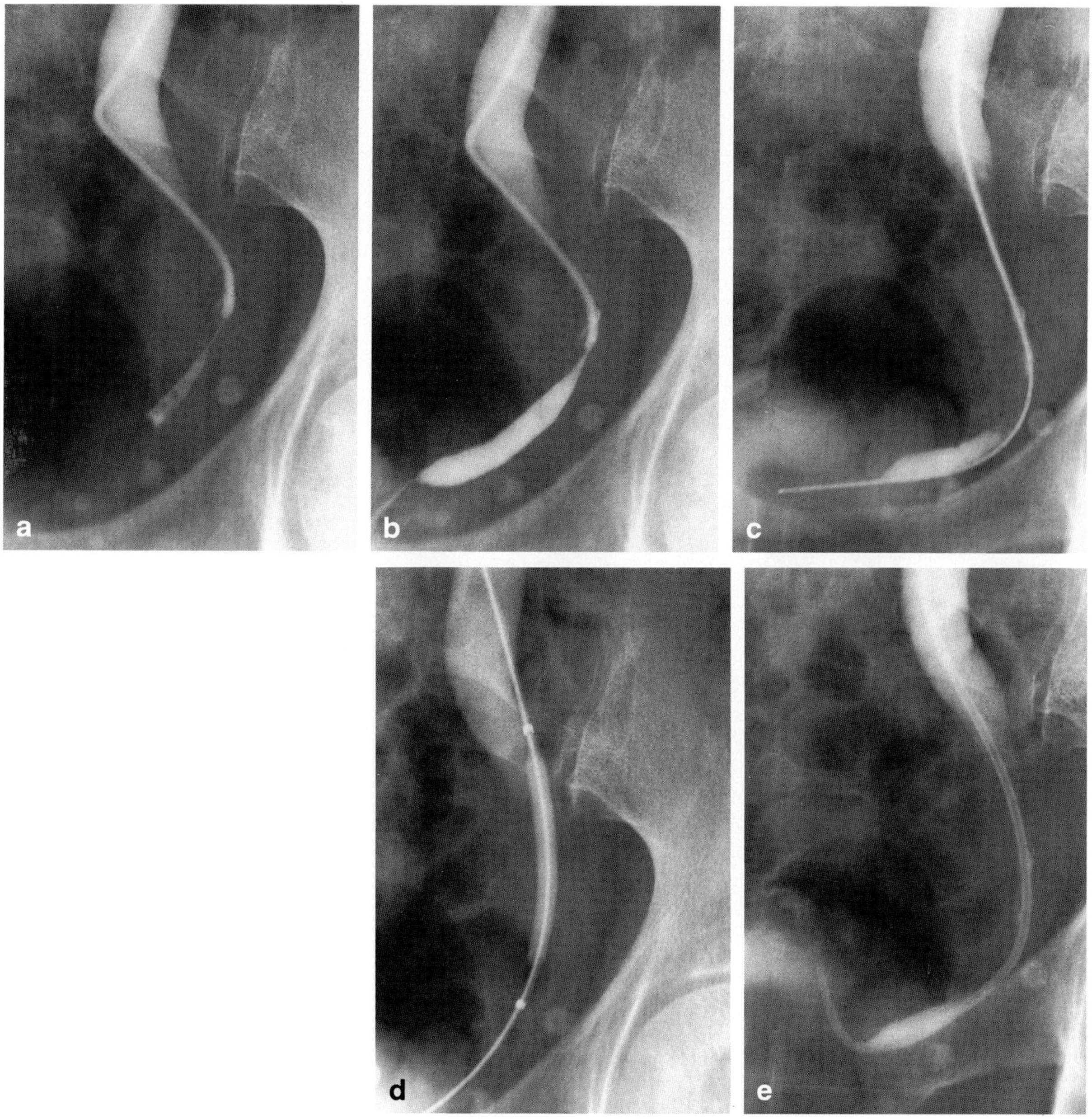

catheter. The flexible wire can be left distal to the stricture as a "safety" wire. The advantage of the Lieberman catheter is that it allows the placement of two guidewires and because of the tapering, it provides some dilatation prior to balloon insertion. To prevent recoil or dislodging during inflation of the balloon, the main guidewire must be coiled in the bladder or ileal loop. At times, the guidewire may be passed through the stoma of the ureteral ileal anastomosis. Control of both ends of the guidewire affords a more secure seating of the balloon and use of much greater force when

Fig. 3.2. **a** A slightly curved tip catheter has been engaged into the eccentric orifice of the stricture. The injection phase characterizes the stricture. **b** A forceful injection of dilute contrast medium serves to hydrodilate the stricture. **c** A guidewire has now been advanced through the stricture into the bladder. **d** A balloon has been placed across the stricture extending at least 0.5 cm to either margin of the stricture. The inflated balloon no longer shows any waist, nor was there recurrence of a waist when deflating the balloon. This indicates a salutary response to the transluminal dilatation. **e** Finally, an 8.5-F stent is placed across the stricture; this will be replaced by a 9-F stent in 2 weeks to minimize cicatricial narrowing. (LANG 1987)

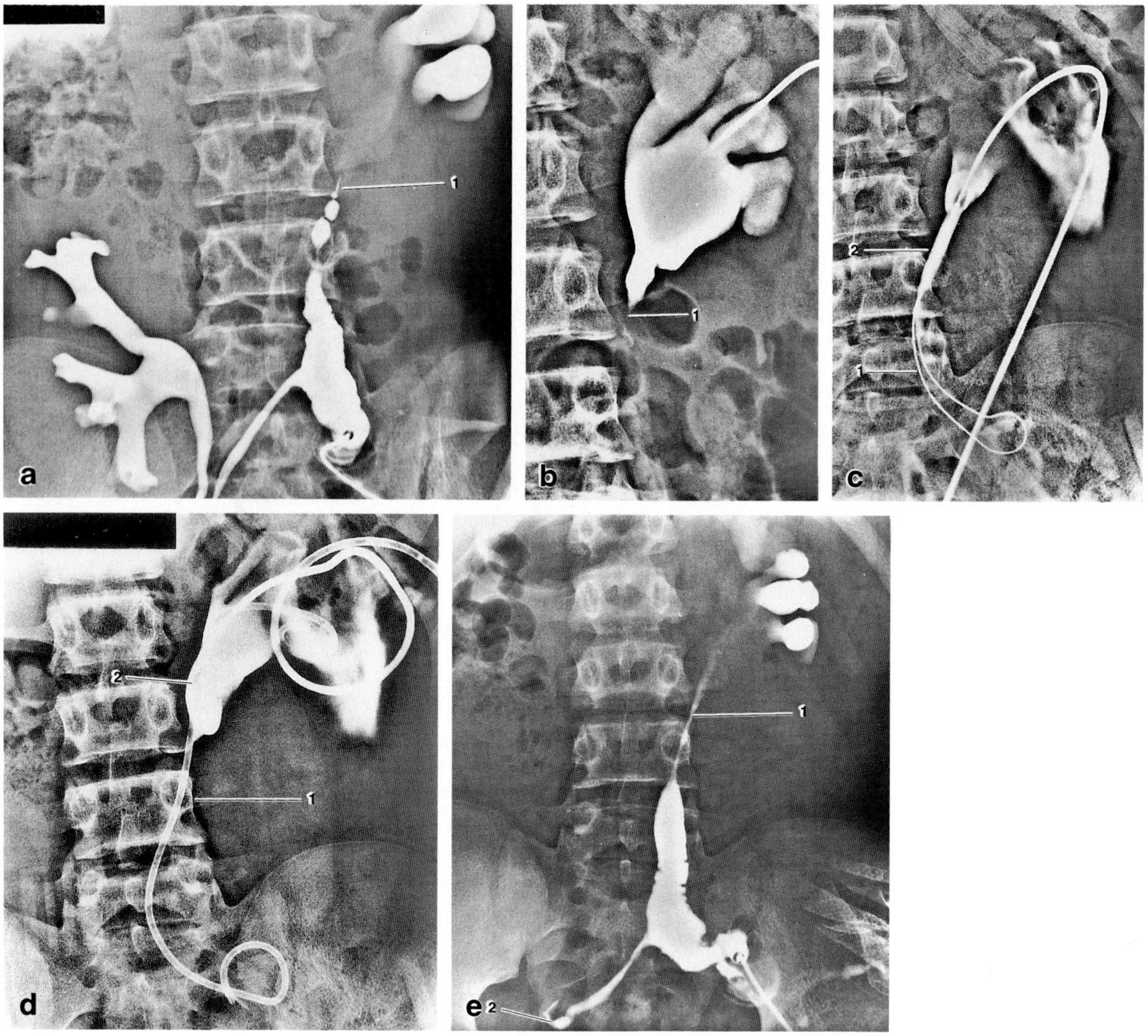

Fig. 3.3a–e. Postsurgical stricture following ileal conduit for dysfunctional bladder and posterior ureteral valves. **a** Loopogram demonstrates areas of dilatation and multiple stenosis and left ureter (*1*) with proximal ureterectasis and pelvic caliectasis. Reflux into the transplant kidney in the right lower quadrant is also noted. **b** Following percutaneous nephrostomy, the nephrostogram shows moderate pelvic caliectasis and proximal ureterectasis secondary to stricture (*1*) in the proximal ureter. **c** A guidewire (*1*) has traversed the stenosis and is in the loop of the ileum. A high pressure balloon catheter (*2*) is inflated at the stricture site without evidence of an indentation following 60 s of pressure. **d** A double pigtail stent catheter (*1*) traverses the stricture with a proximal pigtail in the dilated pelvis and the distal pigtail in the ileum. A nephrostomy catheter with the pigtail near the ureteral pelvic junction (*2*) has been left in place. **e** Postdilatation loopogram 6 weeks later shows tapered narrowing of the ureter (*1*) with less pelvic caliectasis than on the predilatation loopogram. Reflux into the transplanted kidney in the right lower quadrant (*2*) is again noted

utilizing a tapered van Andal catheter or tapered coaxial Teflon dilators. Any uncovered segment of the guidewire exiting from stoma or flank must be protected by a sheath to avoid a saw action upon the soft tissues.

For balloon dilatation of ureteroenteric strictures, a transconduit retrograde approach may be preferable (Banner et al. 1989; Shapiro et al. 1988) (Fig. 3.3).

The length of the balloon is determined by the proceeding diagnostic study. The balloon extends to either side of the stricture by a margin of at least 0.5 cm (Fig. 3.2d). Balloons either 4 or 6 mm in diameter are matched to the adjacent normal ureter for ureteric strictures, 8–12 mm in diameter for ureteropelvic junction strictures, and 8–10 mm in diameter for strictures occurring at ureteral ileal anastomoses. The balloon is advanced over the rigid wire until it is centered at the stricture. High pressure balloons are then inflated to the maximal diameter with diluted contrast material for 2–3 min. Inflation is repeated until a stricture no longer makes an impression or "waist" on the inflated balloon. Lack of reformation of a waist configuration when the balloon is deflated is the accepted criterion for complete and successful dissolution of the stricture (Figs. 3.2d, 3.4). However, if no impression is noted on the initial balloon inflation, it is necessary to use a balloon 1 mm larger in diameter. If antegrade urography demonstrates persistence of the stricture, it can be redilated immediately and then again a few days later with a larger balloon. Each stricture is dilated until the waist disappears.

After successful dilatation, a C-Flex (Cook) or Percuflex (Medi-tech) ureteral stent is placed across the stricture (Mitty et al. 1987). The stent catheters may be left in place for between several days and 3–4 months (Coleman et al. 1984; Glanz et al. 1983; Lang 1984, 1987; Murphy 1972; Pingoud et al. 1980; Voegeli et al. 1988). The underlying etiology of the stricture determines the duration of the stent retention. In some cases, it may be advisable to exchange the stents for progressively larger ones to assure maintenance of an acceptable lumen at the time of maximal fibrotic reaction (Fig. 3.2e). Internal stents are preferred by some and are then removed by cystoscopy (Voegeli et al. 1988). The nephrostomy catheter should be retained at least until stent function is ascertained and sometimes until the ureteral stent is removed since there is risk of obstruction due to ureteral edema whenever the stents are removed (Lavine et al. 1982).

An indication of the effectiveness of the transluminal dilatation of the ureteral stricture is given by comparison of predilatation and postdilatation urodynamic studies if a nephrostomy has been left in place. The postdilatation urodynamic studies must be undertaken after edema attendant upon the use of indwelling stent has subsided. The Whittaker test and radionuclide renal plasma flow studies provide assessment for residual obstruction. If the nephrostomy tube is not in place, then the dilatation is evaluated by morphologic detail on sonograms, intravenous urograms, and nuclear renal scans.

In cases of postsurgical strictures, transluminal dilatation can be entertained within 1 week after surgery. Reabsorbable sutures tend to loosen 1–3

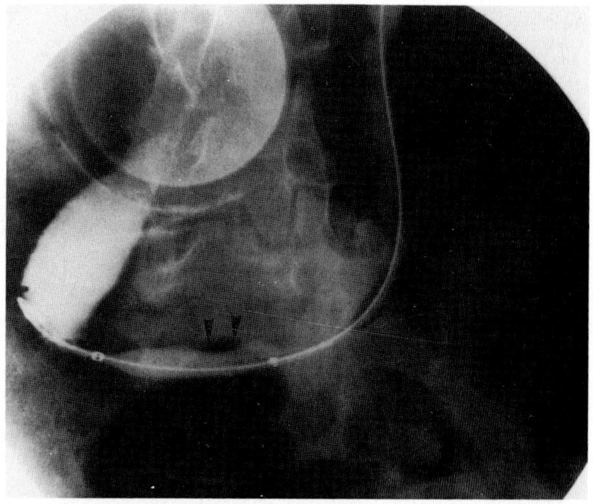

Fig. 3.4. Note the residual waist of the inflated balloon (*arrowheads*) indicating that this stricture proximal to the ureteroileostomy has as yet not yielded

weeks after placement and any resultant stricture will readily respond under the pressure of a dilating balloon (Kaplan et al. 1982) (Fig. 3.5).

Providing the ureter has not been devitalized by stripping during a surgical procedure, damaged by prior radiation therapy, or compromised by recurrent tumor, excellent results can be expected with transluminal dilatation (Lang 1988). Poor results encountered in patients with underlying neoplastic disease are due to devitalization of the ureter rather than recurrent neoplasm. Radical pelvic surgery, retroperitoneal node dissection, and other cancer operations strip the adventitia of the ureter to remove lymphatics and commonly compromise the vascular supply with ensuing fibrosis. Similarly, radiation therapy to the pelvis will frequently cause thrombosis of supply vessels to the ureter and subsequent devascularization of the ureter may result. The poor results of transluminal dilatation in inflammatory strictures are attributable to devascularization of segments of the ureter attendant upon endarteritis obliterans.

To perform endopyelotomy or endoureterotomy, a tract to the kidney pelvis is developed in a fashion akin to the procedure for percutaneous pyelolithotomy (LeRoy et al. 1984). After a rigid guidewire (Lunderquist, Cook, or Amplatz superstiff wire, Medi-Tech) has been advanced into the bladder, a 10-mm Olbert balloon catheter (Bard, Billerica, MA) or Amplatz dilators (Cook, Blooming, IN) are used to dilate the tract to accept a 28-F Amplatz sheath. A flexible ureter-

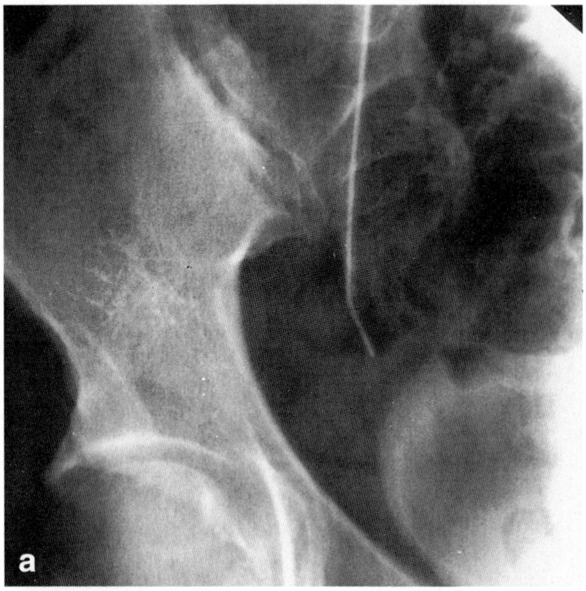

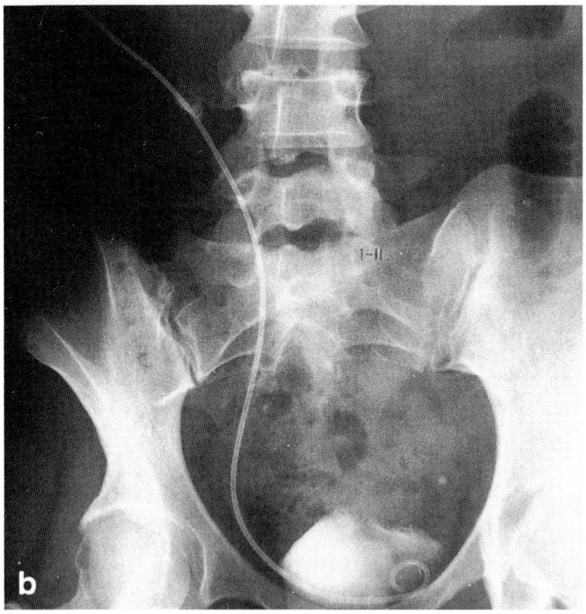

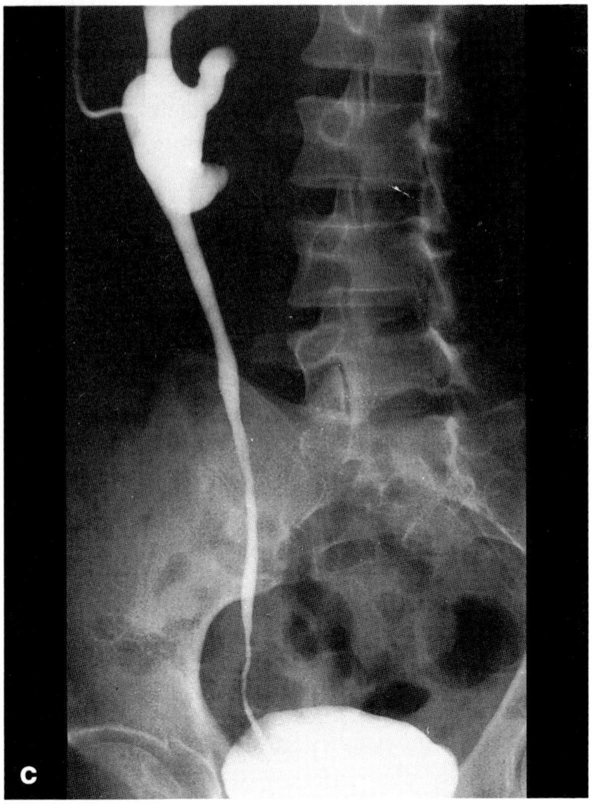

Fig. 3.5. **a** A guidewire is forced through a stricture caused by a suture transfixing the ureter. **b** Bougie dilatation is carried out to a French size 9 and an indwelling stent left in position for 3 weeks. **c** An antegrade pyelogram following removal of the stent demonstrates irregularity of the ureter attributable to edema. This appearance normalized within 48 h. (LANG 1987)

oscope or choledochoscope is then introduced and the stricture at the ureteropelvic junction or in the ureter is visually identified. A laser or electrocautery incision is made over the length of the stricture at the ureteropelvic junction or of the ureter, at 9 o'clock extending into the periureteric or peripelvic fat (BUSH et al. 1989; LANG and THOMAS 1992). Additional dilatation with a balloon catheter (12-mm balloon at the level of the ureteropelvic junction, 8-mm balloon in the ureter) may then be carried out. A double J stent is then placed and retained for 4 weeks. In endopyelotomy patients, a nephrostomy tube is usually retained for 3–4 days. Antegrade pyelograms, obtained immediately after the endopyelotomy, will invariable show extravasation into the peripelvic fat.

3.3 Results

Percutaneous transluminal dilatation of ureteral strictures is successful in 50% of patients in most series (BANNER et al. 1983; BECKMANN et al. 1989; GOTHLIN et al. 1988; LANG 1984, 1987; LANG and GLORIOSO 1988; O'BRIEN et al. 1988; REIMER and OSWALT 1981). Transluminal dilatation of ureteral strictures has proved most effective in the management of short strictures caused by trauma and without historical information suggesting vascular compromise. Transluminal balloon dilatation has been successful in up to 91% of such patients with fresh strictures (LANG 1986, 1987; LANG and GLORIOSO 1988; LANG and THOMAS 1992). However, in at least two other series, the interval between injury and transluminal dilatation did not affect the rate of success (O'BRIEN 1988; VOEGELI et al. 1988).

Results with strictures in transplanted ureters have been less predictable (BANNER and POLLACK 1984). Dilatation was successful in 11 of 14 strictures in transplanted ureters. In 4 of 11 successful cases, the strictures were diagnosed from 6 to 13 years after transplantation (VOEGELI et al. 1988). The findings suggest the dilatation should be attempted regardless of age of the stricture (LIEBERMAN et al. 1982; LIST et al. 1983; KIM et al. 1993).

Strictures that are easily negotiated have been reported to be more likely treated effectively with dilatation and stenting (O'BRIEN et al. 1988). Response to dilatation may also be related to severity and length of the stricture. Previous infection, urinary extravasation, and vascular compromise may be factors in the formation of long ureteral strictures and their resistance to dilatation.

Fresh inflammatory strictures tend to respond readily to transluminal dilatation (LANG 1986, 1987; LANG and GLORIOSO 1988). It is important to remove the underlying cause of the inflammatory response, such as retroperitoneal abscesses, to avoid repeated stricture formation.

Strictures of the ureteropelvic junction or long strictures of the ureter are best treated by endopyelotomy and endoureterotomy followed by transluminal dilatation and stenting for approximately 4 weeks. Endopyelotomy is credited with a success rate of up to 87.5% in the treatment of secondary ureteropelvic junction strictures while the success rate of transluminal balloon dilatation of such lesions reaches only 37.5% (BUSH 1989; LANG and THOMAS 1992). Endoureterotomy is reported to have a success rate of up to 90% in the management of ureteral strictures of 5 cm or greater whereas transluminal balloon dilatation of strictures of this length has a 50–80 percentile success rate (BECKMAN et al. 1989; LANG and THOMAS 1992). For these reasons endopyelotomy and endoureterotomy via an antegrade approach are advocated for the management of such lesions.

Devascularized ureteral strictures pose a particular problem since these strictures respond poorly to transluminal dilatation. Vascular compromise of the ureter is common in patients with underlying neoplastic disease, those with previous radiation or radical surgery, and also those with transplanted ureters. Even if there is temporary reprieve with the transluminal dilatation, strictures caused by devascularization will redevelop and be refractory to further transluminal dilatation (LANG and GLORIOSO 1988).

Patients with strictures caused by known or suspected tumor recurrence are best handled by placement of a permanent or semipermanent stent catheter since transluminal dilatation is unlikely to provide long-term results.

3.4 Complications

Complications of transluminal dilatation of strictures and stent placement are relatively rare. Some believe that long-term ureteral stent may lead to mucosal irritation and recurrent stricture formation. Others think that large diameter stents may cause ureteral ischemia and contribute to recurrent stenosis (BANNER et al. 1983). Rupture at the stricture site during balloon dilatation has been reported (BANNER et al. 1983). Pressure erosion by an indwelling stent can result in ureteral arterial or ureteral bowel fistula (ADAMS 1984; KAR et al. 1984; WHEATLEY et al. 1981). The common iliac artery, being closely related to the base of an ileal conduit, is particularly susceptible to pressure erosion and fistula formation from an indwelling ureteral stent (ADAMS 1984). Lethal complications appear to be attributable primarily to sepsis (WALTER et al. 1985).

Metalic stents combining rigid maintainance of lumen with a degree of flexibility have recently been introduced in the management of extrinsic or intrinsic compromise of the ureteral lumen (PAUER 1992; TOPOROFF 1992).

References

Adams PS (1984) Iliac artery-ureteral fistula developing after dilatation and stent placement. Radiology 153: 647–648

Banner MP, Pollack HM (1984) Dilatation of ureteral stenoses: techniques and experience in 44 patients. AJR 143:789–793

Banner MP, Pollack HM, Ring EJ, Wein AJ (1983) Catheter dilatation of benign ureteral strictures. Radiology 147:427–433

Banner MP, Amendola MA, Pollack HM (1989) Anastomosed ureters: fluoroscopically guided transconduit retrograde catheterization. Radiology 170:45

Barbaric ZL, Gothlin JH, Davies RS (1977) Transluminal dilatation and stent placement in obstructed ureters in dogs through the use of percutaneous nephropyelostomy. Invest Radiol 12:534–536

Beckmann CF, Roth RA (1987) Secondary ureteropelvic junction stricture: percutaneous dilatation. Radiology 164:365

Beckmann CF, Roth RA, Bihrle W III (1989) Dilatation of benign ureteral strictures. Radiology 172:437

Bigongiari LR, Lee KR, Moffat RE, Mebust WK, Foret S, Weigel J (1979) Percutaneous ureteral stent placement for stricture management and internal urinary drainage. AJR 133:865–868

Coleman CC, Clayman RV, Reddy P et al. (1984) Interventional techniques in the ureter. Semin Intervent Radiol 1:24

Bush WH, Brannen GE, Lewis GP (1989) Ureteropelvic junction obstruction: treatment with percutaneous endopyelotomy. Raddiology 171:535–540

Coleman CC, Clayman RV, Reddy P et al. (1984) Interventional techniques in the ureter. Semin Intervent Radiol 1:24

Cornūd FE, Gasanova JMP, Bonnel DH et al. (1991) Impossible ureteral strictures: management with percutaneous ureteroneocystostomy. Radiology 180: 451–456

Deweerd JH, Fassund T, Burke EC (1969) Ureteral neocystostomy. J Urol 101:520–526

Dixon GD, Morre JD, Stockton RI (1982) Successful dilatation of ureteroileal anastomotic stenosis using Gruntzig catheter. Urology 19:555–558

Glanz S, Gordon DH, Butt K, Rubin B, Hong J, Sclafani SJA (1983) Percutaneous transrenal balloon dilatation of the ureter. Radiology 149:101–104

Gothlin JH, Gadeholt G, Farsund P et al. (1988) Percutaneous antegrade dilatation of distal ureteral strictures and obstructions. Eur J Radiol 8:217

Gruntzig A, Hopff H (1974) Perkutane rekanalisation chronischer arterieller Verschlüsse mit einem neuen Dilatationskatheter. Modification der DotteTechnik. Dtsch Med Wochenschr 99:2505–2510

Johnson CD, Oke EJ, Dunnick NR et al. (1987) Percutaneous balloon dilatation of ureteral strictures. AJR 148:181–184

Kadir S, White RIK, Engle R (1982) Balloon dilatation of a ureteropelvic junction obstruction. Radiology 143:263–264

Kaplan JO, Winslow OP, Sneider SE, Pryor TH, Caplan LH, Messinger NH (1982) Dilatation of a surgically ligated ureter through a percutaneous nephrostomy. AJR 139:188–189

Kar A, Angwafo FF, Shunghunwala JS (1984) Uretero-arterial and ureterosigmoid fistula associated with polyethylene indwelling ureteral stents. J Urol 132: 755–757

Kim JC, Banner MP, Ramchandani P, Grossman RA, Pollack HM (1993) Balloon dilatation of ureteral strictures after renal transplantation. Radiol 186:717–721

Lang EK (1984a) Antegrade ureteral stenting for dehiscence, strictures and fistulae. AJR 143:795–801

Lang EK (1984b) Management of strictures of the ureter by dilatation with balloon or bougie catheters. Current concepts of uroradiology. Williams and Wilkins, Baltimore, p 220

Lang EK (1986) Transluminal dilatation of ureteropelvic junction strictures, ureteral strictures and strictures of the ureteroneocystostomy sites. Radiol Clin North Am 24:601–613

Lang EK (1987) Percutaneous management of ureteral strictures. Semin Intervent Radiol 4:79–89

Lang EK, Glorioso LW (1988) Antegrade transluminal dilatation of benign ureteral strictures: long-term results. AJR 150:131–134

Lang EK, Thomas R (1992) Advantage of endopyelotomy and endoureterotomy over transluminal dilatation of ureteropelvic junction strictures and long strictures of the ureter. J Vasc Intervent Radiol (in print)

Lavine RS, Pollack HM, Banner MP (1982) Transitory ureteral obstruction after ureteral stenting. AJR 138:323

Leroy AJ, May GR, Segŭra JW et al. (1984) Rapid dilatation of percutaneous nephrostomy tracks: AJR 142:355–359

Lieberman SF, Kellet FS, Barry JM, Rosch J (1982) Percutaneous antegrade transluminal ureteroplasty for renal allograft ureterostenosis. J Urol 128:122

List AR, Blohme I, Bryuger H, Nilson AE (1983) Balloon dilatation for ureteral strictures in graft kidney, a viable alternative to further surgery. Transplantation 35:105

Lugmayr H, Pauer W (1992) Self expanding metalic stents for palliative treatment of malignant ureteral obstruction. AJR 159:1091–1094

Martin EC, Fankuchen EI, Casarella WJ (1982) Percutaneous dilatation of ureteroenteric strictures or occlusions in ileal conduits. Urol Radiol 4:9–21

Mitty HA, Dan SJ, Train JS (1987) Antegrade ureteral Stents: technical and catheter related problems with polyethylene and polyurethane. Radiology 165:439

Murphy LJT (1972) The history of urology Charles C. Thomas, Springfield, Ill., p 281

O'Brien WM (1988) Ureteral stricture: experience with 31 cases. J Urol 140:737–740

Pauer W (1992) Metallic wall stent a new therapy for extrinc ureteral obstruction. J Urol Aug 148-2:281–284

Pingoud EG, Bagley DH, Zeman RK, Glancy KE, Pais OS (1980) Percutaneous antegrade bilateral ureteral dilatation and stent placement for internal drainage. Radiology 134:780

Reimer DE, Oswalt GC Jr (1981) Iatrogenic ureteral obstruction treated with balloon dilatation. J Urol 126:689–690

Shapiro MJ, Banner MP, Amendola MA, Gordon RL, Pollack HM, Wein AJ (1988) Balloon catheter dilatation of uretero-enteric strictures: long-term results. Radiology 168:385

Toporoff B (1992) Percutaneous antegrade ureteral stenting as an adjunt for treatment of complicated ureteral injuries. J Trauma 32:534–538

Van Schaik JPJ, Herrera MA, Vcinich JL (1987) Code blue catheter for retrograde internal stenting of ureteroileal anastomatic strictures. Urol Radiol 9:191

Voegeli DR, Crummy AB, McDermott JC, Jensen SR (1988) Percutaneous dilatation of ureteral strictures in renal transplant patients. Radiology 169:185–188

Walter PJ (1985) Lethal complications of standard self-retaining ureteral stents in patients with ileal conduit urinary diversion. J Urol 133:851–853

Wheatley JK (1981) Ureteroarterial fistulae. Urology 18:498–502

Witherington R, Shelor WC (1980) Treatment of post-operative ureteral stricture by catheter dilatation: a forgotten procedure. Urology 16:592–595

4 The Postoperative Ureter

DAVID B. SPRING

CONTENTS

4.1 Introduction

The ureters, nestled snugly in their retroperitoneal course, lie close to many abdominal and pelvic structures. Primary ureteral as well as secondary abdominal and pelvic, nonureteral, surgical procedures may result in alterations in ureteral appearance. Evaluation of the postoperative ureter may involve many imaging modalities, including plain radiography, intravenous urography, retrograde ureteropyelography, antegrade pyeloureterography, angiography, radionuclide imaging, ultrasonography, computed tomography (CT), and magnetic resonance imaging (MRI) PFISTER and NEWHOUSE 1978).

Ureteral strictures, sometimes a result of these processes, are discussed elsewhere in this volume (see Chap. 3). Shock wave lithotripsy with its inherent trauma to urinary calculi also may injure the kidneys, ureters, and other retroperitoneal structures. These alterations lie beyond the scope of this chapter.

DAVID B. SPRING, M.D., Associate Professor, Department of Radiology, Kaiser Permanente Medical Center, The Permanente Medical Group Inc., 280 West MacArthur Boulevard, Oakland, CA 94611-5693, USA

4.2 Ureteral Anatomy

The ureters conduct urine from the renal pelvis to the urinary bladder. It is self-evident that "a good kidney is dependent on a good ureter" (BERGMAN 1967). About two-thirds of each ureter is "abdominal," following a course to the iliopectineal line at the pelvic brim; the "pelvic" ureter, or lower-third ureter, follows a course to the posterolateral bladder wall. Adult ureters are each approximately 25 cm long. Surgical procedures that alter the ureters or nearby structures may affect the appearance and function of the ureters. In addition to the description of ureteral anatomy given here, the reader is referred to THOREK (1985).

4.2.1 Abdominal Ureters

The right abdominal ureter follows a retroperitoneal course from lateral to the inflerior vena cava and posterior to the second portion of the duodenum. It passes anterior to the right psoas muscle which traverses from medial to lateral as it passes caudad, resulting in a ureter that crosses from lateral to medial surface of the psoas muscle. The right abdominal ureter ends at the right common iliac bifurcation, where, after passing anterior to the vessels, it becomes the pelvic ureter.

The left abdominal ureter lies lateral to the abdominal aorta, also descending anterior to the psoas muscle. The left ureter usually reaches the pelvic brim anterior to the left common iliac vessels, 1–2 cm before the bifurcation, where it turns into the left pelvic ureter.

4.2.2 Pelvic Ureters in Males

The male pelvic ureters pass downwards near the lower border of the internal iliac arteries, soon reaching the ischial spines. There they turn anterior and medial above the levator ani muscles, reaching the posterolateral bladder wall, where they enter the bladder at the trigone. The seminal vesicles lie caudad, extending upwards from the bladder and prostate bases which abut one another. The vasa deferentia pass lateral to the bladder and then onward to meet the seminal vesicles at the base of the prostate and ejaculatory ducts. The ureters form slings, passing under the vasa. When the bladder floor is elevated, as it often is with prostatic hyperplasia in older males, the vasa hook the distal pelvic ureters.

4.2.3 Pelvic Ureters in Females

The course of the pelvic ureter in the female is more complex than in the male because of its relationship to the pelvic genital organs. There are three portions: (a) a pars posterior, in the uterosacral ligament, (b) a pars intermedia, in the cardinal ligament, and (c) a pars anterior, in the vesicouterine ligament. The pars posterior passes downwards near the posterior margin of the ovary, forming the posterior boundary of the ovarian fossa. The uterine artery, a branch of the internal iliac, passes nearby anterolaterally.

In the pars intermedia the ureter passes in the cardinal ligament to the vesicouterine ligament. Here the ureter passes 1–2 cm from the uterine cervix, where obstetric and gynecologic surgical procedures may injure the ureter. The course

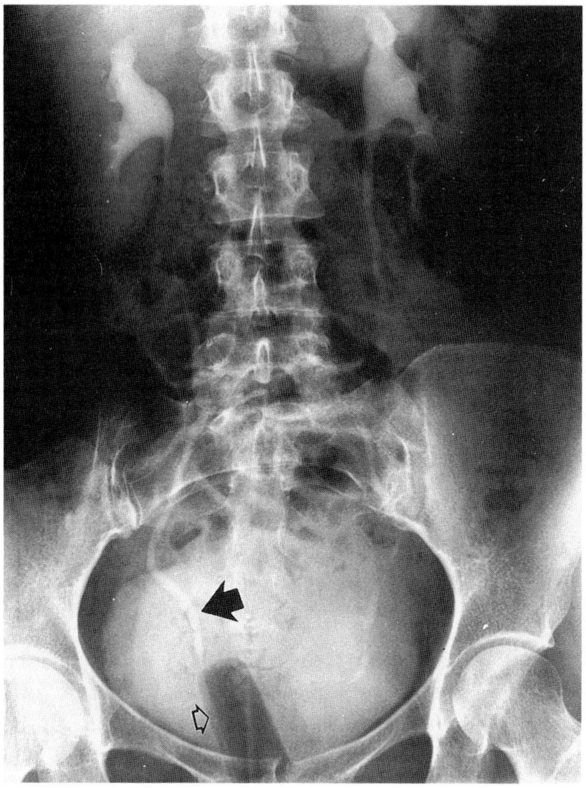

◁

Fig. 4.1. Intravenous urogram demonstrating medial placement of right pelvic ureter, a common normal variant (*arrow*). Tampon (*arrowhead*) is directed towards right vaginal fornix

Fig. 4.2. Diagram of the pelvis, seen from anterior and left, shows course of the three parts of the pelvic ureters in a patient with the uterus centered slightly to the left, resulting in a medially placed right pelvic ureter similar to that in Fig. 5.1

▽

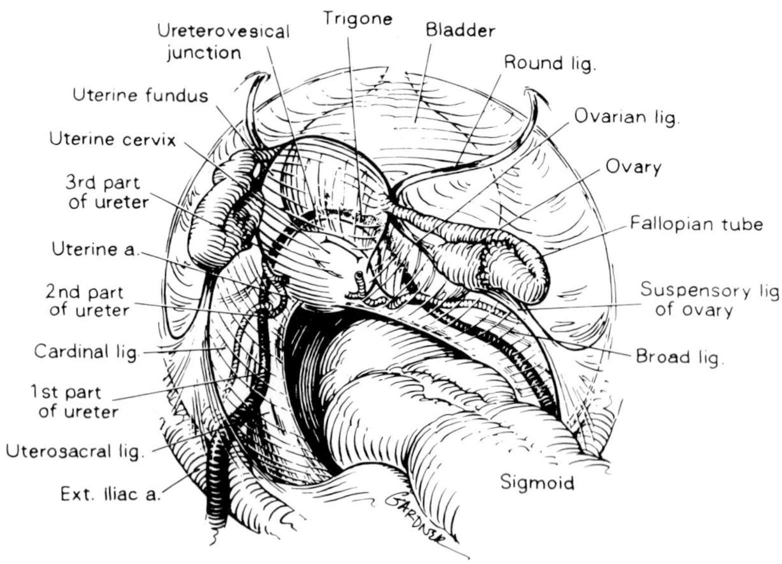

of the pars intermedia varies radiographically, depending upon the position of the uterus within the pelvis (GLAZER HB et al., unpublished data) (Figs. 4.1, 4.2). The pelvic ureters in women frequently are asymmetric, with the right most often having a more medial course (KABAKIAN et al. 1976; APTER et al. 1984).

The pars anterior passes in the vesicouterine ligament lateral to the vesicovaginal space and medial to the vesical venous plexus. The distal ureter enters the posterolateral urinary bladder about 1.5 cm below the level of the anterior lip of the uterine cervix. Distal pelvic ureteral calculi may sometimes be palpated at this site through the vaginal wall. Ureterovesical junction injuries from surgical procedures may communicate with the vagina at this site.

4.3 Primary Ureteral Surgical Procedures

4.3.1 Abdominal Ureter

4.3.1.1 Ureteropelvic Junction Reconstructive Procedure

Idiopathic ureteropelvic junction (UPJ) obstruction is one of the commonest causes of hydronephrosis and obstructive uropathy at all ages (TALNER 1990). The cause and diagnosis of UPJ obstruction has been debated. Most often it has been associated with an extrarenal pelvis of the ampullary type. Indications for surgical intervention include pain, recurrent infection, symptomatic calculus disease, and deteriorating renal function (LINDELL et al. 1991).

Renal pelvic size does not specifically reflect the presence of significant UPJ obstruction. Diuretic urography, diuretic radionuclide urography (KOFF 1982; THRALL et al. 1981), and perfusion pressure flow studies (WHITAKER 1978; DECAMPO and FOWLER 1989; PFISTER and NEWHOUSE 1979) have all been advocated for preoperative and occasional postoperative evaluation of UPJ obstruction. Each has limitations.

There are several surgical procedures commonly used for correction of idiopathic UPJ obstruction. The commonest is dismembered pyeloplasty of the Anderson-Hynes type (Fig. 4.3), in which the adynamic UPJ segment is resected along with a portion of the redundant renal pelvis. Another surgical procedure, pyeloureteroplasty (e.g., Foley Y-V plasty), reconstructs the renal pelvis to form a funneled renal pelvic outlet. A third procedure, calycoureterostomy, anastomoses the deformed calyceal system directly to the proximal ureter.

Postoperatively, after conventional procedures such as Anderson-Hynes dismembered pyeloplasty, the appearance of the calyces may change very little. Calyceal distortion reflects renal parenchymal loss as well as loss of normal compliance secondary to pyelocalyceal muscle hypertrophy and fibrosis. Thus, surgical reconstructive procedures are most often followed by only minor changes in the appearance of the calyces themselves. More rapid radiographic appearance of urine in the ureter correlates best with clinical improvement (CHERRIE and KAUFMAN 1983) (Fig. 4.3). Earlier appearance time of contrast medium in the ureter, however, may simply reflect the decreased size of the surgically trimmed renal pelvis. Increased renal plasma flow rate is another reliable indicator of clinical improvement.

Postoperative improvement of renal function in patients with UPJ obstruction and chronic renal failure traditionally depends upon many factors,

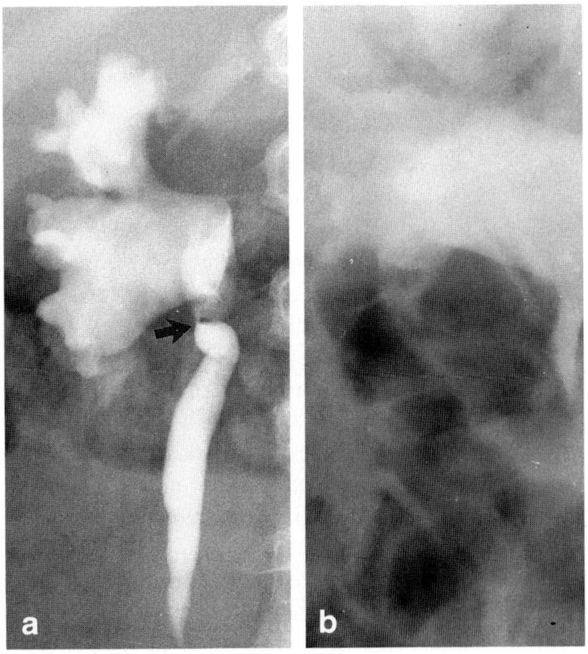

Fig. 4.3. **a** Preoperative retrograde pyelogram in a 2-year-old boy with recurrent urinary tract infections and mild hydronephrosis suggested by sonography and confirmed by excretory urography. Tight UPJ obstruction is seen (*arrow*). **b** Six months postoperatively, after Anderson-Hynes type pyeloplasty, remodeled right UPJ funnels without obstruction

including severity of renal injury and the presence or absence of infection (KUMAR et al. 1988). Gross inspection of the kidney, function as assessed by IVP, and kidney biopsy are all poor predictors of recovery potential. Radionuclide scanning before and after decompression by percutaneous nephrostomy (LANG et al. 1973; LUPTON et al. 1979) has been useful in assessing recoverability, as have serial creatinine clearances. Even failed pyeloplasties may be objectively improved with secondary surgical procedures (BRATT and NILSSON 1984).

4.3.1.2 Ureteroureteral Anastomosis

When a segment of the abdominal or upper pelvic ureter is injured it is most often repaired with a simple end-to-end anastomosis. All common modes of urinary tract imaging, including intravenous urography, radionuclide renal imaging, sonography, and CT, show little if any evidence of ureteroureteral anastomosis. If there is stenosis, frank hydronephrosis, complete obstruction, urinary extravasation, or fistula formation, each of these examinations may prove useful. Images which confirm clinical impressions of postoperative complications of ureteroureterostomy are similar to those noted elsewhere in this section when there has been ureteral injury.

4.3.1.3 Ureteral Diversions (BANNER et al. 1984; SPRING and DESHON 1990)

Surgical variations in urinary tract diversions have blossomed in the past decade with efforts to decrease long-term morbidity from renal reflux and to increase patient acceptance and convenience with continent diversions. The postoperative radiographic appearance of these diversions varies with underlying pathology, residual renal function, chronicity, and type of diversion. A classification of supravesical ureteral diversions is provided in Table 4.1.

Cutaneous ureterostomies are encountered much less frequently since the advent of percutaneous ureterostomies (MOR et al. 1992). Stenoses of these end-cutaneous ureterostomies are less frequent when there is a protruding nipple-like stoma and a preoperative ureteral diameter exceeding 8 mm (FEMINELLA and LATTIMER 1974).

Transureteroureterostomy (TUU) is a procedure best suited for end-to-side anastomosis of

Table 4.1. Ureteral diversions. (After SPRING and DESHON 1990)

A. *Directly to skin*: cutaneous ureterostomy
B. *To the contralateral ureter*: transureteroureterostomy, with or without cutaneous ureterostomy
C. *To bowel*:
  1. Intact anal sphincter: ureterosigmoidostomy (with or without signmoid colostomy)
  2. To redirected bowel (with cutaneous stoma)
     a) Conduits: ureteroileal cutaneous (ileal loop); sigmoid; other colon conduits (ileocecal, transverse colon)
     b) Continent urinary diversions (reservoirs): Kock pouch; Mainz pouch; LeBag (ileocolonic pouch); Indiana pouch
  3. To urethral sphincter through bowel segment (bladder replacement)
     a) Bladder replacement; ileocystoplasty (Camey procedure; hemi-Kock pouch; Melchior ileal pouch)
     b) Ileocecocystoplasty (modified LeBag)

the middle-third ureters (UDALL et al. 1973) (Fig. 4.4). The success rate for TUUs is high, with otherwise normal ureters tending to remain so. Large-field radiotherapy for bladder, bowel, and gynecologic carcinomas is a relative contraindication for TUU, as is urolithiasis, urinary tract tuberculosis, and other chronic renal infections.

Postoperative urographic evaluation of the uneventful ureteral diversion can probably be delayed until approximately 3 months after surgery. Fever, decreased renal function, flank pain, or other symptoms should prompt earlier evaluation which may also include ultrasound (CRONIN et al. 1986), radionuclide (WOODSIDE et al. 1978), CT (SPRING and MOSS 1984), and retrograde studies where appropriate.

Interpretation of these studies requires familiarity with the specific ureteral diversion. Gas, for example, may be seen in the pyelocalyceal system of ileal loops because of the patency of the ureteroileal anastomoses. Migration of ureteral calculi in the ureters requires knowledge of the anatomy of a specific diversion (Fig. 4.5).

Ureteroileostomies have been among the commonest of the ureteral diversions and remain the comparison basis for all other diversions. In addition to the conventional urogram, the retrograde ileostoureterogram ("ileal loopogram") is often useful in evaluating the ileal loop. Because the ileal loop refluxes its infected contents and increases pelvic pressure, STAMEY has recommended a single intramuscular or intravenous dose of an

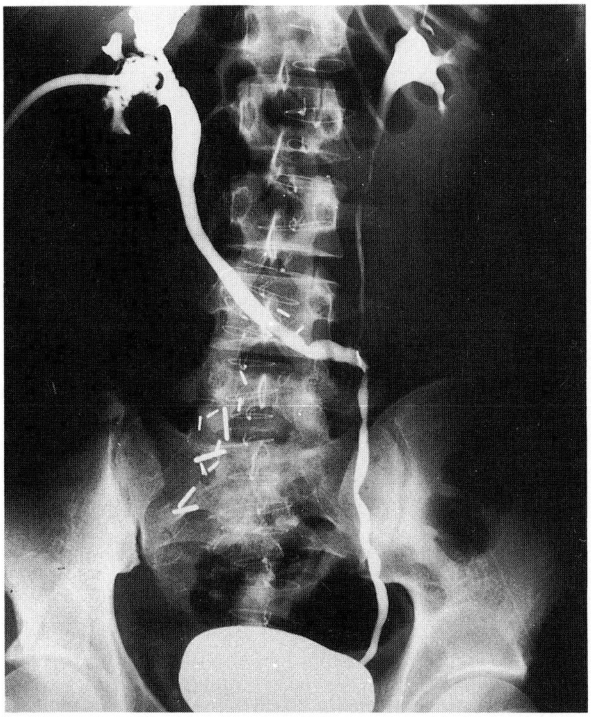

Fig. 4.4. Right-to-left TUU in 23-year-old patient with right ureteral injury from a gunshot wound. Right ureter and iliac vessels were initially repaired. Right-to-right ureteroureterostomy was unsuccessful because distal segment was devascularized

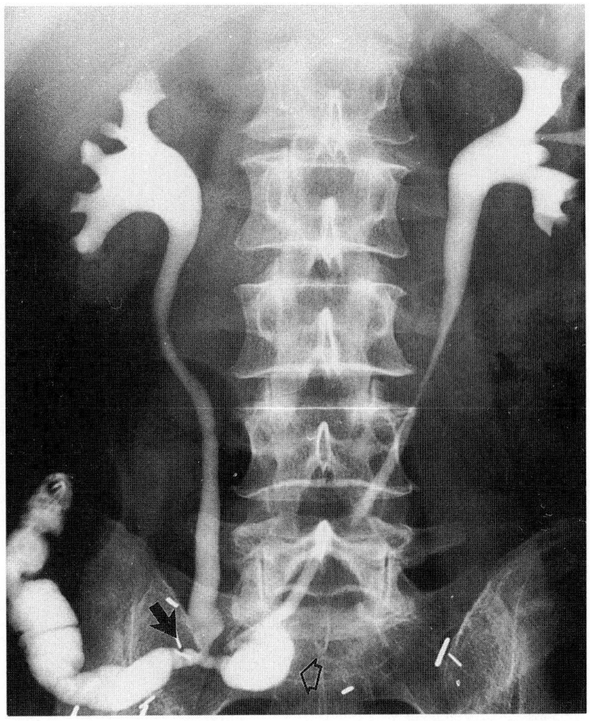

Fig. 4.5. Ileal loop urinary diversion in a 53-year-old man with bladder resection for carcinoma 10 years prior to loopogram. A loop stricture (*arrow*) is present near the ureteroileal anastomoses. A large loop calculus is present, deep to the stricture at the butt end of the ileal loop, obscured here by surrounding contrast material (*arrowhead*)

aminoglycoside when performing an ileal loopogram (STAMEY T, personal communication). Gas loopography (KILCHESKI and POLLACK 1978), radionuclide imaging (WOODSIDE et al. 1978), sonography, and CT loopography (SPRING and MOSS 1984) each may supplement conventional urography and loopography. Retrograde transconduit catheterization of the ureters anastomosed into a ureteroileostomy is advocated for detailed assessment of strictures or obstructions involving the ureters or ureteroileostomy site (BANNER et al. 1989). Rarely, sinography is necessary to assess ureteroileal anastomotic leaks (Fig. 4.6).

MOGG (1967) introduced the sigmoid urinary conduit to avoid the problems of the ileal conduit emanating from loop–kidney reflux. Long- and short-term complications are similar to those of the ileal loop except for complications related to reflux of infected urine. Indeed, sigmoid loopography should confirm patency of the ureterosigmoid anastomoses (YODER and PFISTER 1978).

Continent urinary diversions may be socially and psychologically preferable for some patients. Their long-term advantages and disadvantages remain to be assessed, however. KOCK (1969) initially developed a continent ileostomy for patients undergoing proctocolectomy for ulcerative colitis. SKINNER and associates (1987) have reported results on 250 patients undergoing modified Kock continent ileal reservoir, most often for pelvic malignancy. RALLS and colleagues (1986) have described the postoperative evaluation of the Kock pouch. They perform Kock pouch cystography 3 weeks after surgery to exclude reservoir–ureteral reflux. Gravity infusion of the pouch is performed through a No. 30 Medina tube held 36 in. above the patient. Infusion is stopped when patients sense fullness, usually after 100–300 ml of contrast medium has been instilled. A "mature" pouch has a capacity of as much as 1000 ml, although 500 ml of contrast medium is routinely used. Such studies are performed after 6 months. CT of Kock pouches has been described (MIRVIS et al. 1987).

The Mainz pouch utilizes the cecum and two ileal loops (THUROFF et al. 1988). This mixed augmentation provides a large reservoir with low

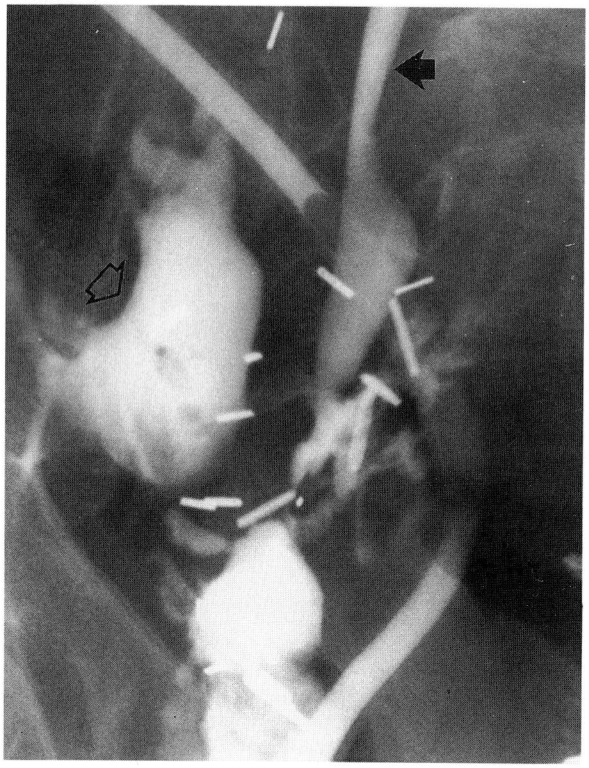

Fig. 4.6. Sinogram in a periloop abscess shows communication with right ureter (*arrow*) at site of leaking ureteroileal anastomosis. Ileal loop (*arrowhead*) also fills partly

pressure. Its evaluation parallels that of the Kock pouch.

Another continent reservoir, the Indiana pouch, also utilizes the cecum and part of the ileum (ROWLAND et al. 1987). The diverted ureters are tunneled into the taeniae of the cecum while the terminal ileum is used as a continence mechanism. The modified Indiana pouch can be accomplished safely and effectively in any patient formerly requiring an ileal conduit (AHLERING et al. 1989).

Uretero-appendicocystostomy combined with psoas hitch is yet another modification to create or enlarge reservoir capacity and compensate for loss of ureteral length (YOKOYAMA et al. 1992).

Another variant, the ileocolonic pouch (LeBag) uses sigmoid clon with nonrefluxing ureterocolonic anastomoses (LIGHT and ENGELMANN 1986). Ileum also adds to the volume of this reservoir. If the urethral sphincter remains intact this reservoir may be used to create a neobladder. It too has a large volume with low internal pressure. CAMEY has utilized a 40-cm segment of terminal ileum to create a continent bladder substitute (LILIEN and CAMEY 1986). The abdominal ureteral remnants are anastomosed to the laterally placed limbs of the isolated ileum. The midpoint of the antimesenteric border of the ileal neobladder is anastomosed to the urethral stump after cystoprostatectomy for bladder carcinoma in males.

MELCHIOR has modified the Camey ileocystoplasty (MELCHIOR et al. 1988). Intussuscepted ileum at the ureteroileal anastomoses prevents reflux.

4.3.2 Pelvic Ureter

4.3.2.1 Ureteral Stone Manipulations

Ureteral calculi may be extracted by ureteroscopy or nephroscopy. Complications of transureteral stone manipulations vary with size and location of calculi. Both transvesical and transrenal ureteral stone manipulations may be associated with ureteral injury – perforation or avulsion – and eventual stricture formation. Ureteroscopic ureteral injuries may be more serious than nephroscopic renal injuries because of the more tenuous ureteral blood supply (CHANG and MARSHALL 1987). In most instances ureteral injuries are immediately recognized and treated with no radiographically evident sequelae.

Transmural ureterolithotomy may be required for patients who fail to respond to expectant, manipulative, or shock wave lithotripsy. Regardless of the approach to the ureter, radiographic changes are subtle in the absence of procedure complications. The scarred, diseased, ischemic ureter, however, is far more likely to appear abnormal after surgical procedures than an otherwise normal ureter.

4.3.2.2 Ureterovesical Reimplantation (QUIOGUE and LEBOWITZ 1990)

One of the most common surgical procedures involving the pelvic ureter is ureterovesical reimplantation (Fig. 4.7). The Politano-Leadbetter ureteral reimplantation for vesicoureteral reflux or ureteral injury consists of creating a new submucosal bladder channel for the ureter more caudad and medial. Obstruction or persistent vesicoureteral reflux is among the commonest postoperative complications of ureteroneocystos-

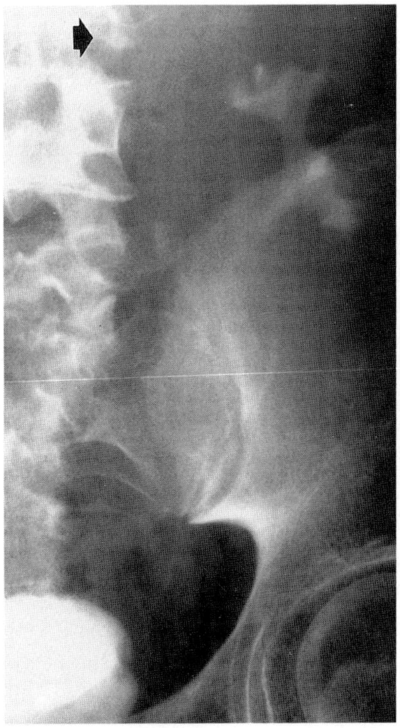

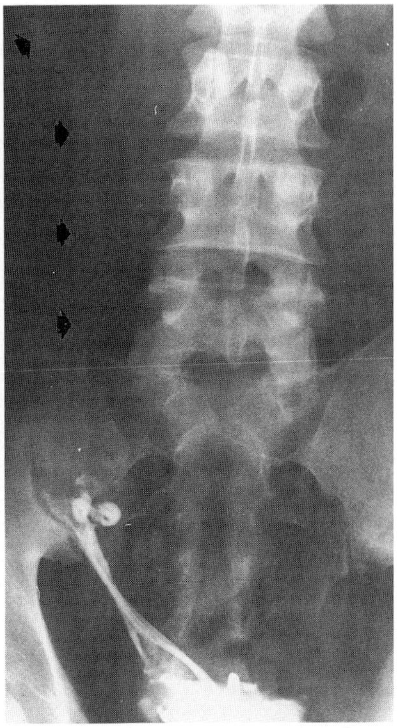

Fig. 4.7 (*left*). Complete ureteral duplication in a left iliac fossa renal transplant. Upper moiety collecting structures (*arrow*) overlie lower lumbar spine on left. Both ureters enter the urinary bladder with separate ureteroneocystostomies. (Courtesy of Dr. ALPHONSE PALUBINSKAS)

Fig. 4.8 (*right*). Stricture in right ureterovesicoplasty (Boari flap) seen during retrograde cystogram. Air is present in the upper urinary tract (*arrowheads*) from nephrostomy tube

tomy. QUIOGUE and LEBOWITZ believe early postoperative intravenous urography is preferable to ultrasound for follow-up because of the subtlety of obstructive changes which may be superimposed upon previously dilated upper tracts. The presence of ureterovesical reflux may be indicated by turbulence seen with submerged ureteric jets and presenting as flow reversal on pulsed or color flow doppler images (ADLER et al. 1991; BURNS et al. 1991). This criterion is exceedingly sensitive and is advocated to identify early and subtle vesicoureteral reflux.

Implantation of the pelvic ureter from the transplant kidney utilizes a modified Politano-Leadbetter ureteroneocystostomy (DAFOE and BARKER 1990; WITHERINGTON et al. 1988).

To prevent persistent ureterovesical reflux the dilated pelvic ureter must be of a caliber to pass through the bladder wall in a tunnel whose length is four to five times that caliber (EHRLICH 1985). Reduction ureteroplasty, performed by infolding and suturing redundant ureter ("imbrication") over a ureteral stent, thus remodels the distal pelvic ureter.

If the distal 3–5 cm of the pelvic ureter is injured, the surgeon may suture the mobilized bladder to the ipsilateral psoas minor muscle tendon, making possible an anstomosis under less tension ("psoas hitch") (KOONTZ et al. 1986). Less commonly, the bladder itself may also be tubularized ("Boari flap"), creating additional length, allowing for a more proximally placed ureteroneocystostomy (Fig. 4.8) (YOKOYAMA et al. 1992).

4.3.2.3 Ureteral Stump

After nephrectomy the distal ureteral remnant may rarely be a source of new or recurrent symptoms (POLLACK et al. 1982). Chronically infected, obstructed, or refluxing ureters may give rise to delayed complications. Retrograde urography is usually the best method of assessment.

4.4 Secondary Ureteral Involvement in Common Surgical Procedures

One encounters ureteral radiographic changes from nearby surgical procedures more often than from primary ureteral surgery. The common forms of ureteral involvement from extraurinary tract surgery are (a) obstruction, sometimes by ligation, (b) displacement or movement, (c) leakage, with pooled urine (urinoma) or fistula formation (e.g., ureterocutaneous or ureterovaginal fistulas), (d) infection from communication with the intestinal tract or from seeding to pooled urine collections, and (e) pipestem narrowing reflecting avascular necrosis of the ureter (LANG 1988).

The most common surgical procedures to involve the ureters are retroperitoneal lymph node dissection, aortoiliac surgery, obstetric and gynecologic procedures, and colonic surgery. This section will examine these.

4.4.1 Abdominal Ureter

4.4.1.1 Retroperitoneal Lymph Node Surgery

Pelvic lymphadenectomy remains the most accurate way to assess lymph node involvement for cancer of the prostate. Operative disruption of the retroperitoneal lymphatics may cause lymphocele formation with medial and anterior displacement of the pelvic ureters near the pelvic brim (SOGANI et al. 1981). Most often lymphoceles can be seen sonographically in the pelvis lateral to the urinary bladder abutting the pelvic brim. Their anterior surfaces are usually within 3 cm of the anterior abdominal wall (SPRING et al. 1981).

4.4.1.2 Abdominal Aortic Surgery

As many as 50% of ureteral injuries in male patients have been reported to be secondary to vascular surgery (HIGGINS 1967). Aneurysmorrhaphies, bypass procedures, vena caval ligations, and lumbar sympathectomies account for most of these injuries (SCHAPIRA et al. 1981).

Due to the close anatomic relationship of the aortoiliac vessels, reconstructive vascular surgical procedures sometimes injure the abdominal ureters. *Aortofemoral and aortoiliac bypass grafts*, when placed anterior to the ureters at the level of

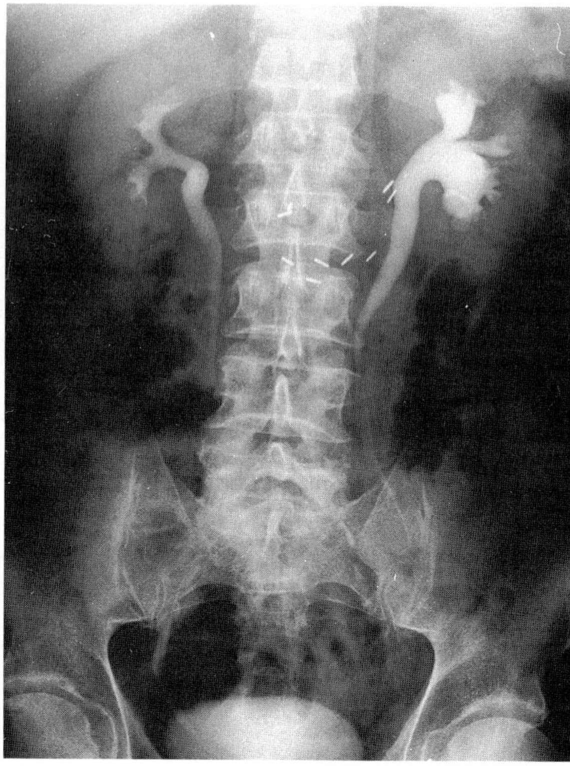

Fig. 4.9. Intravenous urogram showing mild-to-moderate left hydroureteronephrosis in patient after aortofemoral bypass graft placement. Abdominal ureters are drawn medially by periaortic fibrosis

the common iliac arteries, may cause ureteral compression with resultant hydroureteronephrosis. SANT and colleagues, reviewing the literature, however, showed that ureteral obstruction occurred both when the graft passed anterior (28% of reports) and when it was placed posterior to the ureter (49% of reports); they concluded, "the anatomic relationship of the ureter to the graft does not appear to be the major factor in the pathogenesis of the development of ureteral obstruction" (SANT et al. 1983).

Perigraft fibrosis makes the graft more rigid with time. This reaction akin to retroperitoneal fibrosis is another known complication to grafts. Insidiously, ureteral compression may develop (Fig. 4.9). GOLDENBERG and colleagues, using early sonographic screening for hydronephrosis in patients after aortoiliac reconstructive surgeries, showed mild-to-moderate hydronephrosis in 12% of patients and in 8% of kidneys 1 week after operation (GOLDENBERG et al. 1988). At 3 months only a single case of hydroureteronephrosis remained.

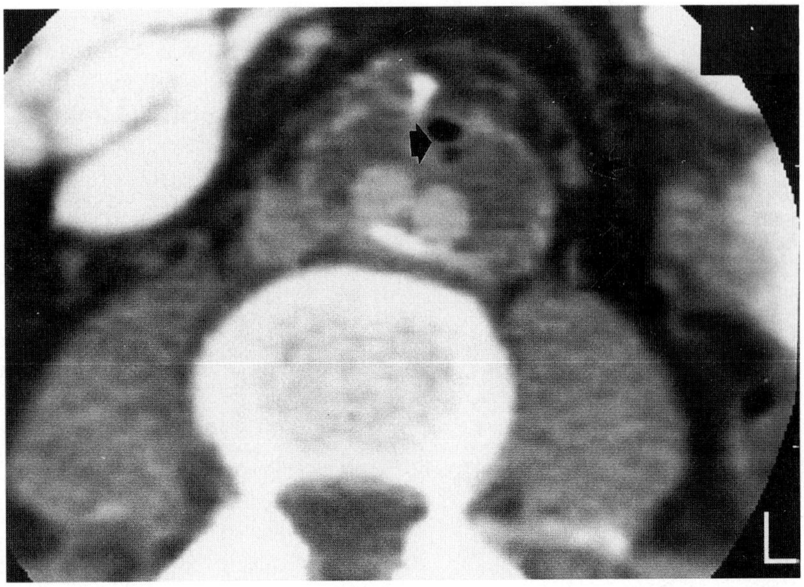

Fig. 4.10. Postoperative aortofemoral bypass graft with graft limbs seen in wrap of patient's native aortic aneurysm bed. Perigraft postoperative gas (*arrowhead*) may be seen in the first two postoperative weeks after surgery, as shown here. The left ureter (*arrow*) lies close to the surgical site and may be engulfed by periaortic postoperative fibrosis

Importantly, however, hydronephrosis may predict more serious vascular complications, including graft infections, anastomotic aneurysm, graft thrombosis, and amputation (Schubart et al. 1985). Wright and colleagues, in a more recent series, confirmed that patients with postoperative ureteral complications were at more than a fourfold greater risk of other graft complications than their fellow patients without ureteral complications (Wright et al. 1990).

Hydroureteronephrosis usually is secondary to periureteral fibrosis or to unintentional ureteral ligation. Periureteric fibrosis after graft replacement is indistinguishable from classic retroperitoneal fibrosis associated with ergot, α-methyldopa, and other sympathetic blocking drugs (Fourcroy et al. 1980). Most often there is plaque-like fibrosis at the sacral promontory, extending laterally and craniad for varying distances (Fig. 5.9).

Hydroureteronephrosis may precede aortoiliac or aortofemoral vascular surgery. Periaortic fibrosis may distort the retroperitoneum, sometimes causing ureteral obstruction or displacement. Contralateral ureteral traction by fibrosis has been a useful sign of an abdominal aortic aneurysm (Peck et al. 1973). The coexistence of aortic aneurysm and retroperitoneal fibrosis is well known (Brock and Soloway 1980; Abbott et al. 1973). Iliac artery aneurysms themselves may obstruct the ureters (Peterson et al. 1977).

Apparent sonographic dilatation of the renal collecting structures does not always indicate hydronephrosis, of course. False-positive dilatation may be encountered with extrarenal pelves, calyceal clubbing, and congenital megacalyces (Talner et al. 1981).

Magnetic resonance imaging may help distinguish perigraft fibrosis from infection. After the early postoperative period when infection and benign perigraft fluid cannot be distinguished, MRI can distinguish low signal fibrosis from a high intensity (T2) zone, suggestive of perigraft infection (Auffermann et al. 1989).

While hydronephrosis in the early postoperative period is common and unlikely to persist if asymptomatic, screening ultrasonography may be warranted to identify the high risk group among patients having vascular reconstructive procedures (Schubart et al. 1985). Long-term vascular surgical and ultrasonographic follow-up may be essential. Hydronephrosis may, in some, be associated with loss of renal function, fistulization, sepsis, and death. Most would agree that symptoms such as flank pain warrant renal sonography to detect hydronephrosis.

Aortic aneurysm surgery may result in ureteral obstruction or injury. Most often the aneurysm is repaired with the aneurysm itself wrapped around

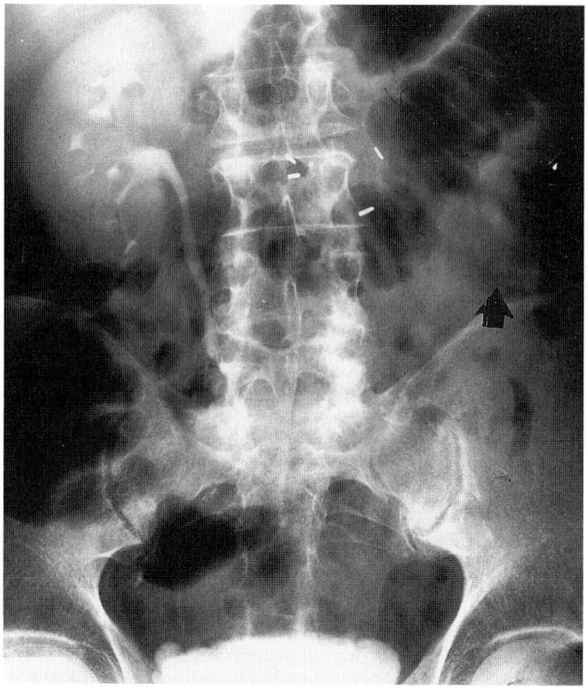

Fig. 4.11. The left kidney functions poorly after injury during emergency surgery for ruptured aortic aneurysm. A tube nephrostomy preserved function for several months but was discontinued when renal function steadily declined

the graft (Fig. 4.10) (Hilton et al. 1982). Ureteral injury recognized in the early postoperative course should be repaired after diverting the urine stream more proximally with a nephrostomy or after stenting the ureter. Continued leakage of urine around the graft itself causes pooling of urine which, if it becomes infected, may necessitate graft removal. Other important vascular complications of endoaneurysmorrhaphy which must be considered in the differential diagnosis of ureteral injuries include retroperitoneal hemorrhage, major vessel occlusion, postoperative pancreatitis, distal anastomotic pseudoaneurysm formation, graft infections, and psoas and vertebral infections.

In *emergency aortic surgery* for leakage or rupture of aortic aneurysm, slow, meticulous dissection is impossible. Blood may obscure anatomic landmarks. Ureteral injury is the most frequently injured part of the urinary tract in the course of such emergency surgery, while the bladder and kidney are less frequently involved (Fig. 4.11). Follow-up sonography, radionuclide renal studies, or intravenous urography may be useful to monitor the status of the upper urinary tract.

Preoperative placement of ureteral catheters has been advocated as an adjunct to aortoiliac graft surgery as it aids in recognition of the ureters in the retroperitoneum (Spirnak et al. 1989). Spirnak and colleagues believe midureteral injuries are best managed by a water-tight ureteroureterostomy with ureteral stenting while distal ureteral injuries are managed with ureteroneocystostomy, with psoas hitch if necessary. Stent placement itself, however, has been associated with ureteral injury. Sacks and Miller (1988) reported ureteral leakage occurring after placing a stent 12 days after aortoiliac bypass graft surgery. They postulated pressure necrosis as the cause, with the injured ureter lying between the pulsating aortic graft and a stiff ureteral stent.

Bilateral lumbar sympathectomy may be performed for nonreconstructible lower extremity vascular disease. When neither angioplasty nor vascular surgical techniques are successful the second, third, and fourth lumbar ganglia have been excised to increase blood flow, ease symptoms, and protect skin areas from gangrene (Schapira et al. 1981). Ureteral injury has been reported during excision of sympathetic ganglia (Higgins 1967).

4.4.2 Pelvic Ureter

4.4.2.1 Pelvic Ureteral Injury from Obstetric and Gynecologic Surgery

The close embryologic relation of the urinary and genital tracts places the pelvic ureters at risk during gynecologic surgical procedures. The incidence of ureteral injury from hysterectomies for benign conditions varies between 0.02% and 3% (Freda and Tacchi 1962). The incidence for vaginal hysterectomy is 0.12%–4.76% (van Nagall and Roddick 1972). For radical hysterectomy for malignancy the incidence of ureteral injuries is predictably higher (12.5%) (Green et al. 1962).

Transient ureteral dilatation develops in most instances during the first 24 h after both radical and simple hysterectomies (Symmonds 1981); it is maximal at about the third postoperative week (Talbert et al. 1965). Persistence or worsening of hydronephrosis on ultrasound, then, should alert the physician to significant ureteral obstruction.

During obstetric procedures the ureters may also be injured. Cesarean section and cesarean hysterectomy place the pelvic ureter at risk. During vaginal delivery the ureter may be injured during repair of high vaginal or cervical injuries with forceps or suture trauma (SCHAEFER and GRABER 1981).

Risk factors which appear to increase the likelihood of ureteral injury during pelvic surgical procedures include endometriosis, pelvic adhesions, distorted pelvic anatomy, bladder repair, ovarian neoplasm, and previous pelvic surgical procedures (DALY and HIGGINS 1988). Despite the greater risk in such circumstances the routine, easy hysterectomy has usually accounted for most ureteral injuries (SYMMONDS 1981).

Because bleeding is a common problem during pelvic surgical procedures, inadvertent ureteral injury with cautery or ligation may occur. Suture or clamp trauma readily leads to ureteral injury from crush injury and/or partial transection. Overrepair, likewise, can devitalize the ureter (SYMMONDS 1983).

Ureteral injuries often occur near the pelvic brim along the infundibulopelvic ligament and ovarian vessels. More often they occur at the level of the uterosacral ligament, uterine artery, or lateral vaginal angle (Fig. 4.12) (SYMMONDS 1983). These injuries may be more readily overlooked because of the greater difficulty seeing or palpating the distal pelvic ureter (Fig. 4.2). Treatment varies with location. In the abdomen or upper pelvis ureteroureterostomy can usually be accomplished, often with stenting. Deeper in the pelvis ureteroneocystostomy is more appropriate. If the length of injured ureter is too great for a simple ureteroureterostomy, a bladder flap (psoas hitch), transureteroureterostomy, or autotransplantation may be necessary. Good results have been obtained with percutaneous ureterocystostomy and ureteroneocystostomy (LANG 1988).

Hydronephrosis is most often a reflection of obstruction, which may be partial or complete. Strictures may develop at the site of injury (see Chap. 3). Antegrade or retrograde stenting may be adequate therapy. Poor function or nonfunction of a kidney should raise the question of ureteral severance, ligation, or leak.

In a series of 600 genitourinary fistulas 95 (16%) involved the ureter (SYMMONDS 1981). A retrospective study of ureterovaginal fistulas indicated that 80%–90% were secondary to gynecologic surgical procedures, most often total abdominal hysterectomy (70%–75%). GREEN et al. (1962) reported that the incidence of uretero-

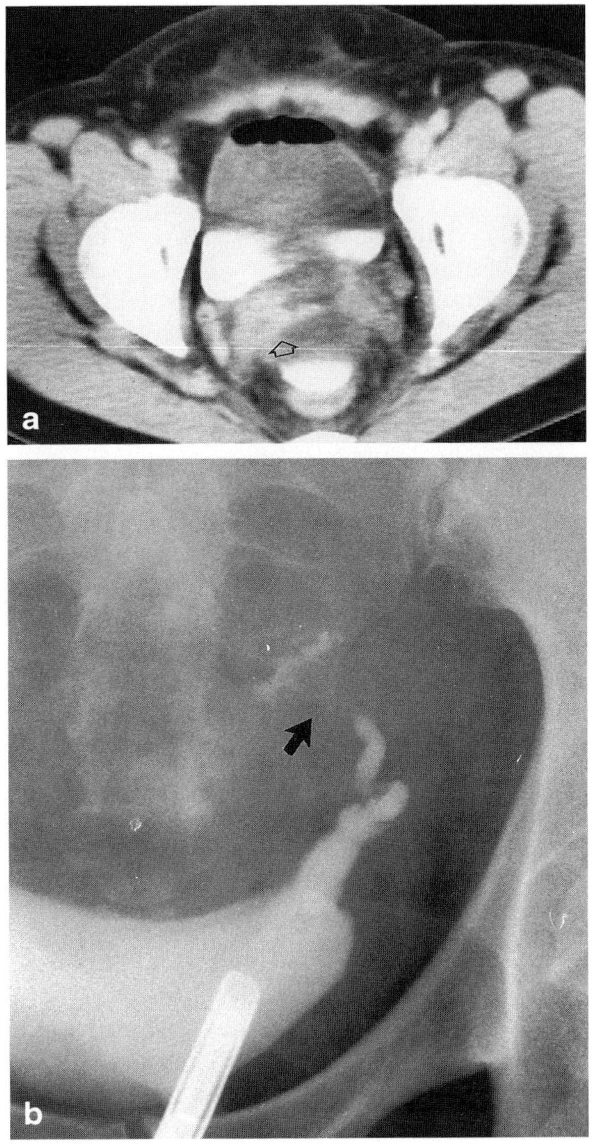

Fig. 4.12. a Computed tomogram performed for early postoperative fever after abdominal hysterectomy. Contrast material can be seen in the cul-de-sac (*arrowhead*). **b** Retrograde ureterogram confirms site of ureteral injury and leak in the pelvic ureter (*arrow*)

vaginal fistula after radical hysterectomy was 8.5%. The close course of the distal pelvic ureter to the vaginal fornix explains its relative vulnerability. While symptoms of a leak may begin as early as the first 24–48 h after surgery, they usually present in the second postoperative week with urinary incontinence.

"The venial sin is injury to the ureter, but the mortal sin is failure of recognition" (HIGGINS 1962). Diagnosis of the site of a possible genitourinary fistula can be aided by placing a tampon in the vagina and performing the "two-dye test" (SCHAEFER and GRABER 1981). Methylene blue is then instilled in the urinary bladder. If the tampon is then stained blue, a vesicovaginal fistula is likely. If not stained, a second tampon is placed in the vagina. Indigo carmine is injected intravenously. If the tampon now stains, a ureterovaginal fistula is likely.

Preoperative intravenous urography prior to routine hysterectomy should not be done (MUSHLIN and THORNBURY 1989). It may be, however, appropriate to request urography before hysterectomy to evaluate women with large pelvic masses or known pelvic cancers. SIMEL suggests selective use of preoperative urography in nonmalignnant disease such as those instances in which there is uterine size of 12 weeks' gestational age or larger and an adnexal mass 4 cm or larger (SIMEL et al. 1989). Instances of severe endometriosis, known extensive pelvic adhesive disease, and known müllerian anomalies also are considered by some to be appropriate indications for preoperative urography.

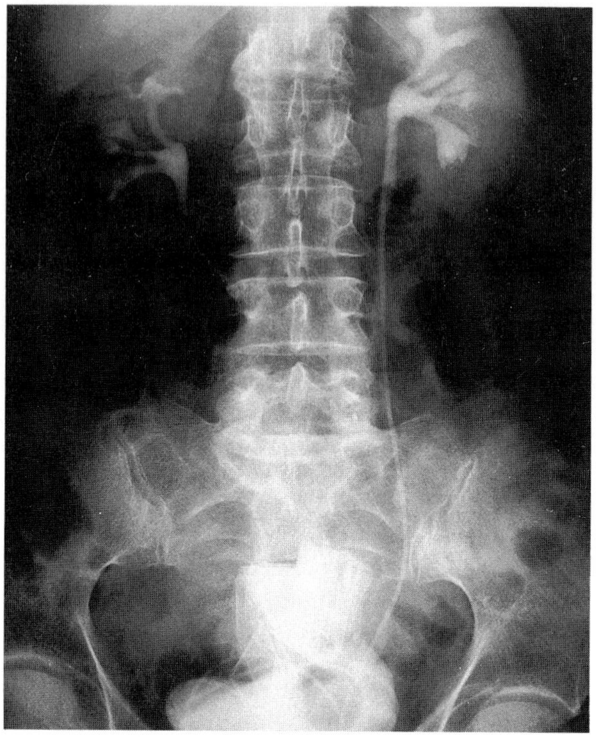

Fig. 4.13. Left ureter is stented following injury to ureter during resection of low sigmoid colon carcinoma. Stented ureteral course often lies medial in the pelvis after mobilization during anteroposterior resection of distal colorectal carcinomas. (Courtesy of Dr. LESLIE PREGER)

4.4.2.2 Postoperative Pelvic Ureteral Changes from Colonic Surgery

The colon surgeon operating on the intestine near the pelvic brim may also injure the ureter. The incidence of ureteral injuries during colon surgery is reported to be 0.3%–6% (CASS and BUBRICK 1981). Surgery for invasive carcinoma of the middle or upper rectum places the ureters, particularly that on the left, at high risk. Abdominoperineal or low anterior rectosigmoid resection are the surgical procedures most often associated with these injuries. Injury to the left ureter often occurs during mobilization of the sigmoid or during ligature of the inferior mesenteric vessels; either ureter may be injured during take-down of the lateral rectal ligaments or reperitonealization of the pelvis.

When intraoperative ureteral injury is suspected one may inject 5 ml indigo carmine intravenously to identify the site of urine leakage (PERSKY 1975). The dye, filtered by the kidney much like urographic contrast, stains the operative field about 20 min after injection.

When injury is suspected postoperatively, sonography, radionuclide imaging, and excretory urography are most useful. Anuria, flank pain and tenderness, fever, chills, nausea, and vomiting are all symptoms which raise suspicion postoperatively of ureteral injuries from colonic surgery. Both excretory urography and retrograde ureteropyelography help to define the site of ureteral injury. When the location of a pelvic urine leak is unclear, cystography with contrast material or indigo carmine may help in identifying and localizing vesical injuries. Once identified, ureteral injuries may be treated with open surgical techniques. End-to-end ureteroureterostomy over a stent is usually the preferred surgical repair for abdominal and upper pelvic ureteral injuries (CASS and BUBRICK 1981). Surgical techniques include most often ureteroureterostomy and transureteroureterostomy. Rarely, when large segments of the ureter have been injured a renal autotransplantation may be performed. Nephrectomy occasionally is the procedure of choice when a patient's age or physical condition precludes other procedures. In selected instances interventional techniques including percutaneous nephrostomy, antegrade catheterization and stenting of partial

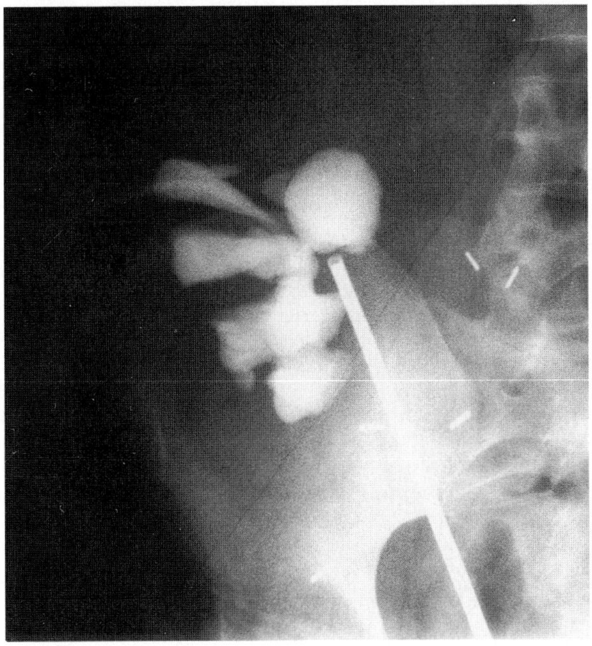

Fig. 4.14. A rigid ureteroscope has been advanced into the native ureter and brought into proximity of a dilated calyx of the transplant kidney. A percutaneous ureterocalycostomy (i.e., anastomosis of the native ureter to the calyx) will be performed. A stent will be seated for 4–6 weeks to ensure coverage by uroepithelium. (LANG 1988)

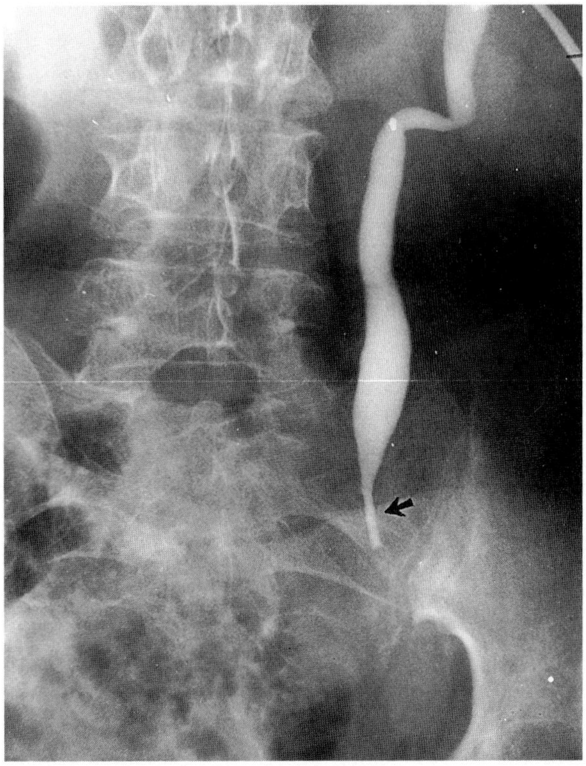

Fig. 4.15. Antegrade ureterogram demonstrating pipestem narrowing of the distal portion of the left ureter and ultimately a complete cut-off (*arrow*). This is a fairly typical appearance of avascular necrosis due to excessive radiation therapy via external ports to the pelvic ureters. (LANG et al. 1973)

ureteral injuries, and antegrade ureteroneocystostomy may be most appropriate.

The course of the pelvic ureter is often more medial after abdominoperineal resection (SPILLANE et al. 1951). Inward bowing of the ureters at the midsacrum or promontory is commonly seen after resection of the rectum (Fig. 4.13).

4.4.3 Leakage from Reimplanted Ureter of a Transplant Kidney

Leakage at the ureteroneocystostomy site of a transplanted kidney and ureter is a not uncommon complication (LANG 1988; MATALON et al. 1990). Since this is not infrequently caused by and associated with avascular necroses of the transplant ureter, correction by surgical ureterocalycostomy or ureteropyelostomy, using the native ureter and anastomosing it to segments of the transplant kidney, or by an identical procedure utilizing interventional radiologic techniques, is advocated (Fig. 4.14).

4.5 Radiation-Induced Injury of the Ureters

Though megavoltage therapy has reduced the incidence of radiation-induced injury to the ureters attendant upon therapy of pelvic neoplasms (most often carcinoma of the cervix), late stricture and stenosis of the ureter remain a dreaded complication of radiation therapy. The changes usually afflict the pelvic and distal ureters over an approximately 15-cm segment equating to the size of the radiation therapy ports. Avascular necrosis caused by endarteritis obliterans leads to pipestem stenosis of long ureteral segments (Fig. 4.15) (LANG et al. 1973)). Short strictures are sometimes the consequence of excessive radiation delivered by radium (or cesium) implants in treatment of carcinoma of cervix (Fig. 4.16) (LANG

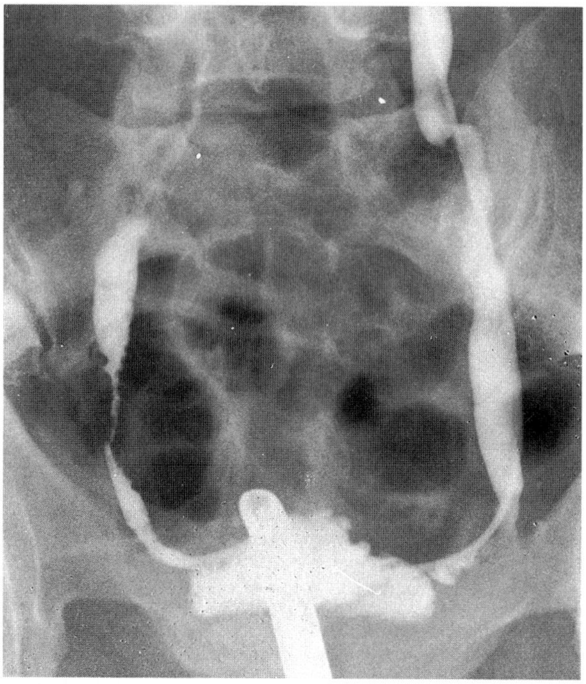

Fig. 4.16. Retrograde ureterogram demonstrating strictures in both pelvic ureters. These are the result of excessive interstitial radiation therapy delivered by a radium implant in treatment of carcinoma of the cervix. (LANG et al. 1973)

et al. 1973). Though a patent lumen usually remains, these strictures are dynamically damaging. Lack of peristalsis increases back pressure and ultimately progressive loss of renal function results. Stenting can lessen the ill effects of such strictures. Transluminal dilatation is not effective, because of the presence of avascular necrosis and reduced vascular perfusion of the involved segments. Ureteroneocystostomies are prone to failure for the same reason. Diversion procedures sacrificing the lower ureters are often the only intervention capable of remedying the condition.

References

Abbott DL, Skinner DG, Yalowitz PA, Mulder DG (1973) Retroperitoneal fibrosis associated with abdominal aortic aneurysms: an approach to management. J Urol 109:987–989

Adler RS, Rubin JM, Price CI (1991) Interpretation of submerged laminar jets: ureteric jet phenomenon. Radiology 178:888

Ahlering TE, Weinberg AC, Razor B (1989) A comparative study of the ileal conduit, Kock pouch and modified Indiana pouch. J Urol 142:1193–1196

Apter S, Rubinstein ZJ, Hertz M (1984) CT demonstration of urinary bladder displacement causing medial deviation of the distal ureter. J Comput Assist Tomogr 8:294–295

Auffermann W, Olofsson PA, Rabahie GN, Tavares NJ, Stoney RJ, Higgins CB (1989) Incorporation versus infection of retroperitoneal aortic grafts: MR imaging features. Radiology 172:359–362

Banner MP, Pollack HM, Bonavita JA, Ellis PS (1984) The radiology of urinary diversions. Radiographics 4:885–913

Banner MP, Amendola MA, Pollack HM (1989) Anastomosed ureters: fluoroscopically guided transconduit retrograde catheterization. Radiology 170:45–52

Bergman H (1967) The ureter. Hoeber Medical Division, Harper and Row, New York, p xv

Bratt C-G, Nilsson S (1984) Late results after surgical correction of pyeloplasty failure in idiopathic hydronephrosis. J Urol 132:231–233

Brock J, Soloway MS (1980) Retroperitoneal fibrosis and aortic aneurysm. Urology 15:14–16

Burns PN, Jequier S, Paltiel H, Lafortune M (1991) Interpretation of submerged laminar jets: ureteric jet phenomenon. Radiology 178:889

Cass AS, Bubrick MP (1981) Ureteral injuries in colonic surgery. Urology 18:359–364

Chang R, Marshall FF (1987) Management of ureteroscopic injuries. J Urol 137:1132–1135

Cherrie RJ, Kaufman JJ (1983) Pyeloplasty for ureteropelvic junction obstruction in adults: correlation of radiographic and clinical results. J Urol 129:711–714

Cronin JJ, Amis ES, Scola FH, Schepps B (1986) Renal obstruction in patients with ileal loops. Radiology 158: 647–648

Dafoe D, Barker C (1990) Renal transplantation – clinical considerations, In: Pollack HM (ed) Clinical urography, vol 3. W.B. Saunders, Philadelphia, p 2647

Daly JW, Higgins KA (1988) Injury to the ureter during gynecologic surgical procedures. Surg Gynecol Obstet 167:19–22

deCampo J, Fowler R (1989) Volume related configurational changes in the aetiology of pelvi-ureteric junction obstruction. Australas Radiol 23:60–63

Ehrlich EM (1985) The ureteral folding technique for megaureter surgery. J Urol 134:668–670

Feminella JG Jr, Lattimer JK (1974) A retrospective analysis of 70 cases of cutaneous ureterostomy. J Urol 106:538–540

Fourcroy JL, Azoury B, Miller HC (1980) Bilateral ureteral obstruction as a complication of vascular graft surgery. Urology 15:556–558

Freda VC, Tacchi D (1962) Ureteral injury discovered after pelvic surgery. Am J Obstet Gynecol 83:406–408

Goldenberg SL, Gordon PB, Cooperberg PL, McLoughlin MG (1988) Early hydronephrosis following aortic bifurcation graft surgery: a prospective study. J Urol 140:1367–1369

Green TH, Meigs JV, Ulfelder H, Curtin RR (1962) Urologic complications of radical Wertheim's hysterectomy. Obstet Gynecol 20:293–312

Higgins CC (1962) Ureteral injuries. JAMA 182:225–229

Higgins CC (1967) Ureteral injuries during surgery. A review of 87 cases. JAMA 199:82–88

Hilton S, Megibow AJ, Naidich DP, Bosniak MA (1982) Computed tomography of the postoperative abdominal aorta. Radiology 145:403–407

Kabakian HA, Armenian HK, Deeb ZL, Rizk GK (1976) Asymmetry of the pelvic ureters in normal females. AJR 127:723–727

Kilcheski TS, Pollack HM (1978) Gas contrast radiography of ileal conduits. Radiology 129:242–244
Kock NG (1969) Intra-abdominal "reservoir" in patients with permanent ileostomy. Preliminary observations on a procedure resulting in fecal "continence" in five ileostomy patients. Arch Surg 99:223–231
Koff SA (1982) Ureteropelvic junction obstruction: role of newer diagnostic methods. J Urol 127:898–901
Koontz WW, Klein FA, Smith MJV (1986) Surgery of the ureter. In: Walsh PC, Gittes RF, Perlmutter AD, Stamey TA (eds) Campbell's urology. W.B. Saunders, Philadelphia, pp 2595–2597
Kumar A, Sharma SK, Vaidyanathan S (1988) Results of surgical reconstruction in patients with renal failure owing to ureteropelvic junction obstruction. J Urol 140:484–486
Lang EK (1984) Antegrade ureteral stenting for dehiscence, strictures, and fistulae. AJR 143:795–801
Lang EK (1988) Percutaneous ureterocystostomy and ureteroneocystostomy. AJR 150:1065–1068
Lang EK, Price EW (1983) Redefinition of indications for percutaneous nephrostomy. Radiology 147:419–426
Lang EK, Wood M, Brown R et al. (1973) Complications in the urinary tract related to treatment of carcinoma of the cervix. South Med J 66:228–236
Light JK, Engelmann UH (1986) Le Bag: total replacement of bladder using ileocolonic pouch. J Urol 136: 27–31
Lilien OM, Camey M (1986) 25-year experience with replacement of the human bladder (Camey procedure). J Urol 132:886–891
Lindell O, Makinen J, Salo J, Pitkaranta P, Lehtonen T (1991) Intramural ureteric injuries due to acute dilatation. Annals Chir Gynedol 80:402–404
Lupton EW, Testa HJ, Lawson RS, Charleton Edwards E, Carroll RNP, Barnard RJ (1979) Diuresis renography and the results of pyeloplasty for idiopathic hydronephrosis. Br J Urol 51:449–453
Matalon TAS, Thompson MJ, Patel SK, Ramos MD, Jensik SC, Merkel FK (1990) Percutaneous treatment of urine leaks in renal transplantation patients. Radiology 174:1049–1053
Melchior H, Spehr C, Knop-Wagemann I, Persson MC, Inenemann KP (1988) The continent ileal bladder for urinary tract reconstruction after cystectomy: a survey of HH patients. J Urol 139:714–718
Mirvis SE, Whitley NO, Javadpour N, Young JD (1987) Computed tomography of Kock and modified Kock continent ileal reservoir. Urology 29:361–367
Mogg RA (1967) The treatment of urinary incontinence using the colon conduit. J Urol 97:684–692
Mor Y, Ramon J, Rabiv G, Herz M, Golwasser B, Jonas P (1992) Low loop cutaneous ureterostomy and subsequent reconstruction: 20 year of experience. J Urol 147:1595–1597
Mushlin AI, Thornbury JR (1989) Intravenous pyelography: the case against its routine use. Ann Intern Med 111:58–70
Peck DR, Bhatt GM, Lowman RM (1973) Traction displacement of the ureter: a sign of aortic aneurysm. J Urol 109:983–986
Persky L (1975) Iatrogenic ureteral and vesical injuries. In: Karafin L, Kendall AR (eds) Urology. Harper and Row, Hagerstown, MD, Chap 5, p 1
Peterson LJ, McAninich JW, Weinerth JL (1977) Ureteral obstruction of solitary kidneys by iliac artery aneurysms. Urology 9:17–21
Pfister RC, Newhouse JH (1978) Radiology of ureter. Urology 12:15–39
Pfister RC, Newhouse JH (1979) Interventional percutaneous pyeloureteral techniques. I. Antegrade pyelography and ureteral perfusion. Radiol Clin North Am 17:341–350
Pollack HM, Banner MP, Popky GL (1982) Radiologic evaluation of the ureteral stump. Radiology 144:225–230
Quiogue T, Lebowitz RL (1990) Postoperative uroradiological appearances in the child. In: Pollack HM (ed) Clinical urography, vol 3. W.B. Saunders, Philadelphia, pp 2539–2569
Ralls PW, Barakos JA, Skinner DG, Boswell WD Jr, Rodin DR, Colletti PM, Halls JM (1986) Radiology of the Kock continent ileal urinary reservoir. Radiology 161:477–483
Rowland RG, Mitchell ME, Bihrle R, Kahnoski RJ, Piser JE (1987) Indiana continent urinary diversion. J Urol 137:1136–1139
Sacks D, Miller J (1988) Ureteral leak around an aortic bifurcation graft: complication of ureteral stenting. J Urol 140:1526–1528
Sant GR, Heaney JA, Parkhurst EC, Blaivas JG (1983) Obstructive uropathy – a potentially serious complication of reconstructive vascular surgery. J Urol 129: 16–22
Schaefer G, Graber EA (1981) Complications in obstetric and gynecologic surgery. Harper $ Row, Philadelphia, pp 428–429
Schapira HE, Li R, Gribetz M, Wulfsohn MA, Brendler H (1981) Ureteral injuries during vascular surgery. J Urol 125:293–297
Schlegel JU, Lang EK (1980) Computed radionuclide urogram for assessing acute renal failure. AJR 124: 1029–1034
Schubart P, Fortner G, Cummings D, Reed D, Thiele BL, Bandyk DF, Radke HM (1985) The significance of hydronephrosis after aortofemoral reconstruction. Arch Surg 120:377–381
Simel DL, Piscitelli J, Matchar DB (1989) Intravenous pyelography before hysterectomy (letter). Ann Intern Med 111:541
Skinner DG, Lieskovsky G, Boyd SD (1987) Continuing experience with the continent ileal reservoir (Kock pouch) as an alternative to cutaneous urinary diversion: an update after 250 cases. J Urol 137:1140–1145
Sogani PC, Watson RC, Whitmore WF (1981) Lymphocele after pelvic lymphadenectomy for urologic cancer. Urology 17:39–43
Spillane RJ, Kaiser TF, Prather GC (1951) Medial deviation of the ureters complicating carcinoma of the rectum and sigmoid, and proctosigmoidectomy. Surg Gynecol Obstet 93:273–282
Spirnak JP, Hampel N, Resnick MI (1989) Ureteral injuries complicating vascular surgery: Is repair indicated? J Urol 141:13–14
Spring DB, Deshon GE Jr (1990) Radiology of vesical and supravesical urinary diversions. In: Pollack HM (ed), Clinical urography, vol I. W.B. Saunders, Philadelphia, pp 296–310
Spring DB, Moss AA (1984) Computed tomography of ileal loop urinary diversion in adults. J Comput Assist Tomogr 8:866–870
Spring DB, Schroeder D, Babu S, Agee R, Gooding GAW (1981) Ultrasonic evaluation of lymphocele formation after staging lymphadenectomy for prostatic carcinoma. Radiology 141:479–483

Symmonds RE (1981) Urologic injuries. In: Schaefer G, Graber EA (eds) Complications in obstetric and gynecologic surgery. Prevention, diagnosis, and treatment. Harper & Row, Philadelphia, pp 412–429

Symmonds RE (1983) Unrecognized clamping of ureter at hysterectomy, In: Nichols DH, Anderson GW (eds) Clinical problems, injuries, and complications of gynecologic surgery. Williams & Wilkins, Baltimore, pp 1–3

Talbert LM, Palumbo L, Shingleton H, Bream CA, McGee JA (1965) Urological complications of radical hysterectomy for carcinoma of the cervix. South Med J 58:11–17

Talner LB (1990) Ureteropelvic junction obstruction. In: Pollack HM (ed) Clinical urography, vol II. W.B. Saunders, Philadelphia, pp 1637–1651

Talner LB, Scheible W, Ellenbogen PH, Beck CH Jr, Gosink BB (1981) How accurate is ultrasonography in detecting hydronephrosis in azotemic patients? Urol Rad 3:1–6

Thorek P (1985) Anatomy in surgery, 3rd edn. Springer, New York Berlin Heidelberg, pp 614–619

Thrall JH, Koff SA, Keyes JW Jr (1981) Diuretic radionuclide renography and scintigraphy in the differential diagnosis of hydroureteronephrosis. Semin Nucl Med 11:89–104

Thuroff JW, Alken P, Riedmiller H, Jacobi GH, Hohenfellner R (1988) 100 cases of Mainz pouch: continuing experience and evolution. J Urol 140:283–288

Udall DH, Hodges CV, Pearse HM, Burns AB (1973) Transureteroureterostomy: a neglected procedure. J Urol 109:817–820

van Nagall JR, Roddick JW (1972) Vaginal hysterectomy, the ureter and excretory urography. Obstet Gynecol 39:784–786

Whitaker RH (1978) Clinical assessment of pelvic and ureteral function. Urology 12:146–150

Witherington R, Benson DC, Humphries AL Jr (1988) Ureteroneocystostomy in renal transplantation: a simple transvesical technique. J Urol 140:270–272

Woodside JR, Boorden TA, Damron JR, Kiker JD (1978) Isotope loopography, a new test: comparison with standard loopography and its relationship to renal function in patients with ileal conduit urinary diversion. J Urol 119:31–34

Wright DJ, Ernst CB, Evans JR, Smith RF, Reddy DJ, Shepard AD, Elliott JP Jr (1990) Ureteral complications and aortoiliac reconstruction. J Vasc Surg 11:29–37

Yoder IC, Pfister RC (1978) Radiology of colon loop diversion: anatomical and urodynamic studies of the conduit and ureters in children and adults. Radiology 127:85–92

Yokoyama N, Iio S, Iwata H, Takeuchi H (1992) Bilateral ureterovaginal fistula treated by psoas hitch and uretero-appendicocystostomy. J Urol 147:1102–1104

5 Inflammatory Lesions of the Ureter: Congenital, Calculous, and Inflammatory Lesions of the Bladder

WALTER HRUBY, M. URBAN, H. MOSSER, W. ANZBÖCK, and W. KRAMPLA

CONTENTS

5.1 Inflammatory Lesions of the Ureter

Inflammatory changes of the ureter are not to be regarded as isolated lesions. They usually occur in association with cystitis or pyelonephritis (PUTSCHAR 1934). Various forms of ureteritis may be distinguished according to their etiology:

1. Infectious excretory ureteritis (pyelitis): In this form descending infections occur. Infectious excretory ureteritis occurs in patients with various infectious illnesses or saprophytic infections.
2. Toxic (abacterial) excretory ureteritis.
3. Ascending ureteritis (pyelitis): This form is seen in gonorrhea, prostatitis, and cystitis.
4. Autochthonous pyelitis and ureteritis based upon predisposing local factors such as concrements, tumors, parasites, coagula, and foreign bodies. In these cases there is usually a secondary infection by *E. coli, Streptococcus, Straphylococcus*, or *Proteus mirabilis* (KASS 1985; LATHAM and STAMM 1984).

Pathoanatomically, distinction can be made between (ZOLLINGER 1966):

1. Catarrhal inflammation
2. Fibrinous pseudomembranous inflammation
3. Diphtheroid inflammation
4. Necrotizing and ulcerous inflammation

5.1.1 Acute Lesions

Acute secondary infections following blockage of the ureter by concrements, tumors, or foreign bodies can result in acute inflammatory lesions of the ureter. Congenital megaureter or vesicoureteral reflux (VUR) can also lead to pyoureter in the presence of preexistent hydroureter.

Acute inflammatory lesions lead to a striate pattern of the renal pelvis and ureter due to swelling of the mucosa (e.g., as occurs with acute purulent ureteritis or VUR in children) (Figs. 5.1, 5.2). Such a pattern may also occur after trauma and submucosal bleeding affecting the renal pelvis and ureter, with leukoplakia, or with metastasizing cancer of the ovaries or testes or Wilms' tumors (NIEH and ALTHAUSEN 1979). Similar morphologic structures also can be found in healthy children; however, in these cases the findings are usually more clearly circumscribed and the striations are thinner.

5.1.2 Chronic Lesions

Chronic inflammatory lesions of the ureter have various origins:

WALTER HRUBY, M.D., Professor and Chairman; M. URBAN, M.D.; H. MOSSER, M.D.; W. ANZBÖCK, M.D.; W. KRAMPLA, M.D.; Department of Radiology, Danubehospital, Langobardenstraße 122, 1220 Wien, Austria

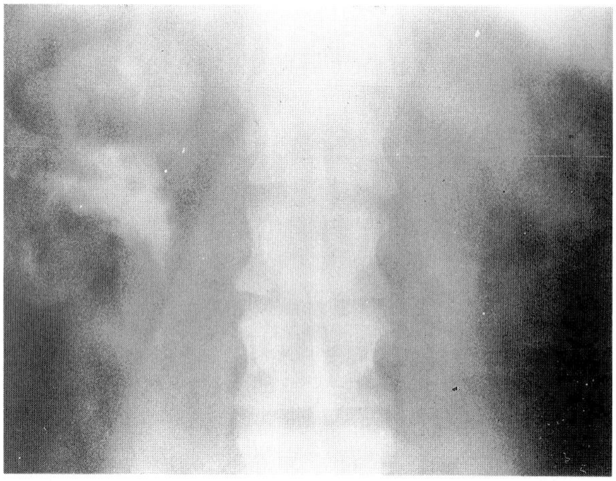

Fig. 5.1. Pyelitis granulomatosa (Courtesy of Dr. C. Türk, KA-Rudolfstiftung, Vienna)

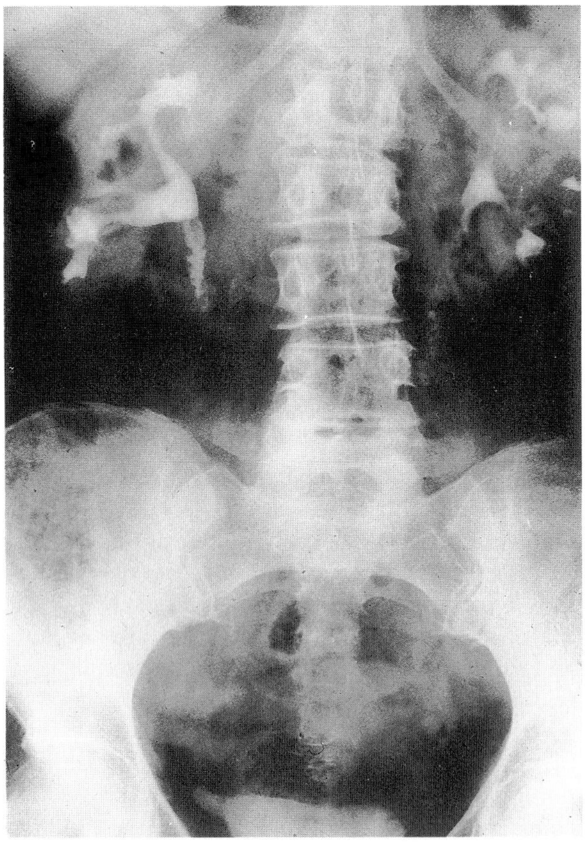

Fig. 5.2. Ureteritis granularis. (Courtesy of Dr. C. Türk, KA-Rudolfstiftung, Vienna)

1. Tuberculosis (Ten Cate 1971; Moonen 1958; Christensen 1974)
2. Schistosomiasis (Forsyth and MacDonald 1966)
3. Worm infections
4. Fungal infections
5. Recurrent bacterial infections which appear morphologically as malacoplakia or ureteritis cystica (Sotoropoulos et al. 1957)

5.1.2.1 Tuberculosis

Tuberculosis usually occurs in young adults; it is less common in children. During the earlier stages, tuberculous ureteritis causes edema; later there is cellular infiltration and mucosal ulceration. These early changes present as spiculations from the ureteral lumen (Cos and Crockett 1977).

The inflammatory changes disable ureteral peristalsis and lead to dilatation of the ureter. Periureteritis and multiple strictures may develop in the area of these ulcerations (Lattimer and Wechsler 1978). Single strictures are usually located at the ureteropelvic junction, at the ureterovesical junction, or at the crossing with the iliac vessels. The strictures are usually short, though they also may be long and straight, and sometimes the whole ureter including the renal pelvis is involved (pipestem ureter) (Birnhaum et al. 1990). Patchy discontinuous ureteral calcifications may also occur. A corkscrew or pipestem ureter should be taken as indicative of tuberculosis until proven otherwise.

5.1.2.2 Chistosomiasis

In most cases of schistosomiasis, terminal hematuria is found. Usually it is accompanied by pain, urgency, and frequency. In order to make the correct diagnosis the characteristic ova have to be discovered in the urine.

Radiologically, symmetrical and parallel calcifications are seen in the distal ureter (railroad track ureteral calcifications) which, in severe cases, can involve the entire collecting system. Initial changes usually can be seen at the ureterovesical junction, where strictures result in dilatation and tortuosity (Thelen 1949).

The ova can infiltrate the wall of the ureter, especially the muscular layers, where they weaken the wall. Fibrosis then develops, further weakening the wall (UMERAH 1977). The vasa vasorum of the ureter can be occluded, causing ischemia of the muscular layer. Coexisting endarteritis obliterans increases ischemia. All of the aforementioned factors lead to muscular atrophy followed by dilatation, lengthening, and tortuosity without obstruction. In cases where obstructions occur, muscular hypertrophy develops above the obstruction. The ureter then becomes trabeculated and sacculated. In chronic cases, fatty and fibrous tissue may form large periureteral tumefactions. Furthermore, polyps, ureteritis cystica, or ureteral concrements can be seen above the stricture (MAKER 1948).

5.1.2.3 Worm Infections

Isolated worm infections of the ureter occur rarely. They cause spastic pains and sometimes hematuria. Some ureteral obstructions are caused by *Dioctophyma renale*.

5.1.2.4 Fungal Infections

Candidiasis. Candidiasis usually occurs in patients with diabetes mellitus (FORLAND et al. 1977), after long-term therapy with steroids, antibiotics, or chemotherapeutic or immunosuppressive agents, in renal transplant patients, in premature infants, and in people suffering from AIDS. Urinary tract candidiasis is very rarely an ascending infection; much more often it is caused by hematogenous spread (MARGOLIN 1971).

Candida albicans can be gas forming and produce "air pyelograms" or gas in the bladder on an intravenous pyelogram. Both acute and chronic inflammation can be caused by *Candida albicans* (BIGGERS and EDWARDS 1980; DEMBNER and PFISTER 1977; WISE et al. 1976).

Actinomycosis. Actinomycosis usually spreads from the gastrointestinal tract or from the lungs through the diaphragm to the kidneys and can cause perirenal abscesses or fistulas between the collecting system and the gastrointestinal tract or lungs. Sinus formations and multiple fistulas are characteristic.

5.1.2.5 Rare Forms of Inflammation

Pyeloureteritis Cystica. Invaginations of the transitional epithelium (Brunn's nests) are observed. Sometimes these nests undergo cystic changes and multiple small fluid-filled cysts develop in the mucosa. Nests also can often be seen in the renal pelvis, urethra, and bladder.

Radiologically, submucosal lesions appear as multiple filling defects usually located at the pyeloureteral junction. An association exists between uretritis cystica and recurrent urinary tract infections by *E. coli*.

Cystitis cystica is quite often considered the response of the urinary system to recurrent and long-term urinary tract infections. There is also an increased incidence of carcinoma of the bladder.

Pyeloureteritis Follicularis and Granularis. The lesions are similar to those of pyeloureteritis cystica but smaller. As a result of chronic inflammation, nodules occur which consist of lymphoid follicles or granulation tissue (Fig. 5.1).

Malacoplakia. Malacoplakia is a histiocytic proliferative disease which can occur in the distal two-thirds of the ureter as well as in the bladder (ELLIOT et al. 1972; NIEH and ALTHAUSEN 1979).

Radiologically, multiple shallow filling defects are observed. They sometimes obstruct the ureter, which can lead to hydronephrosis.

5.2 Congenital Diseases of the Bladder

5.2.1 Embryology (MARSHALL and MÜCKE 1968)

The cloaca, as a transient structure, drains both the intestinal and the urinary tract. Initially, the cloaca extends from the origin of the allantois to the cloacal membrane. It then divides into a ventral and a dorsal chamber. The ventral chamber develops into the urogenital sinus whereas the dorsal chamber develops into the rectum (FRIEDLAND 1983). These two chambers are separated by the urorectal septum, which, if open, communicates the urogenital sinus and the rectum. In late stages of development this opening becomes progressively smaller as the walls of the urorectal septum grow. The ventral and dorsal wall of the cloaca grow at different speeds (the ventral wall grows much faster than the dorsal). As a result of this difference in rate of growth, the urogenital sinus becomes much larger than the dorsal chamber, and the cloacal membrane, which in the early stages of the development faces ventrally, comes to face inferiorly. At this stage there is only a small channel left (Reichel's cloacal duct) through which the urogenital sinus and the dorsal chamber communicate.

During the next stage the cloacal membrane is completely shut and there is no longer a connection between the frontal and the dorsal chambers. After this fusion the cloacal tubercula become the genital tubercula, which in the male form the penile and distal bulbous ureter. The lowermost portion of the urorectal septum forms the floor of the proximal bulbous ureter. The urogenital membrane subsequently breaks down, causing loss of the roof of the phallic portion of the urogenital sinus. The genital folds then fuse in the midline to form the penile ureter.

The bladder is formed from the upper part of the urogenital sinus and also from the allantois. The cranial portion of the bladder subsequently narrows and forms the urachus (vesicoumbilical ligament in adults) (Jaramillo et al. 1990; Rubenstein et al. 1961; Gruber 1934).

5.2.2 Agenesis and Hypoplasia

Agenesis is sometimes associated with a congenital small pelvic outlet and absence of kidneys. Hypoplasia and agenesis usually accompany sacral agenesis (hypoplasia as part of the abdominal muscular deficiency syndrome – prune belly syndrome).

5.2.3 Duplications of the Bladder

Seven types of bladder duplication can be distinguished:

1. Complete duplications of the bladder: Complete duplications are always associated with duplications of the urethra and usually also with duplications of the penis, uterus, and vagina (Senger and Santare 1952; Witzleben et al. 1965). Very often there are malformations of the rectum, especially rectal and ureteral fistulas (Wehrbein 1940).
2. Incomplete duplications: Two bladders are found which unite at the base, but there is a single ureter.
3. Hourglass bladder: The bladder is divided into an upper and a lower portion by a partial muscular and fibrous septum.
4. Complete sagittal septum: Separates the bladder into two halves. One part is separated from the urethra. On this side hydronephrosis and renal dysplasia are inevitable. The obstructed and separated portion forms tumefactions which may compress the contralateral ureter and lead to hydronephrosis.
5. Incomplete sagittal septum.
6. Complete frontal septum.
7. Multiseptate bladder (Caldwell et al. 1991).

5.2.4 Urachal Anomalies

Partially and completely patent urachi have to be distinguished (Cherry 1950). There are two forms of partially patent urachus: (a) urachal diverticulum, in which the urachus is closed at the umbilicus but not at the bladder, and (b) urachal cyst, in which the urachus is closed at the umbilicus and the bladder but not in between. Completely patent urachus is very often associated with ureteral atresia and obstructive posterior ureteral valves.

Urachal fistulas can be observed on lateral radiographs (Jaramillo et al. 1990; Nagasaki et al. 1991). Cystography will demonstrate urachal diverticulum. Urachal cysts are best demonstrated by ultrasonography, double contrast cystography, or computed tomography (Jaramillo et al. 1990; Steinhart et al. 1989; Mandel et al. 1991).

5.2.5 Vesical Exstrophy

Vesical exstrophy is very often associated with epispadias, agenesis of the ureter, malformations of the rectum, and other congenital abnormalities. In exstrophy of the bladder the lower abdominal wall and the anterior bladder wall are absent (showing the inner surface of the posterior wall of the bladder) and malformations of the pubic bones are usually present (Marshall and Mücke 1962). Exstrophy is associated with a significantly higher incidence of adenocarcinoma of the bladder (Meglin et al. 1990; Jaramillo et al. 1990). Persistent cloacal membranes are seen as the reason for vesical exstrophy (Harvard and Thompson 1951; Spence 1966).

5.2.6 Congenital Vesical Diverticula

True diverticula – involving all layers of the wall – are usually localized at the hiatus uretericus, the cranial part of the torus uretericus, the lateral bladder wall, or the fundus (Fig. 5.3) (LURZ 1925).

Paraureteral (Hutch) diverticula usually occur with VUR and are reversible. Concrements or tumors are quite often found (AMAR 1972).

Congenital diverticula hardly ever occur in girls. Usually they do not cause obstructions, but they can extend downward into the pelvis and obstruct the urethra (LEADBETTER and LEADBETTER 1959).

5.3 Calculous Diseases of the Bladder

Calculi of the bladder are much more often found in men than in women. They can be solitary or multiple and are either spherical or oval (EMMETT and WITTEN 1971; SMITH 1968). Their chemical structure may be of five types:

1. Urate calculus: mere urate, sodium urate, or ammonium urate
2. Oxalate calculus
3. Phosphate calculus: apatite, potassium carbonite, brushite, struvite, or aragonite
4. Cystine calculus
5. Xanthine calculus (BRESSEL et al. 1968)

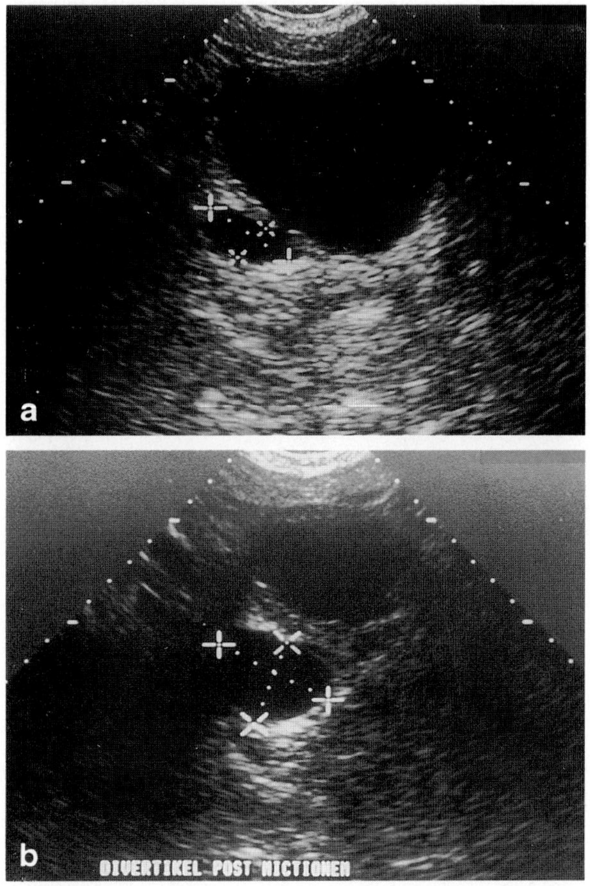

Fig. 5.3 a,b. Bladder diverticulum: **a** prevoiding, **b** postvoiding

5.3.1 Origin of the Calculi

Primary formation of calculi in the bladder may occur for the following reasons:

1. Obstruction of the bladder due to prostatic hypertrophy ureteral strictures, neurogenic cystoparalysis, or diverticula.
2. Bacterial infections of the urinary tract. Bacteria such as *Proteus vulgaris*, *Streptococcus*, *Staphylococcus*, *Pseudomonas*, and *E. coli* can produce urease, which alkalify the urine and subsequently leads to the formation of phosphate calculi (BOSHAMER 1961; ROCHA and SANTOS 1969).
3. The presence of foreign bodies such as suture material, catheters, or coagula, which offer a nidus for the formation of the calculi (VARDI et al. 1991; STRAFFON and HIGGINS 1970).

Calculi may also appear in the bladder secondary to descent from the renal pelvis or ureter.

5.3.2 Complications (STAEHLER 1959)

1. Ulcerous cystitis and perforation
2. Ascending pyelonephritis
3. Peridiverticulitis and diverticulitis with concrements in diverticula
4. Contracted bladder
5. Hypoplasia of the m. detrusor vesicae

5.3.3 Methods of Detection

Bladder calculi may be detected by ultrasound, intravenous urography, cystography, pyelography, cystoscopy (Figs. 5.4, 5.5, 5.6), and computed tomography (VOGLER 1974; GÜNTHER 1952).

Stones composed of uric acid or urates are often invisible on radiographs (EDLING 1952). Calcium oxalate stones may resemble a tesselated stone (Fig. 5.5) (SCHREYER 1974). Stones

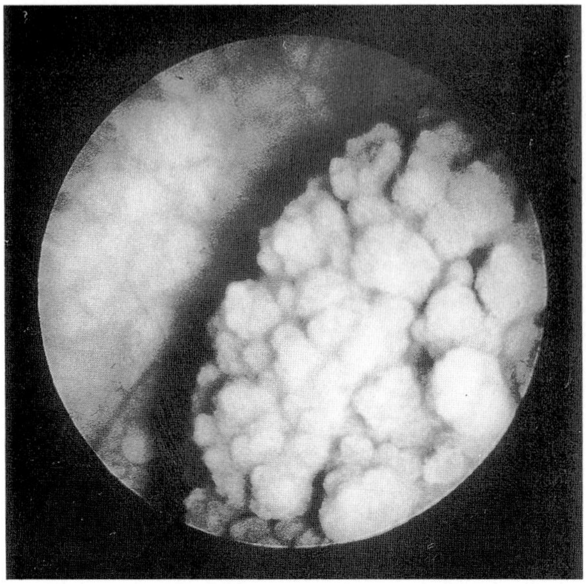

Fig. 5.4. Endoscopic view of bladder calculi. (Courtesy of Dr. P. PORPACZY, SMZO, Vienna)

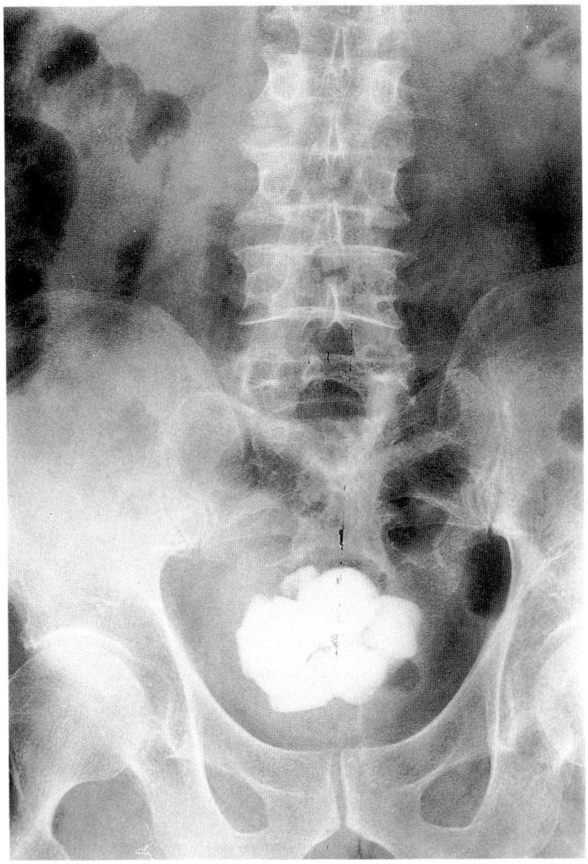

Fig. 5.5. Bladder calculi (plain film)

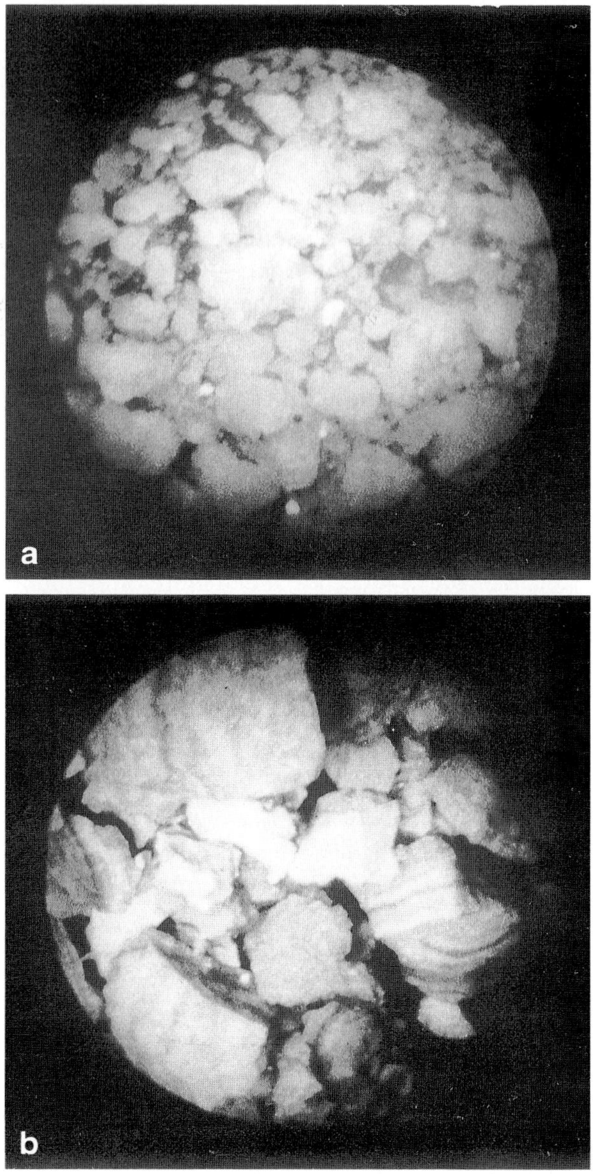

Fig. 5.6 a,b. Bladder calculi; the bladder wall is thickened

occupying the entire lumen of the diverticulum can protrude into the bladder; the orifice of the diverticulum then constricts around the stone and causes a characteristic shelf (KNEISE and SCHOBER 1963).

In order to distinguish small stones lying on the bladder base from calcifications of the prostate, the patient is rolled onto the right side and a lateral decubitus view is obtained. Prostatic calcifications will remain fixed whereas bladder stones will roll to the most dependent part of the bladder (MURPHY et al. 1990; HENNING 1961).

Bladder calculi can become so big that they mimic a bladder filled with contrast medium. When performing ultrasound studies, fecal material may mimic sigmoid–vesical fistulas.

5.4 Therapy

As most bladder calculi are caused by subvesical obstruction, it is essential to treat this predisposing factor first. Bladder calculi should be disintegrated in situ by means of ultrasound, lithotripsy, laser lithotripsy, or mechanical fragmentation (Fig. 5.7).

5.4 Inflammatory Diseases of the Bladder

5.4.1 Etiology

1. Bacterial inflammation: the most common bacteria causing inflammation of the bladder are *E. coli*, *Streptococcus*, *Staphylococcus*, *Neisseria*, *Enterobacter aerogenes*, and *Mycobacterium* (Kunin and Halmagyi 1962; Cyr et al. 1973).
2. Paracytic inflammation, e.g., due to *Schistosoma*, *Trichomonas*, or *Amoeba* (Sanjurjo 1970).
3. Inflammation caused by chemical substances, e.g., cantharidin, bismuth, barium, aniline derivatives.
4. Inflammation caused by physical agents, e.g., electrocoagulation, radiation.

5.4.2 Routes of Infection

1. Descending
2. Ascending from the urethra, the prostate, the seminal vesicles, or catheterization (Martin and Brookrajian 1962)
3. Lymphogenous from the colon, rectum, prostate, seminal vesicles, or parametrium
4. Hematogenous: tonsillitis, dental foci, endocarditis (Friedland et al. 1983)

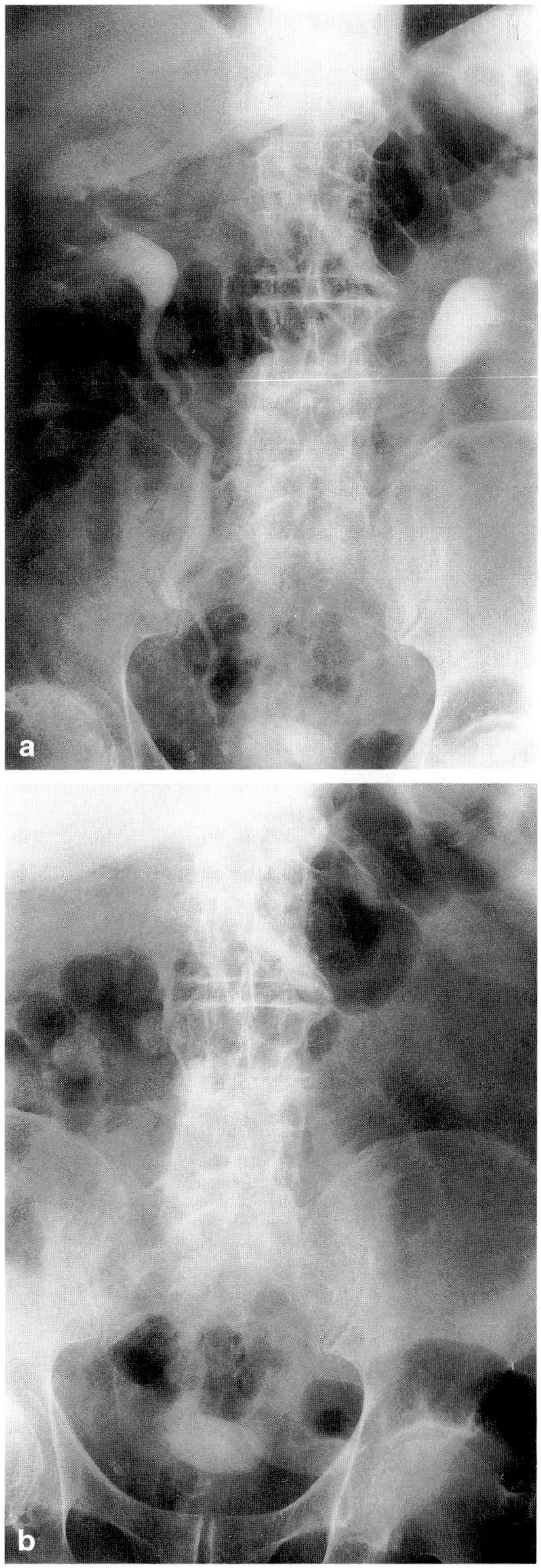

▷

Fig. 5.7a,b. Disintegration of bladder calculi by ultrasonic lithotripsy. (Courtesy of P. Porpaczy, SMZO, Vienna)

5.4.3 Predisposing Factors

1. Inflammation of the bladder is much more common in patients with predisposing factors, e.g., diabetes mellitus, septicemia, or AIDS (Vejlsgaard 1973; Stamey 1983).
2. Urination disorders, e.g., infravesical obstructions, neurogenic bladder, diverticula, VUR.
3. Congenital anomalies such as exstrophy posterior stenosis of the urethra, and vesicoureteral or vesicovaginal fistulas (Vogler and Schreyer 1974; Aabeck and Lien 1982; Mufson et al. 1973; Bodian 1957; Burns et al. 1947).

5.4.4 Cystitis

5.4.4.1 Acute Cystitis

1. Cystitic catarrhalis sive dequamativa: Only the superficial layers of the mucosa are involved.
2. Purulent cystitis: Inflammatory infiltration of the submucosa and submucosal bleeding are found (Tung and Papanicolaou 1990). Sometimes deeper layers of the bladder wall are involved, which can lead to phlegmon and pericystitis (Smith and Dehner 1972).
3. Pseudomembranous (fibrinous) cystitis and gangrenous cystitis (Stirling and Hopkins 1934): These forms are usually found with cystoplegia, diphtheria, typhoid, or diabetes; they may also be caused by chemical substances or irradiation. Gangrenous cystitis can become chronic and is also sometimes found after injuries or due to extravesical pressure (pregnancy).
4. Cystitis bullosa sive emphysematosa: Emphysematous cystitis is caused by gas-forming organisms (*E. coli* or *Enterobacter aerogenes*) (Bailey 1961; Bojsen and Lewis-Jonsson 1954; Blight 1978). It usually appears in middle-aged women but is also found in infants (Diller 1963; Feingold et al. 1953; Francke and Lane 1956). Diabetic patients have a higher incidence of emphysematous cystitis (Datta and Seminario 1978; Hawtrey et al. 1974; Maliwan 1979).

5.4.4.2 Chronic Cystitis

Chronic cystitis leads to thickening of the bladder wall, edema and hyperemia, and lymphocytic infiltration of the mucosa. Sometimes there is destruction of the muscular layer with subsequent fibrosis leading to shrinkage of the bladder or complete atony.

There are various forms of chronic cystitis:

1. *Interstitial cystitis*: Middle-aged women are most commonly affected (Oravisto 1975). Interstitial cystitis is characterized by edema of the mucosa, lymphocytic infiltration, proliferation of connective tissue, and shallow ulcerations which often calcify (Parsons 1987). Interstitial cystitis has to be considered precancerous (Fall et al. 1985; Gordon et al. 1973; Hanash and Pool 1970; Holm-Bentzen et al. 1987).
2. *Malacoplakia*: The etiology is unknown. Recurrent *E. coli* infections seem to play an important part. Proliferation of granulation tissue in the mucosa is characteristic. The lesions generally measure only about 5 mm in diameter but can grow to a size of almost 3 cm and may then mimic bladder cancer. Histologically Michaelis-Gutmann bodies can be found in macrophages and histiocytes.
3. *Cystitis follicularis and granularis*: Proliferations of lymphatic follicles and granulation tissue bulge at the trigone.
4. *Cystitis glandularis sive cystica*: Invaginations of transitional epithelium called Brunn's nests frequently occur in the renal pelvis, ureter, and bladder (Brogdon et al. 1965; Lin et al. 1980). Some of these nests may undergo cystic changes (cystitis cystica); multiple small fluid-filled cysts measuring 2–7 mm in diameter develop in the mucosa. The changes are most often found in the trigone but can involve all parts of the bladder (Kittredge and Braman 1958; Lin et al. 1980).
5. *Tuberculous cystitis*: Infection usually spreads via either the descending or the hematogenous route. In men, ascending infections from genital tuberculosis are also found (Moonen 1958; Speirs et al. 1990; Cafeten 1971; Kelalis et al. 1962). Characteristically, tuberculous cystitis leads to a small and smooth, often asymmetrically contracted bladder (Kneise and Schober 1963). Mucosal edema and granulomas impart a cobblestone appearance on radiographs. Filling defects can be caused by

large granulomas, sometimes simulating carcinoma. In rare cases very patchy calcifications of the bladder can be found, simulating schistosomiasis. As the disease progresses the bladder continues to shrink and VUR develops (MAY 1968).

6. *Fungal cystitis*: *Candida albicans* sometimes leads to gas formation in the bladder. Actinomycosis can lead to the formation of fistulas (GOLDMAN et al. 1960; MCDONALD and FAGAN 1972; KING and LAM 1978; SAKAMOTO 1978).
   Schistosomiasis is discussed in Sect. 5.1 (see also PALUBINSKAS 1960; AREAN 1966; ATAAH 1976). Schistoso miasis in the bladder leads to submucosal calcifications which show up as symmetrical eggshell calcifications on radiographs (SANJURJO 1970). These calcifications nearly always occur in combination with symmetrical calcifications of the ureters (AL GORAB et al. 1978).
7. *Cystitis caused by irradiation*: Cystitis following irradiation may be primary or secondary in nature. When it is primary, edema and bullous cystitis are seen (HIETALA et al. 1975); when secondary, ulcerations and atrophy of the mucous membrane and squamous metaplasia can be found. Irradiation-induced cystitis leads to VUR, hydroureter, and contracted bladder (BECKER and ZUM WINKEL 1961).

5.5 Future Aspects – Digital Techniques in Uroradiology

Radiology is primarily a service-rendering specialty which has, during its almost 100-year history, evolved from a merely diagnostic imaging method to become part of an interdisciplinary and integrated clinical approach; moreover it is also moving increasingly into the therapeutic field through the application of minimally invasive techniques, especially in uroradiology.

In addition to the production and interpretation of image-dependent diagnosis, a chief goal is the presentation of the results in a timely manner to the referring colleague to enable him/her to decide upon the patient's therapy. Since many different modalities are used, being applied singly or in combination according to the clinical problem, there is a need to present the results in an integrated fashion.

Computers are not new in uroradiology; for example, the digital imaging modalities such as ultrasound and computed tomography are well-established methods. Also, the indications for magnetic resonance imaging are becoming clearer as the number of scientific publications in this field increases (Cox et al. 1988). The aforementioned digital methods are responsible for about 25%–40% of uroradiologic examinations, according to the nature and the utilization of digital equipment in the radiology department. Nevertheless, the majority of examinations still consist in "conventional" radiography (images of the chest and abdomen as well as contrast media examinations of the genitourinary tract).

Through the introduction of digital radiography with storage phosphor disks and the digital image intensifier, the field of conventional imaging is now also utilizing computerization (TEMPLETON et al. 1987). The main advantages lie in the reduction of exposure and thereby a reduction of the dose by elimination of reexaminations secondary to exposure errors.

References

Aabeck HS, Lien EN (1982) Cystitis cystica in childhood: clinical findings and treatment procedures. Acta Paediatr Scand 71:247

Al Gorab MM, El-Rfiaie M, Abou El Azm T, Saad SM, Rahmann MA, Hanafy HM, Arafa A (1978) Radiologic findings of bilharzial (schistosomal) contracted bladder. Urology 11:303

Amar AD (1972) Vesicoureteral reflux associated with congenital bladder diverticulum. J Urol 107:966

Arean VM (1966) Schistosomiasis: a clinicopathologic evaluation. In: Summer S (ed) Pathology annual, vol 1. Appleton-Century-Crofts, New York, p 68

Ataah EB, Nkposong EO (1976) Schistosomiasis and carcinoma of the bladder: critical appraisal of causal relationship. Trop Geogr Med 28:268

Bailey H (1961) Cystitis emphysematosa. AJR 86:850

Becker J, zum Winkel K (1961) Strahlentherapie akuter Erkrankungen der Niere und ableitenden Harnwege. Radiologie 1:115

Biggers R, Edwards J (1980) Anuria secondary to bilateral ureteropelvic fungus balls. Urology 15:161

Birnbaum BA, Friedmann JP, Lubat E et al. (1990) Ureter CT extrarenal genitourinary tuberculosis: CT appearance of calcified pipestem ureter and seminal vesicle abscess. J Comput Assist Tomogr 14:653

Blight EM Jr (1978) Case profile: gonorrheal pelvic inflammatory disease presenting as bullous cystitis. Urology 11:196

Bodian M (1957) Some observations on the pathology of congenital idiopathic bladder-neck obstruction (Marion's disease). Br J Urol 29:393

Bojsen E, Lewis-Jonsson J (1954) Emphysematous cystitis. Acta Radiol 41:269

Boshamer K (1961) Morphologie und Genese der Harnsteine. In: Alken CE, Dix VW, Weyrauch HM, Wildbolz E (eds) Handbuch der Urologie, vol X. Springer, Berlin

Bressel M, Hoppe-Seyler G, Dorn H (1968) Diagnostik und konservative Therapie der Urolithiasis. Internist 9:184

Brogdon BG, Silbinger ML, Colston JAC Jr (1965) Cystitis glandularis. Radiology 85:470

Burns E, Cummins H, Hyman J (1947) Incomplete reduplication of bladder with congenital solitary kidney; report of case. J Urol 57:257

Cafeten HW (1971) Tuberculosis of the genitourinary tract. In: Emmett JL, Witten DH (eds) Clinical urography. W.B. Saunders, Philadelphia

Caldwell B, Gambrino J, Dietrich RB, Walot I, Greensite F, Kangarloo H (1991) Genitourinary system, abnormalities. MR evaluation of congenital anomalies of the pediatric genital tract. RSNA Scientific exhibit

Cherry JW (1950) Patent urachus; review and report of case. J Urol 63:693

Christensen WI (1974) Genitourinary tuberculosis. Medicine (Baltimore) 53:377

Cos LR, Crockett ATK (1980) Genitourinary tuberculosis revisited. Urology 20:11

Cox GG, Arenson RL, Bosco HL (1988) Current status of radiology image management systems. Invest Radiol 23:656–663

Cyr WL, Johnson H, Balfour J (1973) Granulomatous cystitis as a manifestation of chronic granulomatous disease of childhood. J Urol 110:357

Datta NS, Seminario O (1978) Emphysematous cystitis presenting with subcutaneous emphysema. Urology 12:701

Dembner AG, Pfister RC (1977) Fungal infection of the urinary tract: demonstration by antegrade pyelography and drainage by percutaneous nephrostomy. AJR 129:415

Diller WF (1963) Ungewöhnliche Zystitisformen im Röntgenbild (Cystitis emphysematosa und Cystitis clacarea). Fortschr Röntgenstr 98:316

Edling NPG (1952) Untersuchungen der Harnorgane. In: Schniz HR, Bänsch WW, Friedl E, Vehlinger E (eds) Lehrbuch der Röntgendiagnostik. Thieme, Stuttgart

Elliot GB, Moloney PJ, Clement JG (1972) Malacoplakia of the urinary tract. Am J Roentgenol Radium Ther Nucl 16:830

Emmett JL, Witten DM (1971) Calculous disease of the genitourinary tract. In: Emmett JL, Witten DM (eds) Clinical urography, vol II. W.B. Saunders, Philadelphia

Fall M, Johannsson SL, Vahine A (1985) A clinicopathological and virological study of interstitial cystitis. J Urol 133:771

Feingold JE, Hansen CO, Rigler LG (1953) Cystitis emphysematosa. Radiology 61:346

Forland M, Thomas V, Shelokov A (1977) Urinary tract infections in patients with diabetes mellitus. Studies on antibody coating of bacteria. JAMA 238:1924

Forsyth DM, MacDonald G (1966) Urological complications of endemic schistosomiasis in school children. 2. Done School, Zanzibar. Trans R Soc Trop Med Hyg 60:568

Francke P, Lane VW (1956) Cystitis emphysematosa (case report). AJR 75:921

Friedland GW (1983) Congenital anomalies of the urinary tract. In: Friedland GW et al. (eds) Uroradiology, an integrated approach. Churchill Livingstone, New York

Friedland GW, Filly R, Goris ML et al. (1983) Infections and infestations. In: Friedland GW, Filly R, Goris ML et al. (eds) Uroradiology, an integrated approach. Churchill Livingstone, New York

Goldman HT, Littmann ML, Oppenheimer GD, CGlickman SI (1960) Monilial cystitis: effective treatment with instillations of amphotericin B. JAMA 174:359

Gordon HL, Rossen RD, Hersh EM, Yium JJ (1973) Immunologic aspects of interstitial cystitis. J Urol 109:228

Gruber GB (1934) Die Entwicklungsstörungen der Harnblase. In: Lubarsch O, Henke F (eds) Handbuch der speziellen pathologischen Anatomie und Histologie. Springer, Berlin

Günther GW (1952) Röntgenuroskopie. Thieme, Stuttgart

Hanash KA, Pool TC (1970) Interstitial and hemorrhagic cystitis: viral, bacterial and fungal studies. J Urol 104:705

Harvard BM, Thompson GJ (1951) Congenital exstrophy of urinary bladder; late results of treatment by Coffey-Mayo method of ureterointestinal anastomosis. J Urol 65:223

Hawtrey CE, Williams JJ, Schmidt JD (1974) Cystitis emphysematosa. Urology 3:612

Henning O (1961) Steine der Harnblase, der Harnröhre und der Vorsteherdrüse. In: Alken CE, Dix VW, Weyrauch HM, Wildbolz E (eds) Handbuch der Urologie, vol X. Springer, Berlin

Hietala SO, Winblad B, Hassler O (1975) Vascular and morphological changes in the urinary bladder wall after irradiation. Int Urol Nephrol 7:119

Holm-Bentzen M, Jacobsen F, Nerstrom B, et al. (1987) A prospective double-blind clinically controlled multicenter trial of sodium pentanopolysulfate in the treatment of interstitial cystitis and related painful bladder diseases. J Urol 138:503

Jaramillo D, Lebowitz RL, Hendren WH (1990) Cloacal malformation: radiologic findings and imaging recommendations. Radiology 177:441

Kass EH (1985) Asymptomatic infections of the urinary tract. Trans Assoc Am Physicans 79:56

Kelalis PP, Greene LF, Weed LA (1962) Brucellosis of the urogenital tract: a mimic of tuberculosis. J Urol 88:347

King DT, Lam M (1978) Actinomycosis of the urinary bladder. JAMA 240:1512

Kittredge WE, Braman W (1958) Cystitis glandularis. Trans Am Assoc Gen-urin Surg 50:136

Kneise O, Schober KL (1963) Die Röntgenuntersuchung der Harnorgane. VEB Thieme, Leipzig

Kunin CR, Halmagyi NE (1962) Urinary-tract infections in schoolchildren. II. Characterization of invading organisms. N Engl J Med 266:1297

Latham RH, Stamm WE (1984) Role of fimbriated *Escherichia coli* in urinary tract infections in adult women: correlations with localization studies. J Infect Dis 149:835

Lattimer JK, Wechsler M (1978) Genitourinary tuberculosis. In: Harrison HH (ed) Campell's urology. W.B. Saunders, Philadelphia, p 557

Leadbetter GW Jr, Leadbetter WF (1959) Diagnosis and treatment of congenital bladder neck obstruction in children. N Engl J Med 260:633

Lin JI, Tseng CH, Choy C, Yong HS, Marsidi PS, Pilloff B (1980) Diffuse cystitis glandularis: associated with adenocarcinomatous change. Urology 15:411

Lurz L (1925) Sogenannte angeborene Divertikel der Harnblase. Z Urol Chir 18:287

Maker N (1948) The bilharzial ureter: some observations on the surgical pathology and surgical treatment. Br Jr Surg 36:148

Maliwan N (1979) Emphysematous cystitis associated with *Clostridium perfringens* bacteremia. J Urol 121:819

Mandel J, Blyth BR, Peters CA (1991) Structural genitourinary defects detected in utero. Radiology 178:193

Margolin HN (1971) Fungus infections of the urinary tract. Semin Roentgenol 6:323

Marshall VF, Mücke EC (1962) Variations in exstrophy of the bladder. J Urol 88:766

Marshall VF, Mücke EE (1968) Congenital abnormalities of the bladder. In: Alken CE, Dix VW, Goodwin WE, Weyrauch HM, Wildbolz E (eds) Handbuch der Urologie, vol VII/1. Springer, Berlin Heidelberg New York

Martin CM, Brookrajian EN (1962) Bacteriuria prevention after indwelling urinary catheterization. Arch Intern Med 110:70

May P, König K (1968) Fortschritte und Diagnostik und Therapie der Urogenitaltuberkulose. Internist 9:195

McDonald DF, Fagan CJ (1972) Fungus balls in the urinary bladder. Am J Roentgenol Radiat Ther Nucl Med 114:753

Meglin AJ, Balotin RJ, Jelinek JS et al. (1990) Genitourinary system, abnormalities cloacal exstrophy: radiologic findings in 13 patients, AJR 155:1267

Moonen WA (1958) Stricture of the ureter and contracture of the bladder and the bladder neck due to tuberculosis: their diagnosis and treatment. J Urol 80:218

Mufson MA, Belshe RB, Horrigan TJ, Zollar LM (1973) Cause of acute hemorrhagic cystitis in children. Am J Dis Child 126:605

Murphy WD, Rovner AJ, Nazinitsky KJ (1990) Bladder diseases. Condylomata acuminata of the bladder: a rare cause of intraluminal-filling defects. Urol Radiol 12:34

Nagasaki A, Handa N, Kawanami T (1991) Diagnosis of urachal anomalies in infancy and childhood by contrast fistulography, ultrasound and CT. Pediatr Radiol 21:321

Nieh PT, Althausen AF (1979) Malacoplakia of the ureter. J Urol 122:701

Oravisto KJ (1975) Epidemiology of interstitial cystitis. Ann Chir Gynaecol Fenn 64:75

Palubinskas AJ (1960) Eosinophilic cystitis. Radiology 75:589

Parsons CL (1987) Sodium pentosanpolysulfate treatment of interstitial cystitis: an update. Urology [Suppl] 29:14

Putschar W (1934) Die entzündlichen Erkrankungen der ableitenden Harnorgane und der Nierenhüllen, einschließlich der Pyelonephritis und der Pyenephrose. In: Henke F, Lubarsch O (eds) Handbuch der speziellen pathologischen Anatomie und Histologie, vol VI/2. Springer, Berlin

Rocha H, Santos CS (1969) Relapse of urinary tract infection in the presence of urinary tract calculi: the role of bacteria within the calculi. J Med Microbiol 2:372

Rubenstein M, Meyer R, Bernstein J (1961) Congenital abnormalities of the urinary system. I.A postmortem survey of developmental anomalies and acquired congenital lesions in children's hospital. J Pediatr 58:356

Sakamoto S (1978) Fungus ball formation of *Aspergillus* in the bladder. Eur Urol 4:388

Sanjurjo LA (1970) Parasitic diseases of the genitourinary system. In: Campbell MF, Harrison JH (eds) Urology, vol I, 3rd edn. Saunders, Philadelphia

Schreyer H (1974) Erkrankungen der unteren Harnwege und Genitalorgane. In: Vogler E (ed) Radiologische Diagnostik der Harnorgane. Thieme, Stuttgart

Senger FL, Santare VJ (1952) Congenital multilocular bladder: case report. J Urol 68:283

Smith DR (1968) Allgemeine Urologie. Urban & Schwarzenberg, Munich

Smith BH, Dehner LP (1972) Chronic ulcerating interstitial cystitis. Arch Pathol 93:76

Sotoropoulos C, Karaslima E, Gilmire J (1957) Cystitis and ureteritis emphysematosa. Radiology 68:866

Speirs RT, Raghavendra BN, Rausen A et al. (1990) Ultrasound findings in diffuse granulomatous cystitis in chronic granulomatous disease of childhood. Urol Radiol 12:106

Spence HM (1966) Ureterosigmoidostomy for exstrophy of bladder: results in personal series of thirty-one cases. Br J Urol 38:36

Stamey TA (1983) Urinary tract infections: radiologic aspects of patients at serious risk. In: Friedland GW, Filly R, Goris ML et al. (ed) Uroradiology, an integrated approach. Churchill Livingstone, New York

Staehler W (1959) Klinik und Praxis der Urologie, vol I. Thieme, Stuttgart

Steinhart JM, Kuhn JP, Eisenberg B et al. (1989) Ultrasound screening of healthy infants for urinary tract abnormalities. Radiology 171:288

Stirling WC, Hopkins GA (1934) Gangrene of the bladder. J Urol 31:517

Straffon RA, Higgins CC (1970) Urinary lithiasis and foreign bodies. In: Campbell MF, Harrison JH (eds) Urology, vol. 1. Saunders, Philadelphia

Templeton AW, Dwyer SJ III, Cox GG et al. (1982) A digital radiology imaging system: description and clinical evaluation. AJR 149:847–851

ten Cate HW (1971) Tuberculosis of the genitourinary tract. In: Emmet JL, Witten DM (eds) Clinical urography. W.B. Saunders, Philadelphia

Thelen A (1949) Die Pathologie des Harnleiters im Röntgenbild. Thieme, Stuttgart

Tung HA, Papanicolaou N (1990) Pyocystis with urethral obstruction: percutaneous cystotomy as an alternative to surgery. J Canad Assoc Radiol 41:350

Umerah BC (1977) Evaluation of the physiological function of the ureter by fluoroscopy in bilharziasis. Radiology 124:645

Vardi Y, Moskovitz B, Levin DR et al. (1991) Bladder, calculi stone formation in substitution cystoplasty. Urol Radiol 12:194

Vejlsgaard R (1973) Studies on urinary infections in diabetics. IV. Significant bacteriuria in pregnancy in relation to age of onset, duration of diabetes, angiopathy and urological symptoms. Acta Med Scand 193:337

Vogler E (1974) Erkrankungen der Nieren und der oberen Harnwege. In: Vogler E (ed) Radiologische Diagnostik der Harnorgane. Thieme, Stuttgart

Vogler E, Schreyer H (1974) Besonderheiten in der radiologischen Diagnostik von Erkrankungen der Harnorgane im Kindesalter: In: Vogler E (ed) Radiologische Diagnostik der Harnorgane. Thieme, Stuttgart

Wehrbein HL (1940) Double kidney and ureter and bilocular bladder in child. J Urol 43:804

Wise GJ, Goldberg P, Kozinn PJ (1976) Genitourinary candidiasis: diagnostic and treatment. J Urol 116:778

Witzleben DI, Chir M, Karlafitis CM (1965) Complete frontal septum of the bladder. J Urol 94:427

Zollinger HU (1966) Niere und ableitende Harnwege. In: Dörr W, Vehlinger E (eds) Spezielle pathologische Anatomie, vol III. Springer, Berlin Heidelberg New York

6 Traumatic, Inflammatory, Neoplastic, and Miscellaneous Lesions of the Bladder

LAWRENCE R. BIGONGIARI and HILARY ZARNOW

CONTENTS

6.1 Normal Anatomy

6.1.1 Anatomic Relationships

The urinary bladder is the body's reservoir for urine. It is a muscular bag lined with a mucous membrane and is located in the bony pelvis below a layer of peritoneum. Occupying the anterior half of the pelvis, it is bounded by the symphysis pubis and the diverging walls of the pelvis ventrally and at its sides. The bladder is flattened

LAWRENCE R. BIGONGIARI, M.D., Clinical Associate Professor; HILARY ZARNOW, M.D., M.S. (Renal Pathology), Clinical Associate Professor; Department of Radiology, St. Francis Regional Medical Center, University of Kansas, Medical School at Wichita, 929 North St. Francis Street, Wichita, KS 67214, USA

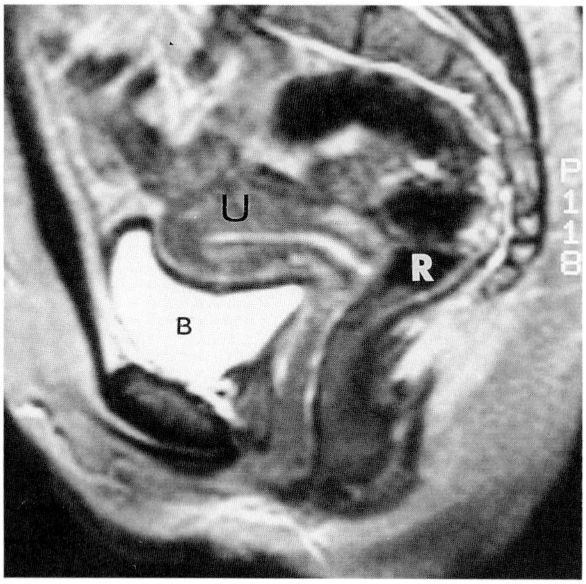

Fig. 6.1. MRI of the bladder in a female: heavily T2-weighted sagittal image; scan performed with fast spin-echo technique. The relationship of the bladder to adjacent organs is shown. *B*, bladder; *R*, rectum; *U*, uterus

superiorly when empty, becomes globular with urine filling, and has a normal capacity of up to 500 ml. It is dorsal and cephalad to the pubis, being separated from it by the retropubic space of Retzius. The urinary bladder does not assume this pelvic position until maturity. It is an abdominal organ in infants and children (CAFFEY 1972). In the male, the rectum is dorsal and caudal to the urinary bladder. The seminal vesicles and the ampulla of the ductus deferens are embedded in endopelvic fascia caudally and dorsally against the fundus of the bladder. In the female, the uterus and vagina lie between the rectum and the bladder (Fig. 6.1). Depending on the state of distention of the bladder, the nongravid uterus and cervix will be dorsal and/or cephalad to the bladder. The vagina is caudal and posterior, its anterior wall loosely attached to the fundus of the bladder (WOODBURNE 1976; PANSKY 1979).

6.1.2 *Reflections, Ligaments, and Fascial Planes*

The superior surface and the uppermost posterior surface of the bladder are covered by peritoneum which extends posteriorly to form the rectovesical pouch of Douglas in the male or the rectouterine pouch (cul-de-sac) in the female. The bladder is firmly attached to the base of the prostate gland caudally in the male and lies on the pelvic floor and urogenital diaphragm in the female.

The urinary bladder is enveloped in the endopelvic fascia, which attaches to the parietal fascia on the back of the pubis and to the superior fascia on the pelvic diaphragm, forming the true ligaments. The pubovesical ligaments are the puboprostatic or lateral ligament of the male and the pubourethral ligament of the female. The rectovesical ligaments extend from the bladder to the sides of the rectum and sacrum. The false ligaments are a group of peritoneal folds extending from the bladder to the abdominal or pelvic walls. They are the medial and lateral umbilical, the lateral ligaments, and the sacrogenital or posterior false ligaments. The medial umbilical ligament extends from the apex of the bladder to the abdominal wall in the midline. This is the vestige of the embryologic urachus (WOODBURN 1976; PANSKY 1979).

The limiting fascial planes of the pelvis are interconnecting and complex. The superior fascia of the urogenital diaphragm fuses with the pelvic fascia, the obturator fascia, and the endopelvic visceral fascia. The inferior fascia of the urogenital diaphragm fuses with Colles' fascia, which continues as Scarpa's fascia anteriorly and as the dartos muscle and fascia inferiorly and fuses inferolaterally with the fascia lata of the thigh. The loose areolar connective tissue which envelops the bladder is continuous with the retropubic space of Retzius (SANDLER et al. 1986; PANSKY 1979).

6.1.3 *Mucosa and Musculature*

The mucosa of the bladder consists of transitional epithelium with an underlying well-developed submucosal layer of connective and elastic tissue. External to the submucosa is the bladder muscle, the detrusor, which is composed of coarse fascicles that do not run in continuous planes but decussate and crisscross, changing direction and level to form a meshwork rather than definable layers. Longitudinally orientated muscle bundles tend to predominate in the outer and inner aspects of the detrusor. Close to the internal meatus, the detrusor assumes three definite layers: inner longitudinal, middle circular, and outer longitudinal (TANAGHO 1992a). The inner layer of muscle shows a tendency to longitudinal convergence on the urethra and much of it is continuous

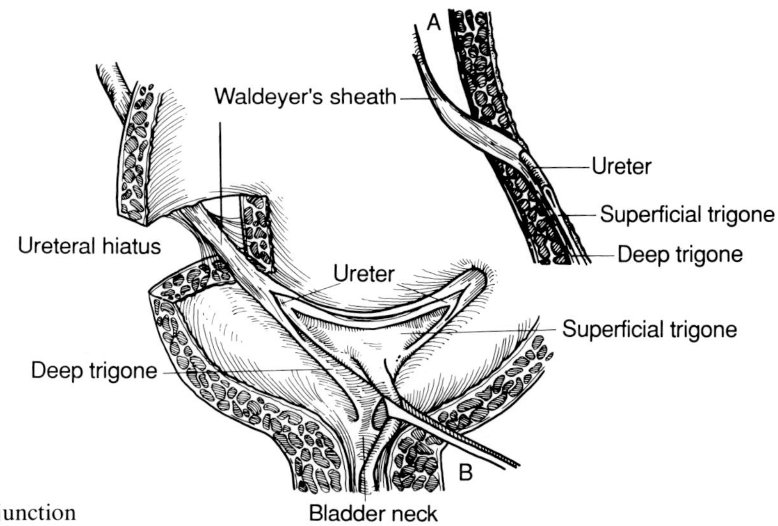

Fig. 6.2. Drawing of the ureterovesical junction

with the internal longitudinal musculature of the urethral wall. In the female, some of the posterior outer longitudinal detrusor muscle bundles extend over the bladder base to merge with the anterior vaginal wall. Anteriorly, some outer longitudinal detrusor muscle bundles continue into the pubovesical ligaments, providing the muscular component of these structures (GOSLING 1985). The internal sphincter or bladder neck is not a true sphincter but rather a thickening formed by interlaced and converging muscle fibers of the detrusor as they pass distally to become the smooth muscle of the urethra. The smooth muscle of the bladder neck is histologically, histochemically, and pharmacologically distinct from that composing the rest of the detrusor (GOSLING 1985). These arching bundles of muscle are derived from the circular layer, extend from just above the trigone down to the area anterior to the internal urethral orifice, and are functionally capable of constricting the urethral aperture. Detrusor contraction squeezes urine toward and out the urethra. The bladder mucosa, which is smooth when the bladder is distended, becomes heaped into numerous folds of rugae when the bladder is contracted. These can be mistaken for muscular trabeculation when demonstrated radiographically (GOSLING 1985; TANAGHO 1988a; WOODBURNE 1976; CAFFEY 1972).

6.1.4 Ureteral Orifices and Trigone

The distal ureter passes obliquely through the muscular layer of the bladder wall and then courses submucosally to its orifice (Fig. 6.2). As the ureters penetrate the bladder wall just lateral to a prominent posterior band of longitudinal detrusor muscle, the superficial fascicles of the detrusor medial to the ureter are elevated and fascicles both medial and lateral to it are separated. The ureter penetrates medially under the deeper layers of detrusor muscle and so traverses the bladder wall. Internal detrusor bundles arch over the ureter as it bulges into the bladder lumen. The ureter then tunnels submucosally for about 1 cm to its aperture. (WOODBURNE 1964, 1976). Approximately 3 cm of the lower ureter is encased in a fibromuscular sheath, Waldeyer's sheath, which is attached to the detrusor by a few small fascicles of muscle. A small separation (Waldeyer's "space" or separation) exists between the distal ureter and the detrusor muscle, allowing motion (WOODBURNE 1964, 1976; TANAGHO 1986, 1992a).

TANAGHO and PUGH (1963) described the anatomy of the ureterovesical junction in detail based on their dissection of 25 normal ureterovesical junctions of adults obtained at autopsy or at surgery. They found that the arrangement of muscle fibers in the ureteral wall changes as the ureter is traced downwards. The juxtavesical segment (the lowermost few centimeters) has mainly longitudinal muscle fibers in the long axis of the lumen but also has fairly well developed oblique and circular fibers. In the intramural segment (which averaged 0.9 mm in length and was entirely surrounded by bladder muscle) and the submucosal segment (which averaged about 0.7 mm in length and lay superficially in the bladder base, covered only by the mucous membrane), the muscle is entirely longitudinal with no circular fibers to be seen. The latter two segments together constitute the intravesical ureter. The circular and oblique fibers do not end in the juxtavesical portion but rather change orientation, becoming longitudinal (TANAGHO 1986). There is nothing about the arrangement of muscle fibers here to suggest the usual active muscular sphincter. Being entirely longitudinal in the intravesical ureter, the muscles cannot even transmit peristalsis. The muscle fibers of the roof of the ureteral orifice split and swing to the side, forming the lips of the ureteral orifice; they then join with the floor fibers, accumulate just distal to the orifice, and fan out into the trigone (TANAGHO 1986). The longitudinal fibers of the roof of the intravesical ureter wrap around the ureteral orifice to join the floor fibers and form the superficial trigone (TANAGHO and PUGH 1963).

Waldeyer's sheath, which consists of fibromuscular tissue, forms an encircling layer around the lowermost 1.5–3 cm or the juxtavesical segment of the ureter. As the sheath is traced cephalad, the amount of muscle gradually decreases and the fibrous tissue becomes more prominent, until at its upper limit it consists only of fibrous tissue that has become continuous with the adventitia of the ureter. TANAGHO (1986) stated that the sheath's muscular element gradually fuses with the ureteral musculature. Dissection of the intravesical portion showed that the sheath follows the ureter through the ureteral canal or hiatus through the detrusor muscle, forming a complete encircling fibromuscular layer around the ureter. At the level of the junction of the intramural and submucosal segments, the muscle fibers encircle the lumen much as the ureteral muscle fibers do, and then form a layer deep to the superficial trigonal muscle.

The trigone is a smooth triangular area above the urethral orifice (cf. Fig. 6.3 for appearance of an edematous trigone). The trigone is both the termination and the attachment of the ureter. The ureter is loose in the bladder wall but firmly attached to the trigone by Waldeyer's sheath (TANAGHO and PUGH 1963). The ureteric terminations form the cephalad corners of the trigone joined by the interureteric ridge. The internal urethral orifice is the trigone's ventral and caudal apex. The trigone shape is formed by the blending of the continuing longitudinal muscles of the ureters across the midline to form

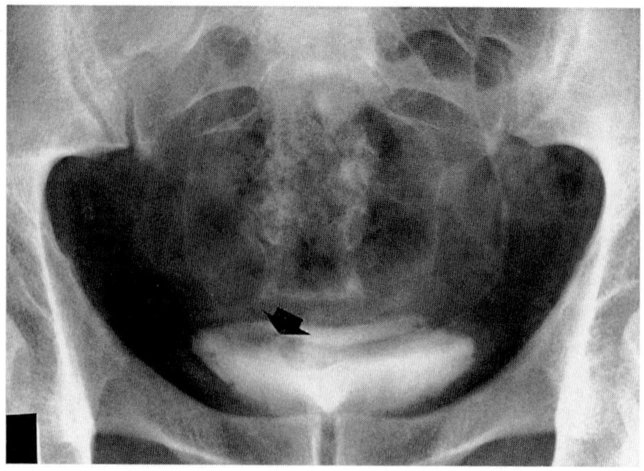

Fig. 6.3. Edematous trigone: 5-min film showing stone (*arrow*) at right ureterovesical junction. The trigone is asymmetric because of the edema on the right. (CUNNINGHAM 1975)

the interureteric ridge plus a fanning downward toward the urethral aperture. The smooth muscle of the superficial trigone is relatively thin but becomes thickened along its superior border as the interureteric ridge. Similar thickenings occur along the lateral edges of the trigone (WOODBURNE 1976; GOSLING 1985). Since the mucosal membrane of trigone is firmly adherent to the underlying muscle, the trigone is smooth whether the bladder is full or empty (TANAGHO 1986).

TANAGHO and co-workers (TANAGHO and PUGH 1963; TANAGHO et al. 1965) demonstrated that the superficial trigonal muscle layer is a direct continuation of the ureteral muscle and the deep trigonal muscle layer a direct continuation of Waldeyer's sheath. The superficial muscle layer is unattached to any structure between the point where the ureter proper ends and the urethra (TANAGHO 1963). These two layers together constitute the trigone of the bladder, which is embryologically, anatomically, and functionally a direct continuation of the ureter. TANAGHO et al. (1965) also referred to the two layers together as the trigonal muscle. TANAGHO (1986) says that the deep trigone forms a dense compact layer in the base of the bladder which fuses to a certain degree with the detrusor muscle and anchors the ureterotrigonal unit. The superficial trigonal muscle is continuous with the smooth muscle of the urethra in both sexes, ending at the verumontanum in the male and just inside the external urethral orifice in the female. The deep trigone ends at the bladder neck (TANAGHO 1992a; GOSLING 1985).

GOSLING (1985) states that the muscle cells of the deep layer are indistinguishable from those of the detrusor and feels the layer is merely the posteroinferior portion of the detrusor muscle proper and should be called the "trigonal detrusor muscle." He goes on to state that the superficial trigonal muscle represents a morphologically distinct component of the trigone that, unlike the detrusor, is composed of relatively small-diameter muscle bundles that are continuous proximally with those of the intramural ureters.

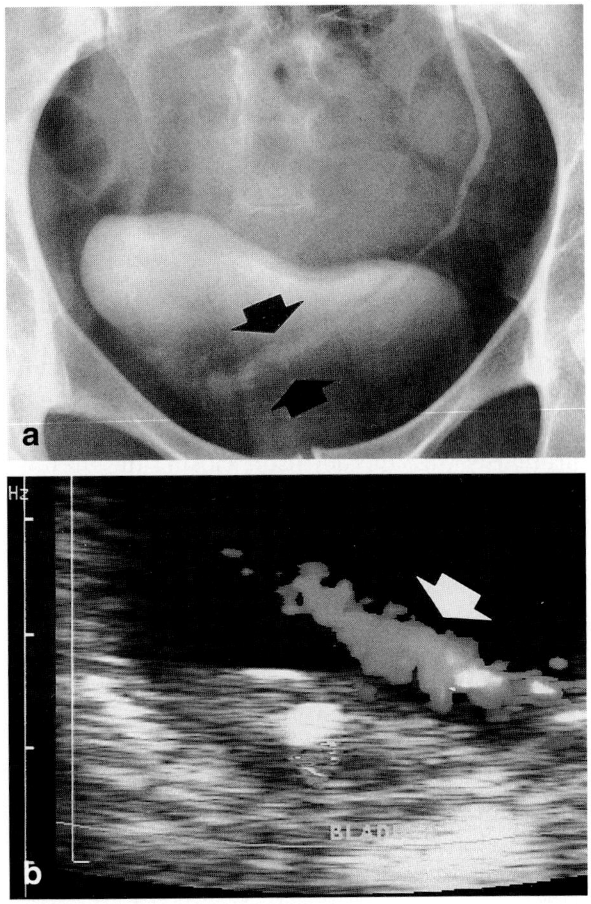

Fig. 6.4 a,b. Ureteral jets. **a** Single jet (*arrows*) splashing against the opposite bladder wall. **b** Doppler ultrasound appearance of ureteral jet (*arrow*)

It was once felt that the ureterovesical junction acts as a flap valve. It was believed that intravesical pressure and perhaps intrinsic ureteral elongation via muscle fibers coursing from the ureteral meatus to attachments in the posterior urethra compress the intramural portion of the ureter so that reflux is prevented but efflux is permitted (LAPIDES and DIOKNO 1976).

Using nonrefluxing dogs, TANAGHO et al. (1965) proved that normal trigonal muscle tone occludes the intravesical ureter. Surgical interruption of the trigone on one side between the ureteral orifice and the urethra 3 mm below the ureteral orifice resulted in shortening of the intravesical ureter and reflux on that side. The reflux ceased when the wound healed. Paralysing the trigone by unilateral sympathectomy resulted in reflux on that side. Focal electrical stimulation of one side of the trigone moved the ureteral orifice caudally, lengthening the intravesical ureter, and increased resistance to flow through the ureterovesical junction to the point that efflux of urine ceased on the stimulated side.

TANAGHO et al. (1965) also demonstrated that shortly before the expected sharp rise in intravesical pressure generated for voiding, the pressure in the intravesical ureter rose sharply and persisted for 20 s after detrusor contraction had ceased. Therefore, ureterovesical competence is independent of detrusor action and is determined by tone of the trigone, which contracts vigorously just before voiding, helping to open and funnel the vesical neck. Simultaneously, the intravesical ureter is pulled down, coapting its lips so that it is occluded while intravesical pressure is high. Therefore, normal ureterotrigonal tone prevents vesicoureteral reflux (TANAGHO et al. 1965; TANAGHO 1992a).

Furthermore, biopsy of the trigone and intravesical ureter in patients with primary reflux demonstrated markedly deficient development of its smooth muscle and suggested that the common cause of reflux, particularly in children, is congenital attenuation of the ureterotrigonal musculature. The theory that ureterovesical competence was maintained by intravesical pressure compressing the intravesical ureter against its backing of detrusor muscle has effectively been disproved (TANAGHO et al. 1965; TANAGHO 1992a).

In summary, the muscle fibers of the roof of the intravesical ureter do not end at the ureteral orifice but sweep around the margins of the ureter to meet the floor fibers of the ureter, then proceed downward with them in the superficial trigonal muscle layer. The muscle fibers of Waldeyer's sheath do likewise and form the deep trigonal muscle. The muscles of the trigone, intravesical ureter, and juxtavesical ureter act as a unit, contracting simultaneously. The downward pull of the contracting trigone approximates the roof and floor of the orifice, closing the orifice to reflux.

The contraction of the intravesical ureter also compresses it against the suppoiting muscles of the bladder wall behind it (TANAGHO et al. 1965). Resting trigonal muscle tone keeps the ureterovesical junction closed except when a ureteral peristaltic wave forces it open, squirting urine into the bladder. These "jets" of urine may occasionally be seen at urography or on ultrasound examination of the bladder (Fig. 6.4) (Cox et al. 1991; BAKER and MIDDLETON 1992). As the bladder fills, the ureteral orifices tethered to the urethra by the stretching trigone are distorted, preventing reflux and eventually even efflux. During voiding, the trigone contracts synchronously with the detrusor, closing the ureterovesical junction to both reflux and efflux (TANAGHO et al. 1965; TANAGHO 1986).

6.1.5 Arterial Supply; Venous and Lymphatic Drainage

The superior and inferior vesical branches of the internal iliac artery and the middle rectal branches of the internal iliac arteries supply the urinary bladder. The branching is variable.

The vesical venous plexus drains to vesical veins, which in turn drain to the internal iliac veins, and to communications with the prostatic venous plexus.

The lymphatic drainage of the bladder is by way of internal iliac (hypogastric) nodes, the posteromedial nodes of the internal iliac group, and the sacral nodes. The lymphatics of the bladder arise from the submucous plexus and form three groups of vessels. The superior and inferolateral surfaces drain to external iliac nodes. The fundus drains to external and internal iliac nodes. The bladder neck joins with lymphatic vessels of the prostate gland and drains to sacral and medial common iliac nodes.

The innervation of the bladder is via inferior hypogastric and vesical plexuses (PANSKY 1979; WOODBURNE 1976).

6.2 Imaging Techniques

6.2.1 Cystography, Single and Double

Cystography obtains a radiographic image of the bladder by radiographing it filled with opaque contrast, usually via urethral catheterization. Preliminary plain film may identify calcification before it is obscured by thė opaque medium. Since the bladder is a sphere, the thickness of the contrast in the middle of the sphere may actually obscure even large filling defects. The best outline of mucosal masses is at the periphery. Multiple views, including oblique views, must be obtained to visualize the periphery optimally. Prone and upright views can also be helpful. They view the bladder from additional angles and give objects within the bladder the opportunity to demonstrate movement. Imaging the bladder with varying degrees of distention may also be helpful, as may monitoring filling by occasional fluorography and spot film. A view of the bladder taken during voiding can provide a urethrogram and a postvoid view may be quite helpful. The addition of air creates a double contrast image which adds another dimension to the examination (Fig. 6.5). While the opaque contrast does not coat the mucosa, additional information can occasionally be gained from distention by air, particularly in visualizing masses (LANG 1968a).

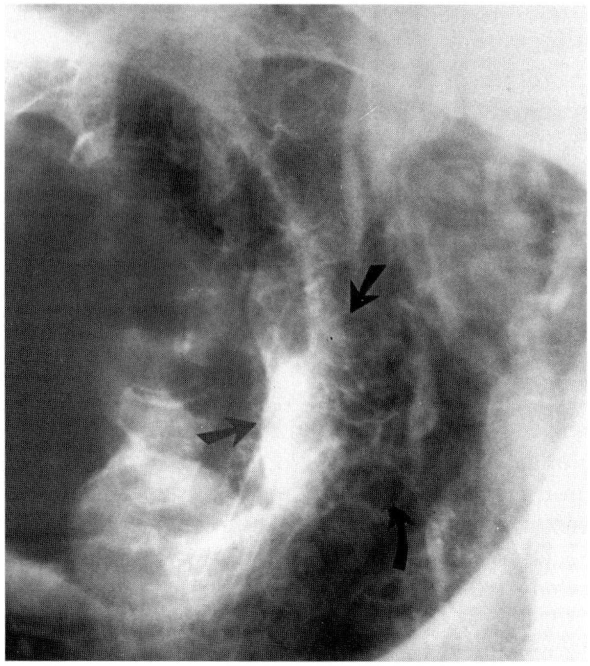

Fig. 6.5. Double contrast cystogram with bladder tumor in the left wall (*arrows*) (triple contrast arteriogram). (Courtesy of Dr. E.K. LANG)

6.2.2 Excretory Urography

Excretory urography, also known as intravenous urography, visualizes the entire urinary system through the use of radiopaque iodinated contrast agents which are excreted via the kidneys. Radiographs are taken during the initial excretion. Plain film laminograms may also be obtained. Modern contrast agents, particularly the nonionic ones, are quite safe in respect to contrast media reactions (PALMER 1988; KATAYAMA et al. 1990) and efficacious (GAVANT et al. 1992). Acute renal failure is rarely induced, this usually in particularly susceptible patients such as diabetics or others with preexisting renal failure (MOORE et al. 1992). Intravenous contrast can be safely administered to myeloma patients when the clinical need arises as long as they are well hydrated (McCARTHY and BECKER 1992). In adequately hydrated low-risk patients with predominately normal initial renal function, no consistent clinical change in renal function was found using either ionic or nonionic contrast even when using two times higher than recommended doses (MILLER et al. 1988). The incidence of acute renal failure after intravenous contrast administration in a large series was found to be 0.15% in the general population (BYRD and SHERMAN 1979). For an optimal study, careful attention must be paid to the details of technique, patient preparation, contrast choice and dosage, filming, and use of compression (HATTERY et al. 1988). Filling of the bladder is not as controlled by the examiner as with cystography and the degree of distention is seldom as great. The excreted contrast that reaches the bladder is diluted by the excreted urine and the residual in the bladder. Urography is an excellent method for screening the urinary tract. Use of a prone film is important in finding lesions on the anterior wall or dome of the bladder (IMRAY and SAIGH 1987). The utilization of urography has been markedly reduced since the introduction of ultrasound, computed tomography (CT), and magnetic resonance imaging (MRI), but urography will have much to offer physicians and patients for many years to come (POLLACK and BANNER 1985).

6.2.3 Angiography

Angiography obtains radiographs during the injection of radiographic contrast material via a catheter in an artery. The blood supply to an organ can thereby be exquisitely demonstrated. The injection can be uncomfortable or painful, requiring sedation. The procedure is invasive with complications directly related to technique. If angiography is performed with the bladder distended with air, bladder masses may be exquisitely demonstrated and wall thickness visualized (Fig. 6.6) (LANG 1968b).

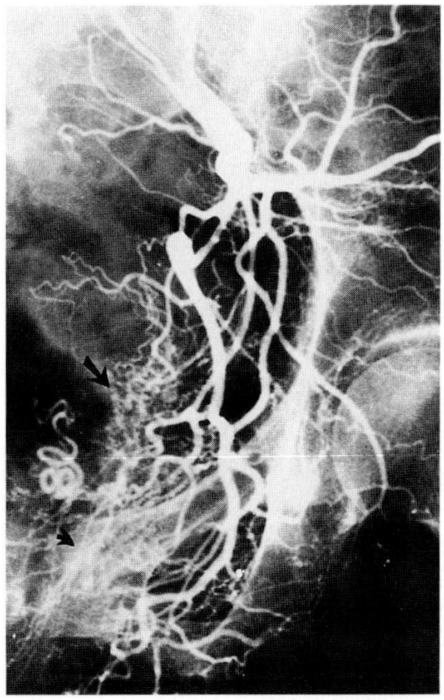

Fig. 6.6. Angiogram of bladder mass. Reconstitution of flow in the hypogastric artery after previous occlusion. Note neovascularity in the bladder (*arrows*), prominently perfused. (Courtesy of Dr. E.K. LANG)

6.2.4 Lymphography

Lymphography is accomplished by cannulating a lymphatic in each foot and injecting oily contrast into the lymph system. After the draining nodes have been thus opacified, radiographs will demonstrate their size and internal architecture (Fig. 6.7) (VON ESCHENBACH et al. 1985). While CT is more accurate in determining the extent of bulky metastases, lymphography can identify small localized foci in normal sized nodes. Defects 5–7 mm in diameter can be detected (VON ESCHENBACH et al. 1985). Enlarged nodes on CT may prove to be only hyperplastic or conglomerates of small nodes on lymphography. Since the nodes remain opacified for at least 6 months, they may be followed by plain abdominal radiographs. The

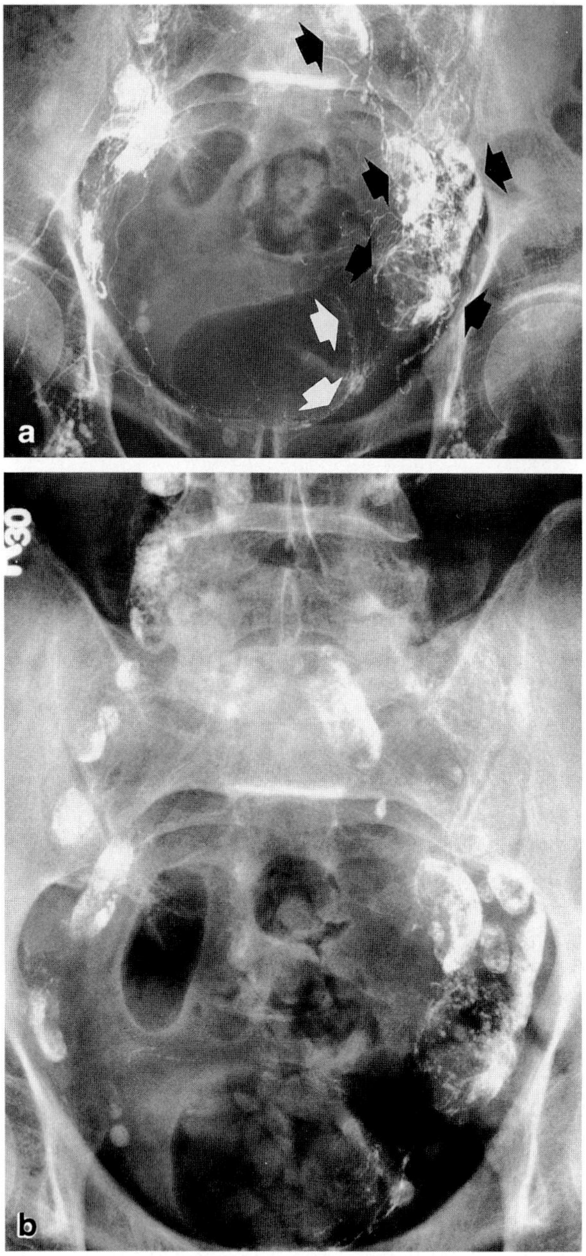

Fig. 6.7. **a** Collateral flow around nodes (*black arrows*) enlarged by metastases. Obstruction has caused retrograde flow into the bladder wall (*white arrows*). **b** Twenty-four hour film showing filling defects in nodes bilaterally

opacified nodes are marked for fine needle biopsy with fluoroscopy and for radiation therapy (North et al. 1992). In staging, the presence or absence of metastases is a more important question than size of the node. Lymphography can have an overall accuracy of more than 90% in staging lymphoma and 91% in determining regional lymph node involvement by urologic tumor (Strijk et al. 1983).

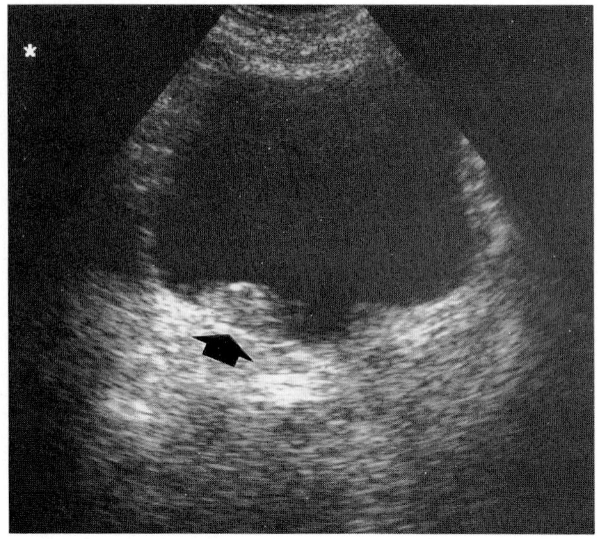

Fig. 6.8. Bladder lesion (*arrow*) found incidentally during pelvic ultrasound. The lesion was subsequently diagnosed as a papillary transitional cell carcinoma stage I

6.2.5 Ultrasound

Sonography produces an image using reflection of high frequency sound wave. The fluid in the bladder makes an excellent sonographic window and is used to survey the pelvis with an ultrasound probe placed on the suprapubic abdominal wall (Rifkin 1985). The urinary bladder and perivesical areas can be well visualized. The procedure involves no ionizing radiation and can be used on pregnant women. The bladder may be filled by diuresis or catheterization. Mucosal masses can be well visualized (Fig. 6.8). Occasionally a clinically silent mucosal bladder mass is found in the course of an ultrasound examination of the pelvis performed for another reason. Transrectal and intravesical probes are also available (Rifkin 1985; Abu-Yousef 1986).

6.2.6 Computed Body-Section Tomography

Computed tomography creates an image by computer reconstruction of radiographic attenuation values in an axial section of the body after an x-ray tube and detector array have encircled the section. The images provide excellent anatomic detail with fine spatial resolution and contrast (Fig. 6.9). The intestines may be opacified with radiopaque material such as dilute barium. Further information may be obtained through the

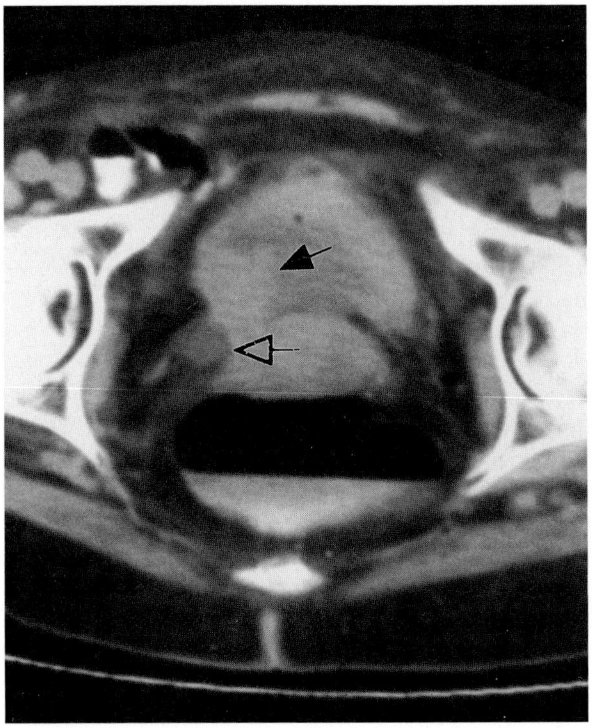

Fig. 6.9. Computed tomogram of papillary bladder cancer (*black arrow*) obstructing the right ureter (*open arrow*). The lesion is at least stage B2 and probably C

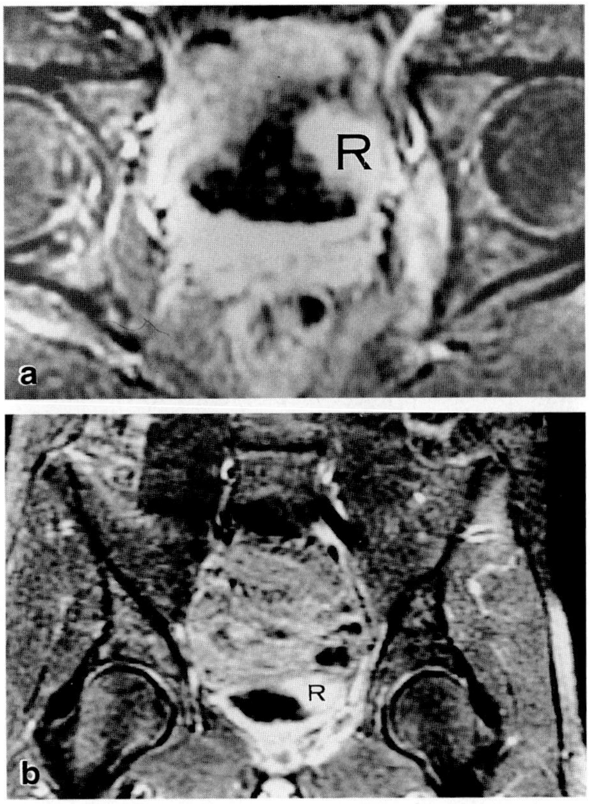

Fig. 6.10. a Axial and **b** coronal MRI demonstrating bladder wall involvement by soft tissue rhabdomyosarcoma (*R*) of the pelvis in a 16-year-old male; T1 weighting with gadolinium enhancement and fat suppression technique

administration of intravenous radiopaque contrast medium to further increase contrast. Images taken rapidly during the administration of intravenous contrast can provide opacification of blood vessels and demonstrate the vascularity of structures. The detail of CT is superb for visualization of lymph nodes but it does not show internal architecture. It can identify enlarged lymph nodes but can suggest the cause only if there is a nearby mass. Microscopic spread of malignancy cannot be detected. The images are degraded by motion and cannot be used in agitated patients without sedation. CT has been quite useful in staging bladder cancer with up to 88% overall accuracy and up to 92% accuracy in evaluating for lymph node metastasis (ARGER 1985; ARGER et al. 1986). CT can be used to guide fine needle aspiration biopsy for cytology of enlarged lymph nodes.

6.2.7 Magnetic Resonance Imaging

Magnetic resonance imaging creates a computed image from the radiofrequency signal coming from hydrogen atoms in body water in a strong magnetic field (HAGGAR and KRESSEL 1985). It is expensive and sometimes time consuming, but uses no ionizing radiation. The patient must lie absolutely still during image generation. The magnetic field precludes the use of most monitoring equipment and the procedure is not for seriously ill or unstable patients. Direct multiplanar imaging can be obtained (Fig. 6.10). MRI can identify blood and blood flow specifically. Since perivesical fat gives a strong signal, MRI is able to detect extension of bladder tumor (HAGGAR and KRESSEL 1985).

6.3 Trauma

6.3.1 Penetrating and Blunt Trauma with Clinical Categorization

Bladder trauma represents about 22% of all urologic injuries. The injury may be penetrating or nonpenetrating. Nonpenetrating is by far the more frequent, accounting for about 86% of bladder injuries (GODEC 1985). Most injuries of the bladder are the result of motor vehicle accidents or sports injuries; there is a definite male preponderance. Occasionally iatrogenic injury may occur. Intraperitoneal and extraperitoneal ruptures of the bladder have been reported to be about equally distributed, with about 10% being combined (BONAVITA and POLLACK 1983). A more recent civilian practice experience revealed one-third intraperitoneal and two-thirds extraperitoneal rupture in blunt trauma (SANDLER 1988, unpublished work). Extraperitoneal rupture of the bladder is associated with pelvic fracture in up to 98% of cases (GODEC 1985; BONAVITA and POLLACK 1983; CORRIERE and SANDLER 1986). The greater the severity of the pelvic fracture, the greater the chance of lower urinary tract injury (PALMER et al. 1983). Extraperitoneal rupture of the bladder occurs in 5%–10% of patients with pelvic fractures, particularly those involving the pubic arch (BONAVITA and POLLACK 1983; FALLON et al. 1984; WOLK et al. 1985). Approximately half of urinary tract injuries in patients with pelvic fracture involve the urethra alone, a third the bladder alone, and about 10% both (BONAVITA and POLLACK). WOLK et al. (1985) reported that most patients (53%–85%) with bladder rupture and pelvic fracture have extraperitoneal bladder rupture. The rest have either intraperitoneal (15%–45%) or combined (0%–12%) intraperitoneal and extraperitoneal ruptures.

The degree of distention of the bladder with urine determines its shape and, at least to some degree, the injury it may sustain from blunt trauma. Pelvic scars or preexisting pelvic pathology may modify the situation. An exceedingly light blow may rupture the fully distended bladder but the empty bladder is seldom injured except by crushing or penetrating wounds.

Penetrating injuries of the bladder are classified simply as intraperitoneal, extraperitoneal, and combined. Bladder injuries due to blunt trauma have been classified as contusions, extraperitoneal ruptures, or intraperitoneal ruptures.

Table 6.1. Blunt injury to the bladder, as classified according to SANDLER

Type I	Bladder contusion
Type II	Intraperitoneal rupture
Type III	Interstitial rupture
Type IV	Extraperitoneal rupture a) Simple b) Complex
Type V	Combined bladder injury

SANDLER (SANDLER et al. 1986; SANDLER 1988, unpublished work) has expanded this basic classification to a more comprehensive and useful one (Table 6.1).

Bladder contusion (type I) is an incomplete or nonperforating tear of the bladder mucosa following blunt trauma to the pelvis. As would be expected, the imaging investigation fails to show extravasation. Most patients will have hematuria. Bladder contusion is considered the most common form of bladder injury, accounting for approximately one-third of injuries. The injury is usually self-limiting and requires no specific therapy. The bladder may be "teardrop," elevated, or deviated by pelvic hematoma. Bladder contusion should not be confused with these configurations.

Intraperitoneal bladder rupture (type II) is the result of a sudden rise in intravesicular pressure from a blow to the pelvis or lower abdomen. In the absence of pathologic changes in the bladder wall, the posterior peritonealized dome is the weakest portion of the bladder. An approximately midline longitudinal tear occurs and intraperitoneal extravasation follows (Fig. 6.11). In experimental work done on cadavers, OLIVER and TAGUCHI (1964) found this portion of the bladder wall to be least well supported, and its muscle fibers most widely separated. This injury requires a distended bladder and need not be associated with a pelvic fracture. It may result from a steering wheel or seat belt injury or a fall onto the abdomen.

Intraperitoneal rupture is much more common in children than in adults because the bladder is primarily an abdominal rather than a pelvic organ in children and when fully distended it is proportionally larger than in the adult. Since urethral catheter drainage is frequently complicated by urethral stricture formation, suprapubic cystostomy is favored (GUERRIERO and DEVINE 1984a).

Spontaneous rupture of the bladder does occur but is most likely the result of unrecognized injury, and is not infrequently associated with preexisting bladder pathology such as inflammation, stones, surgical scars, tumor, tuberculosis, neurogenic dysfunction of the bladder, outlet obstruction such as prostatic enlargement, or posterior urethral valves. In children consideration should be given to the possibility of child abuse (GODEC 1985; GUERRIERO and DEVINE 1984; ZERIN and LEBOWITZ 1989).

Interstitial bladder rupture (type III) applies to an incomplete perforation of the bladder that results in irregularity of the bladder wall on cystograms, but without frank extravasation of contrast material. This injury is uncommon and probably represents an incomplete form of extraperitoneal bladder rupture. Since an identical injury could occur along the peritoneal portion of the bladder wall, it is given a separate category. The term was coined by NOWAK and ZIELINSKI (1977) to describe a dissecting rupture without a complete perforation. It is not a missed rupture but rather an incomplete one.

In *simple extraperitoneal bladder rupture (type IVa)*, the extravasation is confined to the perivesical space. In *complex extraperitoneal bladder rupture (type IVb)*, the extravasation extends beyond the perivesical space. Both are usually, but not always, associated with pelvic fracture. Extraperitoneal rupture may occur in diastasis of the symphysis pubis when stress is transmitted to the bladder wall by the puboprostatic ligaments and/or hypogastric wing (MOREHOUSE and MACKINNON 1969). In 42% of CORRIERE and SANDLERS' (1988) patients the extravasation extended outside the perivesical space and rupture of the urogenital diaphragm commonly occurred, allowing extravasation to extend into the scrotum, thigh, and penis.

Most extraperitoneal ruptures occur at the anterior lateral wall close to the bladder base. The location of the extravasation depends on the site of injury and the amount of disruption of the normal fascial boundaries within the pelvis. The extravasation may extend retroperitoneally, upward to the anterior and posterior perinephric spaces. It may extend into the anterior abdominal wall within the confines of Colles' fascia, into the thigh via the obturator canal, through the greater sciatic notch into the buttocks, or into the scrotum. MOREHOUSE and MACKINNON (1969) postulated the inguinal route to the scrotum.

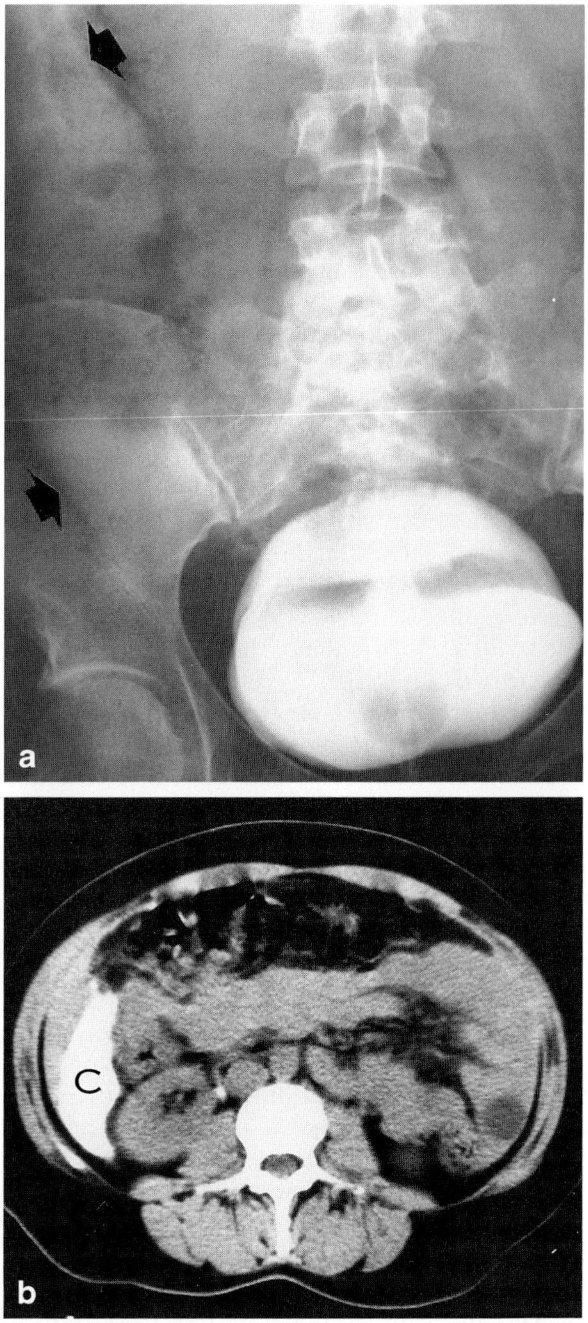

Fig. 6.11a,b. Intraperitoneal bladder rupture. **a** Cystogram demonstrates extravasation into the cul-de-sac and right flank (*arrows*). **b** CT demonstrates contrast (*C*) in the right paracolic gutter

According to SANDLER et al. (1986), however, the path of extravasation more often appeared to extend into the scrotum more medially than the inguinal canal. They postulated that the superior fascia of the urogenital diaphragm had been disrupted, allowing direct extravasation into the scrotum. Extravasation of contrast material into the thigh and penis implies disruption of the inferior fascia of the urogenital diaphragm. Extravasation near the bladder base leading to extravasation below the pelvic floor can be easily confused with urethral injury. Vesicorectal, vesicovaginal, or vesicocutaneous fistulas may occur. Vesicovaginal fistula is the most common, usually presenting as incontinence.

Extraperitoneal rupture of the bladder has long been thought to be most commonly due to laceration or puncture of the bladder by a sharp spicule of fractured bone. Not only may extraperitoneal rupture occur in the absence of rupture of the pelvic ring, but CORRIERE and SANDLER (1988) and CARROLL and MCANINCH (1984) found that only 35% of bladder lacerations are in the area of pelvic fracture. The site of contrast medium extravasation was not in the area of the fracture in 65% of their patients. CARROLL and MCANINCH (1984) noted that the highest percentages of laceration were along the dome in their patients with pelvic fracture. CORRIERE and SANDLERS' (1988) findings suggest that the most common mechanism for extraperitoneal bladder rupture is either a bursting type of injury similar to the intraperitoneal bladder rupture or a shearing injury owing to the forces of the pelvic ring fracture disrupting the ligamentous attachments between the bladder and pelvis. Laceration of the bladder by a transiently displaced bone fragment may occur in some instances. Actual puncture of the organ seems unlikely, since they never found a spicule of bone in the bladder in any of their patients and demonstration of a penetrating spicule is unusual indeed.

In *combined bladder injury (type V)*, both intra- and extraperitoneal extravasation are present. This type of injury is uncommon and one component (usually intraperitoneal rupture) may hide the other. The intraperitoneal contrast may obscure the extraperitoneal contrast or the rent in the dome may be so large that flow is preferentially to the peritoneum rather than out of the extraperitoneal tear.

6.3.2 Evaluation of Bladder Injury

6.3.2.1 Clinical Evaluation

Hematuria is the most common sign of bladder trauma, occurring in up to 100% of patients in one series (CARROLL and MCANINCH 1984). Patients with bladder rupture often have no desire to void and no urine is obtained when a catheter is inserted. They may urinate with difficulty and pass only small amounts of bloody urine. The bladder may be impalpable. With intraperitoneal rupture, bowel sounds are usually abnormal. If unrecognized, the injury may produce hyperkalemia, hypernatremia, uremia, and acidosis as a result of reabsorption of urine from the peritoneal cavity. Because urine may drain from a catheter placed in such a patient, delay in treatment of days and even weeks may occur. With the introduction of infection, the clinical picture of intraperitoneal rupture may eventually become that of peritonitis with boardlike rigidity of the abdomen. In extraperitoneal rupture, there is usually moderate pain low in the pelvis, with spasm of the lower rectus muscle and gradual ascending dullness to percussion over the suprapubic areas up to the level of the umbilicus. The clinical picture is that of cellulitis (SCOTT and CARLTON 1976).

6.3.2.2 Retrograde Cystography

Retrograde cystography is the keystone of evaluation of the injured bladder. Excretory urography is inadequate for this purpose because of dilution of the contrast material within the bladder and because resting intravesical pressure is too low to demonstrate a small tear (BONAVITA and POLLACK 1983).

A Foley catheter should be advanced into the bladder gently and only if there is no suspicion of urethral injury. If any doubt exists, a urethrogram should be performed first. A patient with urethral injury should have a cystogram performed following placement of a suprapubic catheter. BONAVITA and POLLACK (1983) recommend that a 30% concentration of iodinated contrast material be instilled into the bladder under fluoroscopic control until a detrusor contraction is provoked and that multiple films in several projections, including AP and both oblique views, should be obtained. SCLAFANI and BECKER (1985) do not routinely perform oblique or lateral views as part of cystography, particularly on patients with pelvic fractures. With small lacerations in simple extraperitoneal rupture, the extravasated contrast material may be obscured by the otherwise distended bladder. For this reason a postdrainage

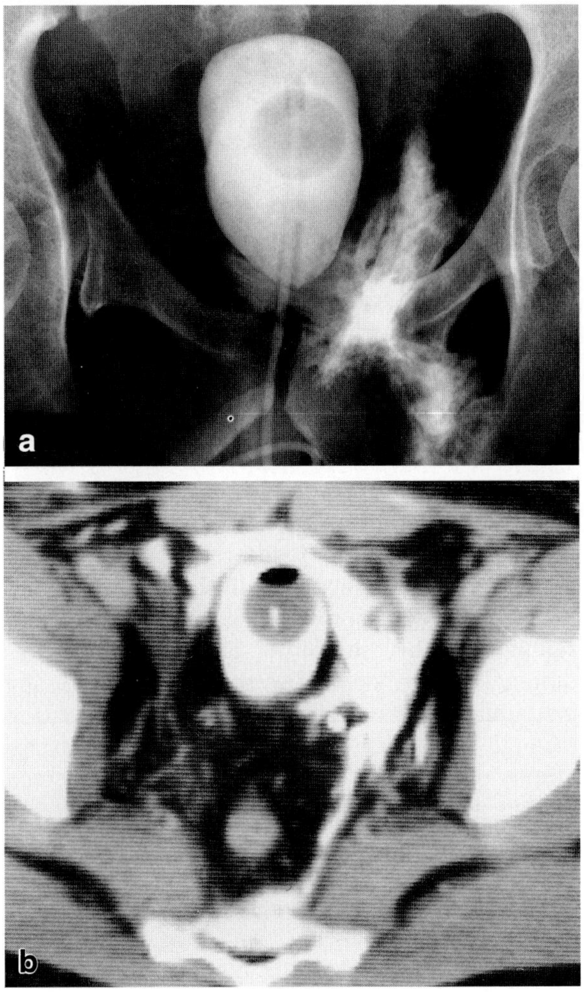

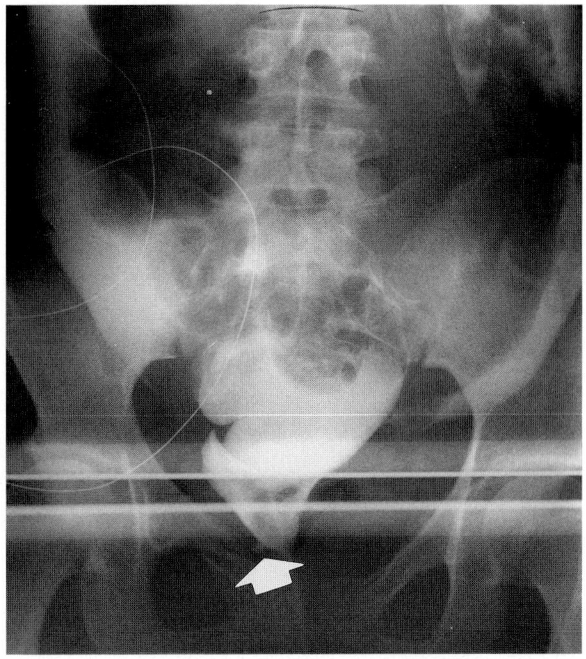

Fig. 6.13. Combined bladder injury with large intraperitoneal extravasation and minor extraperitoneal extravasation (*arrow*) next to the pelvic fracture

◁

Fig. 6.12 a,b. Extraperitoneal bladder rupture: **a** cystogram and **b** CT scan

film is imperative as part of cystography for suspected bladder injury. Godec (1985) utilizes a "stress cystogram," filling the bladder to capacity by gravity and then injecting an additional 60 ml. The key is adequate distention.

The overall accuracy of retrograde cystography has been about 85% in detecting bladder rupture (Carroll and McAninch 1983). A small tear may seal spontaneously, concomitant urethral rupture may interfere with evaluation of the bladder, or inappropriate filming may preclude accurate evaluation (Reisner and Nicholas 1963; Bonavita and Pollack 1983). A film with the bladder fully distended followed by a postdrainage film may be totally adequate. Cass (1976) found cystography 100% accurate when a volume of 400 ml of contrast medium was used. In each of the false-negatives in the series, 250 ml or less was used. Cass (1984) used a post-"washout" rather than a postdrainage film. The bladder is irrigated with 250 ml normal saline and a frontal radiograph obtained to distinguish residual contrast from extravesicular extravasation. Any contrast remaining after washout is considered extravasated.

The diagnosis of intraperitoneal rupture is usually made easily on cystography when contrast enters the peritoneal cavity, fills the cul-de-sac, outlines loops of bowel, extends to the paracolic gutters, and outlines the intraperitoneal viscera. False-negative results in intraperitoneal bladder rupture after blunt trauma are unusual (Sandler et al. 1986). As in penetrating injury from small-caliber bullets, small tears may be plugged by omentum, blood clot, or spasm (Reiser and Nicholas 1963; Bacon 1943). The false-negatives in Reiser and Nicholas' (1963) series occurred in gunshot wounds. They postulated that the heat-searing effect of the bullet, the sharply cut edges, the natural elasticity of the bladder wall, the edema, and the interlacing bundles of detrusor muscle tend to produce some degree of coaptation that prevents extravasation.

In extraperitoneal rupture of the bladder (Fig. 6.12a), the contrast is not free-flowing but will streak in a flamelike fashion as it extends within the narrow confines of the extraperitoneal perivesical soft tissue space. With extensive extravasation the usual streaky appearance may be lost and an intraperitoneal rupture simulated.

Combined intra- and extraperitoneal bladder rupture (Fig. 6.13) will demonstrate both sets of findings. The amount of contrast extravasated depends on the size of the laceration and the volume and rate of contrast material infused. Quantitation of the amount of extravasation is useless. Overzealous injection may actually extend the extravasation.

6.3.2.3 Ultrasound

Although there has been little use of ultrasound in acute trauma, a few points are worthy of discussion. Free fluid from intraperitoneal rupture can be identified in the peritoneal recesses but is indistinguishable from ascites. A pseudomass can be created by extravasated urine which does not disappear on bladder emptying with catheterization. A "bladder within a bladder" appearance can be created on the sonogram when hypoechoic extraperitoneal extravasated blood and urine surround the hypoechoic urine within the bladder. An echogenic ring between the two hypoechoic layers represents the thickened muscular wall of the collapsed bladder (Kauzlaric and Barmeir 1986). Transient cystic and solid bladder filling defects can be created by minor cystography-related trauma. These defects clear after emptying and refilling the bladder. They are often coincident with transient, mild, gross hematuria and are thought to be due to bleeding and clot formation (Markle and Catena 1986).

6.3.2.4 Computed Body-Section Tomography

Computed tomography is clearly the method of choice for evaluation of patients with blunt abdominal and/or pelvic trauma. Horstman et al. (1991) proposed that, if properly performed, CT is as sensitive for detection of bladder injuries as conventional cystography. They reviewed the cystograms and CT examinations of 25 patients who had had both studies as the initial evaluation of blunt abdominal trauma. Five out of 25 patients with blunt trauma examined with both studies had bladder rupture, in three cases extraperitoneal and in two, intraperitoneal. All injuries were detected by both studies. The authors felt that delayed imaging or contrast instillation can provide the bladder distention needed to demonstrate contrast extravasation from the injury site. They continue to perform cystography in patients with compelling evidence of bladder injury but without CT demonstration of extravasation.

Even with a urethral catheter inserted and clamped, routine CT cannot be entirely relied upon to diagnose bladder rupture (Fig. 6.12b). It beautifully demonstrates intra- and extraperitoneal fluid but cannot differentiate urine from ascites. It should theoretically be able to detect blood but attenuation values have not been found reliable in this situation. During routine abdominal and pelvic studies the bladder is usually inadequately distended to cause extravasation through a bladder laceration. Retrograde cystography remains the most reliable test in suspected bladder rupture (Mee et al. 1987).

6.3.2.5 Magnetic Resonance Imaging

Because of the procedure time and the difficulty of monitoring a seriously injured patient in a strong magnetic field, MRI currently has little place in the evaluation of bladder trauma.

6.3.3 Treatment Controversies in Bladder Trauma

Treatment must be tailored to the individual patient, who may also have multisystem injury (Monstrey et al. 1987). The primary goal of therapy is adequate closure of the bladder defect. Contusion and small extraperitoneal tears of the bladder can be managed conservatively without surgical intervention. Conventional surgical wisdom dictates that all other injuries should have operative repair. All penetrating injuries must be explored since the true extent of the damage cannot otherwise be determined. The management of intraperitoneal bladder rupture must be operative and immediate, usually consisting of exploration, closure, and suprapubic cystotomy

(HAYES et al. 1983). The goals are closure of the bladder defect, adequate diversion away from the area of injury, and prompt drainage of extravasated urine (BONAVITA and POLLACK 1983).

CORRIERE and SANDLER (1988) have shown that patients with extraperitoneal rupture of any size and with any amount of extravasation can be safely and successfully treated with simple urethral catheter drainage. HAYES et al. (1983) believe that prompt adequate catheter drainage prevents continued extravasation and hematoma contamination. Furthermore, since the hematoma probably compresses the bladder and promotes self-sealing of the wounds, it is best left untouched.

6.3.4 Long-Distance Runners' Hematuria

Long-distance runners can sustain a unique bladder injury. The patient presents after running with gross hematuria which clears rapidly, often after only one voiding and always within 24 h. On cystoscopy within 48 h, hemorrhagic areas are present at the base of the bladder involving the interureteric ridge and posterior rim of the internal meatus and on the opposite lower posterior wall in mirror image. The mucosa in these areas may even be denuded with deposit of fibrinous exudate. The injury is felt to be a contusion due to the repeated impact of the flaccid posterior wall on the bladder base while the bladder is empty or nearly empty (BLACKLOCK 1977).

6.3.5 Iatrogenic and Obstetric Injury

The bladder may be ruptured during passage of catheters, sounds, and cystoscopes or during transurethral resection of prostate or bladder tumor (SCOTT and CARLTON 1976). Such an injury tends to be small and clean, and is usually immediately recognized. Four of the five cases of intraperitoneal bladder injuries in the literature treated with Foley drainage alone were iatrogenic, secondary to transurethral instrumentation (CORRIERE and SANDLER 1986).

Obstetric injuries may also involve the bladder. Prolonged pressure of the fetal head during a difficult delivery can produce pressure necrosis of the bladder base at the trigone and bladder neck. Typically, the patient sloughs tissue in her urine or leaks urine per vagina on the third to the 14th postpartum day. Rupture of the bladder can be seen along with spontaneous rupture of the gravid uterus (MCDOUGAL and PERSKY 1981).

The most common operative injuries are associated with obstetric manipulations such as forceps deliveries and cesarean sections, gynecologic procedures such as suction D&Cs, laparoscopy and pelvic surgery, and urologic instrumentation of the lower urinary tract. Less common causes include perforation from prolonged indwelling Foley catheter, orthopedic procedures of the hip, and rectosigmoid resections (MCDOUGAL and PERSKY 1981).

6.3.6 Embolotherapy in Pelvic Hemorrhage

Embolotherapy is an effective method to control intractable hemorrhage from trauma to the pelvic organs. The etiology may be traumatic injury, postpartum hemorrhage, hemorrhage complicating transurethral resection of the prostate or orthopedic procedures such as hip replacement surgery. The goal of transcatheter embolization is control of bleeding and stabilization of the patients's condition without permanent disruption of vascular channels. Surgery destroys the fascial barriers which contain and tamponade venous hemorrhage.

The femoral approach to catheterization of the internal iliac arteries is generally favored. The axillary approach may be necessary in patients with massive trauma to the pelvis since large hematomas may form in the groins, precluding arterial entry. Survey studies are obtained with selective injection of the internal iliac arteries.

Short-term or temporary embolic agents are used. Gelfoam pledgets or blood clots are effective in medium-sized vessels 2–4 mm in diameter. If a large vessel is severed, occlusion can most easily and effectively be achieved with an appropriately sized Gianturco coil. Balloon catheters will provide temporary occlusion and detachable balloons may also be used for permanent occlusion (GERLOCK and MIRFAKHRAEE 1985).

High resolution angiography is essential to depict the bleeding site or sites and the supplying vessels. The tip of the delivery catheter should be advanced as close as possible to the bleeding site using subselective techniques as necessary (Fig. 6.14).

Embolization should be limited to the offending vessel or vessels, ideally seating the embolic

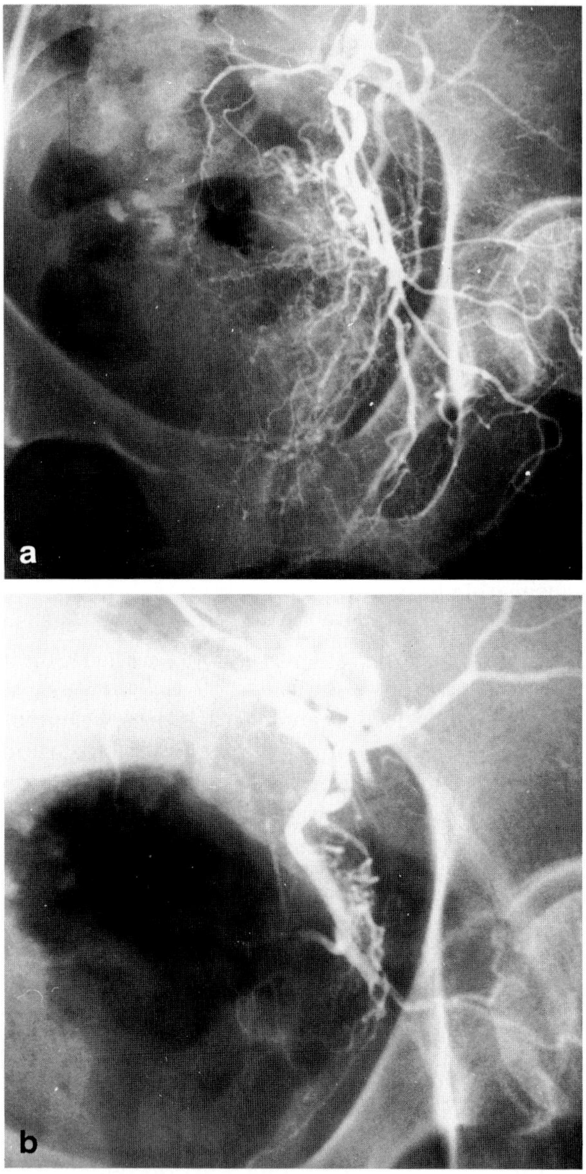

Fig. 6.14a,b. Embolotherapy. **a** Pre- and **b** postembolization high resolution angiography in a patient with a left hypogastric bladder tumor. (Courtesy of Dr. E.K. LANG)

material in muscular vessels only. Perfusion is maintained via the precapillary collateral network (LANG 1981).

Because of the extensive collateral blood supply to the pelvic organs, one or both internal iliac arteries may be sacrificed without producing ischemic necrosis (LANG 1981).

In the internal iliac system, only a relatively peripheral embolic obstruction will reduce pelvic blood flow sufficiently to cause a drop in the distal blood pressure. The extensive intercommunicating network ensures substantial collateral flow to the bleeding site via some major vessel unless the occlusion is set so far peripherally as to eliminate this component of the collateral network. Once the pulse pressure is reduced adequately, intraarterial thrombus formation will occlude the bleeding vessels. Fibroblasts will permeate a clot within 8–24 h. The vessels need be occluded for that length of time only. Thereafter, fibroblastic activity will seal the bleeding site. Material prone to dissolution, such as autologous blood clot, is favored for this reason. Reconstitution of blood flow to nearly all of the affected area is assured, reducing the risk of tissue necrosis (LANG 1981).

Autologous clot tends to fragment on introduction into particle sizes prone to lodge in smaller arteries, thereby causing a substantial reduction in the pulse pressure while retaining collateral perfusion via the precapillary plexus and safeguarding against avascular necrosis. The propensity of clot for lysis within 8–24 h ensures reconstitution of flow. Massive blood transfusions may result in an abnormal clotting mechanism. Addition of Amicar (ε-aminocaproic acid) to the sample will encourage coagulation of the clot. Gelfoam also tends to fragment and therefore may seat in a somewhat smaller vessel. It produces semipermanent occlusion lasting 2–3 weeks with good potential for restoration of vascular continuity.

Particularly in patients with intractable hemorrhage from transurethral resection of the prostate or postpartum bleeding, the precise bleeding site of the bleeding vessels may not be identifiable. In this situation, embolic material is seated in the major branches of the anterior division of the internal iliac arteries bilaterally, hoping that the resulting reduction of pulse pressure and blood flow will permit formation of clots at the often multiple bleeding sites which will later be sealed by fibroblastic activity. This bilateral embolization is tolerated if the occlusion is set at a proximal site, permitting collateral flow from other sources such as the posterior internal iliac branches and presacral, epigastric, and circumflex femoral vessels (LANG 1986).

Pharmacoangiography may be helpful in identifying the bleeding site and in channeling infarct particles selectively into the bleeding vessels. Normal arterioles tend to respond to vasoconstrictive agents and injured vessels do not, making possible almost selective flow into the responsible bleeding vessel group. The elimination of flow to adjacent normal vessels accentuates the bleeding site on the survey study and subsequently siphons particles released into the main branch selectively into the vessel responsible for the bleeding. The peripheral resistance is increased in the normal vessels and decreased in the actively bleeding vessels (LANG 1981, 1986). Direct injection into the involved arterial system maximizes the local effect while minimizing the systemic effect. These vasoactive agents should be used with caution in an hemodynamically unstable patient.

Transcatheter embolization of bleeding sites in the prostate bed after transurethral resection usually requires embolization of the inferior vesical, obturator, and pudendal arteries bilaterally.

LANG (1986) reported success in treating 18 of 19 cases of intractable hemorrhage from pelvic trauma. Initial bleeding was controlled in five patients hemorrhaging from the prostatic bed after transurethral resection. In two of them delayed hemorrhage occurred on the 7th and 10th post-embolization days respectively but was controlled by conservative local measures. Postpartum bleeding responds well to embolotherapy, with Ivalon shavings having proven successful. This is particularly true after low cervical cesarean section. Postpartum bleeding was controlled in all of five patients treated without late sequelae.

Depriving the blood supply of large tissue elements of the pelvis can produce avascular necrosis of the urinary bladder. Patients with trauma, particularly if massive, are already at risk for acute tubular necrosis from shock and myoglobinuria. Devascularizing muscle compounds this danger. Other complications from internal iliac artery embolization include skin, muscle, and bladder necrosis and nerve involvement. Possible sites for neurologic damage during internal iliac artery embolization are the spinal cord, the femoral nerve, the sciatic nerve, and the sciatic roots. Paralysis and paresis may result (LANG 1986; GERLOCK and MIRFAKHRAEE 1985). This complication can be reduced by identification of the bleeding vessels and selective embolization. If this cannot be accomplished, use of emboli not smaller than Gelfoam pledgets $1 \times 1 \times 10$ mm is recommended to preserve peripheral circulation (HARE et al. 1983).

Angiographically placed balloons may be used for proximal control of arterial bleeding during exploration and operative repair (SCALEA and SCLAFANI 1991).

6.4 Bladder Wall Calcification

Bladder wall calcification is an uncommon radiographic finding with few causes. While a few patterns are typical, none are pathognomonic. Correct diagnosis is not possible on the basis of radiographic appearance alone. Firm diagnosis can usually be obtained from a combination of clinical history, physical and radiographic findings, and appropriate laboratory examinations. Cystoscopy and biopsy of the involved tissues are almost always necessary to confirm the diagnosis and to exclude bladder cancer (POLLACK et al. 1981).

The patterns of bladder calcification will be described and illustrated with complete discussion of the disease entities provided elsewhere.

6.4.1 Bladder Neoplasms

Bladder neoplasm may have stippled calcification that is either punctate (finely stippled) or coarse (flocculent). The punctate calcifications tend to be associated with papillary tumors having relatively thin pedicles, characteristic of noninvasive or low grade invasive neoplasms which have been present for a long time, even years. The calcification may also be linear or curvilinear. This tends to occur in large papillary or sessile neoplasms and may develop after radiation therapy. Combinations of these patterns are also possible (Fig. 6.15).

Microscopic calcification is common in bladder neoplasms, but the foci are usually too small to be demonstrated radiographically. The incidence of radiographically demonstrable calcification has

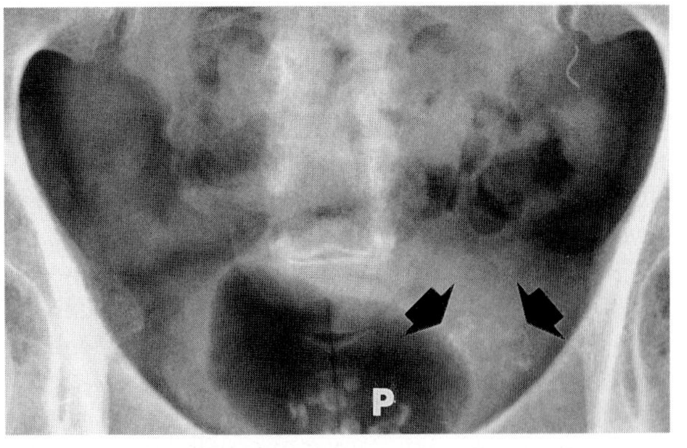

Fig. 6.15. Calcification in bladder neoplasm. Stippled calcification is seen on the plain film (*arrows*); calcification is also present in the prostate gland (*P*)

been estimated at about 0.5% (Miller and Pfister 1974). Calcification is most common in uroepithelial tumors, both transitional and squamous cell, but may also be seen in mesenchymal tumors, including leiomyosarcoma, hemangioma, neuroblastoma, and osteogenic sarcoma. The calcium is usually encrusted on the surface of the tumor but may be within its substance in a subepithelial position in degenerating or necrotic areas. Calcium precipitation is favored by an alkaline urine. A local interaction between the tumor surface and calcium salts in the urine may be operative. Stasis between the fronds may be a factor since the encrustation occurs only on the tumor surface but not on the normal mucosa. The punctate and coarse calcifications usually occur on the tips of the villous fronds of low grade papillary transitional cell tumors, giving a finely stippled appearance. Dystrophic bladder calcification occurs in necrotic tissue either spontaneously or after therapy by transurethral resection and fulguration or radiation therapy (Pollack et al. 1981; Miller and Pfister 1974).

6.4.2 *Schistosomiasis*

The most common inflammatory lesion worldwide causing bladder wall calcification is schistosomiasis. The infestation is caused by any of several species of the parasite genus, *Schistosoma*. Only *S. hematobium* commonly involves the urinary tract, with the worms settling in the prostaticovesical venous plexus. The adult female worm lays her eggs in the subepithelial layers of the lower urinary tract structures, mainly the urinary bladder. The dead ova, which become trapped in the tunica propria, elicit an intense inflammatory reaction with fibrosis and subsequent submucosal calcification (Fig. 6.16). The intensity of the calcification is directly proportional to the number of dead ova. In severe cases, the calcification may also involve the muscularis and adventitial layers of the bladder wall. The ureters and seminal vesicles may also become involved.

Radiographically visible calcification can be identified in about 50% of patients with schistosomiasis of the bladder. Distal ureteral calcification is relatively common, occurring in 15%–37.5% of patients. The vesical calcification is first most apparent and extensive at the base of the bladder, forming a linear opaque shadow parallel to the upper border of the pubic bone. With further calcification, the bladder becomes encircled. The mucosa of the empty bladder is thrown into folds, making the calcification appear as coarse, linear, confluent opacities. Massive calcification of the trigone viewed en face presents a diffuse flocculent pattern which has been likened to cumulus cloud (Umerah 1977).

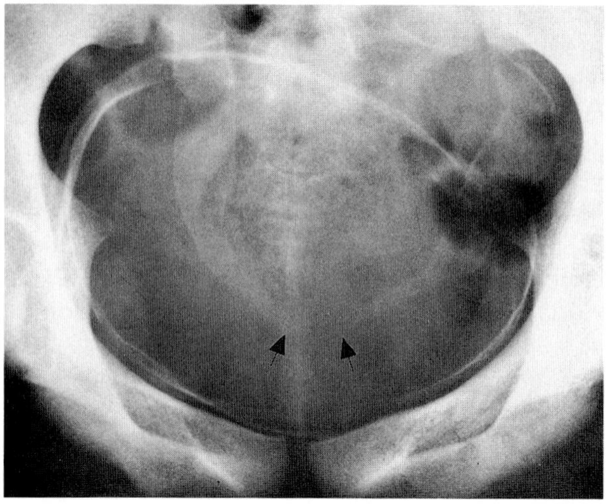

Fig. 6.16. Thin submucosal calcification of the bladder and ureters in schistosomiasis. Note that the ureteral orifices (*arrows*) have been drawn together by fibrosis. (Courtesy of Dr. M. Elkin)

The ureteral calcification of schistosomiasis appears as two thin, roughly parallel lines separated by the caliber of the ureter, with the calcification heaviest in the lower ureter and gradually fading toward the kidneys. With the development of squamous cell carcinoma of the bladder, the continuity of the calcified bladder may be broken in the area of tumor infiltration (Pollack et al. 1981; Al Ghorab 1988).

6.4.3 *Tuberculosis*

Tuberculosis of the bladder usually descends from the kidneys but may ascend from the prostate. The bladder is involved in 10%–20% of patients. Mucosal tubercles form in the bladder which coalesce, producing superficial ulceration. Inflammation progresses to involve the muscularis. Eventually, mural fibrosis occurs, leading to a thickened, markedly contracted bladder. Healing leads to formation of granulation tissue and further fibrosis. A faint irregular rim or nodular speckling of calcification may outline the bladder wall, but radiographically demonstrable bladder

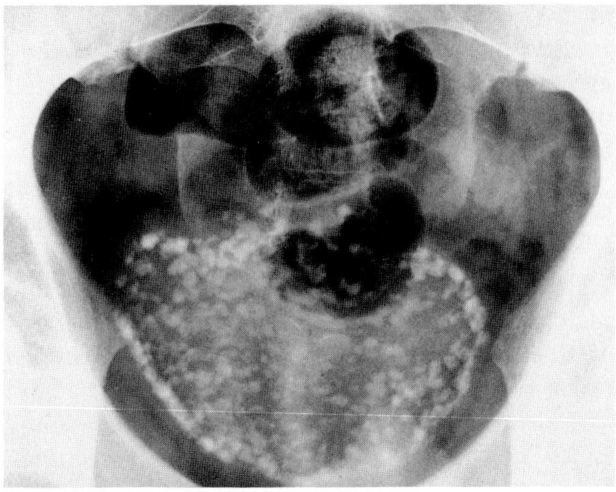

Fig. 6.17. Bladder calcification in tuberculosis. (Courtesy of Dr. M. ELKIN)

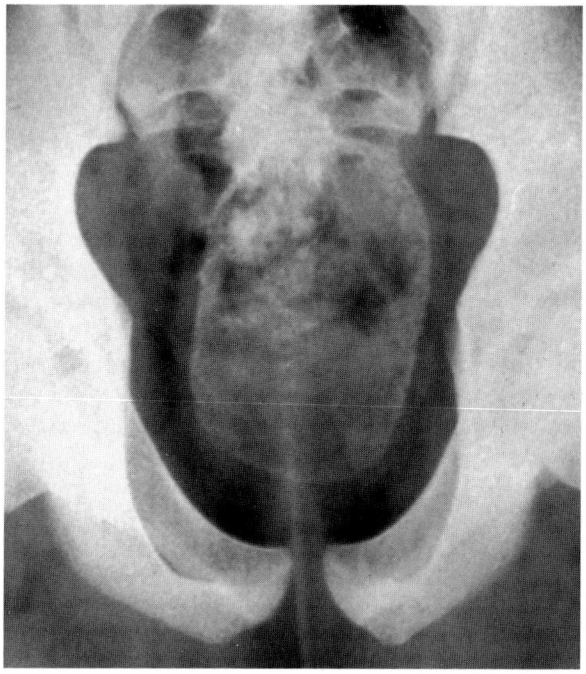

Fig. 6.18. Bladder calcification in a 13-year-old male with chronic *Pseudomonas* infection causing alkaline encrusting cystitis

calcification is rare (Fig. 6.17). When it is present, extensive disease is usually present in the kidneys and ureters and calcification may also be evident in the genital tract (POLLACK et al. 1981; POLLACK 1990; TANAGHO 1992b).

6.4.4 Alkaline Encrusting Cystitis

Bladder necrosis from any cause in the presence of alkaline urine may result in phosphate deposition and calcification which may be radiographically demonstrable (HARRISON et al. 1978). The calcifications of alkaline encrusting cystitis may be linear, flocculent, or nodular (Fig. 6.18) (POLLACK et al. 1981; HARRISON et al. 1978).

6.4.5 Amyloidosis

The calcification described in amyloidosis is submucosal and arranged in sheets and/or diffuse discrete nodules. Localized urinary tract primary amyloidosis is most frequently recognized in the bladder but may involve the upper tracts, prostate gland, seminal vesicles, testes, and kidneys. Biopsy with special staining for amyloid is necessary for diagnosis (POLLACK et al. 1981; THOMAS et al. 1977).

6.4.6 Differentiation

While some patterns are relatively common in a disease, no radiographic appearance or pattern of bladder calcification is pathognomonic of any of the several diseases.

Tubercular and bilharzial calcifications are quite similar, but the latter disease and its calcification usually starts in the bladder and progresses upward, whereas tuberculosis usually starts in the kidney and spreads down. Bladder calcification in tuberculosis is almost always associated with upper tract findings and often with associated prostate calcification. These associations are uncommon in schistosomiasis. The seminal vesicles may calcify in either disease. The calcified bladder of schistosomiasis is unique in that it may retain a relatively normal capacity and distensibility, whereas decreased bladder capacity favors tuberculosis. Both schistosomiasis and amyloidosis can produce submucosal calcification in the distal ureter, but the two have differing radiographic appearances. Intraluminal contrast medium obscures the calcification of schistosomiasis, while in amyloidosis, the uncalcified mucosa clearly separates the submucosal calcified plaques from the opacified ureteral lumen. Cystitis and bladder tumors would not be expected to cause extravesical calcification. Calcification associated with a papillary bladder mass is usually indicative of bladder neoplasm.

History of travel or residence in an area endemic for schistosomiasis favors that etiology of bladder calcification. The diagnosis of tuberculosis or schistosomiasis depends on the demonstration of tubercle bacillus or ova in the urine or tissues of the infected patient. Identification of *Proteus* or appropriate coliform bacillus, especially with alkaline urine, is consistent with a diagnosis of alkaline encrusting cystitis as the etiology for bladder calcification. But the infection may be superimposed on another etiology such as an underlying bladder tumor, cyclophosphamide toxicity, or previous radiation therapy. A persistently alkaline urine is necessary for the formation of encrustation cystitis, whereas tuberculous urine is almost always acid (POLLACK et al. 1981).

6.4.7 Mimics

The following entities may be confused with calcification of the bladder wall radiographically: deposition of calcium salts around an indwelling Foley catheter balloon, which can mimic a calcified bladder tumor; a calcified pelvic hydatic cyst; calcification of the excavated prostatic fossa, especially when due to tuberculosis; calcification on the mucosal surface of an intravesical protrusion of an enlarged prostate; calcification in the wall of a urachal cyst; a large nonopaque vesical calculus with a calcified rim; and pelvic peritoneal calcification after radiation therapy and anterior exenteration for carcinoma of the cervix (POLLACK et al. 1981).

6.5 Inflammatory Conditions (Cystitis)

Cystitis is inflammation of the urinary bladder from any cause. Inflammation of the urinary bladder may be isolated or associated with inflammation of other urinary tract organs or adjacent structures. The inflammation may be due to bacteriologic infection, chemical irritation by substances in the urine, or even external irradiation.

6.5.1 Bacterial Cystitis

Bacterial cystitis is usually acute and caused by coliform organisms, usually by *Escherichia coli*, less commonly by others such as *Staphylococcus albus*, *aureus*, or *saprophyticus*, *Streptococcus faecalis*, *Aerobacter aerogenes*, or *Proteus* or *Pseudomonas* strains. The infection usually ascends from the urethra. Women are afflicted much more often than men and the incidence increases with women's age.

Between 1% and 20% of women will have at least one urinary tract infection in their life, and some will have recurrent infections. Most males with prostatic enlargement will eventually become infected and nosocomial urinary tract infections are the most common hospital-acquired infections (NEU 1983).

Indwelling bladder catheters are the leading cause of nosocomial urinary tract infections. Bacteriuria is always present in patients managed with long-term indwelling Foley catheters and is often polymicrobial and drug resistant (SANT 1987). The presence of indwelling catheters may mechanically remove or inhibit the protective mucous mucopolysaccharide glycosaminoglycans (GAG) layer of the bladder epithelium, allowing increased bacterial adherence, colonization, and infection (SANT 1987; DAIFUKU and STAMM 1986).

Greater than 85% of outpatient urinary tract infections are caused by *E. coli*. Most of the remaining 15% of infections are due to *Proteus mirabilis*, *Klebsiella*, *Streptococcus faecalis*, and *Enterobacter*. Rarely an outpatient may develop urinary infection due to *Serratia*, *Pseudomonas*, *Providencia*, *Morganella*, or *Citrobacter*. These and other unusal organisms are usually seen in hospitalized patients who have had urethral catheters inserted. Patients who are immunosuppressed, on antibiotics or steroids, or otherwise have altered intestinal flora or altered immune response may have a first infection with unusual organisms. Even as a cause of nosocomial infection, *E. coli* is a more fequent organism than *Klebsiella*, *Proteus*, or *Pseudomonas* (NEU 1983; KUNIN 1987). *E. coli* accounts for 80%–95% of all isolates seen in a general hospital setting. *E. coli* can be typed serologically by 150 different O or cell-wall antigens and about 50 capsular (K) and flagellar (H) antigens. The distribution of serotypes of *E. coli* in urinary tract infections closely corresponds to their relative abundance in the gut. Almost any type of *E. coli* can produce urinary tract infection but O types 1, 2, 4, 6, 7, 25, 50, and 75 are the most frequent (KUNIN 1987).

The rectum infects the vagina and periurethral epithelium, which are both enclosed between the labia. The urethra and urinary bladder are then infected (NEU 1983). The bladder is seldom infected from the kidney or hematogenous spread from elsewhere (MEARES 1988). Bacterial receptors have been demonstrated in anterior vaginal epithelium (introitus) of mature women (FOWLER and STAMEY 1977), periurethral epithelium in young girls (KALLENIUS and WINBERG 1978; SVANBORG-EDEN and JODAL 1979), and urethral and bladder epithelium (BEACHEY 1981; SCHAEFFER 1983). The GAG layer protects against bacterial adherence in the bladder (PARSONS et al. 1980). Bacteria also adhere to slime of which Tamm-Horsfall protein is a constituent and are carried out with the urinary stream (SHORTLIFFE and STAMEY 1986b).

The usual bladder infection is caused by the woman's own fecal flora. Bacteria from the colon colonize the anterior vagina, vulva, and periurethral epithelium. FOWLER and STAMEY (1977) demonstrated that *E. coli* adheres more readily to vaginal epithelial cells from women with recurrent urinary infection that to similar cells from control women resistant to urinary infection.

The usual definition of significant bacteriuria is a bacterial count of 10^5/ml of voided urine. A lesser count may be quite significant when collected by suprapubic puncture or catheterization or in the presence of pyuria or appropriate symptomatology (LEBOWITZ and MANDELL 1987; LATHAM et al. 1985). The bacterial count per cubic centimeter may be depressed by urinary frequency in spite of significant infection (SHORTLIFFE and STAMEY 1986a).

Infection occurs when bacterial virulence factors overcome host resistance factors. Bacterial growth is exponential, and a large number of organisms may overwhelm any nonspecific bladder defenses that would be protective against a smaller number. Such growth can also overwhelm other organisms along the pathway from the rectum to the bladder. The ability of the bacteria to adhere to host uroepithelial cells allow them to colonize the region instead of being washed away by urine. This characteristic of some organisms depends on the number and nature of its adhesins, also called fimbriae or pili. They are filamentous, proteinaceous appendages extending from the bacterial cell wall that are able to match up with host epithelial cell receptors. These substances are antigenic and allow characterization and identification of the organism. The more numerous these linkages between the bacteria and the host epithelium, the more likely colonization and invasion of the mucosa. Because bacterial adherence is strikingly specific for certain epithelial cell types and therefore for certain anatomic locations, different species of organisms reside in and infect the oropharynx and the intestine or bladder. The endotoxin of some strains of *E. coli* can actually paralyse the ureteral musculature, interfering with the unidirectional brisk flow of urine that usually washes away unattached bacteria (LEBOWITZ and MANDRELL 1987).

Many specific and nonspecific host resistance factors or defense mechanisms protect the urinary tract and especially the kidney from infection. The epithelial cell receptors in the urinary tract are glycolipids of the globoseries with the number variable from person to person. It seems reasonable to expect that people with increased density of receptor sites would be at greater risk for colonization of their urinary tract. The transitional epithelium of the urinary bladder secretes and binds to its surface a GAG that inhibits the adherence of bacteria (PARSONS et al. 1980). Specific antibodies to an organism or its adhesins would protect the host against bacterial colonization and mucosal invasion. Some children with repeated urinary tract infections have been shown to have lower levels of immunoglobulin A than others the immature immune system of the very young may contribute to the increased susceptibility of infants and young children to bacterial infection of the kidney. Except for neonates, there is a strong gender-related rate of infection, with females much more often affected than boys. This susceptibility is thought to be due to the relative ease of introital contamination and more direct access of bacteria to the bladder. Uncircumcised neonatal males have ten times more urinary tract infections than their circumcised counterparts, perhaps because maternal virulent bacteria are able to colonize the preputial space. The unimpeded unidirectional efflux of urine from the urinary tract is an important nonspecific host defense. The brisk flow of urine is very efficient in washing away unattached bacteria.

Irritative voiding symptoms are the hallmark of bacterial cystitis. Frequency, urgency, nocturia, burning on urination, and dysuria predominate. The patient may complain of low back or suprapubic pain or discomfort. Urge incontinence and hematuria are common, but significant fever is unusual. Suprapubic tenderness may sometimes be elicited, but no specific physical signs are characteristic. The onset in women may follow sexual intercourse ("honeymoon cystitis"). Urinalysis

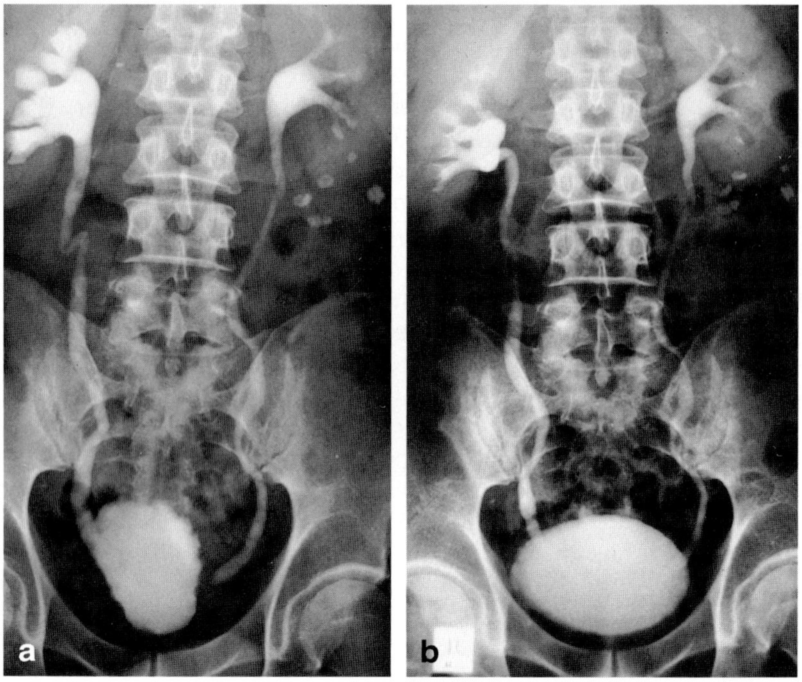

Fig. 6.19 a,b. Nonspecific mucosal edema in bacterial cystitis. **a** Excretory urogram; the right upper tract is dilated. **b** Repeat examination 1 month later demonstrates return to normal after therapy

usually shows pyuria, bacteriuria, and hematuria and urine cultures are positive. Persistent *Proteus* infection suggests the possibility of struvite stone (MACFARLANE 1988b; MEARES 1992).

In the early stages of acute bacterial cystitis, the bladder mucosa typically shows hyperemia, edema, and infiltration by neutrophils. With advanced inflammation, the mucosa is replaced by a friable, hemorrhagic, granular surface focally pitted with shallow ulcers containing exudate. The muscularis mucosa generally is uninvolved (MEARES 1986).

Imaging studies have little place in the workup of the usual bladder infection. They may identify the occasional stone in the bladder or upper tract. Urography may demonstrate the thickened mucosa of cystitis, which may occasionally be quite striking as well as nonspecific (Fig. 6.19). Since edema can be caused by the use of too highly concentrated contrast material, only 15% concentration or less should be used for cystography (IMRAY and KAPLAN 1983).

On ultrasound examination, acute bullous cystitis and chronic cystitis can produce an appearance of diffuse elevation and irregularity of the bladder mucosa (BREE and SILVER 1982). GOODING (1986) suggested an evolution of findings related to degree of involvement. Early mild involvement of the bladder wall may be sonographically normal because the subtle abnormalities from inflamed tissues do not project onto the bladder lumen. In the next stage, tiny irregular excrescences occur on the bladder wall from focal involvement, indistinguishable from early focal transitional cell carcinoma. Progressive inflammation leads to thick bulky vesical wall abnormalities. Intraluminal or intramural gas may be present. A fluid–fluid interface suggests an inflammatory process but can be seen in hemorrhage and occasionally in asymptomatic patients with viscid urine.

Chronic cystitis differs from acute cystitis mainly in the character of the inflammatory infiltrate. It is caused by the same pathogens that cause acute cystitis. In the early stages of chronic cystitis, the mucosa becomes progressively more edematous, erythematous, and friable. The mucosa may ulcerate. In the later stages, the submucosa is infiltrated by fibroblasts, plasma cells, and lymphocytes. The bladder wall eventually becomes thickened, fibrotic, and inelastic. The patient with chronic infectious cystitis may be asymptomatic or have variable symptoms of bladder irritability. The laboratory findings are usually normal except for bacteriuria, with surprisingly little pyuria. The urine culture will usually be positive. The imaging findings will be normal or those of the associated conditions such as obstruction reflux or fistula (MEARES 1992).

6.5.2 Pyocystitis

Acute pyocystitis usually occurs in dialysis patients with low or absent urine output. It usually presents with fever, suprapubic pain, and a palpable mass. Pelvic ultrasound can make the diagnosis by demonstrating the fluid–fluid level or small echogenic densities from floating internal debris (BREE and SILVER 1982). Suspicion warrants bladder aspiration for culture. Management involves drainage and antibiotics (MACFARLANE 1988a).

6.5.3 Emphysematous Cystitis (Cystitis Emphysematosa)

Emphysematous cystitis is an uncommon and peculiar manifestation of urinary tract infection in which gas is present within the wall and/or lumen of the infected bladder. The organism involved is usually *E. coli*, but *Proteus*, *Pseudomonas*, and rarely *Clostridia* may be involved. The organisms have the ability to ferment glucose and the patient is usually a diabetic. Approximately 50% of cases reported in the literature occurred in diabetics. Other cases are related to stasis from outlet obstruction. Other causes of air in the lumen of the bladder are instrumentation and fistula, but air in the bladder wall is almost always due to infection (QUINT et al. 1992; BARTKOWSKI and LANESKY 1988). Symptoms may be minimal and include dysuria, hematuria, or pneumaturia. Pneumaturia must be elicited by specific questioning (MACFARLANE 1988a; IMRAY and KAPLAN 1983).

The appearance of the radiolucent gas-filled vesicles within the bladder wall on plain film, urogram, or CT is characteristic Fig. 6.20 (IMRAY and KAPLAN 1983; NEY et al. 1987; BOHLMAN et al. 1988). The air in the thickened bladder wall blocks the ultrasound beam, causing irregular foci associated with acoustic shadowing (KAUZLARIC and BARMIER 1985).

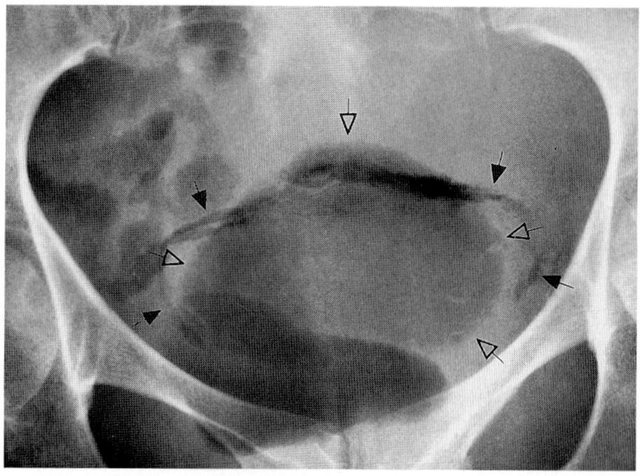

Fig. 6.20. Air in the bladder wall (*closed arrows*) and in bladder lumen *open arrows*) in emphysematous cystitis

6.5.4 Fungal Infections

The three major types of urinary tract involvement by fungus are disseminated, regional, and localized; the most common type is disseminated and deep, usually superimposed upon very severe systemic disease. Urinary tract involvement can occur in histoplasmosis, aspergillosis, actinomycosis, cryptococcoses, and candidiasis. In disseminated disease, the microabscesses are usually too small to be demonstrated on imaging studies. Candidiasis is the most common infection, most frequently involving the bladder and occasionally the renal pelvis and ureter (MARGOLIN 1971).

6.5.4.1 Candidiasis

Fungal infections of the urinary tract are almost exclusively due to *Candida albicans*, a yeast-like fungus that is a normal inhabitant of the respiratory and gastrointestinal tracts and the vagina. Infected patients usually have one or more predisposing conditions.

Fungal infections of the urinary tract are said to be increasing in frequency partly due to an increase in opportunistic infections resulting from more aggressive medical therapy applied in a variety of debilitating conditions. The normal bacterial flora usually keeps its level of growth in check. Infection of the urinary tract may be (a) hematogenous or occur via (b) direct spread from contiguous organs of other systems or (c) a retrograde route through the urethra. The most com-

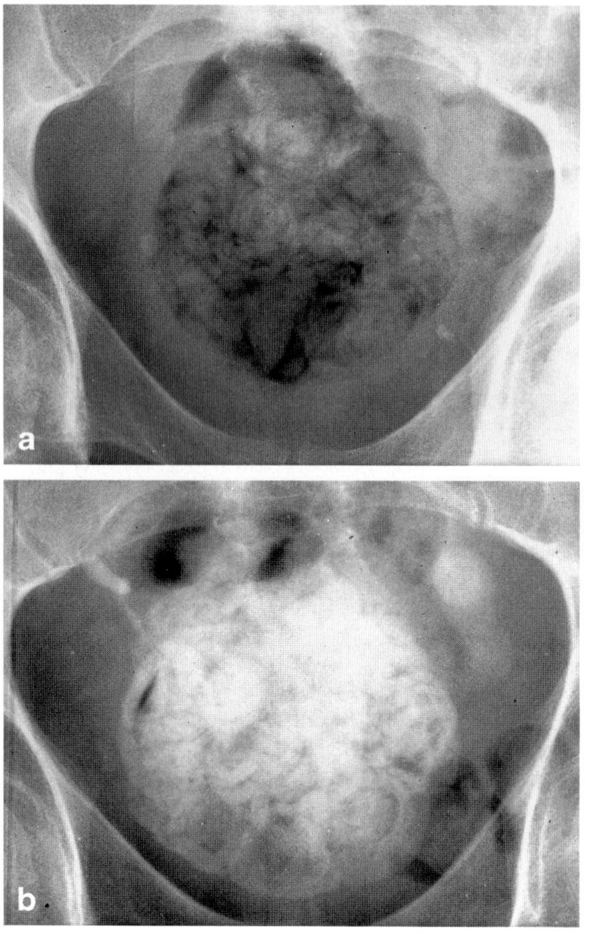

Fig. 6.21 a,b. Fungus balls in the urinary bladder: **a** plain film; **b** after intravenous contrast

mon route of entry in localized involvement of the lower urinary tract is probably retrograde through the urethra (MARGOLIN 1971).

The pseudomycelia tend to cluster, forming bezoars or fungus balls. The mycelia collect in large sheets of colonies which can form fungus balls (Fig. 6.21) (McDONALD and FAGAN 1972). The presence of air in the bladder and in the fungus ball depends on glycosuria and is almost only seen in uncontrolled diabetes. Gas between the layered colonies of fungus creates a characteristic laminated appearance on plain radiographs. Urinary bladder candidiasis may be asymptomatic or present as septicemia. Irritative bladder symptoms are commonly present and pyelonephritis may be associated. Hematuria, pneumaturia, and passage of small clumps of yeast may occur. Cystoscopy usually discloses irregular, slightly raised white or brown plaques or membrane composed of yeast cells and hyphae. The membrane resembles that seen in oral thrush or vaginal moniliasis. Fungus balls typically present as air-containing laminated circular radiodensities varying from 2 to 10 cm and may be single or multiple. Air in the lumen aids identification.

Diagnosis rests upon the demonstration of histologic invasion such as the presence of a large colony of the fungus within an organ or a very large number of organisms in a body fluid.

Without fermented gas, the appearance of a fungus ball in the bladder on CT is that of a solid soft tissue density bladder mass, indistinguishable from any bladder tumor or mass (TRINH et al. 1986). Fungus ball can be mimicked by nonopaque calculus, pus, blood clot, or neoplasm.

Treatment involves alkalinization of the urine with sodium bicarbonate and/or irrigation with amphotericin B. Seriously ill patients may need intravenous amphotericin B. Additional topical administration of amphotericin B via percutaneous nephrostomy will hasten control of the infection. Obstructing fungus balls in the ureter or bladder may require endoscopic or surgical removal. Treatment includes controlling or eliminating any predisposing conditions (MACFARLANE 1988b; MINDELL and POLLACK 1983; McDONALD and FAGAN 1972; MARGOLIN 1971).

6.5.4.2 Actinomycosis

The causative agent of actinomycosis is *Actinomyces israelii* (*A. bovis*), which is a normal inhabitant of the gastrointestinal tract. Marked fibrosis with en bloc involvement and fistulization are characteristic of the infection. These features are similar to the characteristics demonstrated by the more common mandibulocervical and thoracic involvement. The disease can involve the kidney, bladder, or testis by hematogenous spread from a distant primary site of infection. The bladder may also become involved by direct extension from the appendix, bowel, or oviduct.

Microscopically, the organisms are identified as yellow bodies called sulfur granules. They may be recovered from sinus discharge, urine, or needle aspiration of involved tissues. Definitive diagnosis usually requires culture.

Treatment is achieved by parenteral administration of penicillin G 10–20 million units per day for 4–6 weeks. Abscess drainage or surgical removal of the involved organ may occasionally become necessary. Drainage of a granulomatous abscess may lead to the development of a chronic draining sinus (MARGOLIN 1971; TANAGHO 1992b).

6.5.4.3 Tuberculosis

Genitourinary tuberculosis has been seen infrequently in the industrialized countries of the Western world since the introduction of effective antituberculous therapy, but it is still regularly encountered in Third World countries, where it remains poorly controlled. Tuberculosis is now being encountered more frequently in the immune-suppressed population, such as in patients with AIDS, with transplants, or on chemotherapy. It has been considered primarily a disease of young adults, with 60% of patients between the ages of 20 and 40. However, a 10-year review of the experience at the Mayo Clinic up to 1973 found that in 60% of their cases the clinical onset of genitourinary disease was after the age of 40 (KOLLINS et al. 1974). There is a male preponderance and the disease is infrequent in children.

Genitourinary tuberculosis is a secondary infection due to hematogenous spread from the lungs to both kidneys. The prostate may be another possible focus of direct hematogenous spread. The primary lung infection may be inapparent and asymptomatic. In the United States the risk of tuberculosis is greatest in the elderly of both blacks and whites, with black males having a first peak in incidence in age groups 35–45 and 45–55 and a second peak in the oldest age group. Between 1985 and 1987, the largest increase occurred in the 25 to 44-year-old age group, limited primarily to non-Hispanic blacks and Hispanics. By locality, the largest increase was in New York City (RIEDER et al. 1989; BUCKNER et al. 1991).

Tuberculosis can produce one of the specific forms of interstitial cystitis usually secondary to renal infection. The kidneys occasionally appear normal, suggesting that the cystitis is secondary to genital tuberculosis or represents primary bladder involvement. The early findings are nonspecific, comprising only minor irregularities of the bladder contour and increased trabeculation. With progression, the inflammation involves the whole thickness of the bladder, increasing the wall thickness and decreasing the bladder capacity. In the late stages of bladder tuberculosis, bladder capacity may be as little as 25–50 cc. Vesicureteral reflux is common. The thick bladder wall may constrict and obstruct the ureter, producing hydronephrosis (FRIEDENBERG 1971).

Almost 15% of all new cases of tuberculosis in the United Stages involve extrapulmonary sites; of these approximately 30% are in the genitourinary tract. The age and sex incidence parallels that of pulmonary tuberculosis (Cos and COCKETT 1982). Bladder involvement occurs in 33% of cases of genitourinary tuberculosis (DAS et al. 1992).

Most symptoms of genitourinary tuberculosis are vesical in origin. Dysuria, frequency, nocturia, and urgency account for 40% of the symptoms. In males it is relatively common to find a beaded vas deferens, a nodular, rubbery marble-sized epididymis, or a hard prostate (Cos and COCKETT 1982; TANAGHO 1992b).

The most common urographic finding of tuberculous cystitis is a contracted spastic small-capacity bladder as the result of chronic inflammation, cicatrization, and fibrosis. When retrograde pyelography is indicated, it must be remembered that miliary dissemination is a risk after ureteral catheterization in untreated patients. Cystourethrography should be performed in all patients with proved genitourinary tuberculosis in order to search for unsuspected tubercular urethral stricture or prostatic abscess. (Cos and COCKETT 1982).

Sonography can visualize localized and generalized bladder scarring and identify focal nodular lesions, which occur mostly at the base and which may be indistiguishable from bladder neoplasms. The undermining mucosal ulcer of tuberculosis is seen as intravasation of urine into the deeper layer of the bladder wall with overhanging mucosa (DAS et al. 1992).

At cystourethroscopy in acute cases, the posterior male urethra shows a red velvety base with thick longitudinal swollen ridges proximal to the verumontanum. In chronic untreated patients, dilated prostatic ducts, prostatic abscesses, caseation, and sloughing are not infrequently found. Visualization of the bladder may reveal exudates, single or multiple ulcerations, delta-shaped patches of redness below each ureteric orifice, decreased bladder capacity, or rigid ureteral orifices depending on the degree of chronicity of involvement by the disease. A toothpaste-like efflux of caseation may be observed coming from one of the ureteral orifices (Cos and COCKETT 1982).

Definitive diagnosis of genitourinary tuberculosis usually requires the demonstration of

Mycobacterium tuberculosis in the urine. A common practice is to collect three consecutive first voided, morning urine specimens for culture. Sonographically guided fine needle aspiration biopsy of renal lesions may obtain material diagnostic for tuberculosis in patients with negative urine cultures (Das et al. 1992).

The treatment of genitourinary tuberculosis is medical with surgery the last resort (Cos and Cockett 1982).

6.5.5 Alkaline Encrusting Cystitis

Bladder calcification in bacterial urinary tract infection is exceedingly rare. A highly alkaline urine and devitalized mucosal tissue appear to be necessary for the development of mural calcification. Proteus species and several coliform bacteria produce urease which converts urea to ammonia, creating markedly alkaline urine. The precipitation of calcium phosphate and struvite salts is then fostered. A healthy bladder epithelium resists the deposition of calcium but ischemic or necrotic bladder tissue is susceptible, leading to so-called alkaline encrusting cystitis (Pollack et al. 1981). Bladder necrosis from any cause in the presence of alkaline urine may result in phosphate deposition and calcification which may be radiographically demonstrable (Harrison et al. 1978.)

The calcifications of alkaline encrusting cvstitis may be linear, outlining part or all of the bladder wall or either flocculent or nodular.

In addition to appropriate systemic antibiotics, treatment may require bladder lavage and cystoscopic removal of the encrustations with forceps or even suprapubic curettage of the bladder mucosa (Pollack et al. 1981; Harrison et al. 1978).

6.5.6 Interstitial Cystitis (Hunner's Ulcer, Submucous Fibrosis)

Interstitial cystitis is a disorder of the bladder manifested by the complex of irritative voiding symptoms and suprapubic pain relieved by micturition (Fowler 1989). Most patients with interstitial cystitis are middle aged, 80%–90% are female, and the majority are white (Fowler 1989). Oravisto (1975) found that the median duration before diagnosis was 4 years in mild cases, 5 years in medium severity, and 3 years in severe cases.

The history usually discloses uninterrupted dysuria for months or years despite normal urinalysis. Overdistention of the bladder on cystoscopy (usually under general anesthesia) causes typical mucosal petechiae. Transient relief is often given by overdistention. A random biopsy from a healthy-looking site reveals mild fibrosis and edema and often lymphoid aggregates. Interstitial cystitis involves the entire bladder. Antinuclear antibodies are detectable in 50% of such cases.

The histologic hallmark of interstitial cystitis is infiltration of the urothelium and the detrusor muscle by mast cells, the mast cell density roughly correlating with the severity of symptoms (Lynes et al. 1987). Vasoactive amines secreted by mast cells can cause smooth muscle contraction and neurostimulation. Histamine, another secretory product, can produce pain, hyperemia, and fibrosis. The concentration of detrusor muscle histamine and the urinary excretion of histamine metabolites have been found to be increased in interstitial cystitis (Fowler 1989).

Penetration of urinary constituents into the urothelium or suburothelial tissues may be part of the explanation for interstitial cystitis, which has been shown to be associated with a leaky epithelium (Parsons et al. 1991). The bladder epithelium relies primarily on its surface glycosaminoglycans to maintain its impermeablility. Electron microscopy of bladder epithelium of patients with interstitial cystitis showed findings consistent with leakage of solutes through the urothelium and leaky tight junctions (Eldrup et al. 1983). With immunohistochemical techniques, Tamm-Horsfall protein, a normal constituent of urine, has been demonstrated within the urothelium from biopsies of patients with interstitial cystitis but not normal controls (Fowler et al. 1988). This finding supports the possibility that abnormal permeability of the urothelium is associated with, and possibly a cause of, interstitial cystitis. The two currently most popular theories regarding the cause of the histologic changes postulate an autoimmune mechanism or a defect in the bladder mucosal surface lining of glycosaminoglycans (Macfarlane 1988b). Some evidence suggests that interstitial cystitis is an autoimmune collagen disease (Oravisto et al. 1970; Tanagho 1992c).

The symptomatic hallmarks of interstitial cystitis are urinary frequency, urgency, nocturia, and suprapubic pain that is relieved by voiding. Fibrosis with contracture of the bladder is uncommon. Pyuria and microscopic hematuria may be seen but the urinary sediment is usually entirely normal (FOWLER 1989).

As a rule there is gradual aggravation of the symptoms over a period of years without wholly asymptomatic intervals (HANNO and WEIN 1987). The disease is much more prevalent than previously considered (MESSING and STAMEY 1978), the underestimation in part having been due to lack of unanimity as to criteria for diagnosis. The diagnosis is one of exclusion based on clinical and cystoscopic criteria with biopsy.

The cystoscopic findings are characteristic submucosal pinpoint petechial hemorrhages (glomerulations) visualized following repeated bladder distention to 70 cm water pressure under anesthesia (MESSING and STAMEY 1978; MACFARLANE 1988b). The glomerulations, which are currently regarded as the diagnostic hallmark, are red, strawberry-like dots that often coalesce to become hemorrhagic spots which ooze blood from the bladder mucosa on second filling of the bladder under anesthesia (MESSING and STAMEY 1978; HANNO and WEIN 1987). Hunner's ulcers are seldom found. Bladder biopsy and urine cytology must show no evidence of carcinoma in situ, which may masquerade as interstitial cystitis. Interstitial mast cell infiltration is frequently identified and probably plays a role in the inflammatory process (LYNES et al. 1987). Cystometric studies are essentially normal except for small bladder capacity. The diagnosis is confirmed by response to treatment. Urodynamics may quantitate response to therapy (PEREZ-MARRERO et al. 1987).

Cystography and urography are seldom helpful in diagnosing interstitial cystitis since small bladder capacity is a nonspecific finding. Radiologic studies are useful in ruling out other conditions and in establishing a baseline (HANNO and WEIN 1987; MESSING 1987).

The current mainstays of treatment are intravesical installation of dimethyl sulfoxide (DMSO) and hydraulic distention of the bladder (HANNO and WEIN 1987; MEARES 1987; MACFARLANE 1988c; FOWLER 1989).

6.5.7 Eosinophilic Cystitis

Eosinophilic cystitis is an uncommon condition characterized by eosinophilic infiltration of the mucosa and muscularis, particularly the lamina propria of the bladder, accompanied by neutrophils and mast cells (FOWLER 1989; RUBIN and PINCUS 1974; HELLSTROM et al. 1979). Giant cells are usually absent (SIDH et al. 1980; ANTONAKOPOULOS and NEWMAN 1984). It occurs at all ages from neonates to the elderly. It usually occurs in adults with a history of allergies and is thought to be allergic in etiology (FOWLER 1989; RUBIN and PINCUS 1974); it is more common in women than in men.

Eosinophilic cystitis possibly represents a local allergic response to a bacterial, fungal, or viral pathogen or a foreign antigen exposure (BAUER and KOGAN 1991). BAUER and KOGAN (1991) suggested that immune complexes with immunoglobulins A and E precipitating in the bladder wall as a result of local tissue damage may attract an eosinophilic response.

The lesions of eosinophilic cystitis may be focal or scattered throughout the bladder. MELICOW et al. (1974) described a herald lesion which simulates eosinophilic cystitis; this lesion is created by the encroachment of extravesical cancer or inflammatory process upon the urinary bladder in which eosinophils may be prominent.

Eosinophilic cystitis infiltrating the bladder wall may cause erythematous plaques or ulcerated areas but it more often causes tumor mass which may even be palpable. It may imitate chronic inflammation, interstitial and bacterial cystitis, tuberculous cystitis, epithelial tumor, or sarcoma botryoides (SIDH et al. 1980; CASTILLO et al. 1988; FOWLER 1989; THIJSSEN and GERRIDZEN 1990). Imaging studies therefore are nonspecific and findings may be absent. A solitary filling defect, mucosal irregularity, mucosal edema, or restricted bladder volume may be identified.

Eosinophilic cystitis presents with irritative symptoms of frequency, dysuria, urgency, and suprapubic pain (SIDH et al. 1980; FOWLER 1989). The bladder pain may not be relieved by voiding and urinary retention may occur (LITTLETON et al. 1982). Gross hematuria has been called a constant feature (OKAFO et al. 1985). Eosinophilia and eosinophiluria are common (SUTTON 1986). The onset is typically acute and may resolve spontaneously.

In their review of the literature, CASTILLO et al. (1985) found that proteinuria, pyuria, and hematuria are usually present. Hematuria was present in 80% of the reported cases and was gross more than 50% of the time. Radiologic tests, including IVP and VCUG are usually normal, with the most common finding being a small-capacity bladder. Urine cultures were sterile in 70% of the cases. Cystoscopy may reveal hyperemia, raised areas of bladder mucosa with edema, and at times even polypoid lesions. Microscopic findings vary, but in most cases they show mucosal edema and hyperemia, muscle necrosis, and chronic inflammation entailing a predominance of eosinophilic infiltrate with the presence of mast cells, plasma cells, and even giant cells.

Eosinophilic cystitis has occurred in patients after therapy with Tranilast [*N*-(3,4-dimethoxycinnamoyl)anthranilic acid] developed and used in Japan for the treatment of anaphylactic hypersensitivity such as bronchial asthma (NAKADA et al. 1986). The drug was found localized specifically in the transitional epithelial cells of the mucosa and the endothelial cells of venules of the urinary bladder for a fairly long time after oral administration to rats (NISHIGAKE et al. 1990).

Eosinophilic cystitis has been associated with hypersensitivity to food and drugs, respiratory infections, parasitic infestation, and warfarin (SIDH et al. 1980). It has been found in association with eosinophilic gastroenteritis (PETERSON et al. 1989; GREGG and UTZ 1974), Glanmann's thrombasthenia (BOTMA et al. 1987), and chronic rejection of a cadaveric renal transplant (HORNER and WEINGARTEN 1990). It recurred in a 9-year-old girl after antireflux surgery (AXELROD et al. 1991). It has developed in patients treated with instillations of mitomycin C for superficial bladder cancer (INGLIS et al. 1987; GELABERT et al. 1990). An eosinophilic infiltration of the urinary bladder identical to eosinophilic cystitis has been found in children with chronic granulomatous disease involving the urinary bladder (BAUER and KOGAN 1991).

Eosinophilic cystitis has been described as a chronic inflammatory process of unknown causation for which no specific therapy is available (CASTILLO et al. 1988). Symptomatic treatment has been recommended (MARSHALL and MIDDLETON 1974). Antibiotics are given for secondary bacterial infection, corticosteroids may be given if symptoms are severe, and allergens may be identified and removed (GOLDSTEIN 1971; LITTLETON et al. 1982). The heading process is accompanied by fibrosis which can lead to obstruction and renal failure (THIJSSEN and GERRIDZEN 1985).

6.5.8 Chronic Granulomatous Disease

Chronic granulomatous disease is a congenital disorder of neutrophil function which is characterized by the failure of granulocytes to intracellularly destroy bacteria once they are phagocytized. The X-linked recessive enzymatic defect makes the granulocytes unable to produce hydrogen peroxide and superoxide which normally would be released by lysosomes to digest bacteria. Patients are plagued by repeated bacterial and/or fungal infections.

Genitourinary tract involvement is rare in chronic granulomatous disease. The kidney is more usually involved by granuloma formation. An extensive granulomatous reaction may occur in the bladder wall, producing a markedly thickened, asymmetric, and elevated bladder with reduced capacity associated with irritative symptoms (BAUER and KOGAN 1991). Patients with granulomatous cystitis frequently present with hematuria, dysuria, frequency, and enuresis (SPEIRS et al. 1990). Physical examination is generally unremarkable but may reveal a suprapubic mass representing the inflamed and thickened bladder (SPEIRS et al. 1990). Hydronephrosis may develop secondary to inflammation and obstruction at the ureterovesical junction. Cystoscopy may show a raised reddish inflammatory lesion with bullous edema and polypoid changes which may encompass the bladder neck, trigone, and one or both walls of the bladder, sometimes resembling sarcoma botryoides (BAUER and KOGAN 1991). The bladder may have a small capacity and vesicoureteral reflux may be seen (SPEIRS et al. 1990). Ultrasound may demonstrate the involved areas as diffuse thickening with nodularity of the bladder wall and can be used to monitor therapy (SPEIRS et al. 1990). Biopsies of the bladder show acute and chronic inflammation associated with intramural granulomata (SPEIRS et al. 1990). Eosinophilic infiltration of the bladder identical to eosinophilic cystitis has been described in these children (BAUER and KOGAN 1991).

Therapy for granulomatous cystitis in chronic granulomatous disease includes antibiotics to treat identified or suspected infectious agents as well as steroids to suppress the inflammation (Speirs et al. 1990).

6.5.9 Radiation Cystitis

The urinary bladder is included in the radiation therapy fields during the treatment of bladder and pelvic neoplasms. With the advent of supervoltage therapy, complications have become minimal and usually only a mild cystitis ensues (Aron and Schlesinger 1974).

The acute self-limited inflammation of the bladder may cause irritative bladder symptoms and sometimes hematuria. Microscopically the epithelial cells are enlarged with nuclear swelling and pyknosis and edema of the submucosa and detrusor muscle. Anticholinergic medication usually provides symptomatic therapy at this stage (Fowler 1989).

When 3000 R is administered over a 3- to 4-week period, some patients experience mild dysuria and frequency 4–6 weeks after therapy. Bladder tolerance is in the range of 6500–7500 R administered over 6–8 weeks. When 6000–7000 R is applied, a severe acute reaction usually results which lasts for 3–4 weeks (Aron and Schlesinger 1974). Hyperemia, petechiae, ulcers, and connective tissue edema occur and may progress to desquamation.

Urography at this stage may demonstrate small bladder capacity deriving from the increased irritability and contractility. Stasis in the pelvic segments of the ureter may rarely be demonstrated (Aron and Schlesinger 1974).

Chronic cystitis may develop years after treatment in 5%–10% of patients (Fowler 1989). Interstitial fibrosis, obliterative endarteritis, and telangiectasia are frequently found in the irradiated bladder. Ischemia leads to epithelial atrophy or necrosis with the development of ulcers, fissures, and even fistulas (Aron and Schlesinger 1974).

Hemorrhagic cystitis which may develop 2 months to 2 years after treatment seldom shows a bleeding site at cystoscopy. Biopsy will be consistent with radiation cystitis.

6.6 Fistulas

6.6.1 Etiology and Classification

Urinary tract fistulas are rarely fatal but can be extremely uncomfortable and embarrassing for the patient. Fistulas may occur from any part of the urinary tract but most commonly arise from the bladder or urethra. Vesical fistulas are all too common and may communicate with the skin, intestinal tract, or female genital tract. The primary disease is usually nonurologic. The etiologies are: (a) intestinal disease – diverticulitis, 50%–60%; cancer of the colon, 20%–25%; and Crohn's disease, 10%; (b) primary gynecologic disease, pressure necrosis during difficult and prolonged labor, advanced cancer of the cervix; (c) complication of gynecologic conditions, hysterectomy, low cesarean section, or radiation therapy; (d) trauma (Tanagho 1992c).

Direct extension of malignancies of the small or large bowel, uterus, or cervix may perforate the bladder. Inflammation of its adjacent organs may erode the bladder wall. Severe trauma to the bladder may lead to perivesical abscess which may rupture through the skin of the perineum or abdomen. The bladder may be injured during pelvic surgery, leading to a persistent cutaneous fistula (Tanagho 1992c).

Most fistulas after hysterectomy occur in the posterior bladder immediately behind the interureteric ridge and midway between the ureteral orifices. Although these fistulas may result from direct laceration and be immediately obvious, most are the result of devascularization of the posterior bladder wall with necrosis which leads to urine leakage 8–14 days after surgery. This may occur after the patient has left the hospital and even be misinterpreted as stress incontinence (Guerriero and Devine 1984b).

6.6.2 Diagnosis

Diagnosis of vesicovaginal fistula is usually not difficult, but a small pinpoint leak may be hidden in an inflamed bladder. If the fistula is not seen cystoscopically or on vaginal examination, methylene blue, carmine red, or indigo carmine dye can be placed in the bladder following prior placement of pledgets in the vaginal vault. Clear urine in the vagina in this situation indicates ureterovaginal fistula. Vesicovaginal fistula may also be

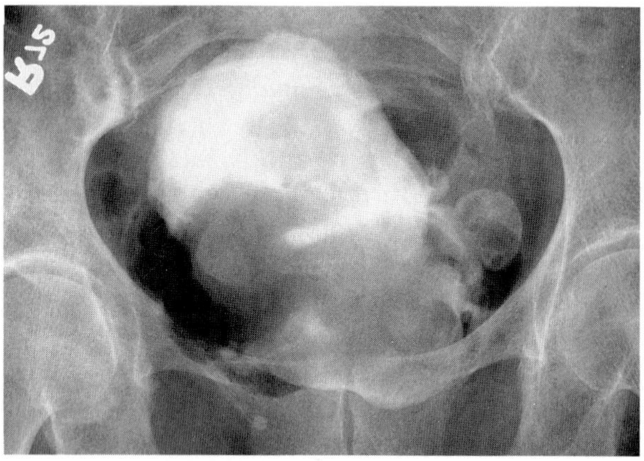

Fig. 6.22. Air in the opacified trabeculated urinary bladder from rectovesical fistula

differentiated from ureterovaginal fistula by the double dye test described by RAGHAVAIAH (1974). The vagina is packed with four sterile wet swabs. One is placed in each fornix, one at the mid vaginal level, and the fourth at the outlet. The bladder is catheterized and filled with carmine red solution. Five minutes later, 5 ml of indigo carmine (blue-green) is injected intravenously. Ten minutes after that, the vaginal packs are removed and their color noted. If the packs are stained red, a vesicovaginal fistula is present at that level. If the packs are deep blue-green, a ureterovaginal fistula is present. The small amount of blue-green urine excreted into the bladder will not significantly dilute the deep red dye in the bladder. If both colors are present in the packs, both vesicovaginal and ureterovaginal fistulas are present. Cystography, vaginography, fistulography, and/or sinus tract injection can be of great help in identifying and locating fistulas (GUERRIERO and DEVINE 1984b).

Vesicointestinal fistula produces bladder irritability, passage of feces and gas per urethra, and usually a change in bowel habits such as obstipation, abdominal distention, or diarrhea caused by the primary bowel disease.

Small bowel follow-through, contrast enema, cystography, or endoscopy may demonstrate the fistula. Plain film demonstration of intravesical gas in the absence of history of catheterization or presence of gas-forming organism is almost diagnostic of the presence of vesical fistula but does not depict its location (Fig. 6.22). CT may show the inflammation but seldom demonstrates the fistula. Cystoscopy finds a severe localized inflammatory reaction from which bowel contents may exude. The fistula itself may be catheterized and contrast injection demonstrates its communication (TANAGHO 1992c).

Vesicovaginal fistula may be secondary to obstetric, surgical, or radiation injury or to invasive cancer of the cervix. Speculum examination of the vagina or cystoscopy often reveals the fistula. Vaginography may be helpful.

An uncommon fistula communicates the uterus and bladder after cesarean section (GUERRIERO and DEVINE 1984b).

6.6.3 Enterovesical Fistulas

Most authorities agree that diverticulitis is the most common cause of enterovesical fistulas and that carcinoma of the colon is the second most frequent cause. The majority of colonic fistulas arise from the rectosigmoid, the cecum being the next most common origin. Crohn's disease is the most common cause of small-bowel fistulas to the bladder and has been reported in 1%–4.6% of patients.

The most common cause of colovesical fistula is diverticulitis (this accounts for 51%–60% of cases). Next most common is colon carcinoma (16%–28% of cases) (GOLDMAN et al. 1984). Other less frequent causes of colovesical fistula include postoperative complications particularly after prostatectomy, trauma, extrusion of a foreign body, bladder cancer, ulcerative or granulomatous colitis, radiation therapy, and pelvic abscess (GOLDMAN et al. 1984).

Clinically, colovesical fistula is most commonly seen in men, with a male to female ratio as high as 5:1; this may be explained by a protective effect of the interposition of the uterus between the colon and bladder (GOLDMAN et al. 1984). Pneumaturia is followed by the development of fecaluria or hematuria. Urine is occasionally passed via the rectum but this is more common with small bowel fistulas or colon fistulas above the sigmoid colon. Pneumaturia is present in up to 87% of cases and fecaluria in up to 46% of cases (ABESHOUSE et al. 1957).

Fistulous communication between bladder and bowel can be difficult to demonstrate. In two large series (NAUCLER and RISBERG 1981; KOVALCIK et al. 1976) only 38% and 55% of all fistulas were demonstrated by extensive workup and imaging studies.

Conventional studies include cystography and barium studies attempting to show the fistulous tract. Radioisotopic techniques (PROKOP et al. 1974), the administration of dyes such as methylene blue, the use of charcoal, and the Bourne test have not gained wide acceptance (GOLDMAN et al. 1985). The Bourne test involves identifying barium in the urinary bladder after a barium enema (AMENDOLA et al. 1984). Evidence of barium or air entering the bladder is proof of the fistula's presence but does not identify its location.

Conventional radiographic techniques are disappointing for diagnosing these fistulas. Gas is seen in the bladder on plain film in only 30% of cases. Urography may show an extrinsic impression on the bladder in the prodromal phase but will demonstrate only 18% of the fistulas. Cystography will demonstrate only 35% of colovesical fistulas, and barium enema, between 20% and 40% (GOLDMAN et al. 1984).

Cystography may show extrinsic pressure secondary to mass effect or irregularity of the bladder caused by an underlying cystitis or bladder invasion by tumor or inflammation.

The diagnosis is usually inferred from finding fecal material in the bladder or the presence of dimpling or focal granulation tissue in the bladder wall. In a survey of enterovesical fistulas, CARSON et al. (1978) reported actual demonstration of the orifice of the fistula tract at cystoscopy in 28 (32%) of 87 patients and findings suggestive of fistula in 35% of cystograms.

Computed tomography is a sensitive, noninvasive method of documenting the presence of such fistulas and can also outline the extravesical component of the primary disease process, thereby localizing the fistula. Air in the bladder is a key finding in the presence of enterovesical fistula. Minute amounts of air can be demonstrated by CT. Iatrogenic air from catheterization and gas due to infection by gas-forming bacteria must be excluded. In 20 enterovesical fistulas identified by CT, other findings were focal bladder wall thickening in 90%, focal bowel wall thickening in 85%, and the presence of an associated soft tissue mass in 75% (GOLDMAN et al. 1985).

The location of the soft tissue mass provides a clue to the etiology of the fistula. The right side anteriorly and/or laterally is affected by cecal, appendiceal, and distal ileal fistulas. The left side of the bladder is affected by rectosigmoid and genitourinary, prostate, or uterine inflammatory and/or neoplastic processes (GOLDMAN et al. 1985).

The ability to demonstrate a soft tissue mass adjacent to the bladder in a patient with enterovesical fistula is a great advantage of CT (GOLDMAN et al. 1985). This information is important in surgical planning, as single-stage procedures may be performed if the adjacent mass is small. Many recommend that CT be the first procedure performed on a patient with suspected enterovesical fistula because it is cost-effective and may obviate the need for other studies such as urography, cystography, and barium enema (GOLDMAN et al. 1985).

The sonographic features of urinary bladder involvement have been described in regional enteritis (BOAG and NOLAN 1988). Sonography can noninvasively demonstrate changes both in the bladder and in the adjacent abnormal bowel. The sonographic findings in regional enteritis are bowel wall thickening, conglomeration of loops, abscess formation and intraperitoneal fluid. Fistulas may sometimes be visible but more often their presence can only be inferred by abnormal bowel adherent to an adjacent organ such as bladder.

6.7 Neoplasm

6.7.1 Primary Epithelial Malignancy

6.7.1.1 Transitional Cell Carcinoma

Cancer of the urinary tract accounts for approximately 10% of cancers in males and 4% of cancers in females. Cancer of the urinary tract causes 5% of the cancer deaths in males and 3% of the cancer deaths in females. There are approximately 50000 new cases of bladder cancer and 10000 deaths a year in the United States. Survival rates for cancer of the bladder are much better for whites than for blacks but are improving for both. The relative 5-year survival in 1963 was 53% for whites and 24% for blacks. In 1987, the relative 5-year survival was 79% for whites and 59% for blacks. Expected 5-year survival rates for all stages, localized disease, regional spread and distant metastases are currently (1992) 79%, 91%, 46%, and 9% for whites and 59%, 81%, 34%, and 4% for blacks. Fortunately, 73% of cancers of the bladder are localized at the time of initial diagnosis. Nineteen per cent have regional involvement and 3%, distant spread. The age-adjusted cancer death rate from bladder cancer in males in the United States has remained fairly stable since 1930, being approximately 6–8 per 100000 population. New cases are predicted at about 50000 per year with 3:1 male-female ratio and deaths at about 10000 per year in the United States (BORING et al. 1992).

Bladder cancer rates in men exceed those in women by about 3 to 1 (BORING et al. 1991; MORRISON 1984). In the United States, the incidence in black males is half that of whites, but in black women the incidence is three fourths that in whites. The mortality figures are about the same. Incidence rates in the northern United States are 30%–50% higher than in the south (MORRISON 1984).

For epidemiologic purposes, the urothelium or transitional cell lining of the renal pelvis, ureter, urinary bladder, and urethra are grouped together as the lower urinary tract. Urothelial tumors display substantial histologic variability. The lesions may be in situ or invasive, papillary or flat, and have a grade that ranges from completely benign to highly malignant (KOSS 1975a). There is controversy as to whether "benign papillomas," which are low grade, noninvasive papillary tumors, are benign or an early malignancy (MORRISON 1984).

The overwhelming majority (98%) of bladder tumors are epithelial in origin and of these most (92%) are transitional cell carcinoma so that bladder cancer and transitional cell carcinoma are almost synonymous. Of the rest, 7% are squamous cell carcinoma and 1%–2% adenocarcinomas. The nonepithelial tumors are mostly sarcomas, pheochromocytomas, malignant lymphomas, mixed mesodermal tumors, and primary carcinoid tumors. Eighty percent of cases occur in people over 50 years old. The average age of patients is 65 years at diagnosis. Fewer than 1% of cases have been reported in patients less than 40 years old. Primary epthelial tumors in the first two decades of life tend to be low grade and low stage with an excellent prognosis (JAVADPOUR and MOSTAFI 1969; BENSON et al. 1983). Primary epithelial malignancy is usually localized at the time of diagnosis with only 9% of cases showing regional metastasis and 6% distant metastasis. Up to 80% of patients develop recurrent tumors. About 30% have increased cellular anaplasia and greater invasiveness on recurrence. The highest incidence is in industrialized countries (JOHNSON et al. 1988).

YOUSEM et al. (1988) reported a large series of 597 patients with transitional cell carcinoma (TCC) of the bladder. Twenty-three (3.9%) developed an upper-tract TCC after a mean delay of 61 months. Synchronous TCCs were found in 2.3% of patients with bladder TCC, 39% of those with ureteral TCC, and 24% of those with renal TCC.

6.7.1.2 Squamous Cell Carcinoma

In their review of 90 cases of squamous cell carcinoma of the bladder, JOHNSON et al. (1976) found that most (90%) were solitary lesions that had developed in patients without prior bladder cancer (82%). They were invariably invasive at the time of diagnosis with ureteral obstruction frequent (42%). There was an almost equal sex distribution. The overall 5 year survival rate was only 10.6%. In another series, the 5-year survival for patients with submucosal and/or muscular invasion was 37%, while for those with perivesical invasion it was 13%; no patient with extravesical disease survived 5 years (FAYSAL 1981).

Pure squamous cell carcinoma of the urinary bladder is usually a devastating neoplasm regardless of stage and histologic grade at diagnosis and the treatment modality selected. Squamous transformation of transitional epithelium can be found associated with high-grade transitional cell carcinomas and may be the result of squamous metaplasia. MOSTOFI (1954) concluded that squamous cell tumors may arise directly from the transitional epithelium, after squamatization and leukoplakia of surface epithelium or through altered differentiation of transitional cell carcinoma. Pure squamous cell carcinoma of the urinary bladder behaves in the same way as a poorly differentiated transitional cell carcinoma with squamous metaplasia. Survival in both is significantly poorer than in the case of poorly differentiated transitional cell carcinoma alone and only radical surgical extirpation can be associated with significant patient salvage (TANNENBAUM et al. 1983). TANNENBAUM (1976) noted a predominance of high-grade lesions at time of diagnosis in squamous cell carcinoma of the urinary bladder.

6.7.1.3 Carcinoma in Situ

Carcinoma in situ (CIS) is a variant of transitional cell carcinoma that is characterized by intraepithelial neoplastic transformation that does not extend into the bladder lumen or penetrate the basement membrane. It may be an aggressive neoplasm that may extend onto the ureters, urethra or prostatic ducts or invade the bladder muscle and disseminate to distant sites (Utz and Zincke 1974; Fowler 1989). Only 2% of transitional cell carcinomas exist as CIS alone when they are initially discovered (Utz and Zincke 1974). The distribution of CIS in the urinary bladder is consistent with the known distribution of invasive carcinoma (Melamed et al. 1964). The large majority of these patients have symptoms of cystitis or prostatitis (Utz and Farrow 1984). CIS is a disease of adults, most having microscopic hematuria and pyuria. Because of anaplasia and decreased adhesiveness, malignant cells can usually be identified on urine cytology and bladder washings are optimal (Fowler 1989; Herr 1983). Cystoscopically CIS often appears as a velvety mucosal erythema. The involved mucosa may also appear normal and random biopsies are required. Carcinoma in situ is responsive to treatment by intravesical administration of chemotherapeutic agents or bacillus Calmette-Guerin (BCG). Extirpative surgery may be needed if response is incomplete (Fowler 1989).

Melicow (1952) reported malignant cells confined to the mucosa in the bladders of patients who had had cystectomy for invasive carcinoma. This process was termed carcinoma in situ. The presence and natural history of CIS have become extremely important in our understanding of bladder cancer because the bladder is often left in place when biopsy shows no invasion or only superficial (lamina propria) invasion. There may be undetected areas of carcinoma in situ elsewhere in the bladder. Therapy is usually directed at maintaining the bladder as a reservoir organ as long as possible. It is recognized that bladder tumors frequently recur, but many patients with low-grade carcinoma will have an indolent clinical course. Cystectomy is usually delayed until muscle invasion has been documented (Cummings 1983).

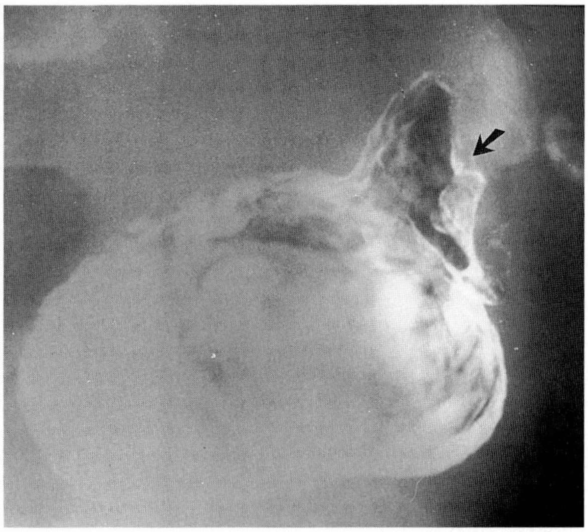

Fig. 6.23. Double-contrast barium-air cystogram demonstrating a scalloped defect in a diverticulum arising from the anterior dome segment of the bladder. This is a classical location for an adenocarcinoma arising from a urachal remnant and projecting into a urachal diverticulum. (Courtesy of Dr. E.K. Lang)

6.7.1.4 Adenocarcinoma

Ward (1971) feels that most adenocarcinomas of the urinary bladder develop from sequential changes initiated by chronic inflammation, that is, from Brunn's nests, to cystitis glandularis and cystica, and, finally, to adenocarcinoma, which is usually mucin secreting. Mostofi (1954) felt that adenomas and adenocarcinomas may arise by the above route or after direct cuboidal or columnar metaplasia of the surface epithelium. Adenocarcinomas of the urinary bladder are usually located in the trigone area. Anderstrom et al. (1983) detailed this process and pointed out that the occurrence of adenocarcinomas of the renal pelvis and ureter along with ureteropyelitis cystica and glandularis of the upper urinary tract favor this totipotentiality-metaplasia theory. Adenocarcinoma may arise in exstrophic bladders or at the dome of bladders with urachal remnants (Rosai 1989) (Fig. 6.23). Adenocarcinoma is the most common malignant tumor arising in the exstrophic bladder and occurs more frequently in areas where schistosomiasis is endemic (Anderstrom et al. 1983).

Advanced cases of adenocarcinoma appear grossly as fungating masses that ulcerate the mucosa and invade the bladder wall. The surface of mucin producing tumors is usually covered with thick, slimy, gelatinous material (THOMAS 1971). Mucus-containing cells and glandular structures are not uncommon findings in predominately transitional carcinomas of the bladder. The diagnosis of adenocarcinoma should be reserved for those malignant tumors in which the glandular component predominates (ROSAI 1989).

The overall prognosis in adenocarcinoma of the bladder is poor. The pattern and frequency of metastases are similar to those in the case of high-grade transitional cell carcinoma. In one series of 64 patients, the 5-year survival rate was only 18% (ANDERSTROM et al. 1983). All the tumors were invasive at the time of diagnosis and 64% penetrated the muscular wall, regardless of the primary tumor location. Two-thirds of the tumors were poorly differentiated. ANDERSTROM et al. (1983) concluded that adenocarcimona of the urinary bladder is a predominantly solitary, poorly differentiated, deeply invasive, large tumor which is consequently associated with an exceedingly poor prognosis. Adenocarcinomas have a more advanced stage at time of diagnosis than transitional cell cancers. In the dome and posterior walls of the bladder, extension of colorectal cancer must be excluded by appropriate studies. Adenocarcinomas of the ovary, prostate, and urethra may also extend through the bladder wall. Adenocarcinoma in the mid anterior dome of the bladder probably derives from urachal remnants.

6.7.2 Etiology

Because of its reservoir function, the urinary bladder mucosa is exposed for long periods to any carcinogens excreted by the kidneys. It follows that most cancers of the bladder involve the bladder base, which is the most dependent portion where carcinogens layer out in highest concentration.

Cigarette smoking and occupational exposure to arylamines are well-established risk factors for the development of bladder cancer. In the United States, it is estimated that more than 50% of cases in men and more than 35% of cases in women are due to either cigarette smoking or industrial exposure (ROSS et al. 1988). DOLL and PETO (1981) have even estimated that 55% of the deaths from bladder cancer are due to cigarette smoking alone.

Smokers develop bladder cancer at two to three times the rate of the disease in nonsmokers and the link is probably causal. There may be genetic factors involved in cigarette induced bladder cancer. Genetically regulated liver *N*-acetyltransferase activity may be involved in carcinogenic detoxification of aromatic amines. People with less detoxifying acetylation activity would then be at higher risk for developing bladder cancer (ROSS et al. 1988).

Occupational exposure in high risk industries is estimated to account for 18%–34% of the bladder cancer in males (COLE et al. 1972; COLE 1973). Arylamines or aromatic amines are the class of chemical carcinogens most strongly related to bladder cancer.

In summary, those at elevated risk for bladder cancer include those who work with dyes, metal, paints, leather, textiles, and organic chemicals, clerical workers, hairdressers, and truck drivers. Cooks, kitchen workers, clerical workers, and employees in aluminum and gas industries may also be at increased risk (COLE et al. 1972; WIGLE 1977). However, many of the studies are inconsistent or contradictory (MORRISON 1984; ROSS et al. 1988). Any association between coffee drinking and risk of bladder cancer is at best weak. Use of analgesics containing aspirin, phenacetin and caffeine may increase risk.

There may be a causal association between urinary tract infections and bladder cancer (OYASU and HOPP 1974; HICKS et al. 1977). In a given case, however, the infection may be secondary due to breakdown of host resistance factors caused by the presence of the cancer. Azo dyes can be broken down into aromated amines by a variety of bacteria, including *E. coli* (OYASU and HOPP 1974). Nitrosamines can be formed from tobacco alkaloids or from ingested nitrites and secondary amines under the acidic conditions in the stomach or by bacterial synthesis.

Artificial sweeteners, especially saccharine, may cause bladder cancer in rodents, but this has not been extrapolated to or proven in humans (ROSS et al. 1988).

Schistosomiasis is strongly associated with squamous cell carcinoma of the urinary bladder after severe and longstanding infestations (GELFAND et al. 1967). In theory the chronic irritation and resultant epithelial proliferation associated with the deposition of ova in the bladder wall is oncogenic (BRAND 1979). The resulting chronic foreign body reaction and fibrosis have been postulated to block lymphatics and thereby permit carcinogenic chemical or metabolites to accumulate (BRAND 1979).

A strong association appears to exist between any chronic irritation or infection of the bladder, besides bilharziasis, and the development of both transitional and squamous cell carcinoma. The association has been predominantly between the existence of a neurogenic bladder, the need for a chronic indwelling catheter, the concomitant presence of chronic infection and a subsequent squamous cell cancer. Squamous cell cancer was found on random biopsy in six of 62 spinal cord injury patients, five of whom had had indwelling urethral catheters for more that 10 years. Squamous metaplasia occurred in 80% of those catheterized for more than 10 years compared to 40% of those catheterized for shorter periods and 20% of those not catheterized at all. In the urethras of the same patients, squamous metaplasia was found in 67%, 36%, and 44% respectively (KAUFMAN et al. 1977).

Bladder cancer has been described as the result of cyclophosphamide therapy (DURKEE and BENSON 1980) and pelvic irradiation (FOKKENS and HOP 1979). Treatment with isoniazid (INH), addiction to opium, and ingestion of bracken fern have also been cited as agents elevating the risk of bladder cancer (JOHNSON et al. 1988).

It is most likely that bladder cancer arises as the result of multiple sequential exposures to low doses of one or more carcinogens perhaps promoted by cofactors not in themselves carcinogenic. The large number of environmental carcinogens and the prolonged latency periods involved support the concept of a multistep process (HICKS 1981).

6.7.3 Staging and Grading Bladder Malignancy

Bladder carcinoma spreads by local extension through the basement membrane of the mucosa to the muscular layer and then to the perivesical fat (Fig. 6.24). It is subsequently disseminated lymphatically and hematogenously (JOHNSON et al. 1988). Local lymphatic spread is into the superior and inferior gluteal, obturator, and external and common iliac node chains. From there, metastases enter the para-aortic chain to the thoracic duct and the general circulation. Should local nodes become obstructed, the tumor cells are shunted onto the vascular compartment. Hematogenous spread is either by the pelvic plexus into the inferior vena cava and general circulation or via the perivertebral veins into the azygos, hemiazygos, intercostal, and other systemic veins. Hematogenously spread metastatic lesions occur in lung, skeleton, liver, and brain (GOLDMAN et al. 1979).

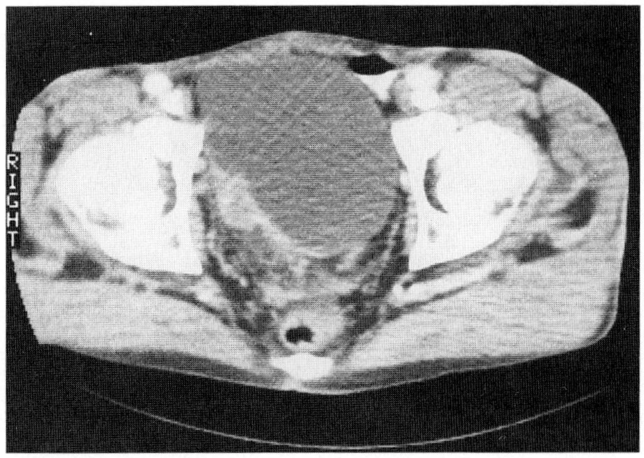

Fig. 6.24. A dynamic computed tomogram demonstrating a small, relatively flat, but infiltrating bladder tumor involving the right lateral bladder wall. Note extension through the entire muscularis and into the perivesical fat. This would be difficult to appreciate by investigations other than CT and MRI. The striate appearance in the abutting perivesical fat is consistent with either lymphatic tumor extension or lymphatic edema. (Courtesy of Dr. E.K. LANG)

Staging describes extent of disease. The higher the stage, the more widespread the disease and the poorer the prognosis. The standard staging systems for bladder cancer are the Jewett-Strong-Marshall classification proposed by JEWETT and STRONG in 1946 then subsequently modified by JEWETT and by MARSHALL in 1952 (JEWETT and STRONG 1946; JEWETT 1952; MARSHALL 1952) and the TNM (WALLACE et al. 1975). The TNM system encompasses the status of the primary tumor (T), the lymph nodes (N), and any metastasis (M) (JOHNSON et al. 1988).

Although the division of stage B according to whether there is extension to one-half the muscular layer or beyond seems arbitrary and difficult to evaluate; it is based on Jewett's (1952) observation that stage B_1 patients had 80% survival but stage B_2 patients only 8% survival (Figs. 6.25–6.27). This extension of the initial staging system was based on 80 patients who had had complete extirpation of the primary tumor. In the same year MARSHALL (1952) extended JEWETT's observations and modified the JEWITT-STRONG system to include stage 0 for those tumors not infiltrating the lamina propria. Preoperative staging was done by careful bimanual examination and biopsy (CUMMINGS 1983).

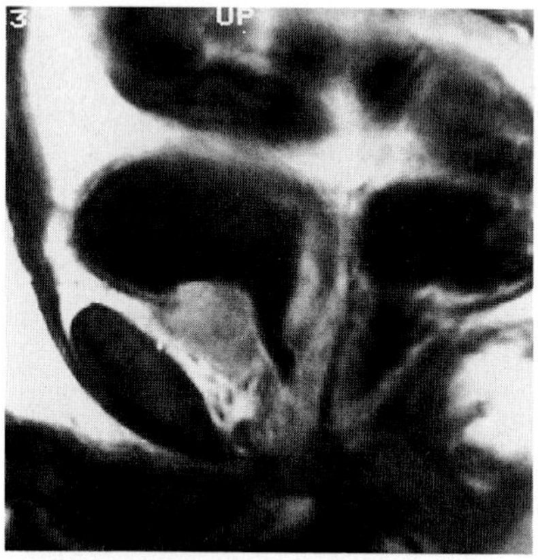

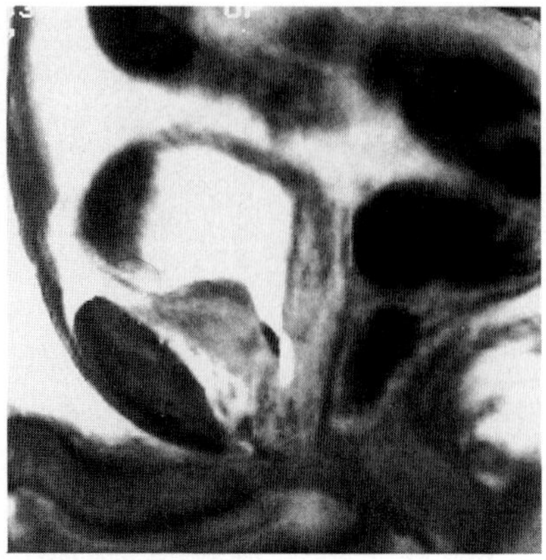

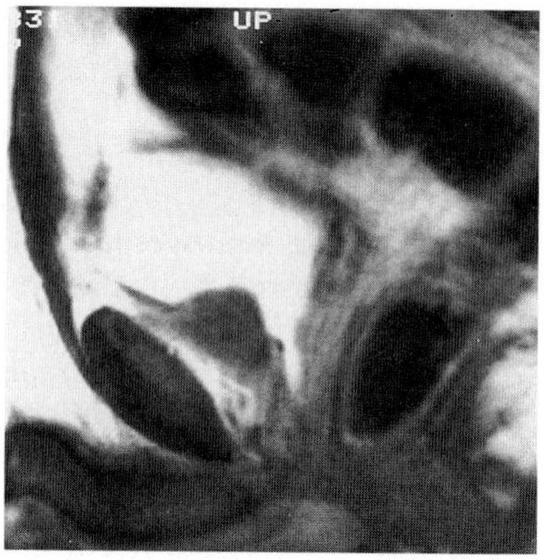

Fig. 6.25 (*left*). A sagittal T1-weighted MRI scan 2 min after administration of gadolinium-DTPA demonstrates a large tumor involving the floor of the bladder and a second relatively flat tumor involving the posterior wall and ascending to the plafond. The perivesical fat appears intact suggesting a B_1 or possibly B_2 type of tumor. As is known from arteriographic studies, hypervascular bladder tumors tend to enhance in capillary transit phase; thus their demonstration on MRI benefits from intravenous administration of gadolinium DTPA. (Courtesy of Dr. D. HAHN)

Fig. 6.26 (*middle*). Same case as Fig. 6.25. A 6-min delayed MRI scan after gadolinium-DTPA administration once again demonstrates the two tumor-bearing areas to advantage. There is now very minimal loss of signal intensity in the perivesical fat along the anterior circumference of the tumor. (Courtesy of Dr. D. HAHN)

Fig. 6.27 (*right*). Same case as Figs. 6.25 and 6.26. A 10-min delayed sagittal MRI scan after gadolinium-DTPA administration shows the bladder to be filled with gadolinium. The intraluminal tumor component contours against the high-signal-intensity bladder urine. (Courtesy of Dr. D. HAHN)

The basis of the Jewett and Strong staging system was their observations in 1944 on autopsy material from 107 cases analyzing the relationship of depth of penetration (stage) to the incidence of local extension and metastases. They concluded that: (a) stage A (submucosal infiltration) was not associated with dissemination; (b) stage B (muscular infiltration) was associated with dissemination in 13% of cases (2 of 15 patients); and (c) stage C (perivesical infiltration) exhibited dissemination in 74% of cases (64 of 89 patients) (JEWETT and STRONG 1946; CUMMINGS 1983).

In JEWETT and STRONG's first series (1946), the primary tumors were segregated into three pathologic stages and the incidence of concomitant lymph node or hematogenous metastases studied for each group. No patient staged A had evidence of metastasis, whereas 13% of those staged B and 74% of those staged C had metastases. JEWETT later (1952) recommended that stage B be divided into superficial and deep categories because B_1 tumors acted much like A tumors and B_2 tumors acted much like C tumors. Of the 80 patients in his report, 14 of the 19 (74%) patients with stage A or B disease survived 5 years, as against only 2 of 61 (3%) in whom the tumor invaded the deep muscle or beyond. Four of the five patients with B_1 disease survived 5 years, compared to one of the 13 with B_2 disease. The total series was 80 and the B lesions were 18 in number (LIESKOVSKY et al. 1988).

MARSHALL (1952) modified the Jewett and Strong system by adding stage 0 to include tumors not infiltrating the lamina propria, patients without tumor in the definitive cystectomy specimen, and patients with carcinoma in situ. He also added stage D to designate metastases. Stage D_1 disease is confined to the pelvis (including invasion of the pelvic walls or rectus muscle below the sacral promontory) (Fig. 6.28). Stage D_2 lesions extend beyond the limits of the pelvis, including distant metastases and lesions above the sacral promontory. The aortic bifurcation was later arbitrarily chosen instead of the sacral promontory to separate stage D_1 from D_2 (SKINNER 1977; LIESKOVSKY 1988). This staging system is summarized in Table 6.2.

The TNM system was originally devised by DENOIX in 1950 and was subsequently adopted by the Union Internationale Contre le Cancer. (UICC) (DENOIX 1978). The classification is based on the assessment of the extent of the primary tumor (T), the condition of the regional nodes (N), and the presence or absence of metastases (M) (LIESKOVSKY et al. 1988).

Table 6.2. Staging of bladder cancer: Jewitt and Strong system as modified by MARSHALL

Stage 0	Tumor is superficial, limited to the mucosa. Includes papillary and in situ lesions
Stage A	Extension into the lamina propria but not into the bladder musculature
Stage B_1	Extension into the musculature but less than half way
Stage B_2	Extension into the musculature more than half way but not invading the perivesical fat
Stage C	Extension through the musculature into the perivesical fat
Stage D_1	Extension beyond perivesical fat but still confined to the pelvis at or below the level of the sacral promontory. Includes extension into contiguous organs, pelvic wall, and lymph nodes below the common iliac bifurcation
Stage D_2	Distant metastases, involvement of organs or lymph nodes beyond the pelvis

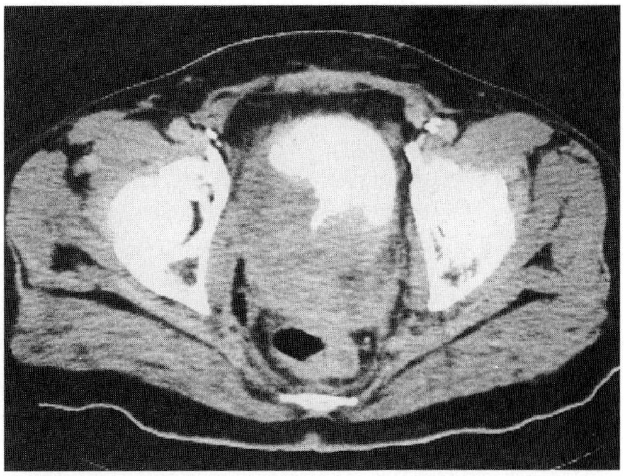

Fig. 6.28. A postenhancement computed tomogram demonstrating an extensive bladder tumor with contiguous extension to and invasion of the right lateral pelvic wall, the prostate, and the posterior elements of the vesical fascia. (Courtesy of Dr. E.K. LANG)

Table 6.3. Staging of bladder cancer: TNM system

Description	TNM stage	JSM stage
No tumor	T_0	0
Carcinoma in situ	T_{1s}	0
Papillary tumor, noninvasive	T_{1A}	0
Papillary tumor, lamina propria invasion	T_1	A
Superficial muscle invasion	T_2	B_1
Deep muscle invasion	T_{3A}	B_2
Perivesical fat invasion	T_{3B}	C
Invasion of contiguous viscera	T_{4A}	D_1
Invasion of pelvic/abdominal wall	T_{4B}	D_1
Single ipsilateral regional adenopathy to bilateral multiple pelvic adenopathy	N_{1-3}	D_1
Juxtaregional adenopathy, above aortic bifurcation	N_4	D_2
Distant metastases	M_1	D_2

JSM, Jewett-Strong-Marshall.

Table 6.4. Grading systems for transitional cell tumors of the bladder. (After ROSAI 1989)

ASH (1940)	MOSTOFI (1960) American Tumor Registry	BERGKVIST et al. (1965)
Transitional cell carcinoma, grade I	Papilloma	Transitional cell tumor, grade 0 Transitional cell tumor, grade I
Transitional cell carcinoma, grade II	Transitional cell carcinoma, grade I	Transitional cell carcinoma, grade II
Transitional cell carcinoma, grade III	Transitional cell carcinoma, grade II	Transitional cell carcinoma, grade III
Transitional cell carcinoma, grade IV	Transitonal cell carcinoma, grade III	Transitional cell carcinoma, grade IV

According to the UICC classification system for bladder cancer, the extent of the primary tumor, T, is assessed by clinical examination, imaging studies, cystoscopy and bimanual examination under anesthesia in addition to biopsy of the tumor. The condition of the regional nodes, N, is evaluated by clinical examination with or without imaging, The extent of metastases M is determined by clinical examination, and imaging (LIESKOVSKY et al. 1988) (Table 6.3).

Several tumor characteristics have predictive value with respect to disease progression including: (a) grade, (b) shape (papillary vs sessile), (c) size (<2 cm vs >5 cm), (d) presence of any degree of invasion, and (e) associated mucosal abnormalities (CUMMINGS 1983).

There are several systems for the grading of transitional cell carcinoma primarily based on the cytologic appearance of the tumor rather that its architecture or invasiveness. All three characteristics are taken into account in grading an individual tumor. The most widely used system was proposed by ASH in 1940. He felt that the most benign-appearing papillary tumors should be classified as carcinoma because of their great tendency to recur locally and also because the microscopic pattern does not always conform with the clinical behavior. The tumors are graded I–IV

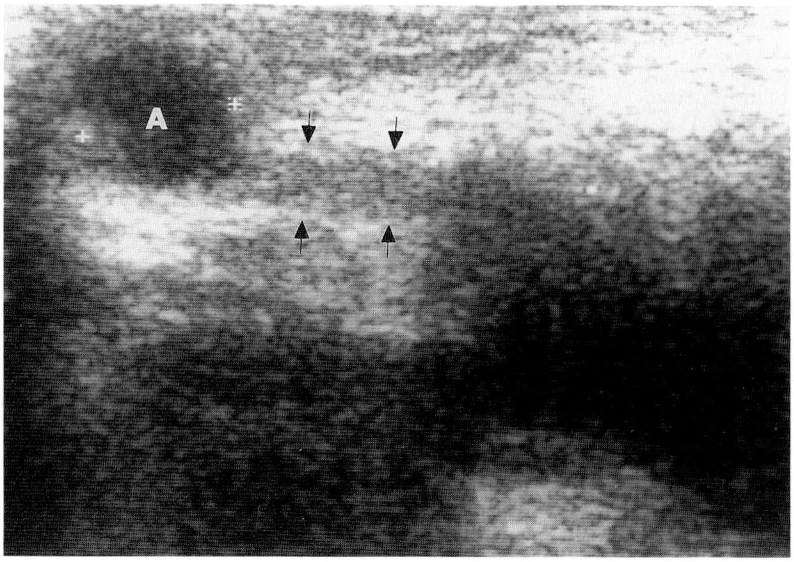

Fig. 6.29. Infected urachal sinus with umbilical abscess. Midline sagittal scan demonstrating umbilical abscess (*A*) and thickened (8 mm) omphalovesical tract (*arrows*). (Avni et al. 1988)

by degree of differentiation, pleomorphism and pattern of organization. In the system proposed by Mostofi (1960) and adopted by The American Tumor Registry, the better differentiated papillary tumors are designated as papillomas. This system is probably the most familiar to clinical urologists. Bergkvist et al. (1965) avoided the distinction between benign and malignant categories by designating all as transitional cell tumors and grading them from 0 to IV (Rosai 1989). These grading systems are summarized in Table 6.4.

Staging and grading assists the clinician in treatment planning and provides prognostic information through evaluation of treatment results (Skinner 1977).

6.7.4 Urachal Remnant and Urachal Carcinoma

Adenocarcinomas of the bladder may be subdivided according to whether they originate from urothelium or from remnants of the allantoic duct or urachus (Nocks et al. 1983).

The urachus represents the remnant of the embryonic allantois and cloaca. It persists in adulthood as a midline musculofibrous tube that can extend from the bladder dome to the umbilicus in the space of Retzius between the transversalis fascia anteriorly and the peritoneum posteriorly. Neoplasm may arise anywhere along its course (Rafal and Markisz 1991). It extends from the dome of the bladder to the umbilicus as the medial collateral ligament (DiSantis et al. 1991). The adult urachus has intramucosal, intramuscular, and supravesical segments with respect to the bladder (Korobkin et al. 1988).

Patent urachus, umbilical urachal sinus, and vesicourachal diverticulum are urachal abnormalities that are usually seen in childhood. Urachal cysts may go undetected until infection occurs or a mass is detected (Fig. 6.29). Percutaneous needle aspiration biopsy can be diagnostic with percutaneous drainage performed if applicable (Spataro et al. 1983).

Cacciarelli et al. (1990) found a small, elliptical, hypoechoic, structure on the middle of the anterosuperior surface of the urinary bladder in 62 of 100 consecutive pediatric sonograms. Surgical removal and pathologic examination in one case disclosed a normal urachal remnant.

Carcinoma of the urachus is situated in the juxta- or intravesical urachus in 90% of cases, in the middle in 6%, and near the umbilicus in 4% (Rao 1986). It accounts for 0.17%–0.34% of all bladder cancers and 20%–39% of all primary bladder adenocarcinomas (Brick et al. 1988).

Almost two-thirds of the patients with urachal cancer are males and two-thirds are between the ages of 40 and 70 years (Korobkin et al. 1988). The reported age range is 4 months to 84 years (Brick et al. 1988). Adenocarcinoma accounts for

85% of these cancers and is most commonly mucinous. Sarcoma, squamous cell carcinoma, transitional cell carcinoma, and signet ring cell carcinomas are also described. In 90% of the cases, the tumor arises from the juxtavesical segment of the urachus. Therefore, the lesion usually arises in a clinically silent location and is usually discovered after it has extended into the bladder lumen or presents with symptoms related to its large size or to its extension into adjacent structures. It is usually high grade and high stage when it is discovered (KOROBKIN et al. 1988).

Urachal carcinomas spread by local extension into the space of Retzius, peritoneum, abdominal wall, or urinary bladder. Metastases occur late and may involve lungs, bone, omentum, liver, regional lymph nodes, skin, and brain (RAFAL and MARKISZ 1991).

The usual presentation is with painless hematuria, occasionally with dysuria and urinary frequency. Less common findings are suprapubic mass or abdominal pain (BRICK et al. 1988). Gross or microscopic mucus is found in the urine of only 25% of patients but is highly suggestive of the diagnosis in the presence of a palpable suprapubic mass. Discharge of blood, mucus or pus from the umbilicus occurs in a few patients (KOROBKIN et al. 1988).

Based on the work of MOSTOFI et al. (1955), the following criteria have been described for classifying a malignancy as a urachal tumor: (a) tumor in the vertex of the bladder, (b) absence of cystitis cystica and cystitis glandularis, (c) invasion of muscle or deeper structures and either intact or ulcerated epithelium, (d) presence of urachal remnants, (e) presence of a suprapubic mass, (f) a sharp demarcation between tumor and normal surface epithelium, and (g) tumor growth in the bladder wall branching into the space of Retzius. JOHNSON et al. (1985) feel these criteria are too restrictive. SCHUBERT et al. (1982) observed intramucosal or intramural urachal remnants in the bladder in only 32% of their autopsy material; of these, the remnants were in the midline on the vertex in 54%, in the posterior wall in 44%, and in the anterior wall in 2%. Since inflammation and cystitis cystica are found together, one should expect occasional areas of cystitis cystica in bladders with urachal carcinoma. The presence of a proliferative variant should not exclude a diagnosis of urachal carcinoma unless a definite transition to malignancy is demonstrated. They therefore proposed the following criteria: (a) location of the tumor in the bladder wall, (b) findings of a sharp demarcation between the tumor and the surface epithelium, and (c) exclusion of a primary adenocarcinoma located elsewhere that has spread secondarily to the bladder.

The exact pathogenesis of urachal carcinoma is not entirely clear. SCHUBERT et al. (1982) found intramural tubular or cystic urachal remnants in the wall of 39 (32%) of 122 autopsy bladders. Development of urachal carcinomas secondary to carcinogens in the urine also seems highly unlikely, as does development of tumors secondary to stasis of urine with calculus formation and inflammation. The cylindrical metaplasia of the transitional epithelium lining the urachal canal found in 31.6% of SCHUBERT et al.'s cases provides a morphologic basis for the formation of urachal adenocarcinomas.

Possible plain film and urographic findings in urachal carcinoma include lateral ureteral deviation, supravesical mass effect, and pelvic calcification (RAFAL and MARKISZ 1991). Less than 5% of plain films show supravesical calcification or, more rarely, soft tissue mass (KOROBKIN et al. 1988).

The anterior location of urachal tumors and their relationship to the bladder make them ideal for detection and characterization by ultrasound. Ultrasound is felt to be sufficient to diagnose urachal cysts, but CT is preferred for solid urachal lesions because of its ability to stage the lesion and detect spread to the umbilicus, peritoneal cavity, liver and lymph nodes (KOROBKIN et al. 1988; LANG 1984b).

Sonography is unaffected by possible interference by bowel loops since the urachus is extraperitoneal. Ultrasound (Fig. 6.30) may show a complex midline mass above the bladder, with or without extension toward the umbilicus. If calcified, the mass may contain high-amplitude echoes with or without shadowing. Invasion of the bladder may sometimes be detected (RAFAL and MARKISZ 1991). AVNI et al. (1988) stress that because of its ease of demonstration, ultrasound should be part of the initial evaluation of any suspected urachal or other midline anomaly. It can also demonstrate thickened omphalovesical tracts. WINSLOW (1989) has described the appearance of urachal carcinoma on endovesical ultrasonography used in preoperative assessment but this technique is not widely available or applied.

Computed tomography can accurately stage a lesion, showing its intra- and extravesical extent

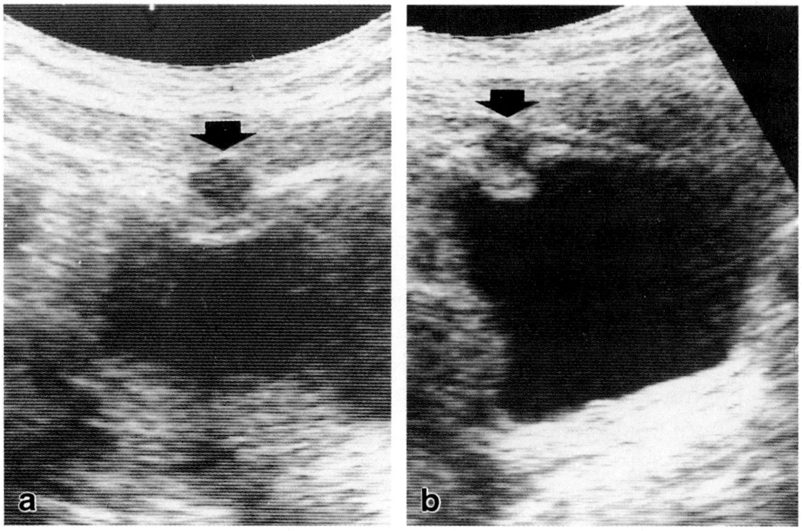

Fig. 6.30 a,b. Urachal remnant. **a** Transverse ultrasound scan demonstrates urachal remnant (*arrow*) in the midline. **b** Sagittal scan demonstrates that the urachal remnant (*arrow*) is anterosuperior to the bladder. (CACCIARELLI et al. 1990)

and can also demonstrate involvement of the lymph nodes, liver, umbilicus, and peritoneal cavity. CT typically shows a solid, cystic or mixed attenuation mass near the midline anteriorly, just beneath the linea alba in intimate association with the anterior and superior aspect of the bladder (Fig. 6.31). About 60% of the time the mass will have regions of low attenuation probably reflecting the high mucin content of most urachal carcinomas. The internal presence of gas or oral contrast material may indicate the presence of an enteric fistula. Calcifications may be demonstrated which are not visible on plain films. The patterns of calcification are variable, including curvilinear, punctate, and peripheral arrangements. With intravenous contrast, a rim may enhance around the supravesical part of the tumor (RAFAL and MARKISZ 1991; LANG 1984b).

KOROBKIN et al. (1988), who reviewed nine cases of urachal carcinoma studied by CT, found that in all cases CT demonstrated a mass in intimate association with the anterior and superior aspects of the bladder, extending in a tubular fashion anterosuperiorly toward the umbilicus. In eight cases, the mass had a soft tissue or inhomogeneous density. In the other, which had been described as cystic, the published picture appeared noncystic. All masses were large, abut 10 cm in greatest diameter. Extension of the mass ventrad and cephalad along the space of Retzius was reflected in an elongated or sausage-like lesion contiguous with or just deep to the rectus abdominus muscles, extending toward the umbilicus. The CT appearance of a lesion extending into the space of Retzius and invading the muscles of the anterior abdominal wall is shown in Fig. 6.32.

In the ten patients reported by BRICK et al. (1988), all tumors were mucinous adenocarcinomas, four were solid, three were cystic, and three were mixed; seven contained calcification on CT examination.

There are few descriptions of MRI findings. In general, the masses have been heterogeneous with increasing signal intensity with increasing T2 weighting. The biggest advantage of using MRI lies in its ability to image in multiple planes. The relationship of the tumor to the bladder and its extension toward the umbilicus can be precisely determined on sagittal images (RAFAL and MARKISZ 1991).

RAFAL and MARKISZ (1991) recommend the use of both CT and MRI in the evaluation of suspected urachal carcinoma.

So then, a solid elongated mass arising in or adjacent to the bladder apex and extending toward the anterior abdominal wall and umbilicus is highly suggestive of urachal carcinoma. But other diagnoses should be considered. An infected urachal cyst may have an attenuation value similar to carcinoma. A primary bladder carcinoma arising in the bladder apex will usually have less of an extravesical component. Ovarian carcinoma is sometimes midline and supravesical but is usually cystic or multiloculated. Ovarian cancer is, obviously limited to females whereas urachal cancer is more common in males. A peritoneal metastasis can occur in the supravesical midline so an adenocarcinoma of the gastrointestinal tract should always be excluded (KOROBKIN et al. 1988).

It is occasionally difficult to distinguish an infected urachal cyst from a urachal carcinoma. The presence of hematuria, mural nodularity, and calcification and the lack of any inflammatory change in adjacent tissues will favor the diagnosis of urachal carcinoma (RAO 1986).

At cystoscopy, the tumor may appear as a bladder wall protrusion, flat epithelioma, or exophytic mass. If present, the urachal orifice may be viewed. The discharge of mucoid material upon pressure application over the suprapubic region is diagnostic (RAFAL and MARKISZ 1991).

Treatment of urachal carcinoma is primarily surgical with many authorities recommending en

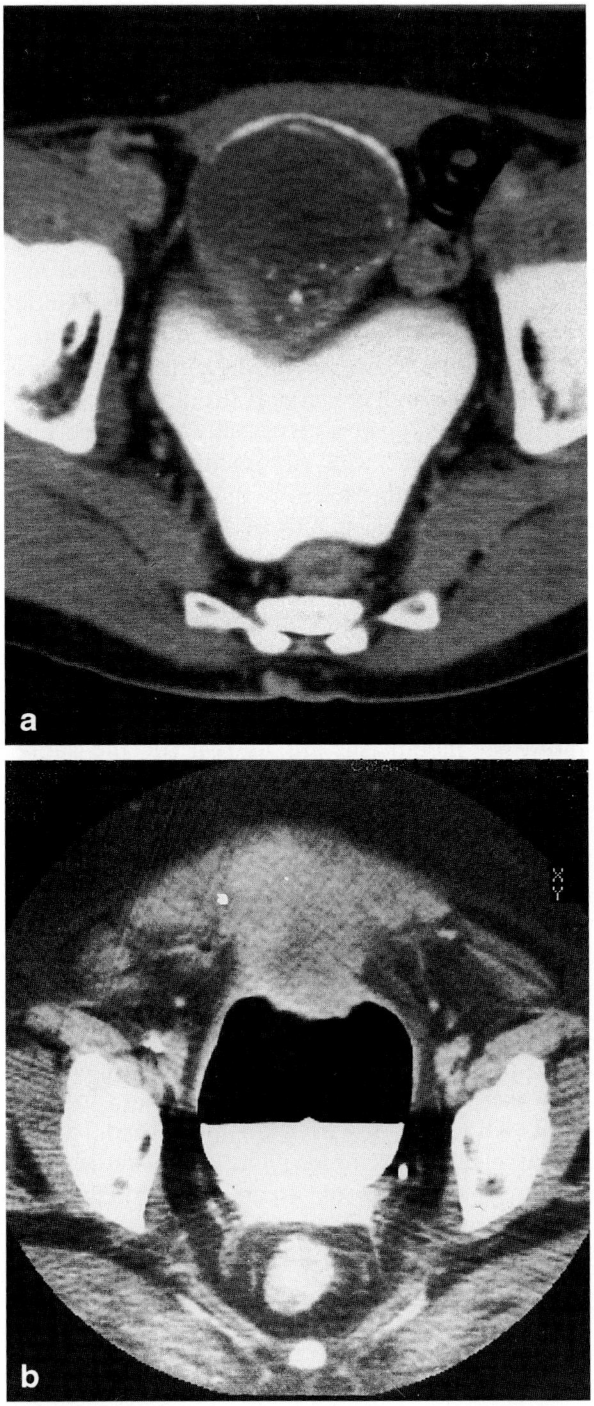

Fig. 6.31a,b. Computed tomography of urachal carcinoma. **a** Cystic anterior midline mass with linear and punctate calcification (courtesy of Drs. L.F. CAMPBELL and S.T. COCHRAN). **b** Solid anterior midline mass with punctate calcification. (Courtesy of Dr. E.K. LANG)

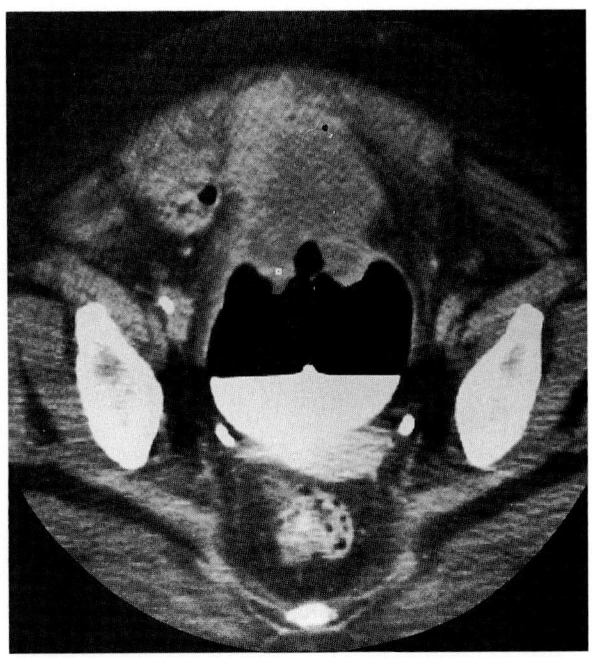

Fig. 6.32. A postenhancement computed tomogram demonstrating contiguous extension into the space of Retzius of a tumor originating from the anterior circumference of the dome of the bladder, with contiguous invasion of muscles of the anterior abdominal wall. (Courtesy of Dr. E.K. LANG)

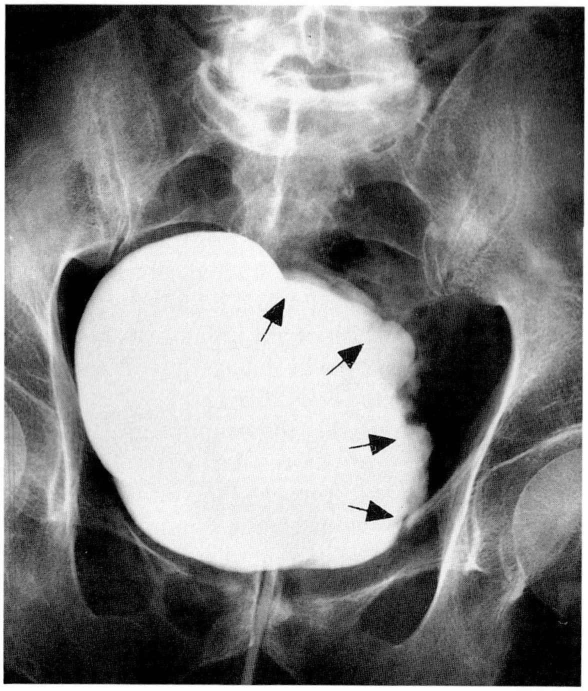

Fig. 6.33. Cystitis glandularis in bladder (*arrows*). (Courtesy of Dr. S.T. Cochran)

bloc partial or total cystectomy with pelvic lymphadenectomy and umbilectomy. Metastases usually appear late, involving lung, omentum, liver, bone, and regional lymph nodes. Local recurrence is common after surgical excision and usually occurs within 2 years (Korobkin et al. 1988). The prognosis is poor and the 5-year survival rates have varied from 6.5% to 15% (Kwok-Liu et al. 1980).

6.7.5 Benign Proliferative Variants

The benign proliferative variants comprise a spectrum of microscopic epithelial changes. The initial microscopic change is focal proliferation of the basal layer of the transitional epithelium, which may produce buds that become solid nodules of tissue (Brunn's nests or islands) located within the lamina propria. Some of these nodules develop a central cystic area filled with accumulated mucin. If the cells lining the cyst maintain a transitional appearance, the condition is called cystitis cystica. If the cells lining the cyst have morphologic features similar to those of colonic epithelium, it is called either cystitis glandularis (Fig. 6.33) or intestinal (glandular, colonic) metaplasia. A mucus-producing colonic type of epithelium may occur. These conditions are felt to represent various stages of manifestation of the same basic process (Rosai 1989).

Mostofi (1954) described the transitional epithelium of the urinary bladder as having multiple potentialities, being capable of nonneoplastic proliferation, metaplasia into squamous, columnar, and cuboidal cells and then neoplasia into not only transitional cell but also squamous cell and glandular tumors. He considered cystitis glandularis and cystica as nonneoplastic proliferation.

Squamous metaplasia most commonly involves the trigone and proximal urethra of women (Fowler 1989). Cystoscopically, it appears as a velvety white well marginated lesion which has been called pseudomembranous trigonitis. Squamous metaplasia may be seen in men treated with exogenous estrogen for metastatic prostate cancer and is unusual in prepubertal females. Estrogenic stimulation of the uroepithelium is thought to potentiate its development (Fowler 1989).

It would follow that patients with extensive intestinal metaplasia are at risk for the subsequent development of adenocarcinoma. Complete replacement of areas of urothelium by benign-appearing intestinal mucosa is rare. All of the 11 documented cases were associated with chronic irritation and/or infection such as indwelling catheters, calculi, and/or bladder outlet obstruction. The condition has been identified most frequently in urinary bladder but has occurred in the ureter and renal pelves. The majority of lesions were described as polypoid or sessile masses or appeared grossly as adenomas. Of the three patients who were observed for more than 2 years, all developed carcinoma. The condition of complete replacement of areas of urothelium by benign-appearing intestinal mucosa appears at least to be a high risk factor for development of adenocarcinoma (Bullock et al. 1987).

Rosai (1989) states that these variable metaplastic changes of the transitional epithelium may result from chronic inflammation or mucosal irritation such as ureteral reimplantation, neurogenic bladder, or bladder exstrophy. Furthermore, the metaplasia may regress completely if the stimulating factor is removed.

Brunn's nests, cystitis cystica and cystitis glandularis can occur anywhere in the lamina propria of the bladder mucosa but are most common in the trigone (Ito et al. 1981). Nonkeratinizing squamous epithelium of the vaginal type may

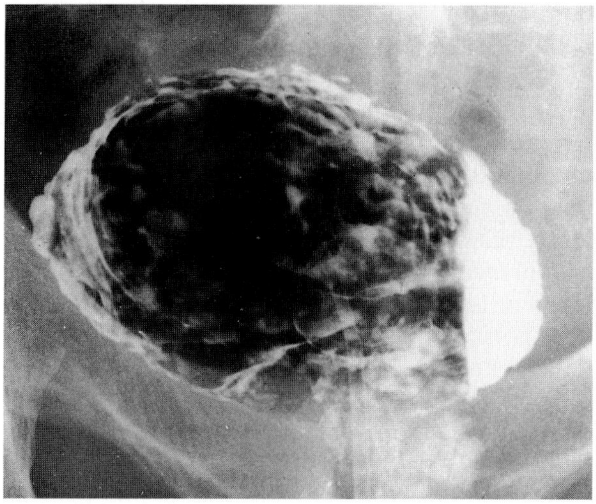

Fig. 6.34. A double contrast barium-air cystogram demonstrating the classical findings of cystitis cystica. (Courtesy of Dr. E.K. LANG)

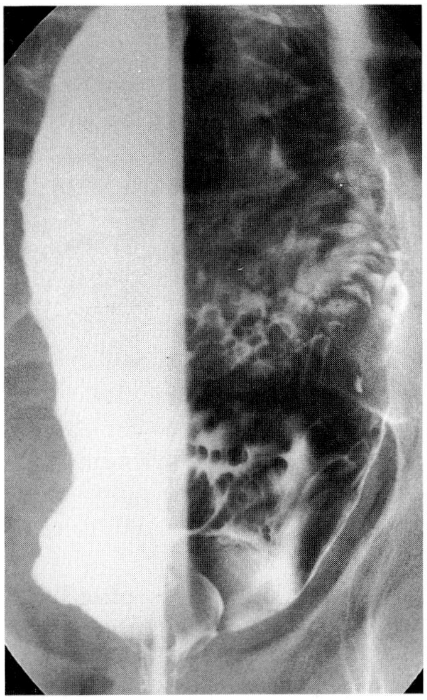

Fig. 6.35. A double contrast barium-air cystogram demonstrating fixation of a massive tumor to the right lateral wall of the bladder. Note evidence of cystitis cystica and cystitis granularis, which are frequently associated with neoplasms. (Courtesy of Dr. E.K. LANG)

occur in the female trigone (WIENER et al. 1979). Cystitis cystica has a female predominance (KAPLAN and KING 1970) which may be related to the female prevalence of urinary tract infections (Fig. 6.34).

Evidence is accumulating that suggests that clinically symptomatic cystitis cystica lesions are a manifestation of a recently appreciated immunologic mechanism by which the urinary tract attempts to react to an infection or irritation within the bladder (WALTHER et al. 1987). HILL (1971) produced the lesions of pyeloureteritis cystica and glandularis by intravenous injection of *E. coli* into rabbits after unilateral ureteral ligation. WALTHER et al. (1987) studied cystitis cystica with electron and immunofluorescence microscopy. The characteristic gland like structures of cystitis cystica are lined by epithelium with features of secretory cells including abundant mitochondria, Golgi apparatuses and rough endoplasmic reticulum. Secretory type granules are seen in the cytoplasm just beneath the luminal membrane of surface columnar cells. Immunofluorescence localizes IgA, IgM, and secretory piece in the epithelium of these cells. These findings may account for the large amounts of IgA and secretory piece found in the urine of some patients with cystitis cystica and urinary tract infection. Brunn's nests may lie dormant until, under the stimulation of infection or irritation, they proliferate and mature in a local attempt to rid the bladder of the offensive agents.

Cystitis glandularis has frequently been found in association with pelvic lipomatosis (CARPENTER 1973; LEVINE et al. 1978; KAUZLARIC et al. 1987; ALLEN and DE KOCK 1987).

In MELICOW et al.'s (1974) review of 910 cases of primary and secondary bladder tumors, hyperplasia of the urothelium and Brunn's nests and the development of cystitis cystica and glandularis were frequently encountered in close proximity to neoplasms, in areas between tumors, in association with foreign bodies, and in infected bladders (cf. Fig. 6.35). Except for the fundus, where remnants of the cloaca may be present, the bladder mucosa of the normal neonate does not display such changes. MELICOW et al. state that squamous cell metaplasia and leukoplakia are often seen in association with chronic irritation. Cancer develops in 15% of cases 15–20 years after discovery of the metaplasia. It may form underneath a plaque of leukoplakia which obscures its presence.

Metaplasia in response to noxious stimuli is the most popular theory to explain this phenomenon of benign proliferative variants of the urothelium. Derivation from embryonic rests of urachus and/or intestinal epithelium in the process of division of the rectum from the urogenital sinus is a less widely held alternative explanation (Erturk et al. 1988; Dann et al. 1972).

The transition of cystitis glandularis into primary adenocarcinoma of the bladder has apparently been well documented by Shaw et al. (1958), Salm (1967), and Parker (1970) and quoted by Erturk et al. (1988) and Dann et al. (1972). Furthermore, O'Brien and Urbanski (1985) reported a case of transitional cell carcinoma in situ of the bladder associated with cystitis glandularis and papillary adenocarcinoma in situ with severe dysplasia in neighboring papillary glandular epithelium. They postulated that the severe dysplasia of the papillary adenomatous component represents an intermediate morphologic pattern between cystitis glandularis and adenocarcinoma of the bladder.

Parker (1970) reviewed 40 cases of cystitis cystica and glandularis, finding glandular metaplasia in eight cases and definite evidence of progression from metaplasia to neoplasm in one. The lesions were found on the trigone in 20 cases, extended to the bladder neck in 14, and were scattered throughout the bladder in the remaining six. Such lesions are characteristically regular and rounded, about 1–5 mm in diameter, translucent with a pearly or yellowish light, and covered by on a thin layer of mucosa. When the cysts are lined by columnar cells, which may or may not secrete mucus, the cysts are more opaque and mucus can sometimes be seen on the surface of red irregular mamillated mucosa. In cystitis follicularis, lymphoid tissue collects beneath the mucosa, forming true lymph follicles with germinal centers. These lesions appear as 2- to 3-mm brownish nodules which are more solid and opaque than the cysts of cystitis cystica. When confluent and in inflamed mucosa, cystitis follicularis may resemble cystitis glandularis and is often wrongly diagnosed. Granular cystitis and bullous edema may also mimic cystitis cystica and glandularis (Parker 1970).

Wiener et al. (1979), who found Brunn's nests, cystitis cystica, and squamous metaplasia in 93 of 100 grossly normal bladders, consider these conditions normal variants and not premalignant. Non-keratinizing squamous metaplasia of the vaginal type was found in 46% of the women but only 7% of the men.

Ito et al. (1981) studied 125 grossly normal-appearing bladders and found some form of benign proliferation or metaplasia to be almost ubiquitous; they concluded that such findings are not premalignant. They can be found anywhere in the bladder but are most common in the trigone.

Morse (1928) found epithelial buds and cell nests of Brunn or cysts in varying numbers microscopically in 108 of 125 (86.4%) almost consecutive bladders at necropsy, of which 63 (58.25%) showed microscopic evidence of inflammation. He concluded they were inflammatory in nature and present in the majority of persons over 25 years of age. He made no comment as to malignant potential.

The benign proliferative variants were once thought to be universally abnormal, and perhaps or probably due to inflammation. Based on the findings of Morse (1928), Wiener et al. (1979) and Ito et al. (1981), that the changes occur with variable frequency in normal bladder epithelium, some (Wiener et al. 1979; Ito et al. 1981; Hahn 1990) feel strongly that they are not premalignant although the conditions may coexist. Wiener et al. (1979) found no satisfactory evidence that inflammation was causally associated with the changes. Others (Mostofi 1954; Shaw et al. 1958; Salm 1967; Erturk et al. 1988) feel they are possibly premalignant (Bell and Wendel 1968; Parker 1970; Dann et al. 1972).

Benign proliferations may remain after the inflammation is gone. When they are found in the otherwise normal bladder, the malignant neoplasia may not have yet manifested itself.

These lesions may produce irregular mamillated masses that may be confused cystoscopically with carcinomas. They can occur anywhere in the bladder, but the area of the trigone is the most commonly affected. In rare instances the entire bladder may be involved (Bell and Wendel 1968). Cystitis glandularis can be seen in any part of the bladder, but most commonly involves the vesicle neck, trigone, lateral recesses, or bladder dome. It has been found involving the entire bladder mucosa and can cause hydronephrosis from ureteral obstruction (Bell and Wendel 1968; Rosai 1989).

It is well known that cystitis cystica and glandularis can produce filling defects on imaging studies, urography, ultrasound, and CT that are indistinguishable from malignancy (Brogdon et al. 1965; Dann et al. 1972; Goff 1983; Manco 1985; Kauzlaric et al. 1987). The affected mucosa may appear thickened and covered by multiple rounded cyst-like elevations and intraluminal mass on sonography (Manco 1985). They may produce single large or multiple small cobblestone masses and even present with hematuria and cause ureteral obstruction (BROGDON et al. 1965; DANN et al. 1972). Cystitis glandularis shares with adenocarcinoma the unique symptom of constant elimination of mucus during and/or following micturition (DANN et al. 1972).

6.7.6 Nephrogenic Adenoma

Nephrogenic adenoma is a rare benign proliferation of the urothelium. The lesion histologically resembles proximal tubules of the nephron, lined by cuboidal or columnar cells. The basement membrane is distinct with rare cytologic atypia. The cells lining the tubules are not capable of the specialized function of either mature nephrogenic tubules or bladder epithelium. The lesion has also been termed "adenomatoid metaplasia," "adenomatoid tumor," and "urothelial metaplasia" (ZIMMERMAN et al. 1989). Some authors prefer to use the term "nephrogenic metaplasia" (YOUNG and SCULLY 1986).

Nephrogenic adenoma is a slow-growing lesion which occurs at any age. The lesion may be found from the renal pelvis to the urethra in papillary, sessile, or polypoid form. It usually occurs in the urinary bladder (ZINGAS et al. 1986).

In an extensive review of the literature, and adding their own cases, YOUNG and SCULLY (1986) found that nephrogenic adenoma has occurred in patients from 4 to 83 years of age with an average of 41 years and a male to female ratio of 2:1. A history of genitourinary operations or procedures such as multiple catheterization was present in 65% of cases, calculi in 14%, trauma in 9%, and renal transplant in 8%. In their reviewed cases, two patients had nonfunctioning bladder, one had schistosomiasis, one had interstitial cystitis, eight had a history of cystitis or chronic urinary tract infection (including tuberculosis in at least three cases), and 11 had prior or concomitant transitional cell carcinoma.

Of YOUNG and SCULLY's (1986) reviewed cases, 60% produced symptoms, including hematuria (59%), frequency (35%), dysuria (24%), nocturia (11%), and irritative symptoms (9%). The rest of the lesions were incidental cystoscopic or microscopic findings. Nephrogenic adenoma involved the bladder in 82% of the cases, the urethra in 13%, and the ureter in 5%. The urethra and bladder were rarely affected together and ureteral involvement was metachronously bilateral in one case. The lesion arose within a diverticulum in 4 of 14 urethral lesions. Bladder occurrence involved the dome, trigone, posterior wall, and lateral wall with approximately the same frequency. Anterior wall involvement was uncommon. The lesions were usually solitary, but two were present in two cases, three in five, five in three, eight in one, and numerous or multiple in ten cases. The lesion was papillary in 61% and polypoid in 15%, and the rest were sessile. The extent ranged from microscopic to involving the whole bladder, but the great majority were small. Of the 40 recorded largest dimensions, 19 were microscopic to 0.5 cm, seven were from over 0.5 to 1 cm, 12 were from over 1 cm to 4 cm, two were 7 cm, and another two were merely described as large.

YOUNG and SCULLY (1986) emphasized that nephrogenic adenoma is most likely to be confused microscopically with adenocarcinoma, particularly the clear cell type. The clinical features of the two are fairly distinctive. Furthermore, nephrogenic adenoma has an antecedent history of intervention, trauma, or chronic infection whereas adenocarcinoma usually does not. Two conditions, schistosomiasis and nonfunctioning bladder, increase the risk of both.

YOUNG and SCULLY (1986) noted that nephrogenic adenoma is almost always encountered in the setting of acute cystitis, chronic cystitis, or both. There is usually a latent period of 1–6 years after tissue injury. When nephrogenic adenoma has been noted in renal transplant recipients, immunosuppression may have contributed to development of the lesion (ZINGAS et al. 1986).

MOSTOFI (1954) felt that metaplasia into epithelial tubules lined by a single layer of cuboidal or low columnar epithelium simulating renal collecting tubules expains the nephrogenic adenoma and that these lesions should be carefully watched for the development of carcinoma. It had been previously postulated that nephrogenic adenoma represents immature mesonephric tubules that are normally seen only during embryologic development of the urinary tract. The trigone is derived from the mesonephric duct, and the lesion occurred frequently the trigonal area in early series. It is now known to be more widespread and this theory would not explain its occurrence elsewhere in the urinary tract.

Nephrogenic adenoma is felt to be papillary or glandular transformation rather than hamartoma or benign neoplasm. Nephrogenic adenoma of

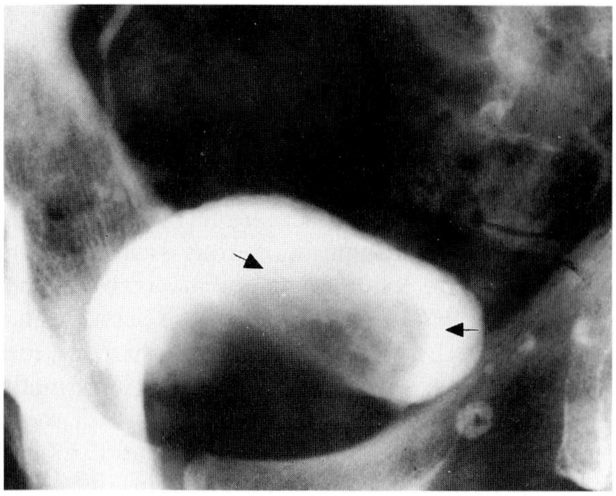

Fig. 6.36. Nephrogenic adenoma presenting as well-defined ovoid mass (*arrows*) arising from an enlarged prostate. (ZIMMERMANN et al. 1989)

the urinary tract is now generally accepted to represent metaplasia of the urothelium in response to chronic inflammation or injury (ZINGAS et al. 1986). Mostofi's theory is supported by the fact that so many of the reported patients with nephrogenic adenoma have an antecedent clinical history of urinary infection or surgery of the lower urinary tract and that inflammatory changes of the bladder frequently accompany nephrogenic adenoma (ZIMMERMAN et al. 1989).

Nephrogenic adenoma has no characteristic appearance and is seen as a mass filling defect or bladder wall irregularity on imaging. The appearance at urography and CT is consistent with the spectrum of gross morphologic appearances from sessile to papillary and polypoid. Of six patients with nephrogenic adenoma of the bladder reported by ZIMMERMAN et al. (1989), three presented with masses in the bladder (Fig. 6.36), two with irregularities of the bladder mucosa on urography and one with no focal abnormalities.

Gross appearance at cystoscopy is variable. Nephrogenic adenoma may present as slightly raised edematous areas. papillary tumors resembling low grade transitional cell carcinoma, or nonspecific flattened masses (ZIMMERMAN et al. 1989). The lesion is not now considered to be premalignant (BERGER et al. 1981; ZINGAS et al. 1986; ZIMMERMAN et al. 1989).

In nephrogenic adenoma, a delicate basement membrane is present beneath the epithelial cells and the tumor remains confined to the mucosa and submucosa. In all cases of mesonephric adenocarcinoma reviewed by SCHULTZ et al. (1984), frank muscle invasion was present.

Nephrogenic adenoma is difficult to eradicate, having a reported recurrence rate of up to approximately 60% (BERGER et al. 1981). Extensive surgery such as cystectomy may be necessary if symptoms become disabling (ZIMMERMAN et al. 1989). In mesonephric adenocarcinoma of the bladder, radical surgery may be required to achieve cure (SCHULTZ et al. 1984).

6.7.7 Inverted Papilloma

Inverted papilloma is a rare, almost uniformly benign lesion of the uroepithelium described and named by POTTS and HIRST (1963). Microscopically, it is composed of cords of urothelial-like cells organized in a fairly characteristic fashion. The cords of epithelium are inverted and exhibit a mosaic pattern separated by a delicate fibrous stroma. ROSAI (1989) describes the most characteristic microscopic feature as invagination of the epithelium without atypical features. The surface of the lesion has urothelium (ANDERSTROM et al. 1982). Most inverted papillomas are polypoid or pedunculated with smooth or lobulated surfaces usually lacking the papillary or filiform appearance of conventional transitional cell papillomas or carcinomas. The lesions are occasionally sessile and at times small surface papillations may occur. Most are smaller than 3 cm (KYRIAKOS and ROYCE 1989).

The majority of the reported lesions have originated in the lower urinary tract, the trigone, the bladder neck or the prostatic urethra. (ANDERSTROM et al. 1982; MULKENS et al. 1990). The bladder is the site of origin in 90% of cases (KYRIAKOS and ROYCE 1989).

Males in the sixth and seventh decades of life account for about 90% of reported patients (KYRIAKOS and ROYCE 1989). Presenting clinical symptoms are obstruction, pain, and/or hematuria. The findings on urography and CT are nonspecific and are those of epithelial mass and/or obstruction. The findings may be subtle (SCHULTZ and BOYLE 1988). Because inverted papilloma is indistinguishable macroscopically from other, more invasive lesions, preoperative frozen or permanent sections are necessary to make conservative surgery possible (MULKENS et al. 1990).

Inverted papillomas are considered to be benign lesions because of their histologic appearance, the low incidence of recurrence, the low incidence of multiplicity, the lack of invasion, and the lack of metastases (MULKENS et al. 1990). Only two cases of local recurrence have been reported (DEMEESTER et al. 1975; SCHULTZ and BOYLE 1988). The inverted papilloma has never demonstrated a clinically malignant behavior. It has never metastasized or recurred as overtly invasive carcinoma (MULKENS et al. 1990). It should, however, be mentioned that several inverted papillomas have been reported to contain on their surfaces a papillary component classified as low grade transitional cell carcinoma (KYRIAKOS and ROYCE 1989).

Inverted papillomas seem to develop in response to a variety of etiologic agents such as chronic irritation and inflammation which may also be responsible for the development of low grade, superficial urothelial tumors.

6.7.8 Neurofibromatosis

HOLT (1978) defines neurofibromatosis (von Recklinghausen's disease) as a hereditary, hamartomatous disorder, probably of neural crest origin, involving not only neuroectoderm and mesoderm but also endoderm, with the potential to appear in any organ system of the body.

The basic lesion is the neurofibroma. Electron microscopic and autoradiographic studies have shown that all cellular elements of a peripheral nerve (Schwann cells, fibroblasts, and perineural cells) play a part in tumor formation. A high concentration of mast cells is characteristic of a neurofibroma (HOLT 1978).

YOUNG et al. (1971) divided neurofibromatosis into three hereditary types: a peripheral form with multiple café au lait spots and subcutaneous nodules but with little central involvement; a central form consisting of multiple central nervous system tumors, primarily neuromas and meningiomas, but with minimal involvement of peripheral nerves and skin; and lastly a mixed form.

The National Institutes of Health Consensus Development Conference on Neurofibromatosis (1987) made a clear distinction between the two most definite categories of neurofibromatosis. NF-1 is the autosomal dominant disorder previously called von Recklinghausen's disease or peripheral neurofibromatosis. This is the most common form of neurofibromatosis. NF-1 is characterized by multiple hyperpigmented macules or café au lait spots; dermal, subcutaneous, and plexiform neurofibromas; iris (Lisch) nodules; axillary freckling; and optic nerve gliomas. NF-2 is the autosomal dominant disorder previously called central neurofibromatosis, bilateral acoustic neurofibromatosis or hereditary bilateral vestibular schwannoma syndrome. NF-2 is characterized by bilateral acoustic neuromas; posterior subcapsular cataracts; meningiomas; trigeminal nerve tumors; schwannomas; spinal cord ependymomas; and dermal, subcutaneous, and plexiform neurofibromas. There are additional variants (ROOS and DUNN 1992).

Cutaneous neurofibromas appear after puberty and are found in only 40% of patients (RINK and MITCHELL 1983). Hemihypertrophy is not uncommon. Focal gigantism can occur in any portion of the body, including the genitalia (RINK and MITCHELL 1983). Approximately 10% of affected children will have mild to moderate mental retardation (HOLT 1978).

The presence of Lisch nodules can establish the diagnosis. Lisch nodules are well-defined, dome-shaped elevations projecting from the surface of the iris and are clear to yellow or brown (LUBS et al. 1991).

The urologic manifestations of neurofibromatosis are: (a) retroperitoneal neurofibromas affecting either the upper or lower urinary tract; (b) hypertension due to renal artery stenosis (primarily in children) or pheochromocytoma (primarily in adults); and (c) a large variety of genital lesions including neurofibromas of the penis, clitoris, vulva, and scrotum (BLUM et al. 1985). As indicated above, enlargement of the penis, clitoris, and/or labia may also occur with or without other lower urinary tract involvement (HOLT 1978; RINK and MITCHELL 1983). Genitourinary neurofibromatosis is usually associated with generalized neurofibromatosis (MILLER et al. 1983b).

Genitourinary tract involvement is rare, the most common site of genitourinary involvement being the urinary bladder (BLUM et al. 1985). Bladder neurofibromas are associated with the syndrome of multiple neurofibromas in 40%–75% of cases. About half of the reported cases of pelvic neurofibromas have occurred in children. The male to female ratio is 2 or 3 : 1 (BLUM et al. 1985).

The mass may extend to involve the prostate, urethra, seminal vesicles, spermatic cords, and testes. The genitals are also involved in 35% of cases of bladder neurofibromatosis (RINK and MITCHELL 1983). Large plexiform neurofibromas

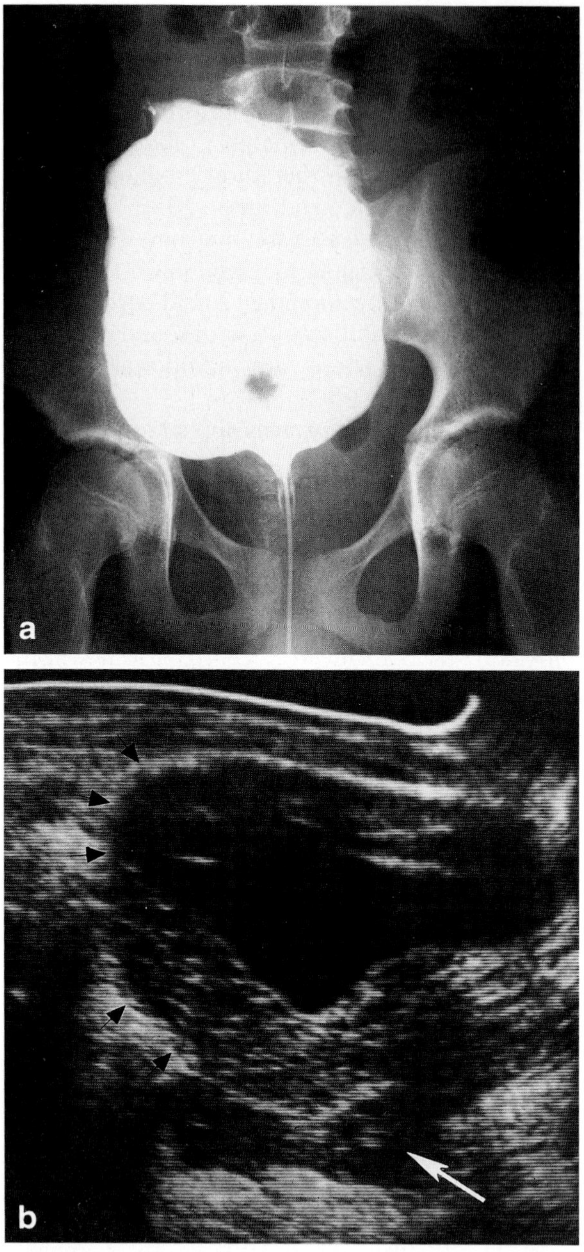

Fig. 6.37a,b. Neurofibroma of the urinary bladder. **a** Cystogram demonstrates irregular scalloping of the contour of the bladder with marked distortion and elevation of the base. **b** Longitudinal midline sonogram of the pelvis demonstrating massive circumferential thickening of the wall of the bladder (*black arrows*). The cervical os (*white arrow*) and uterus are displaced posteriorly. (Miller et al. 1983b)

may arise from the pelvic autonomic nerve plexuses and cause upper tract obstruction. The multicentric origin of these lesions from anatomically contiguous pelvic plexuses explains the occurrence of neurofibromatosis in adjacent pelvic organs (Pessin and Bodian 1964; Blum et al. 1985). Malignant degeneration of neurofibromas has been calculated to occur in about 13%–29% of cases and noted to increase with advancing age (Rink and Mitchell 1983). After sarcomatous change, the tumor grows rapidly and recurs after excision. Metastases are few and occur late. No case of malignant neurofibroma has been found in children with neurofibromatosis (Blum et al. 1985).

The solitary neurofibroma requires only local excision but the plexiform neurofibroma causes urinary obstruction necessitating urinary diversion. Recurrence and malignant degeneration are virtually unheard of in the former but common in the latter (Elliott et al. 1981).

Few patients with genitourinary neurofibromatosis are asymptomatic. Presenting symptoms include hematuria, urinary frequency and urgency, enuresis, pelvic, abdominal, or genital pain, and abdominal or genital enlargement. There is usually a suprapubic or pelvic mass on physical examination and a mass is often palpable above the prostate on rectal examination (Blum et al. 1985).

Treatment is variable and should be as conservative as possible considering the progressive and multiple system nature of the disease. Radical excision may become needed due to diffuse or extensive disease. Urinary diversion may be necessary if upper tract obstruction occurs (Blum et al. 1985).

Urography or sonography may demonstrate hydronephrosis. Radiographic examinations may show elevation, displacement, or distortion of the bladder and/or urethra. The bladder may demonstrate scalloped or irregular contours. Distensibility of the bladder may be markedly limited. Sonography may show massive and diffuse thickening of the bladder wall (Miller et al. 1983b) (Fig. 6.37). CT may show to advantage the local tumor, apposition to tumors in adjacent organs, and the cause of obstruction.

6.7.9 Pheochromocytoma

Pheochromocytomas are paragangliomas which arise from chromaffin cells of the sympathetic nervous system and produce catecholamine. They may rarely produce adrenocorticotropic hormone or dopa and dopamine (Beaser et al. 1986; Robinson et al. 1973).

Pheochromocytomas may arise anywhere from the base of the skull to the urinary bladder. They most often arise in adrenal medullary tissue (RUSSO et al. 1984; GOLDFARB et al. 1989). Extraadrenal locations of pheochromocytomas occur in 10%–20% of cases in adults and 30%–50% of those in children (GOLDFARB et al. 1989). The most common extraadrenal site is the superior para-aortic region (GOLDFARB et al. 1989). Approximately 10% of pheochromocytomas are multiple and 10% are malignant with regional lymph node and distant metastasis (JURASCHECK et al. 1983; RUSSO et al. 1984).

Histology does not allow differentiation of benign from malignant pheochromocytomas since the same features of nuclear irregularity, anaplasia, and hyperchromasia are present in both (RUSSO et al. 1984). Malignancy is determined by the finding of the lesion in organs that normally contain no chromaffin cells, e.g., liver and lymph nodes (RUSSO et al. 1984).

Pheochromocytomas occur with equal frequency in males and females, in all races, and most often in the 30- to 50-year-old age group. Approximately 90% of cases are sporadic and 10% familial. The familial cases are usually intraadrenal, autosomal dominant, and bilateral. Bilateral pheochromocytomas are commonly associated with multiple endocrine neoplasia types II and III, neurofibromatoses, and Hippel-Lindau disease.

Paraganglioma of the urinary bladder has been associated with adenocarcinoma of the kidney, neurofibromatosis, bilateral polycystic disease of the kidney, carcinoma of the urinary bladder, and secretion of parathormone in tumor tissue with clinical hyperparathyroidism. One case of familial and one case of hereditary multiple urinary paraganglioma have been documented (JURASCHECK et al. 1983).

Pheochromocytomas of the urinary bladder are exceedingly uncommon, accounting for 0.06% of all bladder tumors (LEESTMA and PRICE 1971; JURASCHECK et al. 1983), 1% of pheochromocytomas (WARSHAWSKY et al. 1989), and 10% of extraadrenal pheochromocytomas (HEYMAN et al. 1989). They are thought to arise from embryonic rests of chromaffin cells in the sympathetic plexus of the bladder wall (HEYMAN et al. 1989). They are highly vascularized and encapsulated, frequently undergoing hemorrhage, necroses, and cyst formation (HEYMAN et al. 1989). They are usually slow growing, with a long duration of symptoms before discovery and treatment (JURASCHECK et al. 1983). DAS et al. (1983) reviewed the previous 97 cases in the literature along with their own three cases. They found a 3:2 female to male ratio with an average age at diagnosis of 41 years and a range from 11 to 78 years. Tumor size ranged from 0.2 to 10 cm with a mean of 2 cm. Most lesions were solitary but two patients had two lesions and one had four lesions. The lesions are submucosal or intramural with intact overlying epithelium and most often located on the dome of the bladder or in the trigone (DAS et al. 1983; HEYMAN et al. 1989). DAS et al. (1983) found that 15 patients out of the 100 reported had malignant pheochromocytoma of the bladder. MAHONEY and HARRISON (1977) proposed that a clinical course characterized by recurrence be used as evidence of malignancy. Hypertension was the initial symptom in 12 of the 15 (80%) patients with malignant vesical pheochromocytoma, indicating their enhanced potential for hormonal activity (DAS et al. 1983).

Pheochromocytomas of the urinary bladder are most commonly located in the trigone (25%) or in the dome (24%) and are visible at cystoscopy in 84% of reported cases (OCHI et al. 1981).

The classic signs and symptoms of pheochromocytoma in the urinary bladder are headache in connection with micturition and defecation, tachycardia, increased perspiration, and permanent or intermittent hypertension predominantly caused by release of epinephrine and, to a lesser degree, norepinephrine (SCHULTZ and VOGEL 1984). DAS et al. (1983) found hypertension as an initial sign in 65% of reported cases and hematuria in 58%. Micturitional attacks consisted of headaches, palpitations, hypertension, blurred vision, and sweating in 46% of the reported cases, with dysuria and suprapubic pain in only 9%. Serum catecholamine levels were elevated in 67% and urinary vanillylmandelic acid (VMA) was elevated in 63% of reported cases in which they were obtained (DAS et al. 1983; HEYMAN et al. 1989). When the clinical symptoms are present, the diagnosis can be confirmed by serum catecholamine and urinary VMA levels. The tumors are frequently silent with regard to hormonal activity (JURASCHECK et al. 1983) (Fig. 6.38).

With its widespread availability, noninvasiveness, cost-effectiveness and exquisite spatial resolution and detail, CT is the usual method to evaluate a patient for pheochromocytoma. FARRELLY et al. (1984) reported that the CT ap-

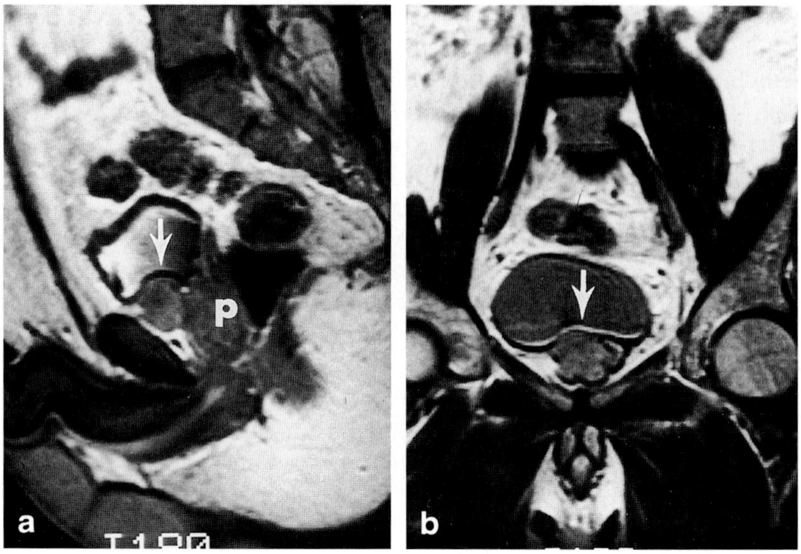

Fig. 6.38 a,b. Pheochromocytoma (*arrow*) in the urinary bladder wall at the base, anterior to the prostate (*P*). **a** Sagittal and **b** coronal T1-weighted MRI. (Courtesy of Dr. I. Yoder)

pearances of pheochromocytoma in children were similar to those in adults. Intravenous contrast should be avoided. CT has been reported to detect 95% of all intraadrenal lesions and has an overall accuracy above 90%, primarily due to its exquisite spatial resolution approaching 1 cm and its tomographic cross-sectional format (Velchik et al. 1989). However, CT provides purely anatomic information but is not capable of differentiating between cortical and medullary masses or between functioning and nonfunctioning lesions (Velchik et al. 1989).

Computed tomography is only slightly less accurate for extraadrenal lesions. In patients with clinical and biochemical evidence of pheochromocytoma, CT is the first study for localization of the tumor (Goldfarb et al. 1989). If thin sections through the adrenals show no mass, the retroperitoneum can be evaluated on abdominal and pelvic CT. Further studies such as chest CT can be obtained if abdominal CT is negative (Goldfarb et al. 1989).

A growing body of information is demonstrating the usefulness of MRI in the identification and localization of pheochromocytoma. Tumors imaged by CT are usually demonstrated by MRI with a fairly specific high signal intensity on T2-weighted spin-echo sequences with a TR of 1700–2500 ms. The clear delineation of vascular structures with MRI on direct coronal and sagittal images helps distinguish tumor margins, and the patency of the renal veins and inferior vena cava can be clearly established without intravenous contrast (Fink et al. 1985). MRI can also identify metastatic deposits, and in the majority of cases of pheochromocytoma may suffice entirely by clearly depicting hepatic, vascular, and renal interfaces (Fink et al. 1985). MRI can identify, localize, characterize, and stage the lesion with one multiplanar examination.

Magnetic resonance imaging is particularly helpful in the imaging of extraadrenal pheochromocytomas because of its ability to yield multiplanar images and tissue characterization of pheochromocytomas (Warshawsky et al. 1989). Since pheochromocytomas usually demonstrate homogeneous and markedly increased signal intensity on T2-weighted spin-echo sequences, MRI is ideally suited for the evaluation of pheochromocytoma in the urinary bladder (Warshawsky et al. 1989). These lesions should be easily distinguishable from bladder carcinomas, the majority of which have been only moderately bright in signal intensity on long TR/TE images (Warshawsky et al. 1989). Since the lesion itself may be obscured by the surrounding, equally bright urine, moderately T2-weighted images (2000/60 ms) are also recommended for delineating the lesion (Warshawsky et al. 1989). The tumor may show enhancement with gadolinium injection. In the patient with appropriate clinical presentation and biochemical studies, MRI can be specific for pheochromocytoma of the bladder (WARSHAWSKY et al. 1989) (Fig. 6.39a,b).

Since it is noninvasive, ultrasound may be attempted but does not provide the fine detail of CT or MRI. If ultrasound examination of the adrenals is negative, the sonographer should image the para-aortic area and pelvis. Bladder masses of more that 0.5 cm should be readily detectable, particularly if they are located in the posterior or lateral walls. Small masses located in the bladder neck or dome may be particularly difficult to detect (GOODMAN and LIPINSKI 1984).

Since pheochromocytomas are vascular lesions, arteriography can be useful to localize extra-adrenal pheochromocytomas. But it is an invasive procedure and contrast medium may precipitate a hypertensive crisis. It should be reserved for tumors that have not been localized by noninvasive means or for large complex lesions in order to define the vascular anatomy for surgical planning (GOLDFARB et al. 1989).

Selective venous sampling from multiple levels in the entire superior and inferior vena cava can be helpful in localization of pheochromocytoma. There are inherent problems with this technique due to variation in venous drainage and dilution of the tumor effluent. Nevertheless, a success rate as high as 97% has been reported. Selective venous sampling like arteriography is reserved for cases where noninvasive techniques have failed to localize the tumor (GOLDFARB et al. 1989). After selective venous sampling has identified the level of the lesion, a CT examination at the identified level with meticulous attention to detail, using thin slices, and with and without contrast may be successful in localizing a mass (MILLER et al. 1983a).

Metaiodobenzylguanidine (MIBG) is a physiologic analog of norepinephrine and guanethidine which can be labeled with iodine-123 or iodine-131 for scintigraphy. In vivo, it is stored in the noradrenergic neurosecretory granules. Since its uptake and storage simulate that of norepinephrine, labeled MIBG is used to image the adrenal medulla and related tumors such as pheochromocytomas, other paragangliomas, and neuroblastomas. The common feature of these lesions is the presence of numerous neurosecretory granules containing catecholamines in the cytoplasm of their cells. Iodine-123 has superior imaging characteristics compared to iodine-131. Iodine-MIBG has proven to be safe, sensitive,

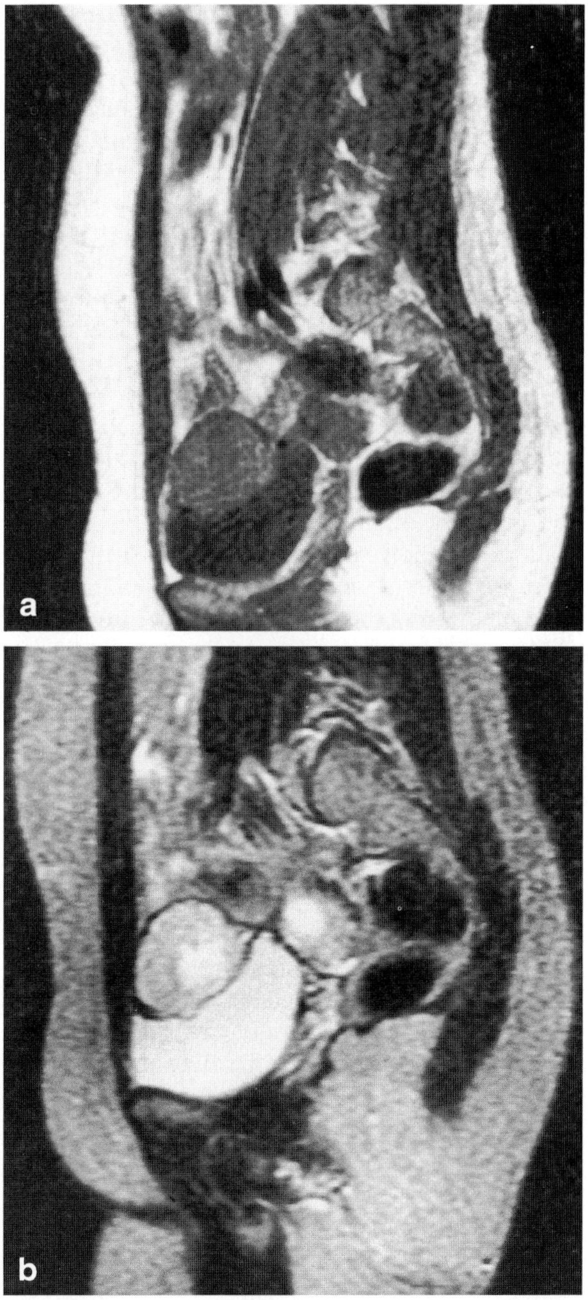

Fig. 6.39. **a** A T1 weighted Magnetic Resonance Image in saggital projection demonstrates a mass indenting the dome of the bladder. (Courtesy E. ZERHOUNI) **b** A T2 weighted MRI Scan in saggital plannar demonstrates the mass with heterogeneous signal intensity. The high signal in the center of the mass suggests an area of necrosis. The mass is characteristic of and was proven to be a pheochromocytoma. (Courtesy of E. ZERHOUNI)

and (most importantly) relatively specific in the detection of pheochromocytoma (BOMANJI et al. 1987; VELCHIK et al. 1989).

Scintigraphy using MIBG and CT have comparable sensitivities for localization of extraadrenal pheochromocytomas. MIBG scintigraphy is noninvasive and allows whole-body imaging covering the whole range of potential extraadrenal sites in one study (GOLDFARB et al. 1989). GOLDFARB et al. recommend that when abdominal CT does not localize a tumor, an iodine-MIBG study should be performed. MIBG provides specific functional information. CT and MRI provide anatomic detail.

Transurethral resection of bladder pheochromocytoma is generally inadequate because the majority of tumors extend into the bladder wall; accordingly, partial cystectomy is the treatment of choice in most cases (JURASCHECK et al. 1983; HEYMAN et al. 1989). Intraoperatively, the ipsilateral hypogastric vein should be ligated before tumor manipulation to decrease catecholamine return to the systemic circulation (JURASCHECK et al. 1983; HEYMAN et al. 1989). The complete excision of the tumor is usually followed by disappearance of all sympathetic symptoms including hypertension. Return of clinical endocrine or biochemical manifestations of pheochromocytoma strongly suggest development of metastases (JURASCHECK et al. 1983).

Extraadrenal pheochromocytoma is generally considered to have a higher malignant potential than the intraadrenal variety, with the incidence of malignancy reported to be between 20% and 40% (GOLDFARB et al. 1989).

MAHONEY and HARRISON (1977) believed three criteria were important for a maximum tumor-free interval: (a) adjunctive lymphadenectomy at the initial operation when one or more lymph nodes contain tumor, (b) close follow-up of all patients with pheochromocytoma by diagnostic biochemical assay for 15 years, and (c) aggressive excision of all single or multiple recurrent pheochromocytomas as soon as a biochemical diagnosis is established. They recommended that all patients with pheochromocytoma have a detailed follow-up every 6 months for 15 years.

6.7.10 Hemangioma

Hemangioma of the bladder is a rare lesion accounting for 0.6% of all bladder tumors. Occurring equally in both sexes, it is most common in the white race and in children, with 65% of cases occurring in patients less than 15 years old (LEONARD et al. 1988).

The lesion probably originates from angioblastic cells that fail to develop into normal blood vessels (PAKTER et al. 1988). Microscopically, the lesion is a collection of thick- or thin-walled blood vessels beneath an intact urothelium. Most lesions are cavernous hemangiomas, but capillary tumors, venous tumors, and even hemangiolymphangiomas are described (GUPTA and BHARGAVA 1987).

One-third of bladder hemangiomas are multicentric and two-thirds are solitary lesions located in the dome or trigone. They rarely involve the bladder neck or ureteral orifices (LEONARD et al. 1988).

Hemangioma of the bladder is primarily an intravesical tumor bulging into the lumen. Two-thirds of the cases involve the muscle layer and the lesion may occasionally extend into the perivesical tissues and invade other pelvic organs, forming pelvic angiomatosis (LEONARD et al. 1988). The lesions may grow either by increasing the size of their original vessels or by forming new vessels (LEONARD et al. 1988).

The most common presenting symptom is gross painless hematuria (PAKTER et al. 1988; LEONARD et al. 1988). The hematuria may be intermittent and the patients are often anemic and may appear quite ill (LEONARD et al. 1988).

Patients occasionally have an associated syndrome such as Klippel-Trenaunay or Sturge-Weber. Approximately 30% of patients with bladder hemangiomas have hemangiomas elsewhere (LEONARD et al. 1988).

Phleboliths are the radiographic hallmark of hemangiomas in soft tissue anywhere. Phleboliths in an area where no normal collection of veins should exist are highly suggestive of hemangioma even in atypical or unusual locations. Otherwise, bladder hemangiomas present on contrast studies as nonspecific filling defects (CACERES et al. 1991).

Hemangiomas have been found to be either hyperechoic or hypoechoic on ultrasound, probably depending on the predominance of blood-containing space or intervening septa (KIM et al. 1991; LEWIS et al. 1986). Ultrasound of bladder hemangioma may demonstrate a thickened bladder wall with multiple serpiginous anechoic spaces. CT may demonstrate diffuse bladder wall thickening with foci of calcification (PAKTER et al.

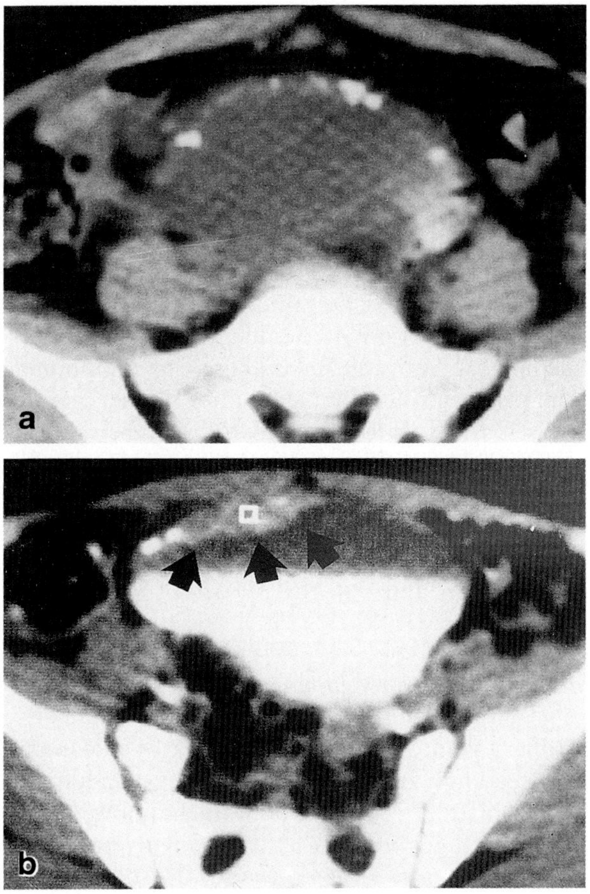

Fig. 6.40 a,b. Hemangioma of the urinary bladder. **a** Unenhanced CT scan of the pelvis demonstrating multiple, round calcifications in focally thickened bladder wall. **b** After intravenous contrast administration, the thickened area enhances (*arrows*). (CACERES et al. 1991)

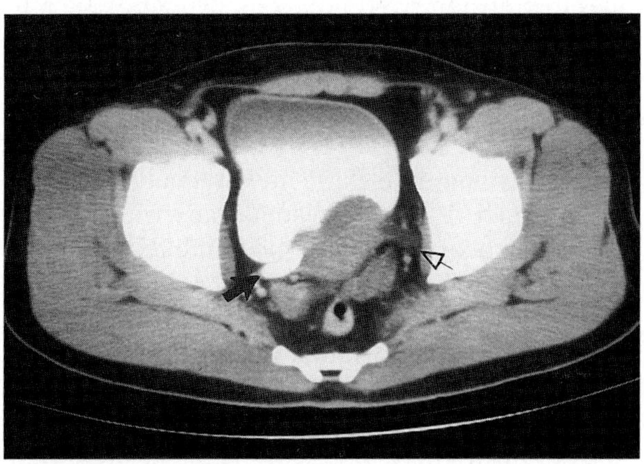

Fig. 6.41. Primary lymphoma of the urinary bladder on CT. A lobulated mass involves the posterolateral aspect of the bladder; both ureters are dilated (*closed arrow on right, open arrow on left*). (BINKOVITZ et al. 1988)

1988) (Fig. 6.40). Characteristics of hemangiomas on MRI have been reported as low signal intensity on T1-weighted images and high signal intensity on T2-weighted images, which can provide excellent contrast with surrounding tissues (KAPLAN and WILLIAMS 1987; KIM et al. 1991).

Cystoscopically, the lesions usually appear sessile, broad based, and lobulated with a bluish red color (LEONARD et al. 1988). As elsewhere, hemangiomas should be compressible but KLEIN and KAPLAN (1975) advise that manipulation be avoided because of the danger of excessive hemorrhage. Angiomatous vessels may be visualized with hyperemic mucosa (CACERES et al. 1991). The size of bladder hemangiomas is often underestimated because of submucosal extension (PAKTER et al. 1988).

Biopsy is to be avoided because of the possibility of intractable hemorrhage.

Bladder hemangiomas may continue to grow at variable rates and may result in chronic illness even though they are not malignant (LEONARD et al. 1988). Partial cystectomy is recommended for large lesions. Transcatheter embolization may offer a viable alternative. For small or diffuse lesions, the current treatment of choice is photocauterization with a laser (HOCKLEY et al. 1989). Periodic follow-up is necessary to detect recurrence or persistent disease (LEONARD et al. 1988).

6.7.11 Lymphoma

Primary lymphoma of the urinary bladder (Fig. 6.41) is quite rare. The origin of this tumor is controversial since normal bladder microscopic sections fail to reveal the routine presence of lymphoid follicles. It has been proposed that primary lymphomas arise as a reaction to the chronic irritation of repeated bacterial cystitis, which may be present in the history of these patients.

The majority of cases of bladder involvement by lymphoma recognized clinically and at necropsy are of the non-Hodgkin's variety (BOCIAN et al. 1982). SUFRIN et al. (1977) found bladder involvement 4 times more often in non-Hodgkin's than in Hodgkin's lymphoma.

Secondary involvement of the bladder with lymphoma is more common than primary involvement and is usually found in patients with advanced or late-stage disease (CHARNSANGAVEJ 1990). SUFRIN et al. (1977) found bladder involvement in 13% of 599 patients who died of malignant lymphoma, including 4% of those with Hodgkin's disease, 18% of those with reticulum cell sarcoma, and 16% of those with lymphosarcoma. Bladder involvement was always a secondary event, being part of disseminated disease. Involvement was usually microscopic although the presence of gross disease was invariably clinically manifest. The bladder dome, posterior wall, trigone, and lateral walls were affected with equal frequency. The foci of involvement were multiple rather that solitary. The randomness and multiplicity of bladder involvement suggest a hematogenous route of extension to the bladder. Grossly visible foci were invariably symptomatic and microscopic foci were usually asymptomatic.

Involvement of the urinary tract in patients known to have lymphoma is uncommon and usually an incidental finding at autopsy (CHAITIN et al. 1984). Premortem diagnosis is unusual without gross invasion of the bladder (BINKOVITZ et al. 1988). Hodgkin's disease has been diagnosed by exfoliative cytology on a single passed urine specimen (BOCIAN et al. 1982).

In CHAITIN et al.'s (1984) review of large autopsy series totalling 1687 cases, secondary involvement of the bladder in patients with lymphoma or leukemia ranged from 1.5% to 13%. Non-Hodgkin's lymphomas and leukemias are far more likely than Hodgkin's disease to affect the lower urinary tract. CHAITIN et al. (1984) questioned whether some reported instances of bladder lymphoma might not be merely extranodal lymphoid infiltrates, which would inflate the actual incidence and apparently unfavorable prognosis of bladder lymphoma.

Primary lymphoma, in contrast, usually presents a distinct clinical picture that gains medical attention. Since it is rare, primary lymphoma is frequently misdiagnosed as some other malignancy. Primary lymphomas have constant clinical and cystoscopic features. In their review, BHANSALI and CAMERON (1960) found that the typical patient is a middle-aged or elderly woman with recurrent gross hematuria, often associated with dysuria and/or frequency. The majority of lesions were large (up to 10 cm), smooth or nodular, submucosal masses. The overlying mucosa is usually intact but occasionally central ulceration may be seen. The vast majority of these neoplasms are confined to the bladder wall; the ureters are usually spared. BHANSALI and CAMERON (1960) felt that suspicion of lymphoma should be raised by a bladder lesion which is smooth, rounded, pink, solid, and essentially submucous, which shows relatively little infiltration compared to its size, and which is not obstructing the ureter or is producing minimal obstruction.

There is nothing specific about the imaging appearance of lymphoma to suggest its diagnosis. Transitional cell carcinoma is a much more likely diagnosis for any bladder tumor. Cystoscopic findings atypical for transitional cell carcinoma such as submucosal multinodular mass without mucosal alteration or hemorrhage may lead to suspicion of an unusual sarcoma or lymphoma. The primary role of imaging after delineating the mass is to exclude disseminated disease and obstruction (BINKOVITZ et al. 1988).

Primary lymphoma of the bladder responds very well to chemotherapy or radiation therapy and rarely requires surgical resection (CHARNSANGAVEJ 1990; AIGEN and PHILLIPS 1986).

6.7.12 *Malignant Melanoma*

Primary genitourinary involvement by melanoma is exceedingly rare, but the frequency of metastasis to the bladder is comparable to the more widely recognized gastrointestinal tract involvement.

Autopsy series have found the bladder involved in 14%–18% of patients with metastatic melanoma (GOLDSTEIN et al. 1974). In their review of 71 patients with malignant melanoma to the urinary tract, GOLDSTEIN et al. found bladder involvement in 20 (28.17%).

Melanoma may spread to the urinary tract by direct extension from adjacent structures such as lymph nodes or via lymphatics. The most common route is probably hematogenous (GOLDSTEIN et al. 1974).

GOLDSTEIN et al. (1974) observed that in all instances when metastatic melanoma involves the urinary tract, it is part of an already widely disseminated process with cure most unlikely. Bladder involvement is usually manifest as one or more nonspecific filling defect at urography (Fig. 6.42). There may be associated ureteral defects. Differential considerations for these lesions include cystitis cystica, bullous edema, and malacoplakia.

The urine may be dark with melanin pigment, especially after standing, and cytologic examination of spun urine may reveal melanocytes. In GOLDSTEIN et al.'s (1974) series, half of the patients with bladder metastases had hematuria.

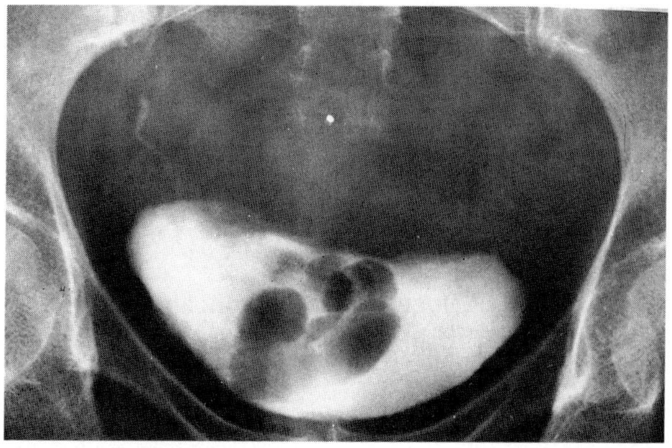

Fig. 6.42. Melanoma of the bladder as filling defects on urogram. (Courtesy of Dr. M. ELKIN)

Cystoscopic findings vary in accordance with the size and configuration of the lesions, which range from tiny black or blue-black areas confined to the mucosa to pedunculated or sessile invasive tumors. When the tumors are large, necrosis and inflammation may obscure the natural blue-black coloration, leading to confusion with primary bladder neoplasm (GOLDSTEIN et al. 1974).

6.7.13 Leiomyoma

Leiomyoma is a rare benign mesothelial tumor of the bladder. Leiomyomas may arise in any organ or structure containing smooth muscle (BELIS et al. 1979). Within the genitourinary system, the renal capsule is the most common location for leiomyoma, but such lesions are often small and only found at autopsy (BELIS et al. 1979). Only 0.7% of leiomyomas are found in the urinary bladder. Leiomyomas represent between 0.1% and 0.5% of bladder tumors (BORNSTEIN et al. 1986). Leiomyomas are the most common mesenchymal tumor of the bladder. They occur in both men and women with a 1:3 ratio (BORNSTEIN et al. 1986).

A leiomyoma is composed of sheets of smooth muscle within a fibrous stroma with which it may imperceptibly blend (KOSS 1975b). It may be submucosal, intramural, or extramural. Submucosal leiomyomas are usually pedunculated or polypoid and are most often symptomatic (BELIS et al. 1979). The patients may present with bladder infection, enuresis, suprapubic or perineal pain, ureteral obstruction, or, in females, prolapse of the lesion through the urethral meatus. Intramural lesions are well encapsulated within the bladder wall and may reach moderate size. They usually present as a pelvic mass but may cause obstructive symptoms when originating near the bladder neck. Extramural leiomyomas can become very large, being attached to the bladder by a pedicle and presenting with symptoms secondary to the mass (BELIS et al. 1979). Extramural tumors may even fill the retrovesical pouch (THURNHER et al. 1992). The submucosal form is the most common and the most likely to cause symptoms such as bladder irritation, urinary tract infection, hematuria, or urinary retention (ILLESCAS et al. 1986). But leiomyoma is frequently asymptomatic and found incidentally (BORNSTEIN et al. 1986).

On cystography, submucosal and intramural leiomyomas of the bladder usually present as smooth filling defects and may be difficult to differentiate from other bladder tumors if they develop an irregular surface because of concomitant cystitis (BELIS et al. 1979). Excretory urography may also show a filling defect without evidence of mucosal ulceration. In males the appearance can be not unlike an enlarged prostate (ILLESCAS et al. 1986). Calcifications suggestive of leiomyoma may be identified within the tumor (THURNHER et al. 1992). Ultrasound demonstrates a well-defined, solid, homogeneous, intramural mass which may be lobulated (BORNSTEIN et al. 1986; ILLESCAS et al. 1986).

Computed tomography shows a well-defined soft tissue mass which may be calcified (THURNHER et al. 1992). Since the mass, like leiomyomas of the uterus, may be pedunculated and may be adjacent to the posteriorly located uterus, its exact relationship to the adjacent organs or its organ of origin may not be evident in the axial plane (ILLESCAS et al. 1986).

The appearance of leiomyomas of the uterus on MRI has been well established. They are imaged with low signal intensity on T1- and T2-weighted images. Leiomyomas free of degenerative changes emit homogeneous signals of low intensity. Leiomyomas with hyaline, myxomatous, or fatty degeneration demonstrate various degrees of inhomogeneity, best seen on images obtained with long TR and TE. They exhibit mixed low and high signal intensity with hypointense degenerative intratumoral zones (HRICAK et al. 1986; THURNHER et al. 1992; KARASICK et al. 1992). Intratumoral architecture may be better demonstrated with use of intravenous contrast (THURNHER et al. 1992). Bladder leiomyomas are expected to follow this pattern.

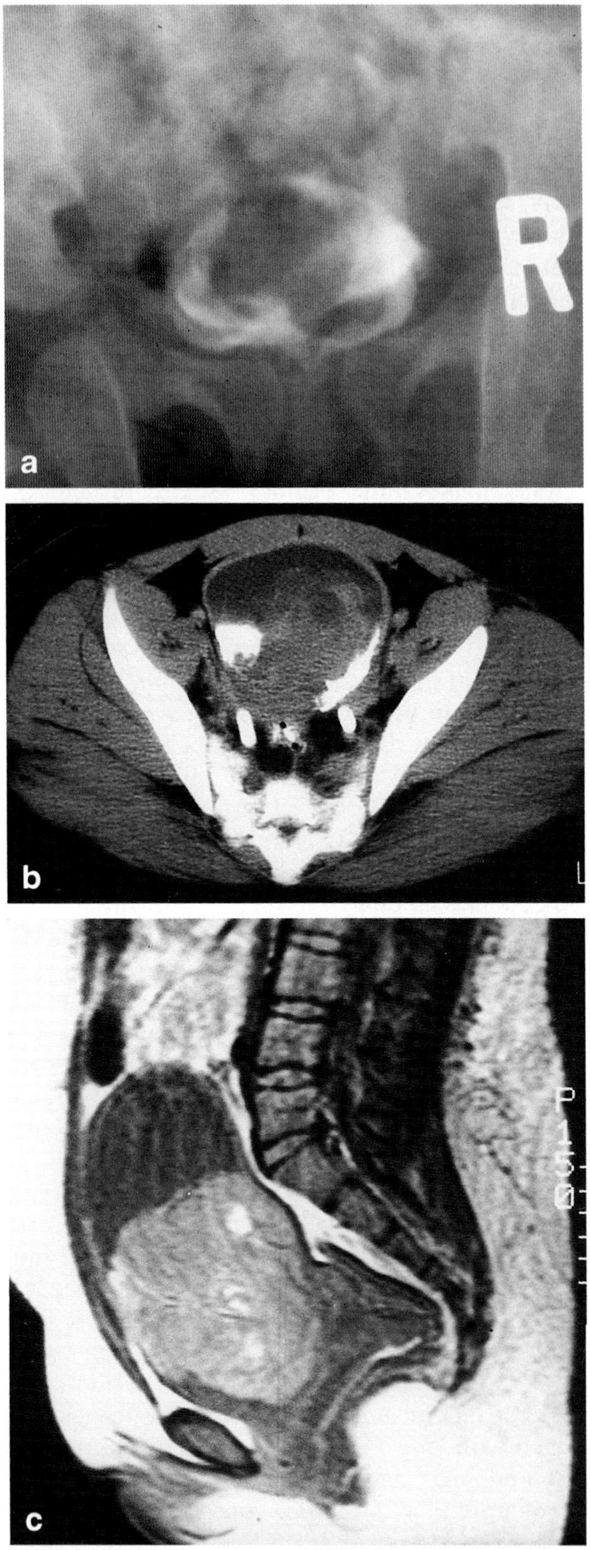

Fig. 6.43a–c. Rhabdomyosarcoma of the bladder. **a** Bulky intraluminal mass on urography in a 5-month-old male. **b** CT and **c** proton density weighted sagittal MRI of pelvis demonstrate bulky inhomogeneous mass in the bladder of a 10-year-old girl. (Courtesy of Dr. M. NEUMAN)

Cystoscopy demonstrates that the mucosa is intact, being stretched over the mass without signs of invasion (BRANT and WILLIAMS 1984; BORNSTEIN et al. 1986).

Differentiation from leiomyosarcoma may be difficult. The absence of mitosis and lack of recurrence indicate a benign histology (THURNHER et al. 1992).

Since leiomyomas are so well encapsulated, the treatment of choice is total enucleation from the bladder wall (ILLESCAS et al. 1986). Only one recurrence has been reported (BRANT and WILLIAMS 1984).

6.7.14 Sarcomas

Sarcomas of the bladder account for only 0.38%–0.64% of all bladder cancers (SWARTZ et al. 1985). In adults, the majority of bladder sarcomas are leiomyosarcomas and in children most are rhabdomyosarcomas (YOUNG and ROSENBERG 1987).

Both leiomyosarcomas and rhabdomyosarcomas arise from the connective tissues of the bladder. Some of the bladder carcinomas contain not only malignant mesenchymal elements but also neoplastic epithelial structures; these are called carcinosarcomas and are presumed to develop from multipotential stem cells. The sarcomatous elements dominate in the majority of carcinosarcomas and they are usually classified with the more common sarcomas. Carcinosarcomas of the bladder in adults have been reported to occur with about the same frequency as leiomyosarcomas and rhabdomyosarcomas (SEN et al. 1985).

Leiomyosarcoma of the bladder has been reported to occur most frequently in middle-aged and older adults, twice as often in men as in women, and typically within the bladder wall away from the trigone (SCHWARTZ et al. 1985). Gross hematuria is almost always the presenting symptom (SEN et al. 1985). No obvious cystoscopic or gross pathologic appearance is noted in adults with bladder sarcomas, in contrast to that of sarcoma botryoides in children (SEN et al. 1985). Wide surgical excision by partial or radical cystectomy remains the curative treatment of choice (SCHWARTZ et al. 1985).

Osteosarcoma is one of the rarest tumors of the urinary bladder, with only a handful of cases reported (YOUNG and ROSENBERG 1987). Most of the reported patients have been male, ranging in age from 41 to 83 years with an average age of 62. The tumors are characteristically large and polypoid and most commonly located in the trigone. It should be distinguished from other bladder tumors that may be associated with bone formation such as carcinosarcomas and transitional cell carcinomas with osseous metaplasia of the stroma, both of which have a better prognosis than osteosarcoma (YOUNG and ROSENBERG 1987).

Rhabdomyosarcoma is the most common tumor of the lower genitourinary tract in the first two decades of life (Fig. 6.43). It occasionally occurs in adults. The annual incidence of genitourinary rhabdomyosarcoma is estimated to be 0.5–0.7 cases per million white children under 15 years of age and it affects boys two times more frequently than girls (BAHNSON et al. 1989). The peak incidence is between 2 and 6 years (BAKER et al. 1985). Since approximately one-third of patients present in the third decade of life, there may be a bimodal distribution (BAKER et al. 1985). Rhabdomyosarcoma of the urinary tract and neurofibromatosis have been reported in association (McKEEN et al. 1978).

Rhabdomyosarcomas are divided histologically into three basic subtypes: embryonal, alveolar, and pleomorphic or undifferentiated (BAKER et al. 1985). Sarcoma botryoides refers to a morphologic characteristic of some embryonal tumors that originate submucosally in a hollow viscus. Polypoid grape-like tumor clusters project into the lumen as it grows. The embryonal subtype is the most common in children. Pleomorphic tumors are quite rare and are generally only found in adults 30–50 years of age.

The bladder is the most common site of occurrence in the genitourinary tract, with the tumors often located in the trigone and most often occurring within the first 3 years of life (BAKER et al. 1985).

Rhabdomyosarcomas are characterized by their bulky nature, propensity for local invasion, and rapid hematogenous and lymphatic dissemination (BAKER et al. 1985). Primary lesions of the genitourinary tract have a statistically higher incidence of lymphatic metastases (19%) than other primary sites of origin (5%). It is particularly high when the primary lesion is in the paratesticular region (40%) (BAHNSON et al. 1989).

Presenting symptoms relate to location. Symptoms of obstruction or frank urinary retention are the most common presentation in children with rhabdomyosarcoma of the lower urinary tract (BAHNSON et al. 1989). Hematuria is unusual.

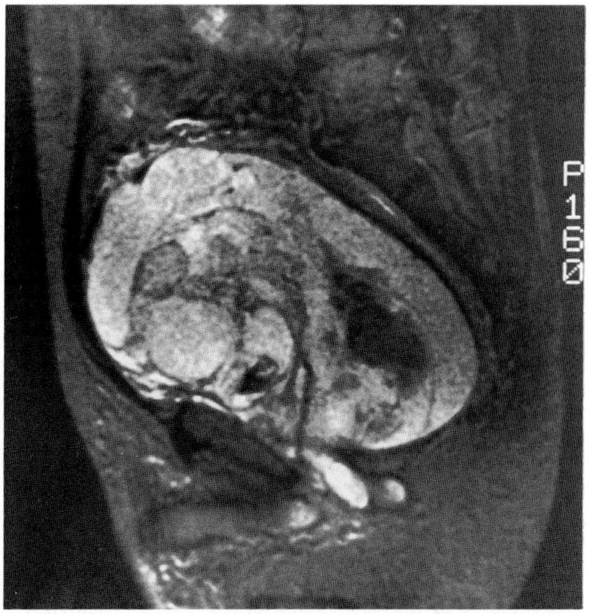

Fig. 6.44. A T2 weighted MRI scan in saggital plan demonstrates a hugh mass with heterogeneous signal intensity and multi-lobulated appearance involving the entire bladder. Extension into the perivesical fat in the dome segment is suggested. The mass proved to be a highly undifferentiated sarcoma. (Courtesy of E. ZERHOUNI)

BAHNSON et al. (1989) recommend preoperative staging evaluation to include excretory urography, voiding cystourethrography, and retrograde urethrography before biopsy for diagnosis, and CT and ultrasonography prior to definitive treatment. BAKER et al. (1985) prefer CT to assess not only the main tumor bulk but also the chest, liver, retroperitoneum, and pelvis. MRI, bone scanning and lymphography can be helpful (Fig. 6.44). Ultrasound is by far the best imaging technique available for lesions of the urinary bladder and those invading the bladder wall in children as it can visualize, measure, and follow these lesions. CT showed the tumor and its relationship to pelvic organs, musculature, and bones to best advantage (TANNOUS et al. 1989).

Ultrasound can be repeated frequently during chemotherapy to appreciate tumor regression and to measure the mass. CT should be performed when tumoral regression seems sufficient to permit complete tumor excision without pelvic exenteration. Both are useful in follow-up to identify local recurrence. Correlation of both ultrasound and CT results with surgical findings is very good (GEOFFRAY et al. 1987).

Transrectal ultrasound can be used to guide needle aspiration biopsy of pelvic masses and its use has been reported in recurrent vaginal rhabdomyosarcoma in a 23-month-old child (MANDELL et al. 1989).

With dramatic improvements in therapy for childhood rhabdomyosarcoma, survival has been prolonged for most patients (BAHNSON et al. 1989; CASSADY 1991). Adults with rhabdomyosarcoma do not fare as well as children with the same diagnosis (PRESTIGE and DONALDSON 1989).

6.7.15 Metastases

The most common secondary tumors of the urinary bladder are extensions of malignancies of adjacent organs such as cancers of the prostate, seminal vesicles, cervix, uterus, sigmoid, etc. (MELICOW 1955). In a review of 1614 cases of tumors of the urinary bladder, MELICOW (1955) found that 108 (6.7%) were local extension to the bladder and 24 (1.5%) were distant metastatic tumors to the bladder. Reviewing 80 cases from the literature, GANEM and BATAL (1956) found that the most common primary cancers which metastasize to the urinary bladder are gastric carcinoma, malignant melanoma, breast carcinoma, and lung carcinoma. Pathways of spread to the bladder include hematogenous, lymphogenous, direct extension, or drop metastasis from other intraabdominal organs.

Imaging may or may not demonstrate a mass in or distortion of the bladder on urography, ultrasound (FORNAGE et al. 1984), CT, or MRI.

6.7.16 Small Cell Carcinoma and Related Neuroendocrine Tumors

The urinary bladder can be the site of neoplasms exhibiting various degrees of endocrine differentiation and secretion. The most common manifestation is the presence of scattered endocrine cells in what is otherwise a typical adenocarcinoma. These behave as other adenocarcinomas and are labeled as such (ROSAI 1989).

Carcinoid tumor of the bladder is exceptionally rare, with typical architectural features and numerous dense core granules on ultrastructural examination (COLBY 1980).

Small cell carcinoma is highly malignant in the bladder and morphologically similar to the varieties found in lung and other organs. Small cell carcinoma arising in the urinary bladder is an aggressive neoplasm that often demonstrates multidirectional differentiation, including the frequent but not invariable expression of neuroendocrine features (MILLS et al. 1987). These tumors may be associated with hypercalcemia (REYES and SONERU 1985), ectopic ACTH secretion (PARTANEN and ASIKAININ 1985), or hypophosphatemia (CRAMER et al. 1981).

6.7.17 Perfusion Chemotherapy and Embolotherapy

Transcatheter intraarterial infusion and occlusion techniques have been applied to selected cancer patients. The rationale of intraarterial infusion of chemotherapeutic agent is to expose the neoplasm to a higher local concentration of chemotherapeutic agent than is possible with intravenous administration, but without increased toxicity. With most cytotoxic agents, the higher the concentration of the drug, the higher the tumoricidal effect will be. A neoplasm that is refractory to systemic chemotherapy may respond to arterial infusion of the same agent at the same dose rate (CHUANG and WALLACE 1981; LANG 1981).

Indications for arterial occlusion include the control of hemorrhage, alleviation of intractable pain produced by tumor bulk, facilitation of surgery by preoperatively decreasing tumor size, vascularity, and blood loss, reduction of tumor hormonal production, and transformation of a vascular neoplasm into an ischemic one (CHUANG and WALLACE 1981; LANG 1981).

Using the Seldinger technique, the catheter tip is placed in the artery as close to the neoplasm as possible so that the infusion bathes the bulk of the tumor but spares the maximum amount of normal tissue, and the catheter is secured to the skin. If perfusion is for longer than 24 h, a conventional radiograph is obtained daily to check the position of the catheter. Contrast injection is sometimes needed. Catheter displacement occurs in approximately 10% of cases and the catheter is repositioned. The patient is allowed limited ambulation during the period of infusion. Ambulation is necessary in prolonged infusion over 24 h and in the elderly (CHUANG and WALLACE 1981).

Agents used in bladder cancer have been cis-diamminedichloroplatinum (cisplatin), mitomycin C, adriamycin, floxuridine, and 5-fluorouracil. Bilateral internal artery infusion is preferred. Reports are scattered and the numbers are usually small. CHUANG and WALLACE (1981) reported a response rate of 60% in 18 patients with stage D_2 disease. Median survival was 52 weeks compared to 13 weeks without chemotherapy. The primary lesion was rarely controlled and pelvic and retroperitoneal lymph nodes seldom sterilized. The primary neoplasm usually caused pain and hematuria. The pain was relieved in 12 of 15 patients and the hematuria controlled in eight of ten patients. Acute renal tubular necrosis occurred in two patients and responded to medical management. An embolus occurred shortly after catheterization in one patient but resolved spontaneously. Transient peripheral neuritis appeared in seven patients. Two patients receiving 5-fluorouracil developed an erythematous skin reaction that accompanied each infusion and persisted for 2 weeks.

Compared to standard intravenous chemotherapy, intraarterial infusion chemotherapy seems to be more effective for local bladder cancer, especially since many of the infusion patients will have had bulky tumors that have been previously irradiated (MALDAZYS and DE KERNION 1986).

The same materials and techniques as are used for control of traumatic hemorrhage can be applied to bleeding from pelvic neoplasms.

6.8 Miscellaneous Conditions

6.8.1 Endometriosis

Endometriosis is defined as the presence of endometrial tissue beyond the endometrium. Infiltration into the uterine muscle is called adenomyosis; outside of the uterus it is classified as endometriosis. Histologically, endometriosis is a benign disease with malignant behavior. It mainly affects white women between 30 and 40 years of age (NETO et al. 1984). Endometriosis affects 10%–20% of actively menstruating women and 30%–40% of infertile women (APPEL 1988).

Although endometriomas are malignant in the sense that they are invasive and metastasize, their aggressive behavior ceases once the ovarian hormonal influence is ended by irradiation, surgical castration, or menopause (KUMAR et al. 1984).

Three mechanisms have been postulated for the pathogenesis of the ectopic endometrium in the urinary bladder. An embryonic theory postulates that endometriosis may arise from the remnant of the wolffian and müllerian ducts. The metaplastic theory suggests that hormonal or inflammatory stimulation may cause bladder epithelial cells to undergo metaplasia, resulting in endometrial tissue formation. The migratory theory proposes that the endometrial tissue originates in the uterine wall and reaches an ectopic position by direct extension, implantation, or metastasis (KUMAR et al. 1984).

Endometriosis has been identified in the urethra, kidneys, ureters, and bladder. The urinary tract is affected in 1.1% of cases of endometriosis and the bladder is the most frequent organ involved, being affected in 84% of cases involving the urinary tract (NETO et al. 1984). The age at onset varies from 18 to 48 years; it is most prevalent in the fourth decade but in theory it may be seen at any time between puberty and menopause (KUMAR et al. 1984). The bladder is usually invaded from without by the endometrial tissue, penetrating the bladder wall and extending into the bladder lumen (KUMAR et al. 1984).

Endometriosis of the bladder presents a variable clinical picture depending on the site and location of the lesion. Its manifestations are influenced by cyclic ovarian hormonal changes. Vesical discomfort expressed as a sense of pressure, heaviness, cramp, or pain in the bladder region is the most common symptom, occurring in 78% of patients (NETO et al. 1984). Other common symptoms are dysuria, urgency, burning, and frequency. Both bladder pain and urinary disturbances tend to be cyclic coinciding with menstruation but may occur before or after the menstrual period. Gross hematuria occurs in only up to about one-third of cases and a mass is palpable in the bladder in about half. Previous abdominal or pelvic surgery is reported in at least half the patients (NETO et al. 1984; KUMAR et al. 1984).

Endometriosis of the bladder is most frequently located along the base or posterior wall of the bladder. It may be a round or lobulated mass ranging from a few millimeters to several centimeters in diameter, with one or more bullae beneath intact bladder mucosa and surrounded by a ring of mucosal edema. The bullae may have a bluish or blue black to dark red discoloration. The size of the mass and bullae increases preceding and during menstruation and may nearly disappear in midcycle. The endometrioma may resemble a chronic inflammatory lesion or an area of infiltrating carcinoma. During menstruation, bleeding and sloughing may be observed. Following radiation or surgical or hormonal castration, the endometrioma becomes fibrotic and disappears (KUMAR et al. 1984).

Sonography shows a filling defect and defines the extent of the tumor. If a mass extends through the wall of the bladder into the uterus, then endometriosis of the bladder should be strongly considered, particularly in a young female with characteristic symptoms (KUMAR et al. 1984). Endoscopic biopsy makes the diagnosis. The appearance of the endometrioma will change depending on the phase of the menstrual cycle, ranging from multiple cysts during menstruation to a purely echogenic mass in midmenstrual cycle (KUMAR et al. 1984).

The differential diagnosis includes mucosal edema, cystitis glandularis, cystitis cystica, papillary transitional cell carcinoma, sarcoma botryoides, leukoplakia, malacoplakia, metastasis, and lymphoma (KUMAR et al. 1984).

In younger women with endometriosis, in whom maintenance of reproductive function is desirable, hormonal management or surgery may be offered. The choice is influenced by the patient's age, marital status, desire for children, extent of disease, severity of urinary symptoms, and menstrual disorders and associated pathology (NETO et al. 1984).

6.8.2 Bladder Hernia

The involvement of the urinary bladder in hernias is not rare: it is said to occur in 10% of all inguinal hernias in men over 50 years of age (LIEBESKIND et al. 1973). The bladder can herniate into any pelvic or abdominal opening within its reach when it is distended. Almost all bladder hernias are inguinal or femoral.

Although only a small portion of the urinary bladder is usually involved, the entire bladder except for the trigone may be found in a hernia. A large bladder hernia into the scrotum is called a scrotal cystocele (LIEBESKIND et al. 1973).

The indirect inguinal hernia protrusion is through the internal inguinal ring, just above the inguinal ligament and just lateral to the deep inferior epigastric artery. The direct inguinal protrusion is into a weak point in the posterior wall of the inguinal canal called Hesselbach's triangle just medial to the deep inferior epigastric artery. Both types of inguinal hernia can traverse the inguinal canal and exit the external ring close to the crest and spinous process of the pubis. The indirect hernia traverses the entire inguinal canal and the direct hernia, only its distal one-fifth. The femoral hernia protrudes through the femoral canal which carries the iliac vessels underneath the inguinal ligament. With the variability in radiographic projection, it is usually not possible to distinguish the type of hernia radiographically (LIEBESKIND et al. 1973).

In the review of LIEBESKIND et al. (1973), females predominated in a ratio of about 2:1 under the age of 50. Over the age of 50, no significant sex predominance existed.

Most bladder hernias are clinically silent. The noted complaints of frequency, urgency, nocturia, dysuria, and hematuria are most likely related to associated conditions such as prostatic hypertrophy or cystitis. Large bladder hernias may produce a specific complaint of two-stage urination in which the patient first empties the abdominal portion of the bladder and then, often with the aid of manual pressure or change in position, reduces the herniated portion of the bladder and voids again (LIEBESKIND et al. 1973).

Visualization of bladder hernia at urography is dependent on patient position. Bladder hernia is located at the lateral inferior wall of the bladder with downward protrusion toward the inguinal region. Therefore the bladder protrusion into a hernia is downward and anteriorly. The small or moderate sized protrusion may not be present with the patient in the supine position, particularly if the bladder is underdistended. The herniated portion may also be pulled out of the hernia in the supine position if the bladder is fully distended or overdistended. Erect and/or prone views of the filled bladder must be taken to demonstrate bladder hernias optimally (LIEBESKIND et al. 1973).

A bladder hernia is distinguished from a cystocele by its inferior-lateral location compared to the inferior-midline position of the cystocele. Also, the cystocele tends to have a triangular shape compared to the rounded balloon shape of the bladder hernia (LIEBESKIND et al. 1973).

Herniation of bowel through an inguinal hernia may cause a fairly characteristic lateral extrinsic impression on the bladder without actual involvement of the bladder in the hernia. The contour defect may require the exclusion of actual bladder pathology (GOLDIN and ROSEN 1975).

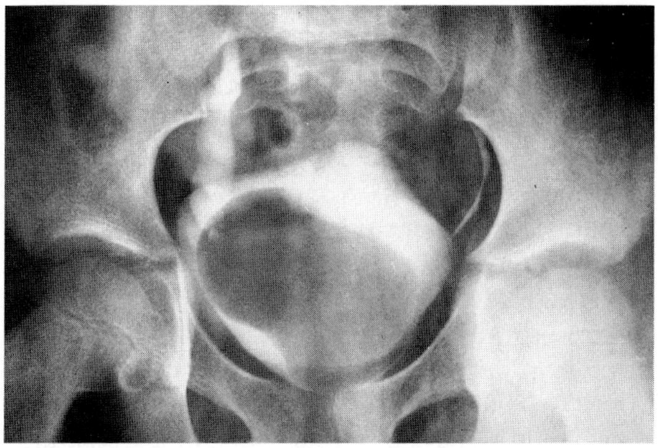

Fig. 6.45. Ureterocele as a mass in the bladder

Scrotal cystocele may present with urosepsis and multiple calculi due to stasis of residual urine in the large herniated portion of the bladder. The identification of bladder calculi in a scrotal soft tissue mass may allow plain film diagnosis (Postma and Smith 1986).

Any anterolateral pointing of the bladder on pelvic CT should prompt a search for contrast or soft tissue in the adjacent inguinal ring. Additional caudal scans or use of prone position may be needed. Coronal CT reconstruction or direct coronal imaging on MRI may be dramatic, particularly in scrotal cystocele (Curry et al. 1988).

Isotope within a bladder hernia may simulate an osseous metastasis when it appears over bone such as pubis and is separated from the bladder (Morano and Burkhalter 1987).

6.8.3 Ureterocele

Ureterocele is a submucosal cystic dilatation of the terminal ureter. The resulting mass can be quite large (Fig. 6.45) and even obstruct the urethra or prolapse through it. Both simple and ectopic ureteroceles may prolapse (Mindell 1990; Fenelon and Alton 1981). The ureterocele may be simple and orthotopically located at the corner of the trigone or ectopically located on a line between the corner of the trigone and the urethra. The ureterocele may be associated with a single or multiple ureter system. The ectopic ureter invariably drains the upper moiety of a duplication according to the Weigert-Meyer rule (Berdon et al. 1968). Between 10% and 20% of ectopic ureters are associated with single or nonduplicated collecting systems (Prewitt and Lebowitz 1976). The ureterocele may be obstructing or nonobstructing and only rarely refluxing (Leong et al. 1980). The ectopic ureterocele may or may not be associated with ureteral or calyceal dilatation (Share and Lebowitz 1989). The etiology of ureteroceles is debated but they are probably congenital (Friedland and Cunningham 1972).

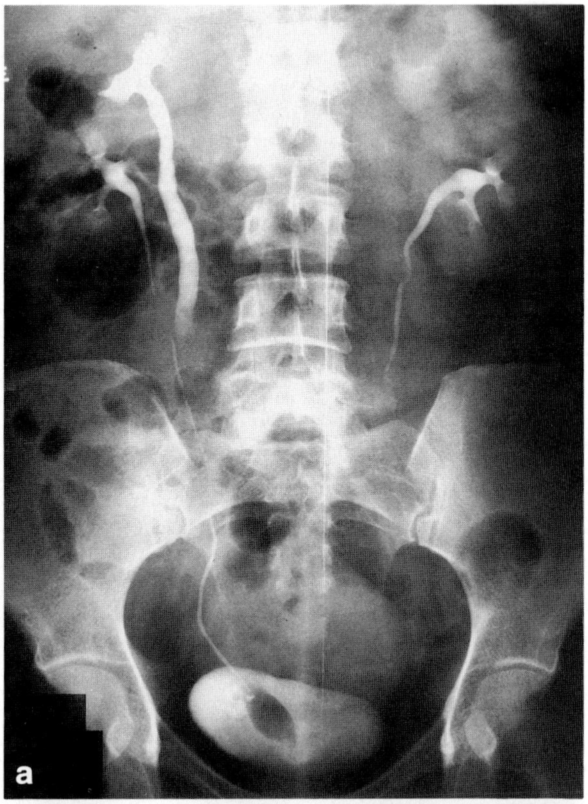

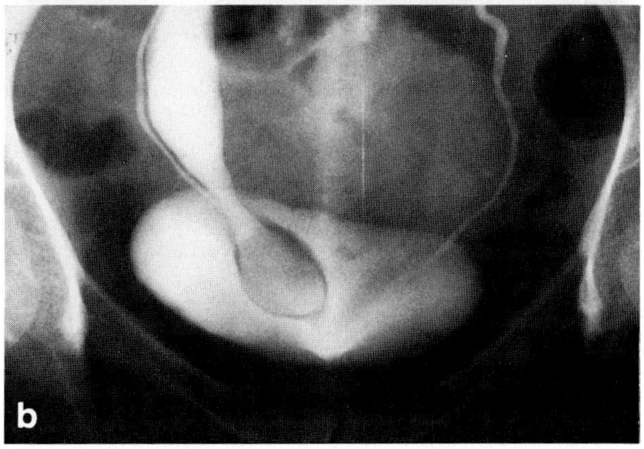

Fig. 6.46 a,b. Obstructing ectopic ureterocele in a young woman. The ureterocele is not filled on an early film (**a**) but is filled on a later film (**b**) with demonstration of its wall

In the adult, simple or orthotopic ureterocele is usually an incidental finding more often found

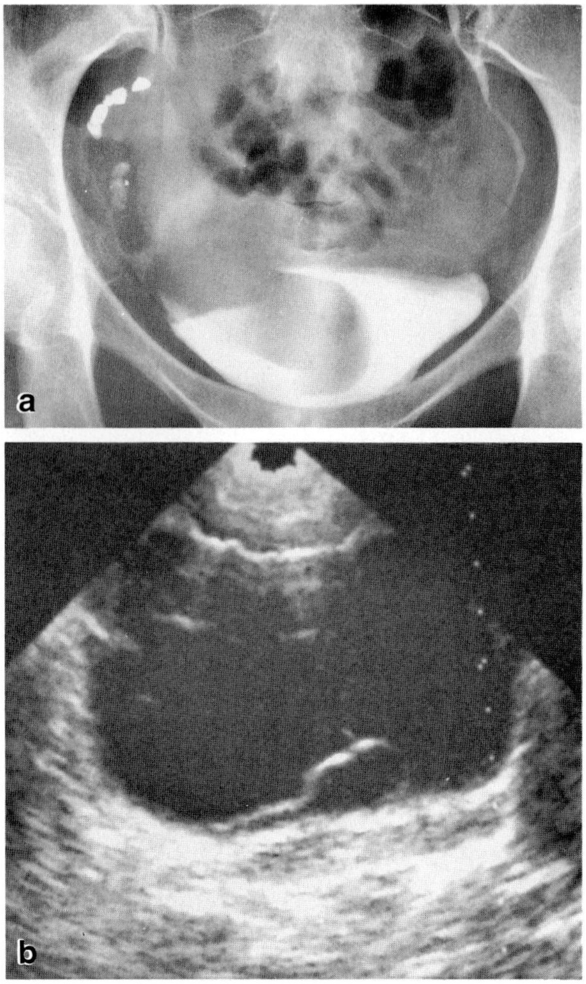

Fig. 6.47a,b. Marked difference in size of ureterocele on **a** urogram and **b** ultrasound performed on the same day

in women than men. It usually has a typical "cobrahead" configuration formed by the outline or halo of its mucosal roof (Fig. 6.46). Large obstructed ureteroceles are not filled with contrast and appear as a mass within the opacified bladder. They can get so large as to fill the bladder and obstruct the opposite ureter. A thickened wall suggests a complication such as tumor or edema from underlying stone or infection. Rarely, a transitional cell carcinoma may arise within a simple ureterocele (FORER and SCHAFFER 1990).

Ureteroceles may intussuscept or evert, that is, collapse and subsequently outpouch through the enlarged ureteral hiatus into the distal ureter (WALLACH and LEBOWITZ 1988; CREMIN et al. 1977). The intussuscepted everted ureterocele can then be seen to be protruding outside the vesical or urethral wall on voiding cystourethrography. KOYANAGI et al. (1980) found this condition in one-third of their cases of ureterocele.

Ectopic ureteroceles in adults have a different clinical presentation than those which present in childhood. Flank pain during voiding is the most common presenting complaint in adults and hematuria is not uncommon. Urinary tract infection is the most common presentation in children (AMITAI et al. 1992).

Ureterocele may be visualized on sonography having an appearance described as "cyst within a cyst" (GRIFFIN et al. 1983). The indentation caused by a dilated ureter outside the bladder may mimic this appearance (NUSSBAUM et al. 1986). Ultrasound may be more useful by evaluating the above kidney for dysplasia, hydronephrosis, or atrophy. NUSSBAUM et al. (1986) noted that ureteroceles are dynamic structures, changing in shape and size according to intravesical pressure (Fig. 6.47).

At cystoscopy, the ureterocele also changes size and shape depending on the degree of filling. It resembles a balloon that fills, then empties and flattens (MITTY and SCHAPIRA 1977). This variability helps explains why a ureterocele may not be seen on all films of a urogram. The cobra shape becomes lost when the ureterocele becomes large (MITTY and SCHAPIRA 1977). When outlined by contrast, the wall of the ureterocele is seen as a thin lucent line on both the inside and the outside of the ballooned mucosa.

A pseudoureterocele refers to outpouching of a previously normal ureteral orifice. With gradual incomplete obstruction of the submucosal or intramural distal ureter by tumor, dilatation of the proximal ureteral segment may assume a cobra shape. The lucency caused by the outlined wall will be more irregular and/or thicker than the thin lucent line of the true ureterocele (MITTY and SCHAPIRA 1977).

Pseudoureteroceles have been reported to be most commonly due to bladder tumor or calculus obstructing the ureteral orifice. They have also been reported to be caused by radiation cystitis, bladder floor invasion by squamous cell carcinoma of the cervix, pheochromocytoma of the intravesical portion of the ureter, obstruction of the orifice after ureteral instrumentation, and "steinstrasse" formation after extracorporeal shock wave lithotripsy (THORNBURY et al. 1977; MITTY and SCHAPIRA 1977; DATTA et al. 1971, 1972; Sherwood and STEVENSON 1969; BARBER et al. 1988).

Incising the wall or removing the ureterocele only converts it from an obstructing ureterocele into a refluxing ureterocele. Complete excision followed by reconstruction and reimplantation is the preferred treatment (TANAGHO 1972; KOYANAGI et al. 1980).

6.8.4 Malacoplakia

Malacoplakia is an uncommon chronic inflammatory granulomatous disease typically consisting of soft, usually yellow or tan mucosal plaques. Originally described as only found in the urinary bladder, it has since been found in practically every organ system in the body. Malacoplakia is believed to be infectious in origin and secondary to a deficiency in intracellular lysosomal digestion. Malacoplakia is composed of foam cells (Hanseman's cells) which have characteristic large intracytoplasmic laminated inclusions (Michaelis-Gutmann bodies) containing iron or calcium. Malacoplakia occurs almost invariably in conjunction with *Escherichia coli* infection. Malacoplakia has a definite female preponderance when it involves the urinary tract with a 4:1 female to male ratio.

In a review of 153 cases of malacoplakia (STANTON and MAXTED 1981), the urinary tract was involved in 58%, the bladder in 40%, the ureter in 11%, the renal pelvis in 10%, and the ureteropelvic junction and urethra in 2% each. The renal parenchyma was involved in 16% of patients. Most of the retroperitoneal involvement was by direct extension of genitourinary involvement (WESTRA et al. 1988).

Grossly, malacoplakia consists of variably sized yellow-brown plaques which are characteristically but not invariably soft and often display central umbilication or ulceration. The peripheral hyperemic epithelium initially remains intact but later erodes and ulcerates. Microscopically, malacoplakia is characterized by dense aggregates of large mononuclear phagocytes or histiocytes, the von Hanseman cells, which are admixed with intracellular and extracellular Michaelis-Gutmann bodies in various stages of maturation, all in a scanty connective tissue stroma and infiltrated by varying numbers of lymphocytes and plasma cells (STANTON and MAXTED 1981).

In early malacoplakia, Michaelis-Gutmann bodies may not be present and in late malacoplakia they may be very few. STANTON and MAXTED (1981) state they are not necessary for the diagnosis of malacoplakia but BAUMGARTNER and ALAGAPIAN (1990) state their presence is generally considered necessary in making the diagnosis.

STANTON and MAXTED (1981) described Michaelis-Gutmann bodies as discrete, sharply demarcated intracellular or extracellular spherical structures ranging in diameter from 5 to 10 μm and usually having a concentric "owl-eye" or "bird's-eye" appearance. They further described a well-recognized morphologic maturation sequence on electron microscopy which begins with a central sphere of calcification, progresses to an outer peripheral calcification giving a target appearance, and culminates in further outer calcification leading to the definitive calcospherule.

Because its onset typically occurs during middle age, malacoplakia is considered to be a manifestation of an acquired defect (STANTON and MAXTED 1981). There is also a strong correlation between malacoplakia and altered host-immune response. Of 153 cases reviewed by STANTON and MAXTED (1981), 62 patients (40%) had either an intercurrent systemic disorder, a carcinoma, an immune deficiency syndrome, or an autoimmune disease. An altered macrophage response to infection by microorganisms may result in impaired digestion within phagolysosomes, creating the lesions of malacoplakia (BAUMGARTNER and ALAGAPPIAN 1990).

STREEM (1984) summarizes that current evidence suggests that affected patients have an abnormality of intraphagosomal digestion that is in most cases acquired rather than genetic. This defect leads to inefficient handling and phagocytosis of bacteria, which is recognized in vitro as diminished mononuclear cell bactericidal activity and clinically as malacoplakia.

Cystoscopically, malacoplakia can appear as flat pink-brown nodules, as yellow and nodular similar to amyloid deposits, or as a soft yellow-brown plaque, often with a central umbilication or ulceration and peripheral hyperemia (STANTON and MAXTED 1981).

ELLIOTT et al. (1972) described the findings on urography, where malacoplakia appears as smooth discrete dome-shaped nodules not more than 5 mm in diameter and studding the mucosal surfaces of the urinary tract. Initially, the overlying epithelium remains intact. The nodules may grow to 2.5 cm in diameter in the bladder, and be either multiple or single. The lesions heal individually, developing an umbilicated, moon-crater

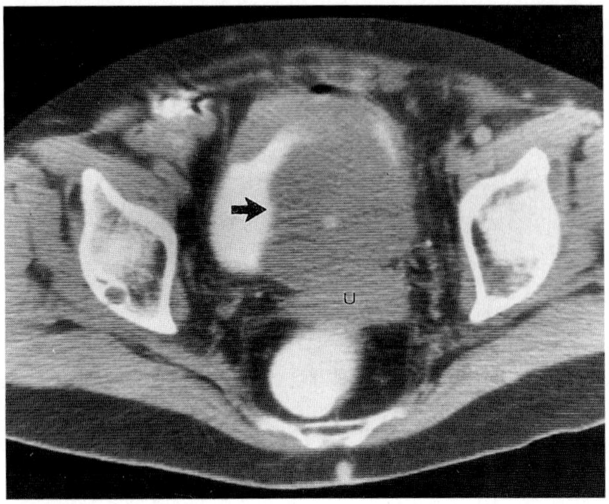

Fig. 6.48. Malacoplakia involving the urinary bladder. A soft tissue mass (*arrow*) involves the posterior-superior aspect of the bladder and is contiguous with the uterus (*U*). (Baumgartner and Alagappian 1990)

appearance which is quite characteristic. Prominent scarring or stenosis is not to be expected.

The findings on CT have been entirely nonspecific. Epstein et al. (1983) found a large solid bladder mass with extension to the left pelvic side wall. Bidwell and Dunne (1987) described a large inhomogeneous mass in the left pelvis that was partially destroying a portion of the left sacrum and left ilium, with encasement of adjacent loops of bowel and internal calcification. Baumgartner and Alagappian (1990) found a 6- to 7-cm mass between the bladder and the uterus in one case and partial right ureteral obstruction with multiple filling defects in another (Fig. 6.48). Both cases were more suggestive of neoplasm than inflammation. CT can help determine the extent of disease and monitor response to therapy. Percutaneous aspiration needle biopsy under CT guidance can provide diagnostic tissue (Bidwell and Dunne 1987).

Malacoplakia is not always a benign or innocuous disease. With vital organ involvement, mortality can exceed 50% and the morbidity can be substantial (Stanton and Maxted 1981). In malacoplakia of the urinary bladder, there are usually associated chronic and unrelenting symptoms of bladder irritability, hematuria, and urinary tract infections (Stanton et al. 1983). Isolated lower tract involvement in nontransplant patients is often benign and self-limiting with apparent cure even after lengthy follow-up intervals (Streem 1984).

Stanton and Maxted (1981) recommended treatment with an intracellularly active antibiotic to which the organism is sensitive in conjunction with bethanechol and ascorbic acid. Surgical treatment may become necessary if the disease progresses.

6.8.5 Xanthogranulomatous Cystitis

Xanthogranulomatous cystitis is a benign chronic inflammatory disorder that may be related to an underlying immunologic defect (Walther et al. 1985). Many believe that malacoplakia and xanthogranulomatous lesions may be different degrees of the same pathologic process (Stanton and Maxted 1981). They are both chronic granulomatous lesions which can occur anywhere in the urinary tract, occasionally occur elsewhere, and can mimic carcinoma. Malacoplakia prefers the bladder and xanthogranuloma the kidney.

Grossly, xanthogranulomas are nodular, focally necrotic, or cystic. They are yellow in color due to large amounts of lipids in the cytoplasm of the macrophages that form them. Microscopically, the mass consists of a large number of macrophages with small round to oval nuclei in a granular or foamy cytoplasm. Acute and chronic inflammatory cells are interspersed in the tissue (Walther et al. 1985).

The xanthomatoses can be divided into three types: (a) lipid infiltration into the cell secondary to hypercholesterolemia (hypercholesterolemic xanthomatoses, (b) lipid accumulation and retention in the cell secondary to increased cellular synthesis and retention (hyperlipidemia), and (c) extracellular precipitation or crystallization of lipid (normocholesterolemic xanthomatoses). The normocholesterolemic xanthomatoses include Hand-Schüller-Christian syndrome and xanthoma cells in inflammatory tissue or true tumors, such as in chronic granulomatous disease, xanthogranulomatous pyelonephritis, and granulomatous cystitis (Walther et al. 1985).

Curiously, the majority of the reported cases of xanthogranulomatous cystitis, 7 of 11 (63.6%), were associated with urachal adenoma and two of these also had a patent urachus (Walther et al. 1985).

Medical management has not been found to be totally effective. Chronic suppressive antibiotic therapy with trimethoprim/sulfamethoxazole (as in the treatment of chronic granulomatous disease) and urinary astringents may be helpful.

6.8.6 Condylomata Acuminata

Condylomata acuminata is a sexually transmitted disease affecting the mucocutaneous surfaces of the anogenital region, with extension to the bladder exceedingly rare.

The condylomata acuminata lesions are typically soft and papillary and usually involve only the external genitalia and mucocutaneous junctions. The disease is typically localized and benign; it is caused by a human papillomavirus. Extension to the bladder may be related to immunosuppression or immune deficiency. Bladder involvement is more virulent and an association with urothelial malignancy has been suggested (MURPHY et al. 1990).

Patients with bladder involvement usually present with nonspecific symptoms associated with other pathologic processes of the bladder such as frequency, dysuria, nocturia, and hematuria.

Imaging examination may localize the lesions to the bladder wall, where they have no distinguishing features.

Treatment is difficult. Fulguration must be repeated and intravesical 5-fluorouracil may be necessary. Most patients come to cystectomy (MURPHY et al. 1990).

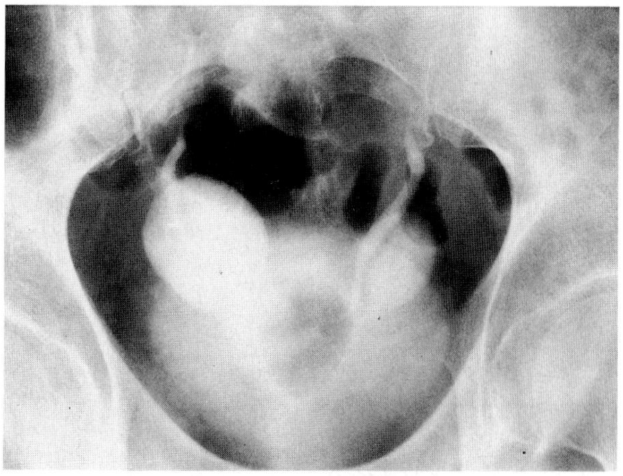

Fig. 6.49. Bilateral Hutch diverticula; medial deviation of the distal ureter is a characteristic of bladder diverticula

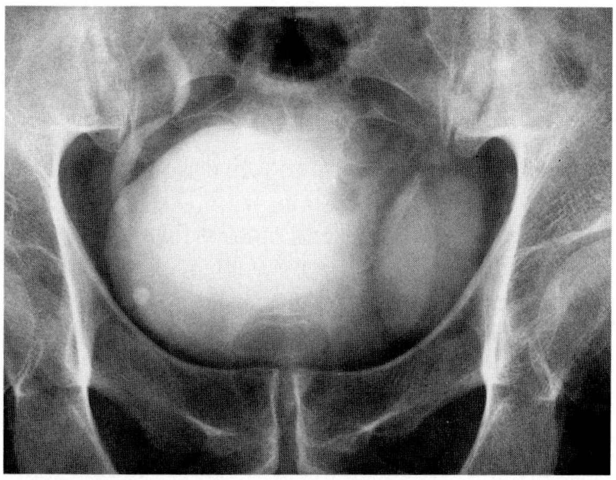

Fig. 6.50. Diverticulum at the left ureterovesical junction in a 64-year-old male; the diverticulum is not obstructing the ureter

6.8.7 Bladder Diverticula

Bladder diverticula are outpouchings of mucosa between the interstices of the detrusor muscle. In the adult they are usually the result of obstruction or upper motor neuron neurogenic bladder. The longstanding increased muscular contractions required to empty the bladder cause thickening of the wall and mucosal herniation in areas of weakness between the hypertrophied detrusor muscle bundles. A common location is just superior to the ureter, which may cause vesicoureteral reflux. This is the so-called Hutch diverticulum (Fig. 6.49) (HERNANZ-SCHULMAN and LEBOWITZ 1985). The diverticula are most commonly located in the posterior wall above the trigone, the region of the ureteral orifices (Fig. 6.50) and the dome at the site of an obliterated urachus (ROSAI 1989). The wall of the diverticulum consists of mucosa, fibrous tissue, and little or no muscle. Without expulsive power, urinary stasis and chronic infection are the rule (ROSAI 1989; TANAGHO 1992c).

Bladder diverticula in infants and children are very similar, yet different from those in adults. The incidence peak in children is at age 10 years and in adults between 61 and 70 years (BAUER and RETIK 1974). BAUER and RETIK (1974) feel that diverticula are secondary to a congenital weakness in the muscular wall with or without the presence of obstruction, and that this weak area is a potential source of diverticulum formation. In children almost all diverticula form at or near the edge of the trigone and are not always associated with distal obstruction.

In a series of 425 bladder diverticula, KNAPPENBERGER et al. (1960) found an incidence of 4% involvement by carcinoma. There were 14

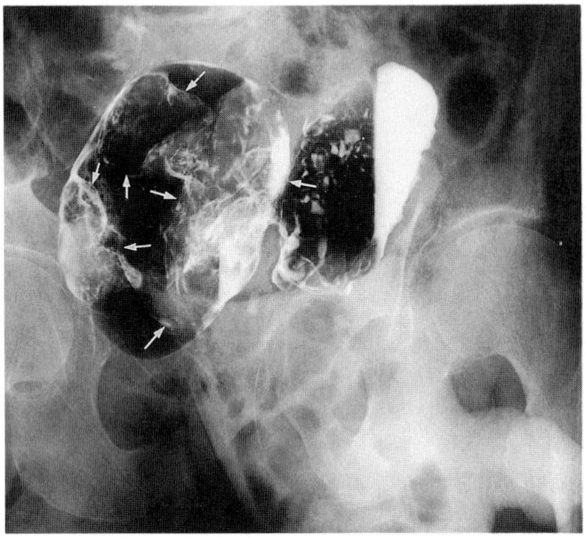

Fig. 6.51. A double contrast barium-air cystogram demonstrates a huge diverticulum with a narrow neck on the right side. Note large filling defects within the diverticulum which represent transitional cell carcinomas (*arrows*). (Courtesy of Dr. E.K. Lang)

transitional cell lesions and two squamous cell lesions. The age range was from 44 to 78 years and all but one patient was male. Melicow (1974) suggested that prolonged stasis of urine in a diverticulum may account for the high incidence of cancer. The incidence of carcinoma in diverticula is reported to reach 10.5%, with the overall incidence from a review of the literature being 3.6% (Das and Amar 1986). The wall of a diverticulum is thinner than that of the bladder and tumors tend to spread rapidly and have a poor prognosis (Gerridzen and Futter 1982; Das and Amar 1986) (Fig. 6.51).

While transitional cell carcinoma is the most common neoplasm found in bladder diverticula, followed by squamous cell carcinoma, paraganglioma and malignant fibrous histiocytoma have also been reported (McCormick et al. 1985). Furthermore, Fig. 6.52 shows a leiomyosarcoma arising in a bladder diverticulum.

Other complications of bladder diverticula include lithiasis (Fig. 6.53) and free perforation into the peritoneal cavity (Rosai 1989).

Diverticula and neoplasms in diverticula can be identified with ultrasound (Saez et al. 1985; Williams and Gooding 1985) or on double contrast barium-air cystography. CT can assess the depth of invasion and the presence of local or distant adenopathy (Lowe et al. 1989). CT stages the disease and aids preoperative planning.

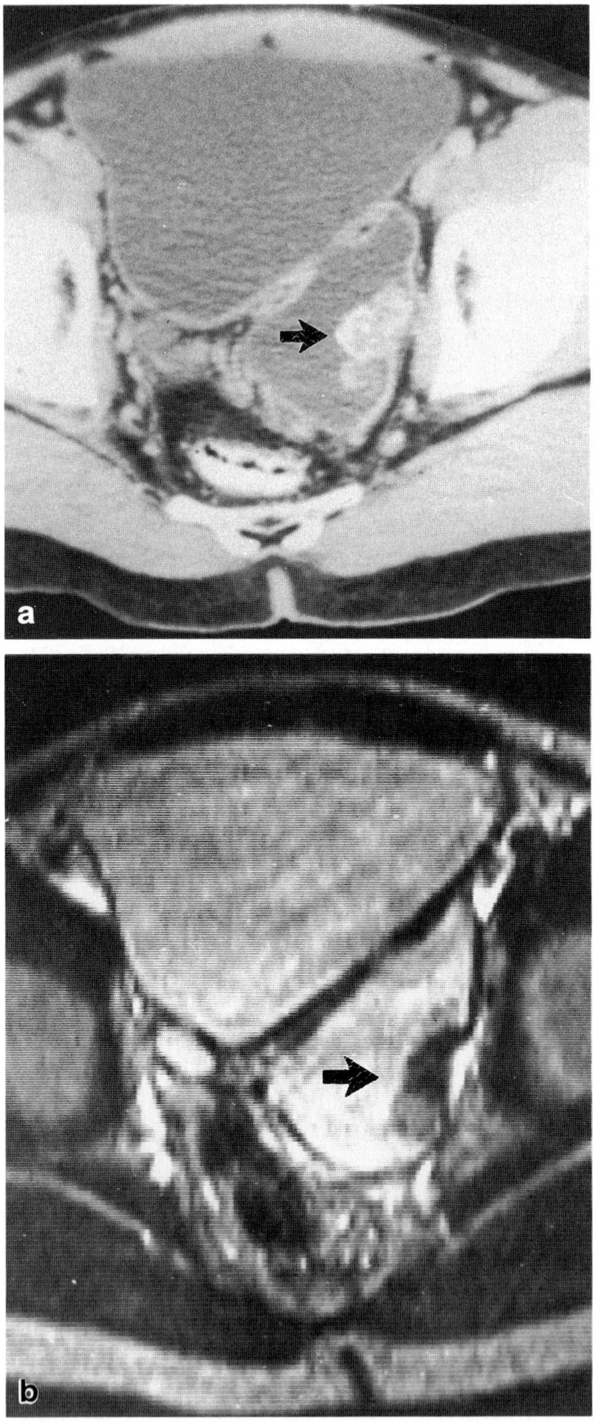

Fig. 6.52 a,b. Leiomyosarcoma (*arrow* or *T*) arising in a bladder diverticulum (*D*). **a** CT; **b** T2-weighted axial MRI. The tumor did not extend through the wall of the diverticulum. (Courtesy of Dr. I. Yoder)

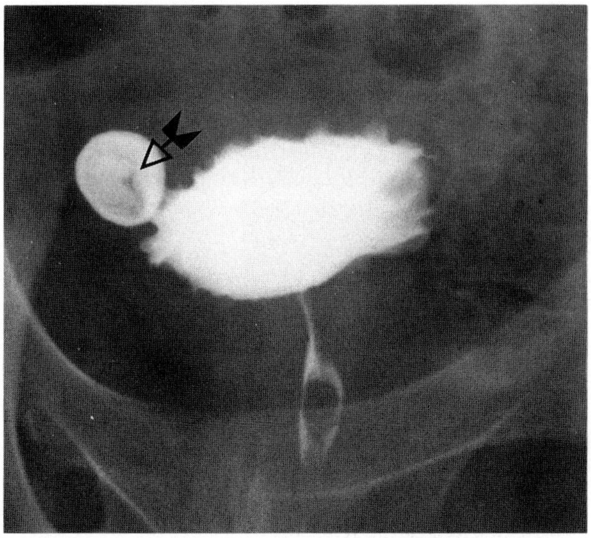

Fig. 6.53. Stone (*arrow*) in bladder diverticulum. (Courtesy of Dr. S.T. COCHRAN)

6.8.8 Amyloidosis

Amyloidosis is best thought of as a disease complex that results in the extracellular deposition of insoluble fibrillar protein material (SCOTT et al. 1986). The protein configuration accounts for the characteristic insolubility of amyloid that promotes its continued accumulation within organs, eventually leading to compromised function (SCOTT et al. 1986). The amyloid fibril proteins present in different clinical types of amyloid have been described and characterized, including those associated with myeloma, so-called primary amyloidosis, secondary amyloidosis, and familial amyloidosis (SCOTT et al. 1986).

Amyloidosis occurs in less than 0.5% of hospitalized patients, and diagnosis depends on biopsy of the involved tissues with appropriate stains (SCOTT et al. 1986).

Systemic amyloidosis accounts for 80%–90% of cases of amyloidosis (Table 6.5). Idiopathic or primary amyloidosis is characterized by the deposition of amyloid in the heart, kidneys, tongue, gastrointestinal tract, blood vessel walls, nerves, skin, muscles, periarticular structures, and carpal ligaments. There is no known cause (SCOTT et al. 1986).

Amyloidosis may be associated with multiple myeloma and other plasma dyscrasia. Males are again more often affected than women, with most patients over 40 years of age (SCOTT et al. 1986).

Table 6.5. Classification of amyloidosis. (After SCOTT et al. 1986)

Systemic
Idiopathic or primary
Related to plasma cell dyscrasias
Reactive or secondary
Familial
Localized
Organ limited: lung, skin, bladder, endocrine, other
Focal
Associated with aging or senility

Reactive or secondary amyloidosis is associated with a disease process other than a plasma cell dyscrasia. In the United States, rheumatoid arthritis, osteomyelitis, and bronchiectasis are the commonest causes (SCOTT et al. 1986). Major sites for reactive or secondary amyloid deposition are the kidneys, liver, spleen and adrenals. The clinical manifestations tend to be renal. After therapy for the underlying disease process, the amyloid deposits may or may not regress (SCOTT et al. 1986).

Approximately 15% of cases of amyloidosis are localized, without systemic amyloidosis ever developing. The usual sites of organ-limited disease are lung, skin, bladder, and larynx (SCOTT et al. 1986). Amyloidosis of the urinary tract may be a manifestation of generalized disease or organ limited. Organ-limited disease may be derived from immunocytes or plasma cells and be either diffuse or nodular (PEAR 1986).

Localized or organ-specific amyloidosis in the urinary tract most frequently occurs in the bladder and most often presents with total gross hematuria, which may be life threatening (THOMAS et al. 1977).

In the bladder, amyloidosis presents as tumorlike masses or diffuse infiltration of the bladder wall (SCOTT et al. 1986). Amyloid lesions in the bladder are grossly similar to an infiltrating neoplasm. They are typically localized, broadbased, and sessile with thickening of the bladder wall and a roughened, nodular surface often with small ulcerations. The amyloid deposits are located in the submucosa and the inner layers of the muscularis with prominent deposits in the media of both arteries and veins (MALEK et al. 1971; STRONG et al. 1974). Amyloid replaces muscle cells and may cause a foreign body reaction with an inflammatory infiltrate of plasma cells and lymphocytes, especially near zones of ulceration (STRONG et al. 1974).

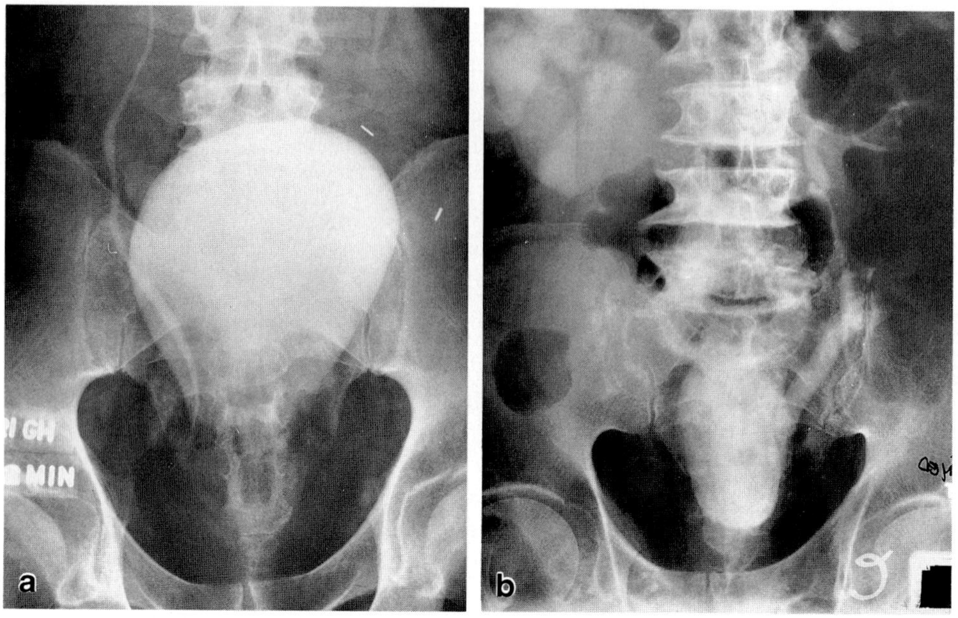

Fig. 6.54 a,b. Pear-shaped bladders from **a** nonobstructing and **b** obstructing pelvic lipomatosis. (Courtesy of Dr. S.T. Cochran)

Cystoscopically, the lesions vary from hemorrhagic ulcers to inflammatory looking excrescences, with most lesions simulating neoplasm (Malek et al. 1971). Cystoscopy may reveal severe localized or generalized inflammation with depositions or nodules. The inflammatory change and bleeding are apparently due to focal necrosis secondary to small vessel occlusion (Thomas et al. 1977). Localized amyloid may be confused with proliferative cystitis (Strong et al. 1974).

Amyloidosis of the urinary bladder seems to occur in men and women about equally, with a mean age of 51 years (Malek et al. 1971).

Symptomatic amyloid in the urinary bladder is most often localized or organ limited. The lower urinary tract lesions of the disseminated forms are rarely if ever symptomatic (Malek et al. 1971), though uncontrollable hemorrhage may also occur in secondary involvement of the bladder (Strong et al. 1974). Localized or organ-specific amyloid of the bladder may be present for a considerable time and seems to run a relatively benign course.

Prolonged follow-up is needed. Small lesions can be treated by transurethral resection and fulguration. Large lesions may require partial cystectomy (Strong et al. 1974). Total cystectomy with ileal diversion may be necessary occasionally (Malek et al. 1971).

There are no pathognomonic radiographic findings although submucosal calcification arranged in sheets or discrete nodules is both extremely suggestive and rare (Pollack et al. 1981). In amyloidosis, epithelial and submucosal atrophy with ulceration is followed by deposition of urate, phosphate, and oxalate crystals. The submucosal intramural calcifications demonstrated radiographically may be mottled and irregular or homogeneous in appearance (Thomas et al. 1977). A nonspecific filling defect or mass is sometimes found (Malek et al. 1971).

History or presence of amyloid in the urinary bladder does not exclude associated neoplasm and every individual lesion must be biopsied carefully (Malek et al. 1971).

6.8.9 Pear-Shaped Bladder

When pressure is applied to the sides of the bladder, a teardrop or pear shape will result. The floor of the bladder may be lifted up as well. The causes are those that symmetrically involve the soft tissues of the pelvis: pelvic lipomatosis (Fig. 6.54), retroperitoneal fibrosis, pelvic hematoma, collateral vessels from inferior vena cava occlusion, and enlarged pelvic lymph nodes usually due to lymphoma. Symmetrically

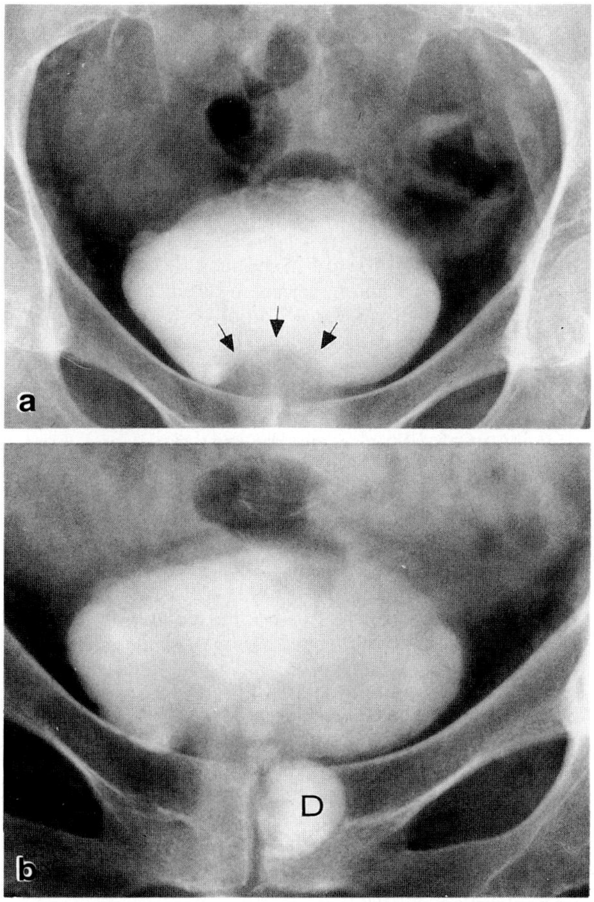

Fig. 6.55. **a** "Female prostate" appearance (*arrows*) from impression by edema due to **b** urethral diverticulum (*D*) demonstrated on post-void film

occurring processes such as bilateral lymphoceles, urinomas, or abscesses can also produce this appearance (Ambos et al. 1977). This bladder deformity can also be seen as a normal variant in a person with iliopsoas muscle hypertrophy and a narrow pelvis (Wechsler and Brennan 1982).

6.8.10 Bladder Base Impression

Mass elevating the base of the bladder is a common finding in males and is almost always due to a prostate enlarged by benign prostatic hypertrophy. A similar appearance may be produced in females by a variety of conditions including symphysis pubis asymmetry, postoperative change, urethral diverticulum (Fig. 6.55), levator ani impression, infiltration of the vesicovaginal septum by tumor, or urethral syndrome (Pope et al. 1981). Urethral syndrome, clinically similar to

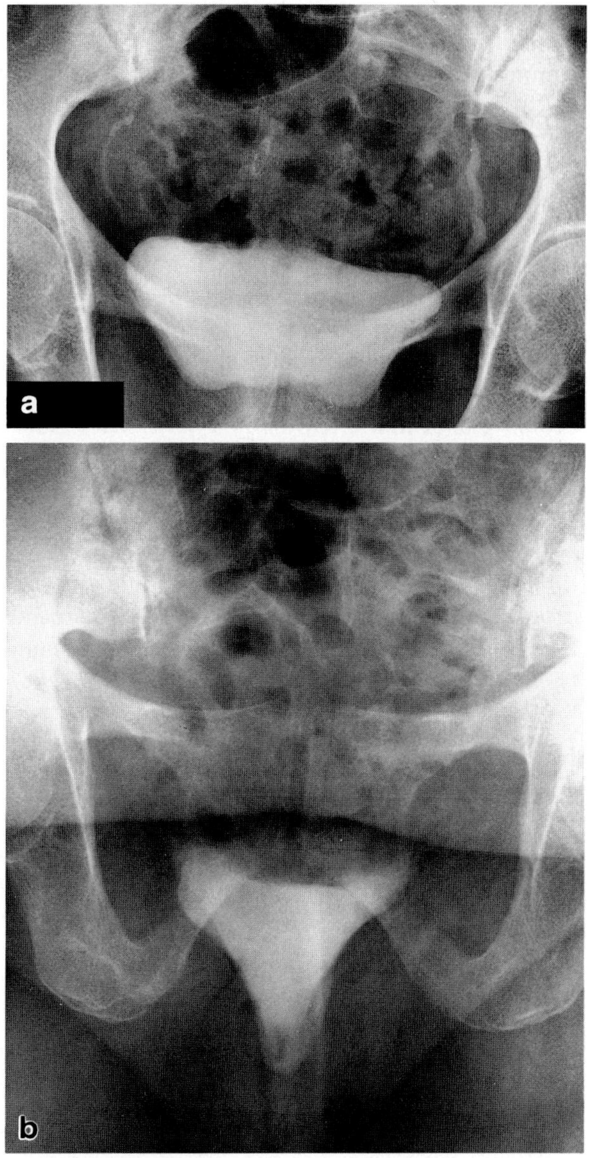

Fig. 6.56 a,b. Spectrum from **a** weakening of the pelvic floor to **b** prolapse

cystitis, is caused by inflammation of the proximal urethra, paraurethral ducts and glands and the bladder neck (Jackson 1976).

6.8.11 Vaginal Prolapse and Cystocele

Vaginal prolapse may be defined as descent of adjacent organs into the vagina and sometimes beyond (Stanton 1983). The urethra, bladder, uterus, and cervix and small bowel and rectum may be involved. Urethrocele refers to urethral prolapse, cystocele to bladder prolapse, enterocele to small bowel prolapse, and rectocele to rectal prolapse. Cysturethrocele is the most common vaginal prolapse and the incidence rises in the elderly. Complete uterine prolapse with a cystocele can cause ureteral obstruction and is potentially fatal. The commonest causes of prolapse are childbirth and menopause. Prolonged and difficult labor, bearing down before full dilatation, multiple births, laceration of the lower genital tract in the second stage of labor, forceful delivery of the placenta during the third stage, and inadequate repair of pelvic floor injuries are factors in childbirth likely to promote prolapse later in life (STANTON 1983). After childbirth, the estrogen withdrawal of menopause is the next most significant factor in the development of prolapse.

The weakening of the pelvic floor can sometimes be demonstrated on an upright film at urography or cystography (Fig. 6.56a). Cystocele and prolapse may be demonstrated in the same fashion (Fig. 6.56b).

References

Abeshouse BS, Robbins MA, Gann M, Salik JO (1957) Intestinovesical fistulas: report of seven cases and review of the literature. JAMA 164:251–257

Abu-Yousef MM (1986) Ultrasound of bladder tumors. Semin Ultrasound CT MR 7:275–286

Aigen AB, Phillips M (1986) Primary malignant lymphoma of urinary bladder. Urology 28:235–237

Al Ghorab MM (1988) Schistosomiasis (bilharziasis). In: Tanagho EA, McAninch JW (eds) Smith's general urology, 12th edn. Appleton & Lange, Norwalk, pp 254–258

Allen FJ, De Kock ML (1987) Pelvic lipomatosis: the nuclear magnetic resonance appearance and associated vesicoureteral reflux. J Urol 87:1228–1230

Ambos MA, Bosniak MA, Lefleur RS, Madayag MA (1977) The pear-shaped bladder. Radiology 122:85–88

Amendola MA, Agha FP, Dent TL, Amendola BE, Shirazi KK (1984) Detection of occult colovesical fistula by the Bourne test. AJR 142:715–719

Amitai M, Hertz M, Jonas P, Apter S, Heyman Z (1992) Ectopic ureterocele in adults with a comparison of the anomaly in children. Urol Radiol 13:181–186

Anderstrom C, Johansson S, Petterson S (1982) Inverted papilloma of the urinary tract. J Urol 127:1132–1134

Anderstrom C, Johansson SL, Von Schultz L (1983) Primary adenocarcinoma of the urinary bladder: a clinicopathologic and prognostic study. Cancer 52:1273–1280

Anichkov NM, Nikonov AA (1982) Primary malignant melanomas of the bladder. J Urol 128:813–815

Antonakopoulos GN, Newman J (1984) Eosinophilic cystitis with giant cells: a light microscopic and ultrastructural study. Arch Pathol Lab Med 108:728–731

Appel RA (1988) Bilateral ureteral obstruction secondary to endometriosis. Urology 32:151–154

Arger PH (1985) Computed tomography of the lower urinary tract. Urol Clin North Am 12:677–686

Arger PH, Coleman BG, Mintz MC (1986) Lower urinary tract computed tomography. Semin Ultrasound CT MR 7:287–297

Aron BS, Schlesinger A (1974) Complications of radiation therapy: the genitourinary tract. Semin Roentgenol 9:65–74

Ash JE (1940) Epithelial tumors of the bladder. J Urol 44:135–145

Avni EF, Matos C, Diard F, Schulman CC (1988) Midline omphalovesical anomalies in children: contribution of ultrasound imaging. Urol Radiol 10:189–194

Axelrod SL, Ring KS, Collins MH, Reiley EA, Hensle TW (1991) Eosinophilic cystitis in children. Urology 37:549–552

Bacon SK (1943) Rupture of the urinary bladder: clinical analysis of 147 cases in the past ten years. J Urol 49:432–435

Bahnson RR, Zaontz MR, Maizels M, Shkolnik AA, Firlit CF (1989) Ultrasonography and diagnosis of pediatric genitourinary rhabdomyosarcoma. Urology 33:64–68

Baker SM, Middleton WD (1992) Color Doppler sonography of ureteral jets in normal volunteers: importance of the relative specific gravity of urine in the ureter and bladder. AJR 159:773–775

Baker ME, Silverman PM, Korobkin M (1985) Computed tomography of prostatic and bladder rhabdomyosarcomas. J Comput Assist Tomogr 9:780–783

Barber L, Amendola MA, Pollack HM, Van Arsdalen KN (1988) Pseudoureteroceles following extracorporeal shock wave lithotripsy. Radiology 167:397–399

Bartkowski DP, Lanesky JR (1988) Emphysematous prostatitis and cystitis secondary to *Candida albicans*. J Urol 139:1063–1065

Bauer SB, Kogan SJ (1991) Vesical manifestations of chronic granulomatous disease in children: its relation to eosinophilic cystitis. Urology 37:463–466

Bauer SB, Retik AB (1974) Bladder diverticula in infants and children. Urology 3:712–715

Baumgartner BR, Alagappian R (1990) Malakoplakia of the ureter and bladder. Urol Radiol 12:157–159

Beachey EH (1981) Bacterial adherence: adhesin-receptor interactions mediating the attachment of bacteria to mucosal surfaces. J Infect Dis 143:325–345

Beaser RS, Guay AT, Lee AK, Silverman ML, Flint LD (1986) An adrenocorticotropic hormone-producing pheochromocytoma: diagnostic and immunohistochemical studies. J Urol 135:10–13

Belis JA, Post GJ, Rochman SC, Milam DR (1979) Genitourinary leiomyomas. Urology 27:424–429

Bell TE, Wendel RG (1968) Cystitis glandularis: benign or malignant? J Urol 100:462–465

Benson RC, Tomera KM, Panayotis PP (1983) Transitional cell carcinoma of the bladder in children and adolescents. J Urol 130:54–55

Berdon WE, Baker DH, Becker JA, Uson AC (1968) Ectopic ureterocele. Radiol Clin North Am 6:205–214

Berger BW, Bhagavan SBS, Reiner W, Engel R, Lepor H (1981) Nephrogenic adenoma: clinical features and therapeutic considerations. J Urol 126:824–826

Bergkvist A, Jyungqvist A, Moberger G (1965) Classification of bladder tumours based on the cellular pattern. Acta Chir Scand 130:371–378

Bhansali SK, Cameron KM (1960) Primary malignant lymphoma of the bladder. Br J Urol 32:440–454

Bidwell JK, Dunne MG (1987) Computed tomography of bladder malacoplakia. J Comput Assist Tomogr 11:909–910

Binkovitz LA, Hattery RR, LeRoy AJ (1988) Primary lymphoma of the bladder. Urol Radiol 9:231–233

Blacklock NJ (1977) Bladder trauma in the long-distance runner: "10,000 metres heamaturia." Br J Med 49: 129–132

Bloedorn FG, Young JD, Cuccia CA, Mercado R, Wizenberg MJ (1962) Radiotherapy in carcinoma of the bladder: possible complications and their prevention. AJR 79:576–581

Blum MD, Bahnson RR, Carter MF (1985) Urologic manifestations of von Recklinghausen neurofibromatosis. Urology 26:209–216

Boag GS, Nolan RL (1988) Sonographic features of urinary bladder involvement in regional enteritis. J Ultrasound Med 7:125–128

Bocian JJ, Flam MS, Mendosa CA (1982) Hodgkin's disease involving the urinary bladder diagnosed by urinary cytology. Cancer 50:2482–2485

Bohlman ME, Fishman EK, Oesterling JE, Goldman SM (1988) CT findings in emphysematous cystitis. Urology 32:63–64

Bomanji J, Levison DA, Flatman WD et al. (1987) Uptake of iodine-123 MIBG by pheochromocytomas. paragangliomas and neuroblastomas: a histopathological comparison. J Nucl Med 28:973–978

Bonavita JA, Pollack HM (1983) Trauma of the adult bladder and urethra. Semin Roentgenol 17:299–306

Boring CC, Squires TS, Tong T (1992) Cancer statistics, 1992. CA 42:19–38

Bornstein I, Charboneau JW, Hartman GW (1986) Leiomyoma of the bladder: sonographic and urographic findngs. J Ultrasound Med 5:407–408

Botma JP, Burger EG, de Kock ML (1987) Eosinophilic cystitis associated with Glanzmann's thrombasthenia: a case report. S Afr Med J 71:533–534

Brand KG (1979) Schistosomiasis-cancer: etiological consideration: a review. Acta Trop (Basel) 36:203–214

Brant WE, Williams JL (1984) Computed tomography of bladder leiomyoma. J Comput Assist Tomogr 8: 562–563

Bree RL, Silver TM (1982) Nongynecologic bladder and perivesical ultrasound. Urol Radiol 4:135–145

Brick SH, Friedman AC, Pollack HM et al. (1988) Urachal carcinoma: CT findings. Radiology 169:377–381

Brogdon BG, Silbiger ML, Colston JA (1965) Cystitis glandularis. Radiology 85:470–473

Buckner CB, Leithiser RE, Walker CW, Allison JW (1991) The changing epidemiology of tuberculosis and other mycobacterial infections in the United States: implications for the radiologist. AJR 156:255–264

Bullock PS, Thoni DE, Murphy WM (1987) The significance of colonic mucosa (intestinal metaplasia) involving the urinary tract. Cancer 59:2086–2090

Byrd L, Sherman RL (1979) Radiocontrast-induced acute renal failure: a clinical and pathophysiologic review. Medicine 58:270–279

Cacciarelli AA, Kass EJ, Yang SS (1990) Urachal remnants: sonographic demonstration in children. Radiology 174:473–475

Caceres J, Mata JM, Lucaya L, Palmer J, Donoso L (1991) General case of the day. RadioGraphics 11:161–163

Caffey J (1972) Section 6: Urinary tract. In: Pediatric radiology, vol I, 6th edn. Yearbook, Chicago, pp 753–812

Cameron KM, Lupton CH (1976) Inverted papilloma of the lower urinary tract. Br J Urol 48:567–577

Carpenter AA (1973) Pelvic lipomatosis: successful surgical treatment. J Urol 110:397–399

Carroll PR, McAninch JW (1984) Major bladder trauma: the accuracy of cystography. J Urol 130:887–888

Carroll PR, McAninch JW (1984) Major bladder trauma: mechanisms of injury and a unified method of diagnosis and repair. J Urol 132:254–257

Carson CC, Malek RS, Remine WH (1978) Urologic aspects of vesicoenteric fisula. J Urol 119:744–746

Case RAM, Hosker ME (1954) Tumour of the urinary bladder as an occupational disease in the rubber industry in England and Wales. Br J Prev Soc Med 8:39–50

Case RAM, Hosker ME, Mc Donald DM et al. (1954) Tumours of the urinary bladder in workmen engaged in manufacture and use of certain dye-stuff intermediates in British chemical industry. Part I. The role of aniline, benzidine, alpha-naphthylamine, and betanaphthylamine. Br J Ind Med 11:75–104

Cass AS (1984) False negative retrograde cystography with bladder rupture owing to external trauma. J Trauma 24:168–169

Cassady JR (1991) Keynote address: contributions of pediatric oncology: examples derived from advances made in the treatment of rhabdomyosarcoma and neuroblastoma. Int J Radiat Oncol Biol Phys 20:1177–1182

Castillo J Jr, Cartagna R, Montes M (1988) Eosinophilic cystitis: a therapeutic challenge. Urology 32:535–537

Chaitin BA, Manning JT, Ordonez NG (1984) Hematologic neoplasms with initial manifestations in lower urinary tract. Urology 23:35–42

Charnsangavej C (1990) Lymphoma of the genitourinary tract. Radiol Clin North Am 28:865–877

Chiang KS, Lamki N, Athey PA (1992) Metastasis to the bladder from pancreatic adenocarcinoma presenting with hematuria. Urol Radiol 13:187–189

Chuang VP, Wallace S (1981) Arterial infusion and occlusion in cancer patients. Semin Roentgenol 16: 13–25

Colby TV (1980) Carcinoid tumor of the bladder. A case report. Arch Pathol Lab Med 104:199–200

Cole P (1973) A population based study of bladder cancer. In: Doll R, Vodopija I (eds) Host environment interactions in the etiology of cancer in man. International Agency for Research on Cancer, Lyon, pp 83–87

Cole P, Hoover R, Friedell GH (1972) Occupation and cancer of the lower urinary tract. Cancer 29:1250–1260

Corriere JN, Sandler CM (1986) Management of the ruptured bladder: seven years of experience with 111 cases. J Trauma 26:830–833

Corrierre JN, Sandler CM (1988) Mechanisms of injury, patterns of extravasation and management of extraperitoneal bladder rupture due to blunt trauma. J Urol 139:43–44

Cos LR, Cockett ATK (1982) Genitourinary tuberculosis revisited. Urology 20:111–117

Cox IH, Erickson SJ, Foley WD, Dewire DM (1991) Ureteric jets: evaluation of normal flow dynamics with color Doppler sonography. AJR 158:1051–1055

Cramer SF, Aikawa M, Cebelin M (1981) Neurosecretory granules in small cell invasive carcinoma of the urinary bladder. Cancer 47:724–730

Cremin BJ, Funston MR, Aaronson IA (1977) "The intraureteric diverticulum", a manifestation of ureterocoele intussusception. Pediatr Radiol 6:92–96

Crowe FW, Schull WJ (1953) Diagnostic importance of cafe-au-lait spot in neurofibromatosis. Arch Intern Med 91:758–766
Cummings KB (1983) Diagnosis, staging and classification of bladder tumors. Semin Urol 1:7–14
Cunningham JJ (1975) Radiographic features of the interureteric ridge. AJR 125:688–691
Curry NS, O'Connor KF, Tubbs CO (1988) Scrotal cystocele diagnosed by computed tomography. Urol Radiol 9:247–248
Daifuku R, Stamm WE (1986) Bacterial adherence to bladder uroepithelial cells in catheter-associated urinary tract infection. N Engl J Med 314:1208–1213
Dann RH, Arger PH, Enterline HT (1972) Benign proliferation processes presenting as mass lesions in the urinary bladder. AJR 116:822–828
Das S, Amar ADA (1986) Vesical diverticulum associated with bladder carcinoma: therapeutic implications. J Urol 136:1013–1014
Das S, Bulusu NV, Lowe P (1983) Primary vesical pheochromocytoma. Urology 21:20–25
Das KM, Vaidyanathan S, Rajwanshi A, Indudhara R (1992a) Renal tuberculosis: diagnosis with sonographically guided aspiratation cytology. AJR 158:571–573
Das KM, Indudhara R, Vaidyanathan S (1992b) Sonographic features of genitourinary tuberculosis. AJR 158:327–329
Datta NS, Singh SM, Bapta BC (1971) False ureterocele: lower ureteral stone simulating ureterocele. Br J Urol 43:301–304
Datta NS, Ito Y, Eisenman JI, Bischoff AJ (1972) "Cobra head" deformity: its relationship to ureterocele "pseudo-ureterocele". J Can Assoc Radiol 23:284–286
Deguchi T, Takeuchi T, Kuriyama M, Sakai S, Shinoda I, Ban Y, Maeda I, Nishiura T (1985) Malakoplakia of urinary bladder following cadaveric renal transplantation. Urology 26:92–94
DeMeester LJ, Farrow BM, Utz DC (1975) Inverted papilloma of the urinary bladder. Cancer 36:505–513
Denoix PF (1978) TNM classification of malignant tumors, 3rd edn. International Union Against Cancer, Geneva
DiSantis DJ, Siegel MJ, Katz ME (1991) Simplified approach to umbilical abnormalities. RadioGraphics 11:59–66
Doll R, Peto R (1981) The causes of cancer: quantitative estimates of avoidable risks of cancer in the United States today. JNCI 66:1191–1308
Durkee C, Benson R Jr (1980) Bladder cancer following administration of cyclophosphamide. Urology 16: 145–148
Eldrup J, Thorup J, Nielsen SL, Hald T, Hainau B (1983) Permeability and ultrastructure of human bladder epithelium. Br J Urol 55:488–492
Elkin M, Urogenital tuberculosis (1990) In: Pollack H, ed. Clinical Urography. Philadelphia, PA; W.B. Saunders Company, pp 1020–1052
Elliott FG, Eid TC, Lakey WH (1981) Genitourinary neurofibromatosis: clinical significance. J Urol 125: 725–727
Elliott GB, Moloney PJ, Clement JG (1972) Malacoplakia of the urinary tract. AJR 116:830–837
Engler RJ, Weber CB, Turnicky R (1986) Hypersensitivity to chromated catgut sutures: a case report and review of the literature. Ann Allergy 56:317–320
Epstein BM, Patel V, Porteous PH (1983) CT appearance of bladder malacoplakia. J Comput Assist Tomogr 7:541–543
Erturk E, Erturk E, Sheinfeld J, Davis RS (1988) Metaplastic cystitis complicated with von Brunn nests, cystitis cystica and intestinal type of glandular metaplasia. Urology 32:165–167
Fall M, Johansson SL, Aldenborg F (1987) Chronic interstitial cystitis: a heterogeneous syndrome. J Urol 137: 35–38
Fallon B, Wendt JC, Hawtrey CE (1984) Urological injury and assessment in patients with fractured pelvis. J Urol 131:712–714
Farrelly CA, Daneman A, Martin DJ, Chan HS (1984) Pheochromocytoma in childhood; the important role of computed tomography in tumour localization. Pediatr Radiol 14:210–214
Faysal MH (1981) Squamous cell carcinoma of the bladder. J Urol 126:598–599
Fenelon MJ, Alton DJ (1981) Prolapsing ectopic ureteroceles in boys. Radiology 140:373–376
Fink IJ, Reinig JW, Dwyer AJ, Doppman JL, Linehan WM, Keiser HR (1985) MR imaging of pheochromocytomas. J Comput Assist Tomogr 9:454–458
Fokkens W, Hop WC (1979) Radiation-induced bladder tumors [letter]. J Urol 121:690
Forer LE, Schaffer RM (1990) Transitional cell carcinoma of a simple ureterocele a specific sonographic appearance. J Ultrasound Med 9:301–303
Fornage BD, Rifkin MD, Lemaire AD, Touche DH (1984) Bladder metastasis of gastric carcinoma: diagnosis by sonography. J Clin Ultrasound 12:578–580
Fowler JE Jr (1989) Nonmicrobial inflammation and noninflammatory disorders. In: Urinary tract infection and inflammation. Year Book Medical, Chicago, pp 291–322
Fowler JE, Stamey TA (1977) Studies of introital colonization in women with recurrent urinary infection. VII. The role of bacterial adherence. J Urol 117:472–476
Fowler JE, Lynes WL, Lau JLT, Ghosh L, Mounzer A (1988) Interstitial cystitis is associated with intraurothelial Tamm-Horsfall protein. J Urol 140:1385–1389
Friedenberg RM (1971) Tuberculosis of the genitourinary system. Semin Roentgenol 6:310–322
Friedland GW, Cunningham JJ (1972) The elusive ectopic ureteroceles. AJR 116:792–811
Ganem EJ, Batal JT (1956) Secondary malignant tumors of the urinary bladder metastatic from primary foci in distant organs. J Urol 75:965–972
Gavant ML, Ellis JV, Klesges LM (1992) Diagnostic efficacy of excretory urography with low-dose, nonionic contrast media. Radiology 182:657–660
Gelabert MA, Arango O, Rosales A, Coronado J, Moreno A (1990) Eosinophilic cystitis and allergy to mitomycin-C. Acta Urol Belg 58:65–72
Gelfand M, Weinberg RW, Castle WM (1967) Relationship between carcinoma of the bladder and infestation with *Schistosoma haematobium*. Lancet I:1249–1251
Geoffray A, Couanet D, Montagne JP, Leclere J, Flamant F (1987) Ultrasonography and computed tomography for diagnosis and follow-up of pelvic rhabdomyosarcomas in children. Pediatr Radiol 17:132–136
Gerlock AJ, Mirfakhraee M (1985) Materials and methods for peripheral visceral embolization. In: Gerlock AJ, Mirfakjraee M (eds) Essentials of diagnostic and interventional angiographic techniques. W.B. Saunders, Philadelphia, pp 209–236
Gerridzen RG, Futter NG (1982) Ten-year review of vesical diverticula. Urology 20:33–35
Godec CJ (1985) Genitourinary trauma. Urol Radiol 7: 185–191

Goff WB (1983) Cystitis cystica and cystitis glandularis: cause of bladder mass. J Comput Assist Tomogr 7: 347–349

Goldfarb DA, Novick AC, Bravo EL, Straffon RA, Montie JE, Kay R (1989) Experience with extra-adrenal pheochromocytoma J Urol 142:931–936

Goldin RR, Rosen RA (1975) Effects of inguinal hernias upon the bladder and ureters. Radiology 115:55–57

Goldman SM, Fajardo AA, Naraval RC, Madewell JE (1979) Metastatic transitional cell carcinoma from the bladder: radiologic manifestations. AJR 132:419–425

Goldman SM, Fishman EK, Gatewood OMB, Jones B, Brendler C, Siegelman SS (1984) The CT demonstration of colovesical fistulae secondary to diverticulitis. J Comput Assist Tomogr 8:462–468

Goldman SM, Fishman EK, Gatewood OMB, Jones B, Siegelman SS (1985) CT in the diagnosis of enterovesical fistula. AJR 144:1229–1233

Goldstein M (1971) Eosinophilic cystitis. J Urol 106: 854–857

Goldstein HM, Kaminsky S, Wallace S, Johnson DE (1974) Urographic manifestations of metastatic melanoma. AJR 121:801–805

Gooding GAW (1986) Varied sonographic manifestations of cystitis. J Ultrasound Med 5:61–63

Goodman A, Lipinski JK (1984) Ultrasound demonstration of a pheochromocytoma of the bladder. J Clin Ultrasound 12:507–508

Gosling JA (1985) Structure of the lower urinary tract and pelvic floor. Clin Obstet Gynecol 12:285–294

Gregg JA, Utz DC (1974) Eosinophilic cystitis associated with eosinophilic gastroenteritis. Mayo Clin Proc 49: 185–187

Griffin J, Jennings C, MacErlean D (1983) Ultrasonic evaluation of simple and ectopic ureteroceles. Clin Radiol 34:55–57

Guerriero WG, Devine CJ (1984a) Bladder trauma. In: Guerriera WG, Devine CJ (eds) Urologic injuries. Appleton-Century-Crofts, Norwalk, pp 73–81

Guerriero WG, Devine CJ (1984b) Fistulas. In: Guerriera WG, Devine CJ (eds) Urologic injuries. Appleton-Century-Crofts, Norwalk, pp 83–107

Gupta AK, Bhargava S (1987) Bladder hemangioma: ultrasonographic demonstration. Urol Radiol 9:181–182

Haggar AM, Kressel HY (1985) Magnetic resonance imaging of the genitourinary tract. Urol Clin North Am 12:725–736

Hahn D (1990) Neoplasms of the urinary bladder. In: Pollack H (ed) Clinical urography. W.B. Saunders, Philadelphia, pp 1358–1380

Haid M, Iganatoff J, Khandikar JD, Graham J, Holland J (1980) Urinary metastasis from breast carcinoma. Cancer 46:229–232

Hall BD (1971) Bladder hemangiomas in Klippel-Trenaunay-Weber syndrome. N Engl J Med 285:1032–1033

Hanno PM, Wein AJ (1987) Interstitial cystitis, parts I and II. AUA Update Series 6:9–10

Hare WSC, Lond FRCR, Holland CJ (1983) Paresis following internal iliac artery embolization. Radiology 146:47–51

Harrison RB, Stier FM, Cochrane JA (1978) Alkaline encrusting cystitis. AJR 130:575–577

Hartge P, Hoover R, Altman R et al. Use of hair dyes and risk of bladder cancer. Cancer Res 42:4784–4787

Hattery RR, Williamson B Jr, Hartman GW, LeRoy AJ, Witten DM (1988) Intravenous urographic technique. Radiology 167:593–599

Hayes EE, Sandler CM, Corriere JN (1983) Management of the ruptured bladder secondary to blunt abdominal trauma. J Urol 129:946–948

Hellstrom HR, Davis BK, Shonnard JW (1979) Eosinophilic cystitis: a study of 16 cases. Am J Clin Pathol 72:777–784

Hernanz-Schulman M, Lebowitz RL (1985) The elusiveness and importance of bladder diverticula in children. Pediatr Radiol 15:399–402

Herr HW (1983) Carcinoma in situ of the bladder. Semin Urol 1:15–22

Heyman F, Cheung Y, Ghali V, Leiter E (1989) Bladder pheochromocytoma: evaluation with magnetic resonance imaging. J Urol:1424–1426

Hicks RM (1981) Carcinogenesis in the urinary bladder: a multi-stage process. In: Connolly JG (ed) Carcinoma of the bladder. Raven, New York, pp 74–89

Hicks RM, Walters CL, Eisebai E, Aasser AB, Merzabani ME, Gough TA (1977) Demonstration of nitrosamines in human urine: preliminary observations on a possible etiology for bladder cancer in association with chronic urinary tract infections. Proc R Soc Med 70:413–417

Hinder RA, Schmaman A (1969) Bilharziasis and squamous carcinoma of the bladder. S Afr Med J 43:617–618

Hockley NM, Bihrle R, Bennet RM III, Curry JM (1989) Congenital genitourinary hemangiomas in a patient with the Klippel-Trenaunay syndrome: management with the neodymium: YAG laser. J Urol 141:940–941

Holm-Bentzen M, Lose G (1978) Pathology and pathogenesis of interstitial cystitis. Urology [Suppl] 29:8–13

Holm-Benzen M, Jacobsen F, Nerstrom B et al. (1987) A prospective double-blind clinically controlled multicenter trial of sodium pentosanpolysulfate in the treatment of interstitial cystitis and related painful bladder disease. J Urol 138:503–507

Holsti LR, Ermala P (1955) Papillary carcinoma of the bladder in mice, obtained after peroral administration of tobacco tar. Cancer 8:679–682

Holt JF (1978) Neurofibromatosis in children. AJR 130: 615–639

Horner SA, Weingarten JL (1990) Eosinophilic cystitis in a renal allograft recipient. J Urol 144:342–343

Horstman WG, McClennan BL, Heiken JP (1991) Comparison of computed tomography and conventional cystography for detection of traumatic bladder rupture. Urol Radiol 12:188–193

Hricak H, Tscholakoff D, Heinrichs L, Fisher MR, Dooms GC, Reinhold C, Jaffe RB (1986) Uterine leiomyomas: correlation of MR, histopathologic findings, and symptoms. Radiology 158:385–391

Hueper WC, Wiley FH, Wolfe HD (1938) Experimental production of bladder tumors in dogs by administration of beta-naphthylamine. J Ind Hyg Toxicol 20:46–84

Illescas FF, Baker ME, Weinerth JL (1986) Bladder leiomyoma: advantages of sonography over computed tomography. Urol Radiol 8:216–218

Imray TJ, Kaplan P (1983) Lower urinary tract infections and calculi in the adult. Semin Roentgenol 17:276–287

Imray TJ, Saigh JA (1987) Importance of prone-position film during intravenous urography in detection of bladder tumors. Urology 29:228–230

Inglis JA, Tolley DA, Grigor KM (1987) Allergy to mitomycin C complicating topical administration for urothelial cancer. Br J Urol 59:547–549

Ito N, Hirose M, Shirai T et al. (1981) Lesions of the urinary bladder epithelium in 125 autopsy cases. Acta Pathol Jpn 31:545–557

Jackson EA (1976) Urethral syndrome in women. Radiology 119:287–291

Javadpour N, Mostafi FK (1969) Primary epithelial tumors of the bladder in the first two decades of life. J Urol 101:706–710

Jewett HJ (1952) Carcinoma of the bladder: influence of the depth of infiltration on the 5-year results following complete extirpation of the primary growth. J Urol 67:672–680

Jewett HJ, Strong GH (1946) Infiltrating carcinoma of the bladder: relation of depth of penetration of the bladder wall to incidence of local extension and metastases. J Urol 55:366–372

Johnson DE, Schoenwald MB, Ayala AG, Miller LS (1976) Squamous cell carcinoma of the bladder. J Urol 115:542–544

Johnson DE, Hodge GB, Abdul-Karim FW, Ayala AG (1985) Urachal carcinoma. Urology 26:218–221

Johnson DE, Swanson DA, von Eschenbach AC (1988) Tumors of the genitourinary tract. In: Tanagho EA, McAninch JW (eds) Smith's general urology, 12th edn. Appleton & Lange, Norwalk, pp 330–434

Jurascheck F, Egloff H, Buemi A, Laedlein-Greilsammer D (1983) Paraganglioma of urinary bladder. Urology 22:659–663

Kallenius G, Winberg J (1978) Bacterial adherence to periurethral epithelial cells in girls prone to urinary-tract infections. Lancet II 26:540–543

Kaplan BW, King LR (1970) Cystitis cystica in childhood. J Urol 103:657–659

Kaplan PA, Williams SM (1987) Mucocutaneous and peripheral soft-tissue hemangiomas: MR imaging. Radiology 163:163–166

Karasick S, Lev-Toaff AS, Toaf ME (1992) Imaging of uterine leiomyomas. AJR 158:799–805

Katayama H, Yamaguchi K, Kozuka T, Takashima T, Seez P, Matsuura K (1990) Adverse reactions to ionic and nonionic contrast media: a report from the Japanese committee on the safety of contrast media. Radiology 175:621–628

Kaufman JM, Jam B, Jacobs SC, Gabilondo F, Yalla S, Kane JP, Rossier AB (1977) Bladder cancer and squamous metaplasia in spinal cord injury patients. J Urol 118:967–971

Kauzlaric D, Barmeir E (1985) Sonography of emphysematous cystitis. J Ultrasound Med 4:319–320

Kauzlaric D, Barmier E (1986) Sonography of traumatic rupture of the bladder: "bladder within a bladder" appearance of extraperitoneal extravasation. J Ultrasound Med 5:97–98

Kauzlaric D, Barmeir A, Campana A (1987) Diagnosis of cystitis glandularis. Urol Radiol 9:50–52

Kessler WO, Clark PL, Kaplan GW (1975) Eosinophilic cystitis. Urology 6:499–501

Kim SH, Lee SE, Han MC (1991) Penile hemangioma: US and MRI imaging demonstration. Urol Radiol 13: 126–128

Klein TW, Kaplan GW (1975) Klippel-Trenaunay syndrome associated with urinary tract hemangiomas. J Urol 114:596–600

Knappenberger ST, Uson AC, Melicow MM (1960) Primary neoplasms occurring in vesical diverticula: a report of 18 cases. J Urol 83:153–159

Kollins SA, Hartman GW, Carr DT, Segura JW, Hattery RR (1974) Roentgenographic findings in urinary tract tuberculosis: a ten year review. AJR 121:487–499

Korobkin M, Cambier L, Drake J (1988) Computed tomography of urachal carcinoma. J Comput Assist Tomogr 12:981–987

Koss LG (1975a) Tumors of the urinary bladder. Atlas of tumor pathology, Second series, Fascicle 11. Armed Forces Institute of Pathology, Washington, DC, pp 9–61

Koss LG (1975b) Tumors of the urinary bladder. Atlas of tumor pathology, Second series, Fascicle 11. Armed Forces Institute of Pathology, Washington DC, p 81

Kovalcik PJ, Beidenheimer MC, Corman ML, Coller JA (1976) Colovesical fistula. Dis Colon Rectum 19: 425–427

Koyanagi T, Hisajima S, Goto T, Tokunaka S, Tsuji I (1980) Everting ureteroceles: radiographic and endoscopic observation, and surgical management. J Urol 123:538–543

Kumar R, Haque AK, Cohen MS (1984) Endometriosis of the urinary bladder. J Clin Ultrasound 12:363–365

Kunin CM (1987) Principles of urinary bacteriology and immunology. In: Kunin CM (ed) Detection, prevention and management of urinary tract infections, 4th edn. Lea & Febiger, Philadelphia, pp 125–193

Kwok-Liu JP, Zikman JM, Cockshott WP (1980) Carcinoma of the urachus: the role of computed tomography. Radiology 137:731–734

Kyriakos M, Royce RK (1989) Multiple simultaneous inverted papillomas of the upper urinary tract. Cancer 63:368–380

Lang EK (1968a) Double contrast cystography. In: Lang EK (ed) Roentgenographic diagnosis of bladder tumors. Charles C. Thomas, Springfield, Ill., pp 36–48

Lang EK (1968b) Arteriography of bladder tumors. In: Lang EK (ed) Roentgenographic diagnosis of bladder tumors. Charles C. Thomas, Springfield, Ill., pp 70–112

Lang EK (1969) Double contrast gas barium cystography in the assessment of diverticula of the bladder. AJR 107:769–775

Lang EK (1981) Transcatheter embolization of pelvic vessels for control of intractable hemorrhage. Radiology 140:331–339

Lang EK (1984a) Transcatheter embolization in the management of intractable hemorrhage from the pelvis and bladder. In: Lang EK (ed) Current concepts of uroradiology. Williams and Wilkins, Baltimore, pp 237–246

Lang EK (1984b) The use of imaging modalities in staging of carcinoma of the prostate and bladder. In: Lang EK (ed) Current concepts of uroradiology. Williams and Wilkins, Baltimore, pp 137–156

Lang EK (1986) Transcatheter embolization in the management of intractable hemorrhage from pelvic organs. In: Lang EK (ed) Percutaneous and interventional urology and radiology. Springer, Berlin Heidelberg New York, pp 201–210

Lang EK (1989) Management of hemorrhagic pelvic neoplasm by transcatheter embolization. J Intervent Radiol 4:113–117

Lang EK, Deutsch JS, Goodman JR, Barnett T, LaNasa JA, Duplessis GH (1979) Transcatheter embolization of hypogastric branch arteries in the management of intractable bladder hemorrhage. J Urol 121:30–36

Lapides J, Diokno AC (1976) Urine transport, storage, and micturition. In: Lapides J (ed) Fundamentals of urology. W.B. Saunders, Philadelphia, pp 190–241

Latham RH, Wong ES, Larson A, Coyle M, Stamm WE (1985) Laboratory diagnosis of urinary tract infection in ambulatory women. JAMA 254:3333–3336

Lebowitz RL, Mandell J (1987) Urinary tract Infection in children: putting radiology in its place. Radiology 165:1–9

Leestma JE, Price EB (1971) Paraganglioma of the urinary bladder. Cancer 28:1063–1073

Leonard MP, Nickel JC, Morales A (1988) Cavernous hemangiomas of the bladder in the pediatric age group. J Urol 140:1503–1504

Leong J, Mikhael B, Schillinger JF (1980) Refluxing ureteroceles. J Urol 124:136–139

Levine E, Farber B, Lee KR (1978) Computed tomography in diagnosis of pelvic lipomatosis. Urology 12: 606–608

Lewis BD, Doubilet PM, Heller VL, Bierre A, Bieger FR (1986) Cutaneous and visceral hemangiomata in the Klippel-Trenaunay-Weber syndrome: antenatal sonographic detection. AJR 147:598–600

Liebeskind AL, Elkin M, Goldman SH (1973) Herniation of the bladder. Radiology 106:257–262

Lieskovsky G, Ahlering T, Skinner DG (1988) Diagnosis and staging of bladder cancer. In: Skinner DG, Lieskovsky G (eds) Diagnosis and management of genitourinary cancer. W.B. Saunders, Philadelphia, pp 264–280

Lipper S, Kahn LB (1978) Amyloid tumor: a clinicopathologic study of four cases. Am J Surg Pathol 2:141–145

Littleton RH, Farah RN, Cerny JC (1982) Eosinophilic cystitis: an uncommon form of cystitis. J Urol 127: 132–133

Lowe FC, Goldman SM, Oesterling JE (1989) Computerized tomography in evaluation of transitional cell carcinoma in bladder diverticula. Urology 34:390–395

Lubs ME, Bauer MS, Formas ME, Djokic B (1991) Lisch nodules in neurofibromatosis type 1. N Engl J Med 324:1264–1266

Lynes WL, Flynn SD, Shortliffe LD, Lemmers M, Zipser R, Roberts LJ II, Stamey TA (1987) Mast cell involvement in interstitial cystitis. J Urol 138:746–752

Macfarlane MT (1988a) Urinary tract infections. In: Macfarlane MT (ed) Urology for the house officer. Williams and Wilkins, Baltimore, pp 85–103

Macfarlane MT (1988b) Interstitial cystitis. In: Macfarlane MT (ed) Urology for the house officer. Williams and Wilkins, Baltimore, pp 111–112

Mahoney EM, Harrison JH (1977) Malignant pheochromocytoma: clinical course and treatment. J Urol 118:225–229

Maldazys JD, de Kernion JB (1986) Urologic applications of regional chemotherapy. In: Lang EK (ed) Percutaneous and interventional urology and radiology. Springer, Berlin Heidelberg New York, pp 217–232

Malek RS, Greene LF, Farrow GM (1971) Amyloidosis of the urinary bladder. Br J Urol 43:189–200

Manco LG (1985) Cystitis cystica simulating bladder tumor at sonography. J Clin Ultrasound 13:52–54

Mandell MJ, Thieme GA, Eggli KD, Ballantine TVN (1989) Transrectal ultrasound guided needle biopsy of recurrent vaginal mass in a 23 month old girl. Pediatr Radiol 20:120–121

Margolin HN (1971) Fungus infections of the urinary tract. Semin Roentgenol 6:323–330

Markle BM, Catena L (1986) Bladder pseudomass following cystography-related bladder trauma. Radiology 159:256

Marshall BR (1952) The relation of the preoperative estimate to the pathologic demonstration of the extent of vesical neoplasms. J Urol 68:714–723

Marshall FF, Middleton AW (1974) Eosinophilic cystitis. J Urol 112:335–337

Marshall VF (1952) Relation of preoperative estimate to pathologic demonstration of extent of vesical neoplasms. J Urol 68:714–723

Marumi Y, Sato T, Kuriyama K et al. (1988) Vesical dome tumors: significance of extravesical extension on CT. Radiology 169:383–385

McCarthy CS, Becker JA (1991) Multiple myeloma and contrast media. Radiology 183:519–521

McCormick SR, Dodds PR, Kraus PA, Lowell DM (1985) Nonepithelial neoplasms arising within vesical diverticula. Urology 25:405–408

McDonald DF, Fagan CJ (1972) Fungus balls in the urinary bladder. AJR 114:753–757

McDougal WS, Persky L (1981) Bladder injuries. In: Libertino JA (ed) Traumatic injuries of the genitourinary system. Williams and Wilkins, Baltimore (International perspectives in urology, vol 1, pp 85–92)

McKeen EA, Bodurtha J, Meadows AT, Douglass EC, Mulvihill JJ (1978) Rhabdomyosarcoma complicating multiple neurofibromatosis. J Pediatr 93:992–993

Meares EM (1987) Guest editorial: interstitial cystitis 1987. Urology [Suppl] 29:46–48

Meares EM (1992) Nonspecific infections of the genitourinary tract. In: Tanagho EA, McAninch JW (eds) Smith's general urology, 13th edn. Appleton & Lange, Norwalk, pp 195–239

Mee SL, McAninch JW, Federle MP (1987) Computerized tomography in bladder rupture: diagnostic limitations. J Urol 137:207–209

Melamed MR, Voutsa NG, Grabstald H (1964) Natural history and clinical behavior of in situ carcinoma of the human urinary bladder. Cancer 17:1533–1545

Melicow M (1952) Histological study of vesical urothelium intervening between gross neoplasms in total cystectomy. Cancer 9:261–279

Melicow MM (1955) Tumors of the urinary bladder: a clinicopathological analysis of over 2500 specimens and biopsies. J Urol 74:498–521

Melicow, MM, Uson AC (1961) The "herald" lesion of the bladder: a lesion which portends the approach of cancer or inflammation from outside the bladder. J Urol 85:543–551

Melicow MM, Uson AC, Stams U (1974) Herald lesion of urinary bladder: a nonspecific but significant pathologic process. Urology 3:140–147

Melicow MM (1974) Tumors of the bladder: a multifaceted problem. J Urol 112:467–478

Messing EM, Stamey TA (1978) Interstitial cystitis: early diagnosis, pathology, and treatment. Urology 12: 381–392

Messing EM (1987) The diagnosis of interstitial cystitis. Urol [Suppl] 29:4–7

Miller SW, Pfister RC (1974) Calcification in uroepithelial tumors of the bladder. AJR 121:827–831

Miller JL, Immelman EJ, Roman TE, Mervis B (1983a) Phaeochromocytoma of the urinary bladder localized by selective venous sampling and computed tomography. Postgrad Med J 59:533–535

Miller WB, Boal DK, Teele R (1983b) Neurofibromatosis of the bladder: sonographic findings. J Clin Ultrasound 11:460–462

Miller DL, Chang R, Wells WT, Dowjat BA, Malinowsky RM, Doppman JL (1988) Intravascular contrast media: effect of dose on renal function. AJR 167:607–611

Mills SE, Wolfe JT III, Weiss MA, Swanson PE, Wick MR, Fowler JE Jr, Young RH (1987) Small cell undifferentiated carcinoma of the urinary bladder. Am J Surg Pathol 11:606–617

Mindell HJ (1990) Transurethral prolapse of a simple ureterocele in a boy: case report. Urol Radiol 12: 103–105

Mindell HJ, Pollack HM (1983) Fungal disease of the ureter. Radiology 146:46

Mitas JA, Thompson T (1985) Ureteral involvement complicating eosinophilic cystitis. Urology 26:67–70

Mitty HA, Schapira HE (1977) Ureterocele and pseudoureterocele: cobra versus cancer. Urology 177: 557–561

Monson RR, Nakano KK (1976) Mortality among rubber workers. I. White male union employees in Akron, Ohio. Am J Epidemiol 103:284–296

Monstrey SJM, VanderWerken C, Debruyne FMJ, Goris RJA (1987) Urological trauma and severe associated injuries. Br J Urol 60:393–394

Monstrey SJM, VanderStaak FHJ, VanderWerken C, Debruyne FMH, Severijnen RSVN, Goris RJA (1988) Urinary tract injuries in children: are they different from adults. Z Kinderchir 43:31–48

Moore RD, Steinberg EP, Powe NR, Brinker JA, Fishman EK, Graziano S, Gopalan R (1992) Nephrotoxicity of high-osmolality versus low-osmolality contrast media: randomized trial. Radiology 182:649–655

Morano JU, Burkhalter JL (1987) Bladder hernia simulating osseous metastatic lesion on radionuclide bone scan. Urol Radiol 9:183–184

Morehouse DD, MacKinnon KJ (1969) Urological injuries associated with pelvic fractures. J Trauma 9:479–496

Morrison AS (1984) Advances in the etiology of urothelial cancer. Urol Clin North Am 11:557–566

Morse HD (1928) The etiology and pathology of pyelitis cystica, ureteritis cystica and cystitis cystica. Am J Pathol 4:33–50

Mostofi FK (1954) Potentialities of bladder epithelium. J Urol 71:705–714

Mostofi FK (1960) Standardization of nomenclature and criteria for diagnoses of epithelial tumors of urinary bladder. Acta Union Int Contra Cancr 16:310–314

Mostofi FK, Thomson RV, Dean AL (1955) Mucous adenocarcinoma of the urinary bladder. Cancer 8: 741–758

Motzkin D (1990) Nonsteroidal anti-inflammatory drugs in the treatment of eosinophilic cystitis. J Urol 144:1464–1466

Mulkens TH, Vereycken HA, Van Nueten JC, Govaerts GC, De Schepper AM, Van Camp KO, Van Marck EA (1990) Bilateral ureteral inverted papillomas in association with bladder carcinoma: a case report and review of the literature. Urol Radiol 12:154–156

Murphy WD, Rovner AJ, Nazinitsky KJ (1990) Condylomata acuminata of the bladder: a rare cause of intraluminal-filling defects. Urol Radiol 12:34–36

Nakada R, Ishikawa S, Sakamota M et al. (1986) *N*-(3′, 4′-dimethoxycinnamoyl)anthranillic acid, an antiallergic compound, induced eosinophilic cystitis. Urol Int 41: 457–464

National Institutes of Health Consensus Development Conference (1988) Neurofibromatosis: conference statement. Arch Neurol 45:575–578

Naucler J, Risberg B (1981) Diagnosis and treatment of colovesical fistulas. Acta Chir Scand 147:435–437

Neto WA, Lopes RN, Cury M, Montelatto NID, Arap S (1984) Vesical endometriosis. Urology 24:271–274

Neu HC (1983) Urinary tract infections in the 1980s. Semin Urol 1:130–137

Ney C, Kumar M, Billah K, Doerr J (1987) CT demonstration of cystitis emphysematosa. J Comput Assist Tomor 11:552–553

Nishigaki R, Mosose Y, Nagata T (1990) Localization of the anti-allergic agent Tranilast in the urinary bladder of rats as demonstrated by light microscopic radioautography. Arzneimittelforschung 40:272–275

Nocks BN, Heney NM, Daly JJ (1983) Primary adenocarcinoma of urinary bladder. Urology 21:26–29

North L, Lindell MM, Jing B, Wallace S (1992) Current use of lymphography for staging lymphomas and genital tumors. AJR 158:725–728

Nowak A, Ziekinski J (1977) Difficulties in bladder rupture diagnostics. Eur Urol 3:351–354

Nussbaum AR, Dorst JP, Jeffs RD, Gearhart JP, Sanders RC (1986) Ectopic ureter and ureterocele: their varied sonographic manifestations. Radiology 159:227–235

O'Brien AME, Urbanski SJ (1985) Papillary adenocarcinoma in situ of bladder. J Urol 134:544–546

Ochi K, Yoshida S, Morita M, Takeuchi M (1981) Pheochromocytoma of the bladder. Urology 27:228–230

Okafo BA, Jones HW, Dow D, Kiruluta HG (1985) Eosinophilic cystitis: pleomorphic manifestations. Can J Surg 28:17–18

Oliker AJ, Harris AE (1971) Endometriosis of the bladder in a male patient. J Urol 106:858–859

Oliver JA, Taguchi Y (1964) Rupture of the full bladder. Br J Urol 36:524–525

Oravisto KJ (1975) Epidemiology of interstitial cystitis. Ann Chir Gynaecol Fenniae 64:75–77

Oravisto KL, Alfthan OS, Jokinen EJ (1970) Interstitial cystitis. Scand J Urol Nephrol 4:37–42

Oyasu R, Hopp ML (1974) The etiology of cancer of the bladder. Surg Gynecol Obstet 138:97–108

Pakter R, Nussbaum A, Fishman EK (1988) Hemangioma of the bladder: sonographic and computerized tomographic findings. J Urol 140:601–602

Palmer FJ (1988) The RACR survey of intravenous contrast media reactions: final report. Australas Radiol 82:426–428

Palmer JK, Benson GS, Corriere JN (1983) Diagnosis and initial managment of urological injuries associated with 200 consecutive pelvic fractures. J Urol 130:712–714

Pansky B (1979) Review of gross anatomy, 4th edn. Macmillan, New York, pp 366–368, 374–375, 390–399

Parker C (1970) Cystitis cystica and glandularis: a study of 40 cases. Proc R Soc Med 63:239–243

Parsons CL, Stauffer C, Schmidt JD (1980) Bladder-surface glycosaminoglycans: an efficient mechanism of environmental adaptation. Science 208:605–607

Parsons CL, Schmidt JD, Pollen JJ (1983) Successful treatment of interstitial cystitis with sodium pentosanpolysulfate. J Urol 130:51–53

Parsons CL, Lilly JD, Stein P (1991) Epithelial dysfunction in nonbacterial cystitis. J Urol 145:732–735

Partanen D, Asikainin U (1985) Oat cell carcinoma of the urinary bladder with ectopic adrenocorticotropic hormone production. Hum Pathol 16:313–317

Pear BL (1986) Other organs and other amyloids. Semin Roentgenol 21:150–164

Perez-Marrero R, Emerson L, Juma S (1987) Urodynamic studies in interstitial cystitis. Urology [Suppl] 29:27–30
Pessin JZ, Bodian M (1964) Neurofibromatosis of the pelvic autonomic plexuses. Br J Urol 25:510–518
Peterson NE, Silverman A, Campbell JB (1989) Eosinophilic cystitis and coexistent eosinophilic gastroenteritis in an infant. Pediatr Radiol 19:484–485
Pollack HM (1990) Clinical urography. W.B. Saunders, Philadelphia
Pollack HM (1988) Long-term follow-up of the upper urinary tract for transitional cell carcinoma: how much is enough? Radiology 167:871–872
Pollack HM, Banner MP (1985) Current status of excretory urography. Urol Clin North Am 12:585–601
Pollack HM, Popky GL, Blumberg ML (1975) Hernias of the ureter – an anatomic-roentgenographic study. Radiology 117:275–281
Pollack HM, Banner MP, Martinez LO, Hodson CJ (1981) Diagnostic considerations in urinary bladder wall calcification. AJR 136:791–797
Pope TL Jr, Harrison RB, Clark RL, Cuttino JT (1981) Bladder base impressions in women: "female prostate". AJR 136:1105–1108
Postma MP, Smith R (1986) Scrotal cystocele with bladder calculi. AJR 147:287–288
Potts AR, Hirst E (1963) Inverted papilloma of the bladder. J Urol 90:175–179
Prestige BR, Donaldson SS (1989) Treatment results among adults with childhood tumors: a twenty-year experience. Int J Radiat Oncol Biol Phys 17:507–514
Prewitt LH, Lebowitz RL (1976) The single ectopic ureter. AJR 127:941–948
Prokop EK, Buddemeyer EU, Strauss HW, Wagner HN (1974) Detection and localization of an occult vesicoenteric fistula. AJR 121:811–818
Quint HJ, Drach GW, Rappaport WD, Hoffmann CJ (1992) Emphysematous cystitis: a review of the spectrum of disease. J Urol 147:134–137
Radin DR, Siskind B, Weiner S, Bernstein R, Ziprkowski M (1984) Retroperitoneal malacoplakia. Urol Radiol 6:218–220
Rafal RB, Markisz JA (1991) Urachal carcinoma: the role of magnetic resonance imaging. Urol Radiol 12: 184–187
Raghavaiah NV (1974) Double dye test to diagnose various types of vaginal fistulas. J Urol 112:811–812
Rao BK (1986) Abdominal case of the day. AJR 146: 1075–1076
Ratner V (1987) Rediscovering a "rare" disease: a patient's perspective on interstitial cystitis. Urology [Suppl] 29: 44–45
Rehn L (1895) Blasengeschwulste bei Fuchsin-arbeitern. Arch Clin Chir 50:588–600
Reisner C, Nicholas E (1963) Rupture of the bladder: unusual features. J Urol 90:53–57
Reyes CV, Soneru I (1985) Small cell carcinoma of the urinary bladder with hypercalcemia. Cancer 56:2530–2533
Rieder HL, Cauthen GM, Kelly GD, Bloch AB, Snider DE (1989) Tuberculosis in the United States. JAMA 262:385–389
Rifkin MD (1985) Ultrasonography of the lower urinary tract. Urol Clin North Am 12:645–656
Rink FC, Mitchell ME (1983) Genitourinary neurofibromatosis in childhood. J Urol 130:1176–1179
Robinson MJ, Kent M, Stocks J (1973) Phaeochrocytoma in childhood. Arch Dis Child 48:137–142
Roos KL, Dunn DW (1992) Neurofibromatosis. CA 42: 241–254
Rosai J (1989) Bladder and urethra. In: Ackerman's surgical pathology. C.V. Mosby, St. Louis, pp 898–922
Ross RK, Paganini-Hill A, Henderson BE (1988) Epidemiology of bladder cancer. In: Skinner DG, Lieskovsky G (eds) Diagnosis and management of genitourinary cancer. W.B. Saunders, Philadelphia, pp 23–31
Rubin L, Pincus MB (1974) Eosinophilic cystitis: the relationship of allergy in the urinary tract to eosinophilic cystitis and the pathophysiology of eosinophilia. J Urol 112:457–460
Russo P, Balfe DM, Weill A, Sicard G (1984) Micturitional hypertension and retropubic mass. Urol Radiol 6:230–233
Saez F, Pena JM, Martinez A, Lopez JA, Marco A, Reyzabal J (1985) Carcinomas in vesical diverticula: the role of ultrasound. J Clin Ultrasound 13:45–48
Salm R (1967) Neoplasia of the bladder and cystitis cystica. Br J Urol 39:67–72
Sandler CM, Hall JT, Rodriguez MB, Corrierre JN (1986) Bladder injury in blunt pelvic trauma. Radiology 158: 633–638
Sandler C (1988) Bladder injuries. Lecture given at The Society of Uroradiology Postgraduate Course on February 3, 1988 in Orlando, Florida
Sandler CM, Phillips JM, Harris JD, Toombs BD (1981) Radiology of the bladder and urethra in blunt pelvic trauma. Radiol Clin North Am 19:195–211
Sant GR (1987) Urinary tract infection in the elderly. Semin Urol 5:126–133
Scalea TM, Sclafani SJA (1991) Angiographically placed balloons for arterial control: a description of a technique. J Trauma 31:1671–1677
Schaeffer AJ (1983) Bladder defense mechanisms against urinary tract infections. Semin Urol 1:106–113
Schubert GE, Pavkovic MB, Bethke-Bedurftig BA (1982) Tubular urachal remnants in adult bladders. J Urol 127:40–42
Schultz RE, Bloch MJ, Tomaszewski JE, Brooks JS, Hanno PM (1984) Mesonephric adenocarcinoma of the bladder. J Urol 132:263–265
Schultz RE, Boyle DE (1988) Inverted papilloma of renal pelvis associated with contralateral ureteral malignancy and bladder recurrence. J Urol 139:111–113
Schutz W, Vogel E (1984) Pheochromocytoma of the urinary bladder – a case report and review of the literature. Urol Int 39:250–255
Sclafani DS, Becker JA (1985) Radiologic diagnosis of extrarenal genitourinary trauma. Urol Radiol 7: 201–210
Scott PP, Scott WW, Siegelman SS (1986) Amyloidosis: an overview. Semin Roentgenol 21:103–112
Scott R, Carlton CE (1976) Traumatic lesions of the urogenital tract. In: Lapides J (ed) Fundamentals of urology. W.B. Saunders, Philadelphia, pp 339–362
Sen SE, Malek RS, Farrow GM, Lieger MM (1985) Sarcoma and carcinosarcoma of the bladder in adults. J Urol 133:29–30
Share JC, Lebowitz RL (1989) Ectopic ureterocele without ureteral and calyceal dilatation (ureterocele disproportion): findings on urography and sonography. AJR 152:567–571
Shaw JL, Gislason GJ, Imbriglia JE (1958) Transition of cystitis glandularis to primary adenocarcinoma of the bladder. J Urol 79:815–822

Sherwood T, Stevenson JJ (1969) Ureteroceles in disguise. Br J Radiol 42:899–901

Shortliffe LMD, Stamey TA (1986a) Infections of the urinary tract: introduction and general principles. In: Walsh PC, Gittes RR, Perlmutter AD, Stamey TA (eds) Campbell's urology, 5th edn. W.B. Saunders, Philadelphia, pp 738–796

Shortliffe LMD, Stamey TA (1986b) Urinary infections in adult women. In: Walsh PC, Gittes RR, Perlmutter AD, Stamey TA (eds) Campbell's urology, 5th edn. W.B. Saunders, Philadelphia, pp 797–830

Sidh SM, Smith SP, Silber SB, Young JD (1980) Eosinophilic cystitis: advanced disease requiring surgical intervention. Urology 15:23–26

Skinner DG (1977) Current state of classification and staging of bladder cancer. Cancer Res 37:2838–2842

Spataro RF, Davis RS, McLachlan MSL, Linde CA, Barbaric ZL (1983) Urachal abnormalities in the adult. Radiology 149:659–663

Speirs RT, Raghavendra BN, Rausen A, Geneiser NB, Ambrosino M (1990) Ultrasound findings in diffuse granulomatous cystitis in chronic granulomatous disease of childhood. Urol Radiol 12:106–108

Stanton MJ, Maxted W (1981) Malacoplakia: a study of the literature and current concepts of pathogenesis, diagnosis and treatment. J Urol 125:139–146

Stanton MJ, Lynch JH, Maxted WC, Chun BK (1983) Malacoplakia of the bladder: a case report of resolution with bethanechol, trimethoprim-sulfamethoxazole and ascorbic acid. J Urol 130:1174–1175

Stanton SL (1983) Vaginal prolapse. In: Raz S (ed) Female urology. W.B. Saunders, Philadelphia, pp 229–240

Stillwell TJ, Segura JW, Farrow GM (1989) Amyloidosis of the urethra. J Urol 141:52–53

Streem SB (1984) Genitourinary malacoplakia in renal transplant recipients: pathogenic, prognostic and therapeutic considerations. J Urol 132:10–12

Strijk SP, Debrune FMJ, Herman CJ (1983) Lymphography in the management of urologic tumors. Radiology 146:39–45

Strong GH, Kelsey D, Hoch W (1974) Primary amyloid disease of the bladder. J Urol 112:463–466

Strube HD, Hofman S (1975) Zur Entartung der Neurofibromatose von Recklinghausen im Kindersalter. Monatsschr Kinderheilkd 123:395–397

Sufrin G, Keogh B, Moore RH, Murphy GP (1977) Secondary involvement of the bladder in malignant lymphoma. J Urol 118:251–253

Sutphin M, Middleton AW Jr (1984) Eosinophilic cystitis in children: a self-limited process. J Urol 132:117–119

Sutton JM (1986) Urinary eosinophils. Arch Intern Med 146:2243–2244

Svanborg-Eden C, Jodal U (1979) Attachment of *Escherichia coli* to urinary sediment epithelial cells from urinary tract infection-prone and healthy children. Infect Immun 26:837–840

Swartz DA, Johnson DE, Ayala AG, Watkins DL (1985) Bladder leiomyosarcoma: a review of 10 cases with 5-year followup. J Urol 133:200–202

Tanagho EA (1972) Anatomy and management of ureteroceles. J Urol 107:729–736

Tanagho EA (1986) Anatomy of the lower urinary tract. In: Walsh PC, Gittes RR, Perlmutter AD, Stamey TA (eds) Campbell's urology, 5th edn. W.B. Saunders, Philadelphia, pp 46–74

Tanagho EA (1992a) Anatomy of the genitourinary tract. In: Tanagho EA, McAninch JW (eds) Smith's general urology, 13th edn. Appleton & Lange, Norwalk, pp 1–16

Tanagho EA (1992b) Specific infections of the genitourinary tract. In: Tanagho EA, McAninch JW (eds) Smith's general urology, 13th edn. Appleton & Lange, Norwalk, pp 240–256

Tanagho EA (1992c) Disorders of the bladder, prostate, and seminal vesicles. In: Tanagho EA, McAninch JW (eds) Smith's general urology, 13th edn. Appleton & Lange, Norwalk, pp 495–514

Tanagho EA, Pugh RCB (1963) The anatomy and function of the ureterovesical junction. Br J Urol 35: 151–165

Tanagho EA, Hutch JA, Meyers FH, Rambo ON (1965) Primary vesicoureteral reflux: experimental studies of its etiology. J Urol 93:165–176

Tannenbaum M (1976) Squamous cell carcinoma and urothelial tumor of the bladder. Urology 7:529–530

Tannenbaum SI, Carson CC III, Tatum A, Paulson DF (1983) Squamous carcinoma of urinary bladder. Urology 22:597–599

Tannous WN, Azouz EM, Homsy YL, Kiruluta HG, Grattan-Smith D (1989) CT and ultrasound imaging of pelvic rhabdomyosarcoma in children. Pediatr Radiol 19:530–534

Thijssen A, Gerridzen RG (1990) Eosinophilic cystitis presenting as invasive bladder cancer: comments on pathogenesis and management. J Urol 144:977–979

Thomas DG (1971) A study of 52 cases of adenocarcinoma of the bladder. Br J Urol 43:4–15

Thomas SD, Sanders SD III, Pollack H (1977) Primary amyloidosis of urinary bladder and ureter. Urology 9:586–589

Thornbury JR, Silver TM, Vinson MD (1977) Ureteroceles vs. pseudoureteroceles. Radiology 122:81–84

Thurnher S, Marincek B, Hauri D (1992) Retrovesical leiomyoma: CT and contrast-enhanced MR imaging findings. Urol Radiol 13:190–193

Tonkin AK, Witten DM (1979) Genitourinary tuberculosis. Semin Roentgenol 14:305–318

Trinh TD, Gatewood OMB, Fishman EK (1986) Candida of the bladder wall: computerized tomography demonstration. J Urol 135:1008–1009

Umerah BC (1977) The less familiar manifestations of schistosomiasis of the urinary tract. Br J Radiol 50: 105–109

U.S. Congress (1977) Office of Technology Assessment: Cancer Testing Technology and Saccharin. U.S. Government Printing Office, Washington, DC

Utz DC, Farrow GM (1984) Carcinoma in situ of the urinary tract. Urol Clin North Am 11:735–740

Utz DC, Zincke H (1973) The masquerade of bladder cancer in situ as interstitial cystitis. Trans Am Assoc Genito-urin Surg 65:64–65

Utz DC, Zincke H (1974) The masquerade of bladder cancer in situ as interstitial cystitis. J Urol 111:160–161

Velchik MG, Alavi A, Kressel HY, Engelman K (1989) Localization of pheochromocytoma: MIBG, CT, and MRI correlation. J Nucl Med 30:328–336

von Eschenbach AC, Jing B, Wallace S (1985) Lymphography in genitourinary cancer. Urol Clin North Am 12:715–723

Wallace DM, Chisholm GD, Hendry WF (1975) T.N.M. classification for urological tumors (U.I.C.C.) – 1974. Br J Urol 54:341–344

Wallach MT, Lebowitz RL (1988) Ectopic ureterocele. Contemp Diagn Radiol 11:1–5

Walther MC, Campbell WG Jr, O'Brien DP III, Wheatly JK, Graham SD Jr (1987) Cystitis cystica: an electron and immunofluorescence microscopic study. J Urol 137:764–768

Walther M, Glenn JF, Vellios F (1985) Xanthogranulomatous cystitis. J Urol 134:745–746

Ward AM (1971) Glandular neoplasia within the urinary tract. The aetiology of adenocarcinoma of the urothelium with a review of the literature. I. Introduction. The origin of glandular epithelium in the renal pelvis, ureter, and bladder. Virchows Arch [A] 352:296–311

Warshawsky R, Bow SN, Waldbaum RS, Cintron J (1989) Bladder pheochromocytoma with MR correlation. J Comput Assist Tomogr 13:714–716

Wechsler RJ, Brennan RE (1982) Teardrop bladder: additional considerations. Radiology 144:281–284

Westra SJ, Verbeeten B Jr, Bots TATM, Tio TL, Tytgat GNJ, Brummelkamp WH, Reeders JWAJ (1988) Urinary tract malakoplakia with extension into the retroperitoneum with secondary gastrointestinal involvement. Urol Radiol 10:181–185

Wiener DP, Koss LG, Sablay B, Freed SZ (1979) The prevalence and significance of Brunn's nests, cystitis cystica, and squamous metaplasia in normal bladders. J Urol 122:317–321

Wigle DT (1977) Bladder cancer: possible new high-risk occupation. Lancet II:83–84

Williams MJ, Gooding GAW (1985) Sonographic diagnosis of a neoplasm in a bladder diverticulum. J Ultrasound Med 4:203–204

Willis AJ, Huang AH, Carroll P (1980) Primary melanoma of the bladder: a case report and review. J Urol 123: 278–281

Winslow DI (1989) Endovesical ultrasonography of urachal carcinoma. Urol Radiol 11:53–54

Wolk DJ, Sandler CM, Corriere JN (1985) Extraperitoneal bladder rupture without pelvic fracture. J Urol 134:1199–1201

Woodburne RT (1964) Anatomy of the ureterovesical junction. J Urol 92:431–435

Woodburne RT (1976) Anatomy of the excretory tract. In: Lapides J (ed) Fundamentals of urology. W.B. Saunders, Philadelphia, pp 1–34

Wydner EL, Onderdonk J, Mantel N (1963) An epidemiological investigation of cancer of the bladder. Cancer 16:1388–1407

Young RH, Rosenberg AE (1987) Osteosarcoma of the urinary bladder report of a case and review of the literature. Cancer 59:174–178

Young RH, Scully RE (1986) Nephrogenic adenoma a report of 15 cases, review of the literature, and comparison with clear cell adenocarcinoma of the urinary tract. Am J Surg Pathol 10:268–275

Young DF, Eldridge R, Nager GT, Deland FH, McNew J (1971) Hereditary bilateral acoustic neuroma (central neurofibromatosis). Birth Defects 7(4):73–86

Yousem DM, Gatewood OMB, Goldman SM, Marshall FF (1988) Synchronous and metachronous transitional cell carcinoma of the urinary tract: prevalence, incidence and radiographic detection. Radiology 167:613–618

Zerhouni EA, Carter HB, Brem RF, Tempany CM, Yang A, Epstein JI, Walsh PC (1991) Non palpable prostate cancer: Detection with MR imaging. Radiology 178: 523–525

Zerin JM, Lebowitz RL (1989) Spontaneous extraperitoneal rupture of the urinary bladder in children. Radiology 170:487–488

Zimmermann K, Amis ES, Newhouse JH (1989) Nephrogenic adenoma of the bladder: urographic spectrum. Urol Radiol 11:123–126

Zingas AP, Kling GA, Crottee E, Shumaker E, Vasquez PM (1986) Computed tomography of nephrogenic adenoma of the urinary bladder. J Comput Assist Tomogr 10:979–982

7 Vesicoureteral Reflux

JOSEPH ORTENBERG and J. CHRISTIAN WINTERS

CONTENTS

7.1 Historical Perspective

Vesicoureteral reflux was recognized by Galen in medieval times (POLK 1965). In 1893, POZZI was the first to identify reflux in a human when urine flowed from a divided ureter during a gynecologic procedure. GRUBER (1929) and SAMPSON (1903) noted the varying appearances of the trigone in certain species and recognized the importance of an oblique course of the ureter, as well as an adequate submucosal tunnel. The clinical implications of vesicoureteral reflux became recognized in the 1950s. At that time, HUTCH (1952) demonstrated that reflux in paraplegic patients could lead to hydronephrosis with renal damage and recommended surgical treatment. The subsequent refinement of surgical techniques to correct vesicoureteral reflux contributed to the development of the specialty of pediatric urology.

Numerous advances have influenced the management of patients with vesicoureteral reflux. With refined radiographic techniques, more cases of reflux are detected and renal growth may be monitored accurately. The greater selection of antibiotics suitable for prophylaxis has decreased the incidence of intercurrent urinary tract infections. These developments have allowed the physician to manage many cases of vesicoureteral reflux nonoperatively, reserving surgery for those children who fail medical management.

7.2 Incidence

The exact incidence of vesicoureteral reflux in asymptomatic infants and children is not known. Several studies have estimated the incidence of reflux in normal children at less than 1%. Reflux is much less prevalent in black children (ASKARI and BELMAN 1982): although the severity of reflux is no different, the time to resolution appears shorter (SKOOG and BELMAN, 1991). The incidence of vesicoureteral reflux in children with urinary tract infections – 14% in females and 29% in males – is much higher than in the general pediatric population (SHOPFNER 1970). Seventy percent of children less than 1 year of age with urinary tract infection have vesicoureteral reflux (BAKER et al. 1976). In siblings of children with known reflux, there is also a higher incidence of reflux, approaching 30% (DWOSKIN 1976; JERKINS and NOE 1982). Siblings with reflux may not have experienced previous symptoms or infection, and are at greater risk of developing renal scarring if compared to a normal aged-matched population. On this basis, it is recommended that siblings of children with reflux should be screened; however, that age range of children who would benefit most from this screening has not been fully established.

7.3 Anatomy and Etiology

The anatomic features that are characteristic of the normal valve mechanism of the ureterovesical junction include an oblique entry of the ureter into the bladder, an adequate length of its submucosal segment, and an appropriate ratio of the

JOSEPH ORTENBERG, M.D., F.A.A.P., Associate Professor, Department of Urology and Pediatrics; J. CHRISTIAN WINTERS, M.D., Resident in Urology, LSU/Ochsner Program; LSU Medical Center, School of Medicine, Louisiana State University, 1542 Tulane Avenue, New Orleans, LA 70112-2822, USA

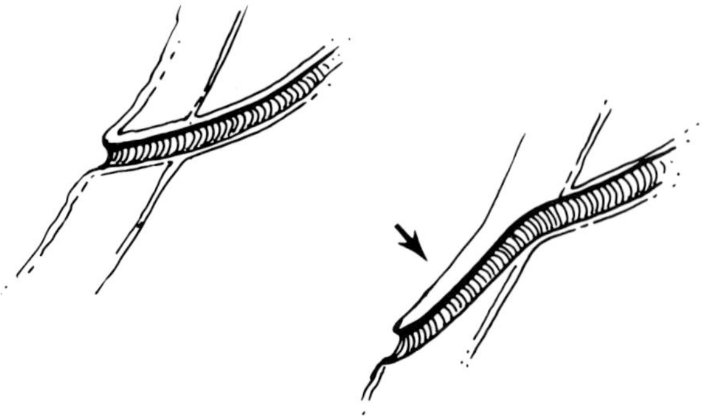

Fig. 7.1. *Above*: deficient submucosal tunnel. *Below*: a normal entry of the ureter with oblique submucosal tunnel

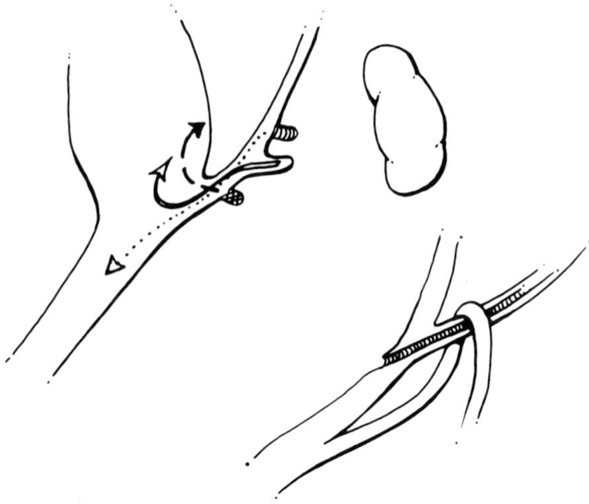

Fig. 7.2. *Above*: possible positions of ureteric bud based on origin from mesonephric duct. *Below*: final location of orifice depends on site of ureteric bud origin

length to the diameter of the ureter (STEPHENS and LENAGHAN 1962; KING et al. 1974; LEVITT and WEISS 1985) (Fig. 7.1). The length of the submucosal tunnel is important for two reasons. First, an adequate length allows compression of the intravesical ureter against the muscle of the bladder wall as bladder pressure increases. This creates a valve effect to prevent retrograde flow of urine. Second, the longitudinal fibers of the intravesical ureter become interspersed with the trigonal fibers, creating one functional unit, which facilitates the propulsion of urine into the bladder (KING and LEVITT 1986).

To understand the anatomy of vesicoureteral reflux one must comprehend the embryology of the ureter and trigonal region of the urinary bladder. The ureter begins development in the 4th week of embryonic life, as a bud arising from the mesonephric (wolffian) duct. Multiple ureteric buds (up to seven) arise from the mesonephric duct; however, most of these involute. The ureteric buds that penetrate the metanephric blastema during the 5th week of gestation produce the collecting system. The portion of the mesonephric duct distal to the ureteric bud is referred to as the common excretory duct. As the common excretory duct is progressively absorbed into the urogenital sinus, the ureter and mesonephric duct become independently joined to the urogenital sinus. As the common excretory duct is incorporated into this expanding urogenital sinus, it forms the trigone (MC C SYNDER 1991) (Fig. 7.2).

The ultimate location of the ureteral orifice in the trigonal region of the bladder is dependent on the initial location where the ureteric bud arises from the mesonephric duct. All ureteral anomalies (bifurcation, duplication, reflux) can be explained by an abnormal origin of the ureteric bud from the mesonephric duct. The abnormal location of the ureteric bud may also be associated with renal anomalies. An aberrant origin of the ureteric bud may contact the nephrogenic cord in a location with less nephrogenic mesenchyme, resulting in varying degrees of renal dysplasia (MACKIE and STEPHENS 1975).

Primary vesicoureteral reflux is classified as congenital reflux resulting mainly from the lateral position of the ureteral orifice. During a normal voiding cycle, the bladder fills at low pressure. At capacity, the detrusor contracts and the continence mechanism relaxes. In children, a common problem is a delay in maturation of the inhibitory control of the detrusor muscle, leading to an "unstable bladder." Bladder instability frequently presents with symptoms of urgency and urge incontinence, as well as urinary tract infection (Fig. 7.3). In some cases, the continence mechanism may fail to relax or strengthen during voiding, creating a functional outflow obstruction (DUCKETT et al. 1986). Children with non-neurogenic bladder dysfunction have a higher incidence of vesicoureteral reflux (KOFF et al. 1979) which may improve when the uninhibited bladder is treated with an anticholinergic medication (KOFF and MURTAGH 1984). Such children are also included in the category of primary reflux owing to the absence of demonstrable neurologic lesions.

Secondary vesicoureteral reflux occurs due to decompensation of the normal valve mechanism

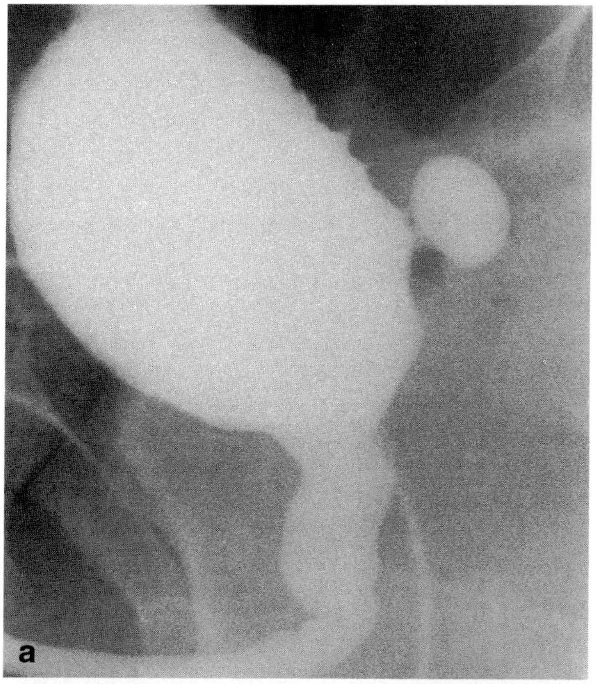

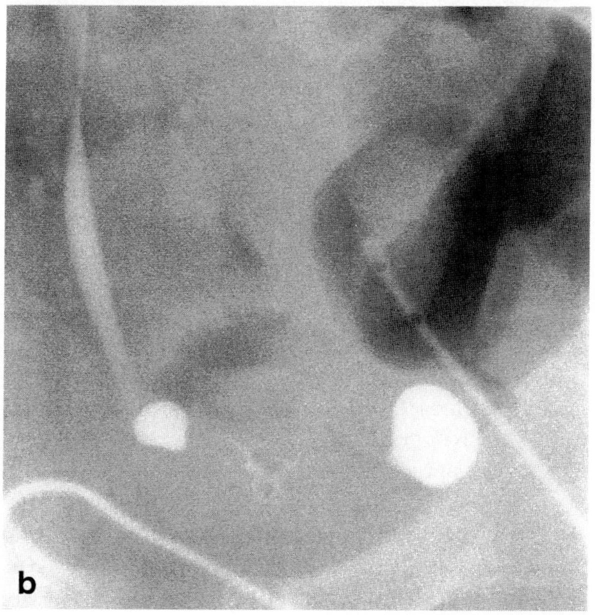

Fig. 7.3. a VCUG of a child with urinary tract infection and bladder instability demonstrating bilateral paraureteral diverticula, one of which is associated with reflux. **b** Post-void view demonstrating empty bladder with two diverticula and reflux

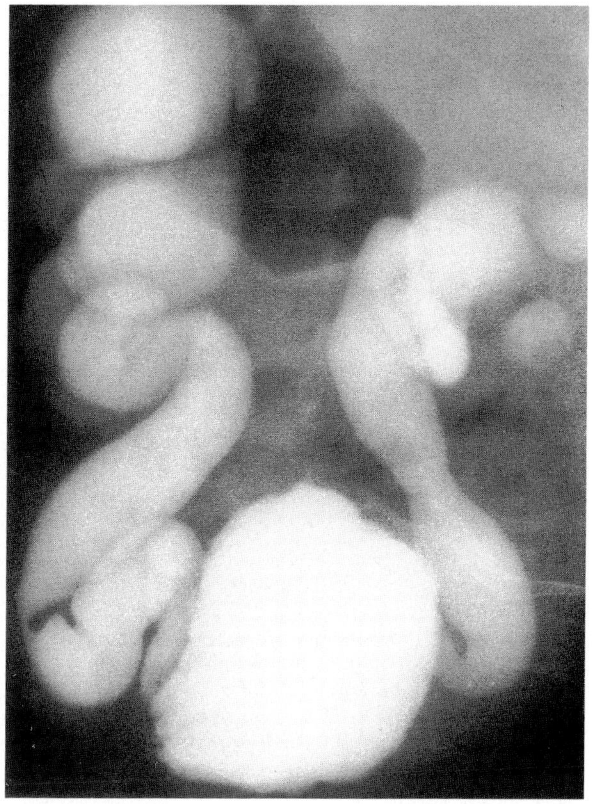

Fig. 7.4. Bilateral high grade vesicoureteral reflux with posterior urethral valves. Bladder trabeculation and a left duplicated system with lower pole reflux

of the uretero-vesical junction. With true neurogenic bladder dysfunction, the combination of detrusor–sphincter dyssynergia, high intravesical pressures, and detrusor decompensation may lead to a loss of the normal flap valve mechanism of the ureterovesical junction (DUCKETT et al. 1986).

The incidence of vesicoureteral reflux in children with myelodysplasia has been estimated at approximately 35%–50% (KAPLAN and FIRLIT 1983; AMI SIDI et al. 1986). Neurogenic bladder may also occur in childhood due to occult spinal dysraphism or neurologic trauma. In these patients, it is important to lower the intravesical pressure with anticholinergic therapy. If detrusor–sphincter dyssynergia is present, bladder emptying by clean intermittent catheterization may be necessary (YIP et al. 1985).

Urethral obstruction from posterior urethral valves or urethral strictures may generate increased intravesical pressure resulting in vesicoureteral reflux (FIRLIT 1986) (Figs. 7.4, 7.5). Reflux may occur when the valvular mechanism has been iatrogenically rendered incompetent owing to failed ureteral reimplant in children or following transurethral surgery in adults (FIRLIT 1986).

Ureteral Duplication. According to autopsy studies, ureteral duplication occurs in approxi-

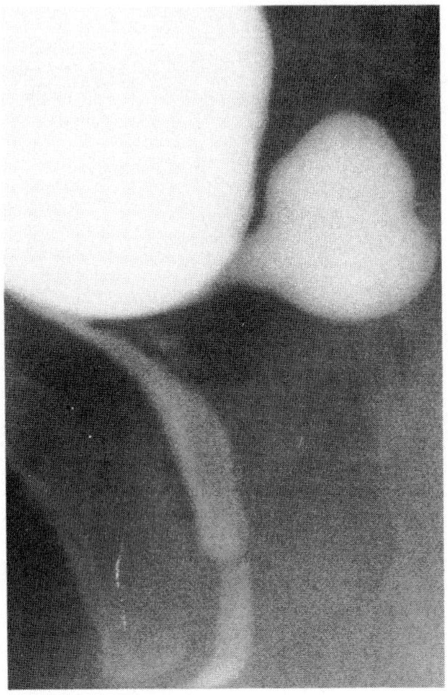

Fig. 7.5. VCUG of patient with posterior urethral valves. Note elongated prostatic urethra and valve leaflets, with the presence of a paraureteral diverticulum

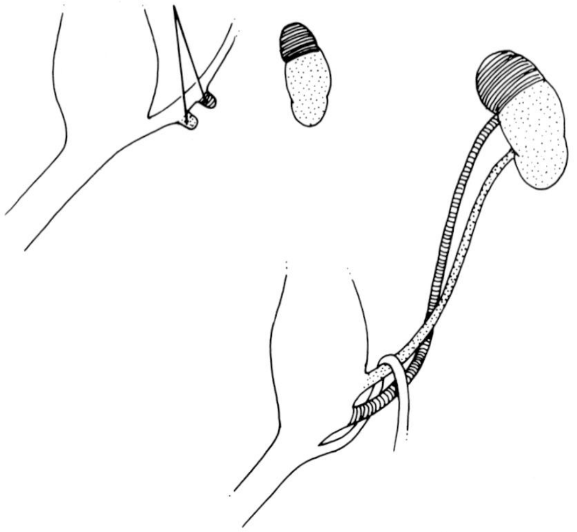

Fig. 7.6. Embryology of duplicated system. The lower bud assumes a more lateral position and is more prone to reflux

mately 1 in 125 patients or 0.8% (Nation 1944; Campbell 1970). In a series of intravenous urograms obtained for urinary symptoms, the incidence of duplication was 2%–4% (Hartman and Hodson 1969). Vesicoureteral reflux was seen in 69% of complete duplex systems and 22% of partial duplex systems in a study of girls with urinary tract infection (Bisset and Strife 1987).

Complete duplication results from two ureteric buds arising from the same mesonephric duct. Both buds migrate to the metanephric blastema and induce renal differentiation. The ureteric buds become incorporated into the trigone, as discussed previously. The lower bud drains the lower pole of the kidney, and this bud is incorporated first into the trigone, assuming a more cranial and lateral position. The upper ureteric bud drains the upper pole and is absorbed into the trigone after the lower bud, with a final position more distal and medial to the lower pole ureter. The embryologic origin and configuration of duplex ureters were described by Weigert (1877) and Meyer (1907) at the turn of the century and their observations remain valid (Fig. 7.6). In some cases, the upper pole ureter may assume an ectopic location due to delayed absorption into the urogenital sinus. Due to the more cranial and lateral location of the lower pole ureter in the bladder, this ureter is more prone to vesicoureteral reflux (Fig. 7.7).

Ureterocele. A ureterocele represents a cystic dilatation of the terminal ureter. The incidence has been reported as from 1 in 500 to 1 in 4000 in pediatric autopsies (Campbell 1952; Uson et al. 1961). The embryologic explanation is not completely understood. Prevalent theories include delayed rupture of Chwalle's membrane (a two-layered membrane between the urogenital sinus and the ureter) or a delay in ureteric bud differentiation causing arrested muscle growth in the terminal ureter. Delayed absorption of the ureter into the urogenital sinus may cause dilatation of the terminal ureter as the urogenital sinus expands to form the trigone (Mc C Snyder 1991).

Ureteroceles may be classified as simple and ectopic. Simple ureteroceles are located on the trigone with the orifice in the usual location, usually occur in adults, and more commonly present with ureteral obstruction rather than reflux. Ectopic ureteroceles are more frequently encountered in children, typically with the upper pole system of ureteral duplication. In duplex systems, an upper pole ureterocele may deform the trigone and lower pole ureterovesical junction, resulting in ipsilateral or contralateral reflux (Fig. 7.8). Ectopic ureteroceles may be further classified depending on the location of the ureterocele and of the orifice of the ureterocele (Fig. 7.9).

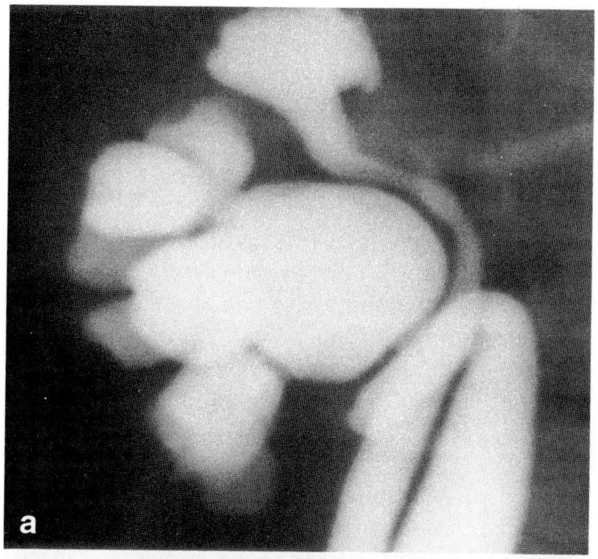

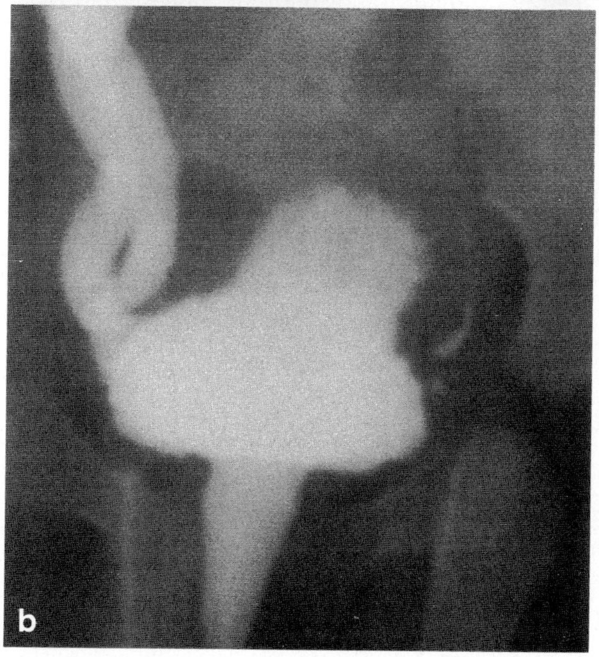

Fig. 7.7a,b. Right complete ureteral duplication with grade III reflux into both ureters. Grade I reflux into left lower pole ureter

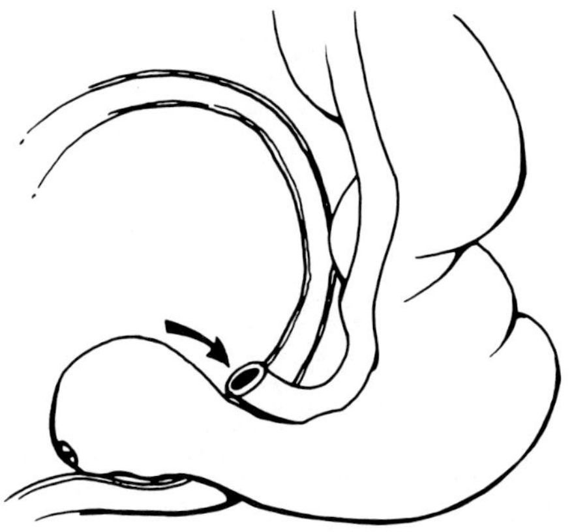

Fig. 7.8. Upper pole ureterocele with reflux into lower pole system

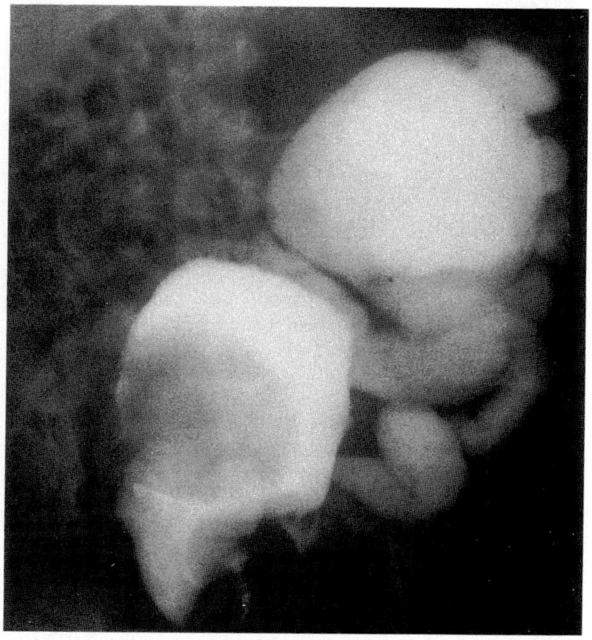

Fig. 7.9. Circular filling defects (×2) in bladder representing ureteroceles. Grade V reflux into left lower pole

Bladder Diverticulum. A congenital diverticulum is a herniation of the bladder wall caused by incomplete muscle formation, in the presence of normal intravesical pressure. An acquired diverticulum represents herniation of mucosa through an area of relatively deficient musculature in the bladder wall, usually in the presence of elevated intravesical pressure. The ureteral hiatus represents a potential weak spot in the posterior lateral wall of the bladder and is the most common site of congenital diverticula (KING and LEVITT 1986). A diverticulum at or near the hiatus predisposes to reflux if it is large enough to impinge upon muscular support of the intravesical ureter. A congenital bladder diverticulum using the same channel through the muscular wall of the bladder as the ureter and associated with vesicoureteral reflux, is known as a Hutch diverticulum (HUTCH 1952) (Fig. 7.10).

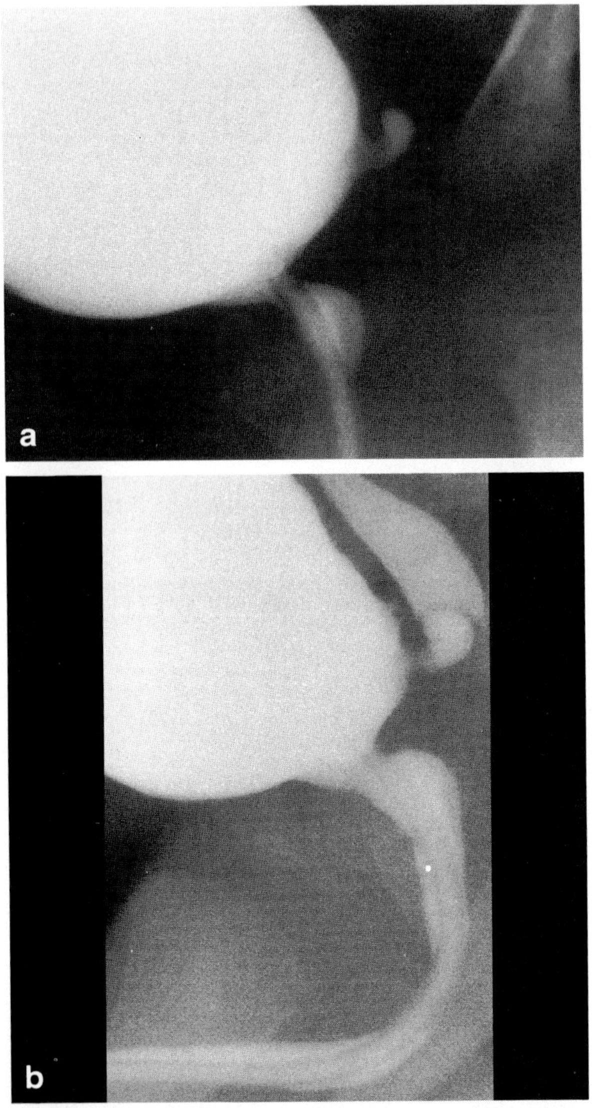

Fig. 7.10. a Cystogram. b Congenital paraureteral diverticulum. Note reflux occurring only with voiding

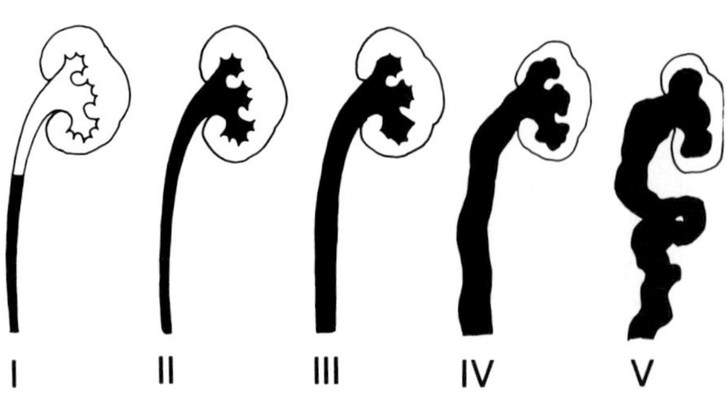

Fig. 7.11. Grading of vesicoureteral reflux according to the International Reflux Study

7.4 Grading

The degree of reflux can be categorized by various grading systems. By grading reflux, the risk of potential renal injury and the rate of spontaneous resolution may be estimated (Arant 1991). Initially, various methods were used to grade vesicoureteral reflux. The International Reflux Study in Children proposed a grading system based on a standardized technique of contrast cystography. In this system the grade of reflux is determined by the degree of reflux present at peak voiding pressure and is based primarily on the appearance of the calyx (Fig. 7.11). Permanent calyceal changes seen on voiding cystourethrography and intravenous pyelography (IVP) should not be interpreted as blunting. If such changes exist, the degree of dilatation of the renal pelvis and ureter determines the grade of reflux (Lebowitz et al. 1985). Intrarenal reflux is the pathologic process whereby urine from the calyx refluxes into the collecting tubules of the nephrons. Although intrarenal reflux may result in scarring, it is rarely detected on contrast cystograms. In reports presenting retrospective data on patients of all ages with vesicoureteral reflux, the distribution of the various grades of reflux was as follows (Arant 1991; Dwoskin and Perlmutter 1973; Bellinger and Duckett 1984):

Grade 1: 5%–8%
Grade 2: 37%–40%
Grade 3: 25%–37%
Grade 4: 14%–24%
Grade 5: 5%

The interpretation of the severity of reflux and dilatation of the collecting system can differ between clinicians. Presently the International Reflux Study Group is conducting a prospective trial to determine the outcomes and rates of resolution of various grades of reflux. The development of a standaridized grading system has enhanced the ability to perform well-controlled, multicenter prospective trials of the management of vesicoureteral reflux.

7.5 Diagnosis

The diagnosis of vesicoureteral reflux usually results from the evaluation of a child with urinary tract infection or by screening siblings of refluxing children. There are several diagnostic modalities employed in the evaluation of these children.

7.5.1 Cystography

7.5.1.1 Voiding Cystourethrography (VCUG)

In a child with prior urinary tract infection, voiding cystourethrography (VCUG) is usually the first test obtained to detect reflux. In comparison with radionuclide cystography, VCUG offers several advantages. First, the grade of reflux may be determined. Second, the urethra and urinary bladder can be accurately visualized. Third, the bladder capacity and adequacy of emptying may be assessed. Fourth, lumbosacral spine views may detect a subtle anomaly such as sacral agenesis or spina bifida occulta which may be associated with neurogenic bladder dysfunction. In order to eliminate technical variation causing changes in the degree of reflux, the technique of voiding cystography should be rigidly standardized. Instillation of contrast material at room temperature, concentrated contrast material, and large urethral catheters may irritate the trigone, producing or exacerbating reflux (FRIEDLAND 1979). Rapid filling, produced with a syringe, may increase detrusor instability and intravesical pressure. Contrast should be instilled into the bladder by gravity from a container, optimally at a height of 60–80 cm and definitely not exceeding 100 cm from the table top (KOFF et al. 1979a). A large bore catheter or a Foley catheter may obstruct voiding; therefore a 6- or 8-F feeding tube should be used.

The use of fluoroscopy reduces the radiation exposure and identifies abnormalities, allowing better positioning and timing for spot films. Routine films include (HOFFMAN 1985):

1. Steep oblique views of each uretero-vesical junction in the filling phase
2. Views of the urethra during voiding
3. A postvoid film of the bladder
4. A film of each renal fossa at the end of voiding or at the time of maximal reflux

In females, only a single anteroposterior view of the urethra is obtained. In males, a steep oblique or lateral view is most useful to visualize the urethra. A study which is terminated prior to voiding is incomplete. If the child is unable to urinate while on the fluoroscopy table, further images should be obtained after voiding to detect reflux during micturition.

In addition to the demonstration of reflux (Fig. 7.12), voiding cystovrethrography can provide

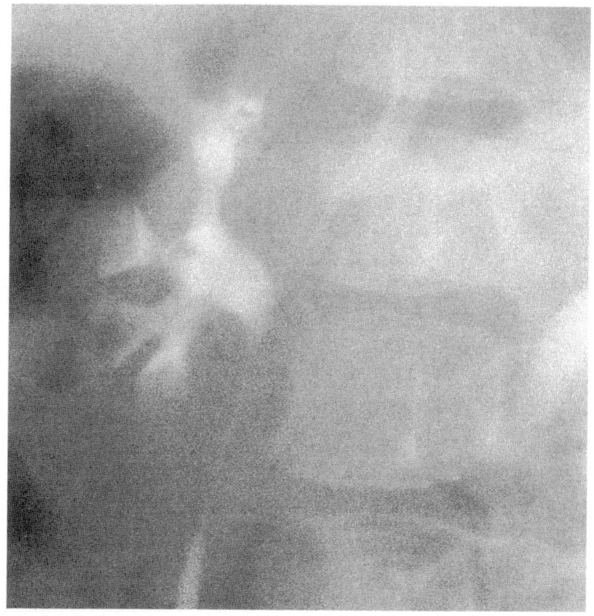

Fig. 7.12. Grade II vesicoureteral reflux

anatomic detail of the bladder and urethra. Trabeculation and thickening of the bladder wall should be assessed. The anatomy of the bladder neck should be reviewed. A persistently open bladder neck suggests neurogenic bladder dysfunction. The location of the ureteral insertion should be in the trigonal region. An aberrant location suggests an ectopic ureter or duplicated system. Ureteral anomalies (megaureter or a paraureteral diverticulum) may be detected on lateral views. If the refluxing renal unit has a "drooping lily" appearance, a duplication with an obstructed upper pole may be present. Urethral pathology is rarely seen in the female. Oblique views of the male urethra will exclude posterior urethral valves, prune belly syndrome, a congenital stricture, or a urethral diverticulum.

With experience, cystography can be readily performed on children in the unsedated state with good cooperation. Only on rare occasions is general anesthesia required for a child who would otherwise be unable to cooperate during routine cystography (LEVITT and WEISS 1985). Reflux has been detected exclusively in the anesthetized state in 20%–30% of patients (WOODARD and FILARDI 1976); however, demonstration of reflux under anesthesia and not on conventional cystography may not reveal the true physiologic competency of the ureterovesical junction. During VCUG, intermittent fluoroscopy and spot films may not

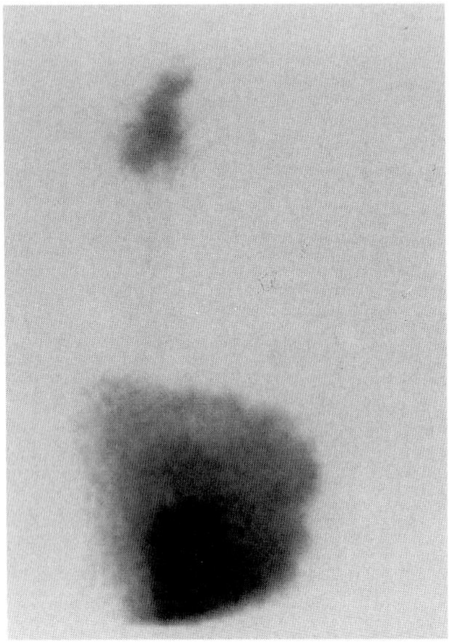

Fig. 7.13. Radionuclide cystogram demonstrating reflux into a nondilated right ureter and kidney

capture fleeting reflux despite meticulous technique; therefore transient vesicoureteral reflux may be missed (KOGAN et al. 1987). In the population of children with pyelonephritis and a negative VCUG, a radionuclide cystogram may detect occult reflux, due to greater sensitivity.

7.5.1.2 Radionuclide Cystography

An alternative technique to diagnose vesicoureteral reflux is radionuclide cystography. Direct radionuclide cystography involves placement of a Foley catheter, followed by a bolus injection of 1 mCi ^{99}Tc pertechnetate. The bladder is then filled to capacity with normal saline. The radionuclide should not be administered in the saline as only a fraction of the dose may be delivered to the bladder if the infusion is stopped prematurely. Nuclear imaging of the bladder and upper tracts is performed continuously throughout the study. Essential to the success of the study is achievement of full bladder capacity. Age-appropriate bladder capacity can be estimated by the formula: normal capacity (ounces) = age (years) + 2 (CONWAY 1983). Permanent images are obtained in the posterior and posterior-oblique projections at full bladder capacity (CONWAY 1983) (Fig. 7.13).

Radionuclide cystography exposes the patient to less radiation. The dosage to the bladder using 1 mCi ^{99}Tc pertechnetate is approximately 1 mrad per minute. During a 20-min study, the bladder receives 20 mrads. The ovaries receive approximately 10% of the bladder dose, while the testicles receive substantially less. Radiation exposure from conventional cystography is 50–100 times greater than that from radionuclide cystography, depending on the fluoroscopy time and number of spot films obtained (BUESCHEN and JOSEPH 1991).

Radionuclide cystrography can provide quantitative information on bladder volume at time of reflux, bladder capacity, refluxed ureteral volume, and postvoid residual. These quantitative data can be measured on sequential studies as parameters of improvement of the reflux. In patients with bladder dysfunction, urodynamic measurements can be obtained at the time of voiding cystography or radionuclide cystography by inserting a double-lumen catheter and recording bladder pressures throughout the study. These data may provide insight into bladder dysfunction and its relationship with vesicoureteral reflux (CONWAY 1983). Radionuclide cystography is more sensitive than conventional cystography in detecting vesicoureteral reflux grades II–V (CONWAY et al. 1975). Due to the continuous monitoring of radionuclide cystography, fleeting vesicoureteral reflux missed by conventional cystography can be detected. Minimal reflux (grade I) may be obscured by the activity in the bladder; thus radionuclide cystography is less sensitive than conventional cystography in detecting grade I reflux (ZHANG et al. 1987).

As radionuclide cystograms do not provide anatomic detail, conventional cystography should be performed as the initial test for vesicoureteral reflux. Subsequently, radionuclide cystography is preferable because of the decreased radiation dose, increased sensitivity, and the ability to quantitate the bladder volume at the point of reflux. Radionuclide cystography should also be used in the postoperative setting to determine whether reflux is present. In asymptomatic siblings, radionuclide cystography should be employed as a screening test owing to the decreased radiation exposure (VAN DEN ABBEELE et al. 1987).

7.5.2 Renal Radioisotope Scanning

Radioisotope studies of renal function may be performed to detect the presence of reflux nephropathy. These studies allow for detection of cortical scarring and assessment of renal function and renal growth. All patients with reflux who are managed medically should be followed with serial renal scans to detect the development or exacerbation of nephropathy.

The major indication for static renography is the detection of renal scars (CARTY 1984) and ^{99}Tc-labeled dimercaptosuccinic acid (DMSA) is most commonly used. ^{99}Tc-DMSA is bound by the protein sulfhydryl groups in renal cortical tubular cells, providing an excellent morphologic image of functioning cortical tissue (Fig. 7.14). Three images of the kidney are made, not less than 2 h after injection, in posterior and oblique views. On oblique views, small peripheral scars can be detected. Regions of interest are drawn around the kidneys, together with background areas of interest. The relative uptake of the kidneys is then calculated. In normal kidneys, the uptake is evenly distributed. Scars are shown as defects in the renal image and represent nonfunctioning tubular cells or fibrous tissue. The scars may be peripheral or central (CARTY 1984). The extent of scarring is better delineated by DMSA imaging than by intravenous urography. ^{99}Tc-DMSA scanning is the method of choice to detect post-inflammatory renal scars (CARTY 1984) as the latent period between the development and detection of a scar on IVP may be prolonged to 8 months to 2 years (COHEN et al. 1990). Acute pyelonephritis may be diagnosed on DMSA scan as a focal defect, particularly if compared to a baseline study. In an animal model, the DMSA scan is highly accurate in the detection of acute pyelonephritic lesions which may progress to scarring (RUSTON et al. 1988).

Other radiopharmaceutical agents such as ^{131}I-hippuran or ^{99m}Tc mercaptoacetyltriglycine (^{99m}Tc-MAG 3) allow determination of individual and total renal function with lower radiation exposure than urography. Morphologic imaging is superior with ^{99m}Tc-MAG 3, and at a lower radiation dose than with ^{131}I-hippuran. However, the clarity of the images does not match that with ^{99m}Tc-DMSA. A good correlation has been demonstrated between glomerular filtration rate, estimated renal plasma flow, parenchymal sonographic volume, and urographic area (TROELL et al. 1988). With skeletal growth, normal children demonstrate a symmetrical increase in glomerular filtration rate and estimated renal plasma flow through puberty. Quantitative renography is thus a sensitive means of monitoring renal growth, as on an annual basis. A decline in the individual or total renal function may occur with pyelonephritis or bladder dysfunctions and warrants further evaluation (ORTENBERG 1989).

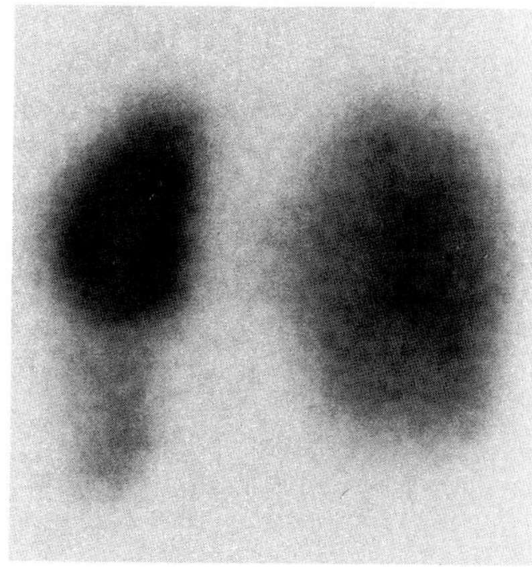

Fig. 7.14. DMSA scan documenting unilateral lower pole scarring

7.5.3 Intravenous Urography and Ultrasonography

In children with urinary tract infection, an imaging study of the upper urinary tract is essential to detect associated anomalies which may influence therapeutic options. Ultrasonography has generally replaced IVP as the initial screening study of the upper urinary tract (LEONIDAS et al. 1985).

To monitor renal growth with reflux on the nephrogram phase of the IVP, renal length is compared to the L1–L3 intervertebral distance (WINSBERG et al. 1979). Other nomograms have been developed to calculate renal growth based on the child's age. Reflux nephropathy may be identified as segmental cortical scarring or thinning, clubbing or splaying of the calyces associated with thinned overlying parenchyma (HODSON and WILSON 1965) (Fig. 7.15). Renal scarring typically affects the upper and lower poles, but may be diffuse, and a decrease in renal length may be seen.

In addition to scarring, IVP may identify hydroureteronephrosis, duplication of the collecting system, or bladder abnormalities. Hydronephrosis may occur as a result of higher grade reflux or secondary ureteropelvic junction or ureteral obstruction. Duplication is suggested if a

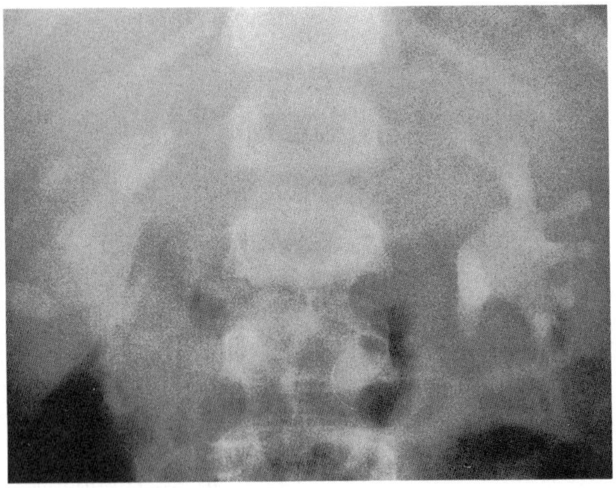

Fig. 7.15. Right calyceal blunting with thin cortex and short kidney length. These are characteristics of scarring on an intravenous urogram

lower pole segment is displaced inferiorly and laterally by a nonfunctioning upper pole segment, resulting in a "drooping lily" sign. Thickening and trabeculation of the bladder wall suggests neurogenic bladder dysfunction or urethral obstruction. The presence of a "cobra head"-shaped filling defect in the bladder suggests the presence of ureterocele. The degree of bladder emptying should be assessed on postvoid films.

Ultrasonography can provide accurate anatomic detail, but reliability is dependent on experience in pediatric imaging. Obviously, it is not possible to diagnose reflux exclusively by ultrasonography or IVP, as dilatation of the calyces and pelvis is not seen with grade I or II vesicoureteral reflux and reflux may be missed. Medullary hyperechogenicity may be shown on ultrasonograms and is considered indicative of intrarenal reflux (Diard et al. 1987). Increased cortical echogenicity suggests the presence of renal dysplasia from reflux and cortical thickness can be assessed by direct measurements.

With the expanded accuracy and use of obstetric ultrasonography, prenatal hydronephrosis is detected with increasing frequency. Ureteropelvic junction obstruction and posterior urethral valves are the two most common causes of obstructive neonatal hydronephrosis (Elder and Duckett 1991). Vesicoureteral reflux is the most frequent nonobstructive cause of hydronephrosis in the neonate. Infants with prenatally diagnosed reflux appeared to differ in three respects from children who present with clinical symptoms of reflux (Gordon et al. 1990):

1. A higher proportion of males
2. A greater severity of reflux
3. A higher coexistence of anomalies

The identification of hydronephrosis in utero allows early detection of vesicoureteral reflux, before the first urinary tract infection. With early antibiotic prophylaxis, reflux nephropathy may be prevented or limited.

7.6 Renal Scarring

Certainly the most feared complication of vesicoureteral reflux is renal scarring, which may alter renal growth, cause a decline in individual or total renal function, or result in hypertension. Children with vesicoureteral reflux should be followed to monitor any scarring. Renal growth should occur commensurate with skeletal growth. Severe reflux nephropathy is characterized by a small, shrunken kidney, with alterations in renal homeostatic function.

The onset of renal scarring with reflux is seen almost exclusively following febrile urinary tract infection. In the absence of infection, high grade reflux does not cause renal scarring except with high bladder pressures caused by urethral obstruction (Olbing 1987). The correlation between reflux and renal scarring was first observed in 1960 by Hodson and Edwards. The upper and lower renal poles were characterized as being most commonly involved (Hodson and Wilson 1965; White 1989). For renal scarring to occur with vesicoureteral reflux, intrarenal reflux must be present (Fig. 7.16). With low pressure reflux, the only segments which are prone to intrarenal reflux contain compound papillae with flattened or concave surfaces and gaping duct orifices (Olbing 1987). An autopsy study of pediatric kidneys demonstrated the presence of compound papillae in 94% of upper poles, 18% of lower poles, and 1% of mid zones (Funston and Cremin 1978). Intrarenal reflux was produced in pigs only in compound papillae located mainly in the upper and lower poles (Ransley and Risdon 1974). Repeated scarring leads to parenchymal contraction which may transform closed orifices into open ones, increasing the papillary surface area prone to intrarenal reflux. Renal scarring was produced in low pressure reflux, only in the presence of infection (Ransley and Risdon 1978). Initiation of treatment of pyelonephritis with antimicrobial therapy during the 1st week after infec-

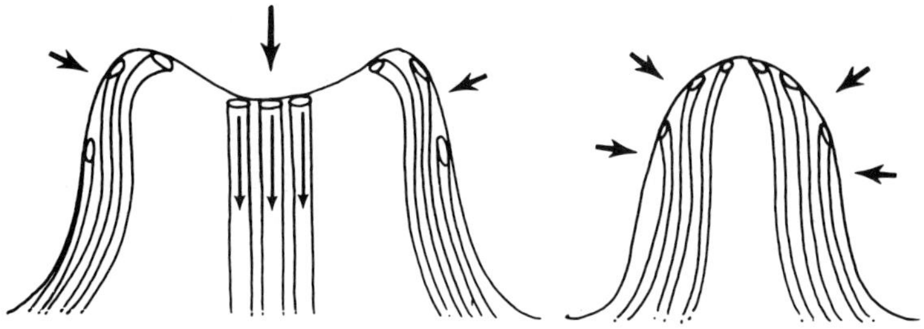

Fig. 7.16. Mechanism of intrarenal reflux with compound papillae

tion decreased the extent of scarring significantly (Ransley and Risdon 1981).

In a review of children with renal scars, all had experienced prior urinary tract infection. In the majority of cases, treatment was delayed following the onset of symptoms of pyelonephritis (Smellie et al. 1985) (Fig. 7.17).

The mechanism of renal damage has been attributed to a direct effect of bacterial inoculation and the resultant inflammatory response. The activated granulocytes aggregate in capillaries, producing ischemia. Further damage may occur from reperfusion with the formation of superoxides and metabolites, which have a direct toxic effect on renal tubular cells (Roberts 1990). The progressive scarring seen with reflux and urinary tract infection leads to small shrunken kidneys with changes of chronic pyelonephritis. Grossly, scarred kidneys contain irregular surfaces with depressed areas. The parenchyma is much reduced in depth, with a net reduction in the ratio of cortical to medullary thickness. Characteristically, the depressed cortex lies over an abnormal, widened calyx (Bouton 1984).

Renal functional alterations can predict reflux nephropathy prior to radiographic diagnosis or pathologic detection. The earliest abnormality associated with reflux is a concentrating defect due to altered renal blood flow or vasopressin insensitivity. The fractional excretion of sodium may be abnormal in children with reflux nephropathy. Reduction of glomerular filtration is a late manifestation of reflux nephropathy. A distal (type I) renal tubular acidosis has been identified in children with reflux, and may impair growth by interfering with calcium homeostasis (Walker 1990). Indeed, Dwoskin and Perlmutter (1973) noted that the physical growth of children with reflux was often impaired.

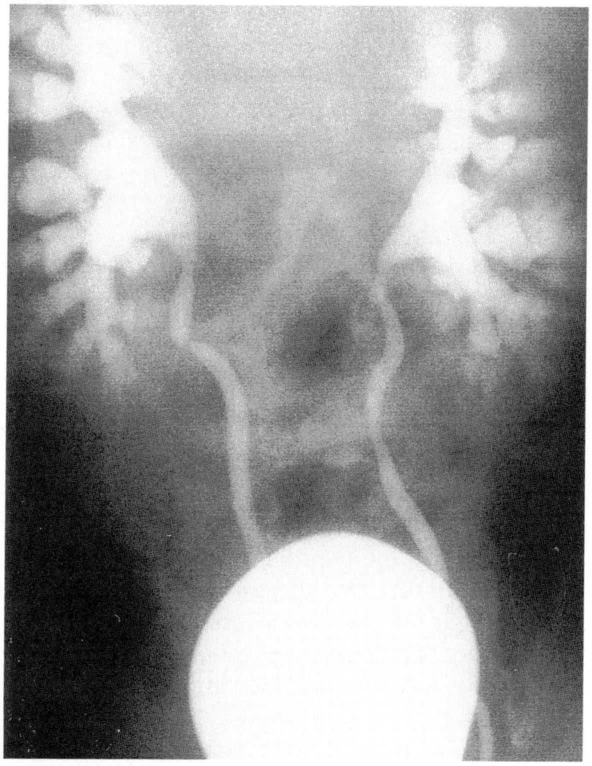

Fig. 7.17. Cystogram demonstrating intrarenal reflux in a child with recurrent pyelonephritis

7.7 Natural History and Management

Following the association of reflux with urinary tract infection and renal scarring, the initial treatment mode was predominantly surgical (Hodson and Edwards 1960). Subsequent observation of spontaneous resolution of reflux prompted nonsurgical management of milder cases (King et al. 1974). Nonsurgical treatment of vesicoureteral reflux is based upon the acceptance that sterile reflux is generally not injurious to the kidney and that vesicoureteral reflux will resolve spontaneously in the majority of instances (Ransley and Risdon 1978). Resolution of vesicoureteral reflux reduces but does not totally prevent further scarring

(Skoog et al. 1987; Smellie et al. 1985). Various parameters used to predict spontaneous resolution of reflux include cystographic and endoscopic observation of grade, tunnel length, and orifice configuration (Skoog et al. 1987). Due to problems with standardization of the cystoscopic assessment, the correlation between favorable orifice morphology and spontaneous resolution of reflux is low, only 50% (Bellinger and Duckett 1984). An accurate cystogram is the most important parameter to predict the rate of resolution, which varies inversely with the grade of reflux (Duckett and Bellinger 1984). Bellinger and Duckett (1984) reported that 87% of grade I, 63% of grade II, 53% of grade III, 33% of grade IV, and 0% of grade V reflux will resolve with observation.

With complete duplication, the natural history of lower pole reflux suggests that spontaneous resolution does occur in a reasonable time frame and a trial of observation is appropriate (King and Levitt 1986; Lee et al. 1991; Ben Ami et al. 1989). With partial duplication, the single ureteral orifice is usually located on the trigone and resolution is comparable to the single system. Reflux into a ureterocele with a duplicated system infrequent but has important surgical implications. Reflux into the ipsilateral lower pole ureter occurs in almost 50% of patients due to lateral displacement of the lower pole orifice by the ureterocele. Contralateral reflux seen with a ureterocele may resolve following decompression of the ureterocele (King and Levitt 1986). Reflux associated with a small paraureteral bladder diverticulum may disappear with growth during childhood; however, spontaneous resolution of reflux in the presence of a larger diverticulum is unusual (King and Levitt 1986).

The major goal in the management of vesicoureteral reflux is the prevention of renal injury. Recent prospective trials support conservative management of mild to moderate reflux with antimicrobial chemoprophylaxis if compliance with therapy is maintained. Three randomized, prospective studies have shown no difference in the rate of new scar formation among patients treated medically or by surgical correction (Birmingham Reflux Study Group 1987; Olbing and Tamminen-Mobius 1989; Arant 1991). Even infants with severe grades of reflux may be managed conservatively in the absence of progressive renal scarring, but such cases will ultimately require surgical correction.

At the initial diagnosis of vesicoureteral reflux, antimicrobial prophylaxis should be instituted. This is usually sulfa-trimethoprim or nitrofurantoin given at one-quarter of the total daily dose. For infants less than 2 months of age, amoxicillin at one-third dosage daily is recommended. The dosage should be given at bedtime to achieve highest levels at night, when urinary stasis is longest. A renal imaging study should be performed at the detection of reflux and at yearly intervals. Intravenous urography or renal scan can be used to detect scarring. Urinalysis should be carried out every 3 months to detect an asymptomatic infection. Urinalysis and a urine culture should be obtained with each febrile illness to exclude possible urinary tract infection. At this institution, radioisotope scans are preferred to intravenous urograms owing to the lower radiation exposure and the quantitative data obtained. Due to the slower rate of resolution, radionuclide cystography should be performed no more frequently than at 18-month to 2-year intervals to assess cessation of reflux. An initial DMSA scan is obtained when the clinical situation suggests a significant risk of prior renal scarring. In clinical practice, a single normal VCUG is considered sufficient to document reflux resolution. In a recent review, the rate of reappearance of reflux after a negative cystogram was as follows: grades I and II 49%, grade III 38%, and grade IV 32%. Two negative VCUGs may be necessary to confirm resolution of vesicoureteral reflux (Tamminen-Mobius 1990).

In recent data from the International Reflux Study, the surgical repair of vesicoureteral reflux was noted to decrease the risk of acute pyelonephritis, although the incidence of cystitis was the same between the two groups (Koskimies et al. 1990). The indications for surgical management of reflux are listed below (Firlit 1986):

1. Persistent or recurrent urinary tract infection despite antibiotic prophylaxis
2. Renal growth arrest
3. Progression of renal scarring
4. Lack of patient or parental compliance with nonoperative therapy
5. Failure of reflux to resolve

Various techniques in ureteral reimplantation employ "opening the bladder" (intravesical technique) or repair of the submucosal tunnel without opening the bladder (extravesical technique). The Leadbetter-Politano reimplantation (Politano

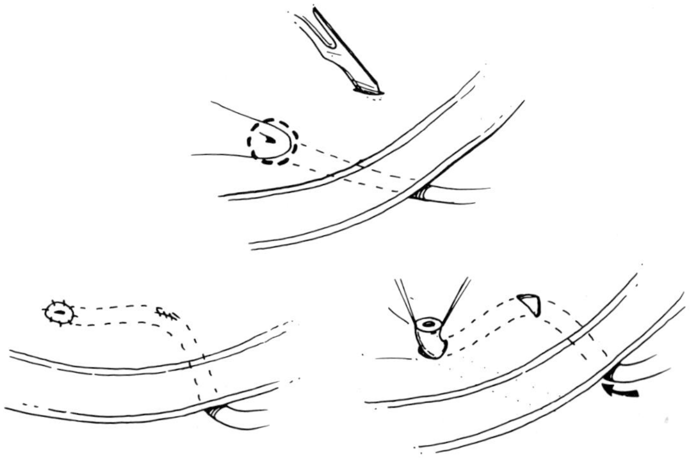

Fig. 7.18. Leadbetter-Politano ureteral reimplant

and Leadbetter 1958) involves mobilizing the ureter after opening the bladder. The ureter is passed outside the bladder and its entry is relocated to a more cranial and lateral position. This maneuver, which is performed without full visualization, carries the risk of inadvertent injury to adjacent organs or excessive angulation or obstruction of the ureter. The new orifice is positioned more caudally and medially on the trigone (Fig. 7.18). Various intravesical ureteral advancement techniques avoid relocating the ureteral entry into the bladder. The Cohen cross-trigonal reimplant involves creating a submucosal tunnel across the trigone from the original hiatus (Cohen 1975) (Fig. 7.19). Unfortunately, this new ureteral meatus is quite difficult to cannulate endoscopically, if stone manipulation is required during adulthood. The Glenn-Anderson advancement technique involves creating a submucosal tunnel inferiorly and medially from the original meatus (Glenn and Anderson 1967) (Fig. 7.20), but this procedure is limited by the proximity of the orifice to the bladder neck. A widened trigone is essential in order to perform this procedure.

Various procedures are employed without opening the bladder (extravesical approach). The Lich-Gregoir method of reimplantation (Lich 1961) involves incising the serosa and muscularis of the bladder above the insertion of the ureter. The ureter is then placed beneath the detrusor muscle, which is then closed over the ureter, increasing the submucosal tunnel. Other techniques of ureteral advancement have been reported in which an extravesical approach is employed (Firlit 1986).

In the management of reflux, several authors have reported good results with endoscopic sub-

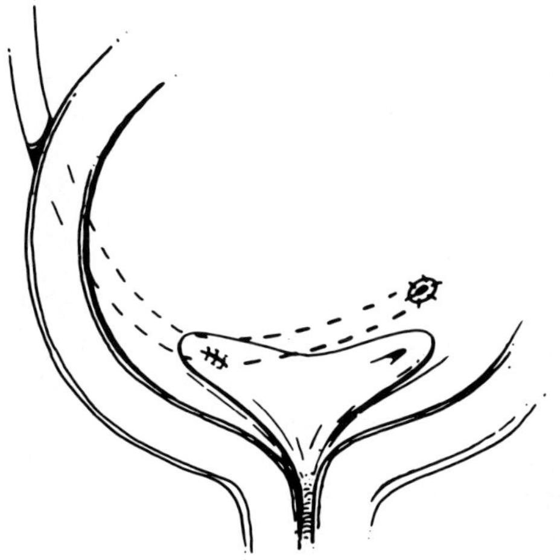

Fig. 7.19. Cohen cross-trigonal ureteral reimplant

ureteral injection of Teflon (Kaplan et al. 1987; O'Donnel and Puri 1986; Blake and O'Connell 1989; Mann et al. 1988), the success rates being as high as 80%. The advantages of this technique are minimal anesthetic time and avoidance of open surgery with decreased hospitalization. Questions have been raised about the results of this procedure as migration of Teflon particles and granuloma formation have been reported, dampening the enthusiasm for this procedure (Malizia et al. 1984). Subureteral injection of bovine collagen has undergone limited clinical trials, with greatest success in low to moderate grade reflux, and may be employed in the future if FDA approval is obtained.

Large dilated ureters may occur with high grade vesicoureteral reflux, rendering the surgery more complex (Fig. 7.21). Although resection of redundant ureteral length may improve drainage,

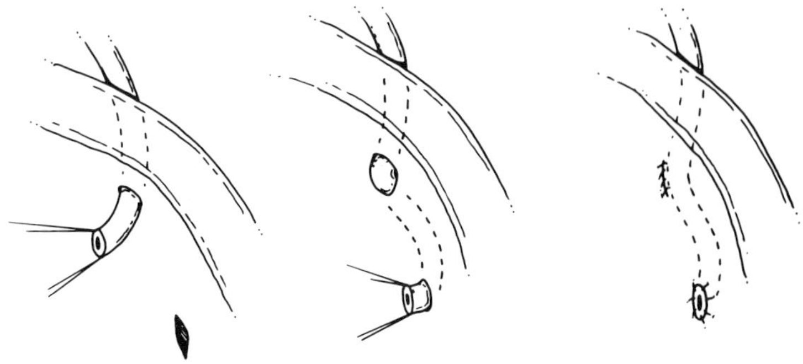

△

Fig. 7.20. Glenn-Anderson submucosal advancement ureteral reimplant

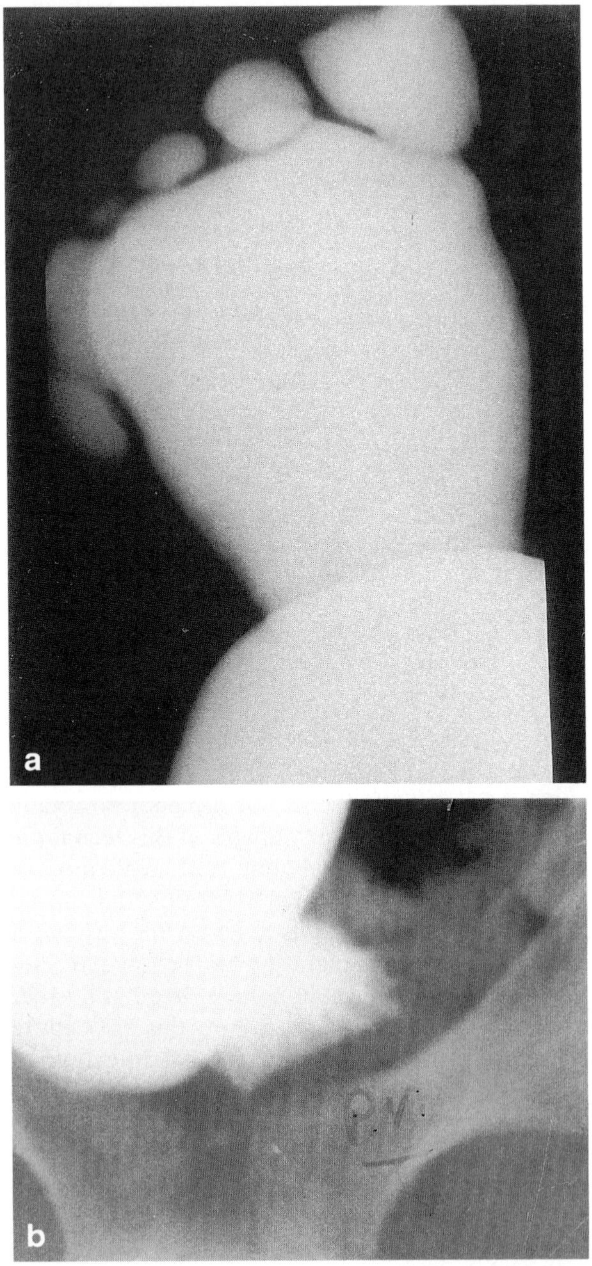

Fig. 7.21. a Grade V vesicoureteral reflux. **b** Empty bladder with massively dilated ureter on post void film

the primary reason for tapering or folding of the new intravesical segment is to secure an adequate submucosal tunnel which will not reflux. A common method employed to taper the distal ureter for reimplantation was first described by HENDREN (1969). The excess ureteral tissue is excised laterally, taking care to preserve the medial blood supply. This excision may extend for several centimeters. An alternative technique involves distal ureteral folding. KALICINSKI's method of modeling uses a continuous absorbable suture to exclude the excess, lateral portion of the ureter from the lumen. This flap of ureter is then rolled and secured underneath the ureter (KALINCINSKI et al. 1977). The ureter is not unduly bulky, but this technique reaches its limitations with a massively dilated ureter where the excisional technique may be required.

Duplicated ureters lie in a common fibromuscular sheath and share a common blood supply. The surgical correction of reflux in one ureter requires reimplantation of both ureters in a common tunnel technique. If one ureter requires excision, as with a partial nephrectomy and ureterectomy for a nonfunctioning renal segment, then the common wall may be left intact to avoid devascularization of the remaining ureter. If only one ureter of a duplicated pair shows reflux, an ipsilateral ureteroureterostomy may be performed. The refluxing ureter is anastomosed to the nonrefluxing ureter in an "end-to-side" fashion. This technique is as reliable as an intravesical common sheath reimplantation and the recovery time is reduced (FIRLIT 1986).

Complications of antireflux surgery have been well described. Persistent ipsilateral reflux occurs in 1.3%–3% of Cohen cross-trigonal reimplantations (CARPENTIER et al. 1982; ERLICH 1982) and in 9% of Leadbetter-Politano reimplantations. Factors contributing to the persistance of postoperative reflux include an improper submucosal tunnel, inadequate muscular support, creation of a fistula by ischemia or operative trauma, and the development of a periureteral diverticulum. In general, postoperative reflux, whether persistent or new, is apt to be of low grade and to resolve spontaneously. Furthermore, it does not seem possible to predict which ureters are at risk for the development of new reflux (Rink and Mitchell 1990).

Postoperative ureteral obstruction may occur as either an early or a late event. Early obstruction is usually transient, secondary to edema or severe bladder spasms caused by a urethral catheter (Gibbons and Gonzales 1983). Late ureteral obstruction is usually more significant. It may be secondary to ureteral angulation extravesically, twisting of the ureter within its submucosal tunnel, or compression from an acquired periureteral diverticulum. Devascularization of the distal ureter may result from excessive dissection of the ureter disrupting the delicate ureteral vessels and producing acute and chronic ureteral obstruction (Rink and Mitchell 1990). Postoperative ureteral obstruction is less likely to occur with advancement techniques such as the Glenn-Anderson and Cohen procedures, and with a nondilated ureter. The most recent data from the International Reflux Study show a 5% incidence of ureteral obstruction (Hjalmas 1990). Although ureteral reimplantation may effectively cure reflux in the vast majority of cases, further radiographic imaging is required to monitor the possibility of silent ureteral obstruction.

Acknowledgments. The authors express their special thanks to Alice Corvers and Helen Sosa for their help in preparing this chapter.

References

Ami Sidi A, Peng W, Gonzalez R (1986) Vesicoureteral reflux in children with myelodysplasia: natural history and result of treatment. J Urol 136:329–332

Arant B (1991) Vesicoureteral reflux and renal injury. Am J Kidney Dis 17:491–511

Askari A, Belman A (1982) Vesicoureteral reflux in black girls. J Urol 127:747–748

Baker R, Maxted W, Maylath J et al. (1976) Relation of age, sex and infection to reflux: data indicating high spontaneous cure rate in pediatric patients. J Urol 95:27–32

Bellinger M, Duckett J (1984) Vesicoureteral reflux: a comparison of non-surgical and surgical management. Contrib Nephrol 39:81–93

Ben-Ami T, Gayer G, Hertz M et al. (1989) Natural history of reflux in the lower pole of duplicated collecting systems: a controlled study. Pediatr Radiol 19:308–313

Birmingham Reflux Study Group (1987) Prospective trial of operative vs. nonoperative treatment of severe vesicoureteral reflux in children. Five year observation. Br Med J 295:237–245

Bisset G, Strife J (1987) The duplex collecting system in girls with UTI: prevalence and significance. AJR 148: 497–500

Blake NS, O'Connell E (1989) Endoscopic correlation of vesicoureteric reflux by subureteric Teflon injection: follow-up ultrasound and voiding cystography. Br J Radiol 62:443–449

Bouton M (1984) The pathology of reflux nephropathy. In: Libertino J (ed) The management of vesicoureteral reflux. Williams and Wilkins, Baltimore (International perspective in urology, vol 10, p 1)

Bueschen A, Joseph D (1991) Nonrenal nuclear medicine in urology. In: AUA Update Series Volume 10, Lesson 39

Campbell M (1952) Ureterocele: a study of 94 instances in 80 infants and children. Surg Gynecol Obstet 93:705

Campbell M (1970) Anomalies of the ureter. In: Campbell M, Harrison J (eds) Urology, 3rd edn. W.B. Saunders, Philadelphia, p 1487

Carpentier P, Bettink P, Hop W et al. (1982) Reflux: a retrospective study of 100 ureteral reimplantations by the Politano-Leadbetter method and 100 by the Cohen technique. Br J Urol 54:230–233

Carty H (1984) Radioisotope studies in the diagnosis of reflux nephropathy and in the assessment of individual kidney function. In: Libertino J (ed) Management of vesicoureteral reflux. Williams and Wilkins, Baltimore (International perspectives in urology, vol 10, p 19)

Cohen S (1975) Ureterozystoneostomie: eine neue Antirefluxtechnik. Aktuel Urol 6:1

Cohen R, Rushton G, Belman A et al. (1990) Renal scarring and vesicoureteral reflux in children with myelodysplasia. J Urol 144:541–544

Conway J (1983) Radionuclide cystography in reflux nephropathy. Contrib Nephrol 39:2–17

Conway J, Belman A, King L et al. (1975) Direct and indirect radionuclide cystography. J Urol 113:689–693

Diard F, Nicolau A, Bernard S (1987) Intrarenal reflux: new cause of medullary hyperechogenicity? Pediatr Radiol 17:154–158

Duckett J, Bellinger M (1984) Cystographic grading of primary vesicoureteral reflux as an indicator of treatment. In: Libertino J (ed) Management of vesicoureteral reflux. Williams & Wilkins, Baltimore (International perspectives in urology, vol 10, p 97)

Duckett J, Mc C Snyder H, Turner R et al. (1986) The dysfunctional voider (Hinman syndrome). In: AUA Update Series, Lesson 11, vol V, p 3

Dwoskin J (1976) Sibling uropathology. J Urol 115:726–727

Dwoskin J, Perlmutter A (1973) Vesicoureteral reflux in children: a computerized review. J Urol 109:888–890

Elder J, Duckett J (1991) Perinatal urology. In: Gillenwater J, Grayhack J (eds) Adult and pediatric urology. Mosby Year Book, New York, p 1171

Erlich R (1982) Success of the transvesical advancement technique for vesicoureteral reflux. J Urol 128:554–557

Firlit C (1986) Vesicoureteral reflux. In: Welch K, Randolph J, Ravitch M (eds) Pediatric surgery, vol 2. Yearbook Medical, Chicago, pp 1184–1193
Friedland G (1979) Pediatric urography. Urol Clin North Am (2) 6:375–393
Funston M, Cremin B (1978) Intrarenal reflux – papillary morphology and pressure relationships in children's necropsy kidneys. Br J Radiol 51:665–667
Gibbons M, Gonzales E (1983) Complications of antireflux surgery. Urol Clin North Am 10:489
Glenn J, Anderson E (1967) Distal tunnel ureteral reimplantation. J Urol 97:623–626
Gordon A, Thomas O, Arthur R et al. (1990) Prenatally diagnosed reflux: a follow up study. Br J Urol 65:407–412
Gruber G (1929) A comparative study of the intravesical ureter in man and experimental animals. J Urol 21:567
Hartman G, Hodson C (1969) The duplex kidney and related abnormalities. Clin Radiol 20:387
Hendren W (1969) Operative repair of megaureter in children. J Urol 101:491–508
Hjalmas K (1990) Complications after anti-reflux surgery. Abstract no. 90. Presented at the American Academy of Pediatrics Urology Section, Boston, Mass.
Hodson C (1965) Coarse pyelonephritis scarring with "atrophic pyelonephritis". Proc R Soc Med 58:785–787
Hodson C, Edwards D (1960) Chronic pyelonephritis and vesicoureteral reflux. Clin Radiol 11:203–219
Hodson C, Wilson S (1965) Natural history of chronic pyelonephritic scarring. Br Med J II:191–203
Hoffman A (1985) Uroradiology: procedures and anatomy. In: Kelalis P, King L et al. (eds) Clinical pediatric urology, 2nd edn. W.B. Saunders, Philadelphia, p 93
Hutch J (1952) Vesicoureteral reflux in the paraplegic: cause and correction. J Urol 68:457
Jerkins G, Noe H (1982) Familial vesicoureteral reflux: a prospective study. J Urol 128:774–777
Kalicinski Z, Kansz J, Kotarkinska B et al. (1977) Surgery of megaureter: modification of Hendren's operation. J Pediatr Surg 12:183–188
Kaplan W, Firlit C (1983) Management of reflux in the myelodysplastic child. J Urol 129:1195–1197
Kaplan W, Dalton D, Firlit C (1987) The endoscopic correction of reflux by polytetrafluoroethylene injection. J Urol 138:953
King L, Levitt S (1986) Vesicoureteral reflux, megaureter, and ureteral reimplantation. In: Walsh P, Gittes R et al. (eds) Campbell's urology 5th edn. W.B. Saunders, Philadelphia, p 2031
King L, Kazmi S, Belman A (1974) Natural history of vesicoureteral reflux: outcome of a trial of non-operative therapy. Urol Clin North Am 1:441
Koff S, Murtagh D (1984) The uninhibited bladder in children: effects of treatment on vesicoureteral reflux resolution. Contrib Nephrol 39:211–220
Koff S, Fischer C, Poznanski A (1979a) Cystourethrography: the effect of reservoir height upon intravesical pressure. Pediatr Radiol 8:21–22
Koff S, Lapides J, Piazza B et al. (1979b) Association of urinary tract infections and reflux with uninhibited contractions and voluntary sphincteric obstruction. J Urol 123:373–376
Kogan S, Sigler L, Levitt S et al. (1987) Elusive vesicoureteral reflux in children with normal contrast cystograms. J Urol 136:325–327
Koskimies O, Jodal U, Olbing H (1990) Surgical repair of vesicoureteral reflux decreases the risk of acute pyelonephritis. Abstract No. 95. Presented at the American Academy of Pediatrics Urology Section, Boston, Mass.
Lebowitz R, Olbing H, Parkkulainen K et al. (1985) International system of radiographic grading of vesicoureteral reflux. Pediatr Radiol 15:105–109
Lee P, Diamond D, Duffy P et al. (1991) Duplex reflux: a study of 105 children. J Urol 146:657–659
Leonidas J, McCanley R, Klauber G et al. (1985) Sonography as a substitute for excretory urography in children with UTI. AJR 144:815–819
Levitt S, Weiss R (1985) Vesicoureteral reflux: natural history, classification and reflux nephropathy. In: Kelalis P, King L et al. (eds) Clinical pediatric urology, 2nd edn. W.B. Saunders, Philadelphia, pp 355–380
Lich R, Howerton L, Davis L (1961) Recurrent urosepsis in children. J Urol 86:554–558
Mackie G, Stephens F (1975) Duplex kidneys. A correlation of renal dysplasia with position of the ureteral orifice. J Urol 14:274
Malek R, Kelalis P, Burke E et al. (1972) Simple and ectopic ureterocele in infancy and childhood. Surg Gynecol Obstet 134:611–616
Malizia A, Reiman H, Myers R et al. (1984) Migration and granulomatous reaction after periureteral injection of Polytef (Teflon). JAMA 251:3277–3281
Mann CI, Jequier S, Patriquin H et al. (1988) Intramural Teflon injection of the ureter for treatment of vesicoureteral reflux: sonographic appearance. AJR 151: 543–548
Mc C Synder H (1991) Anomalies of the ureter. In: Gillenwater J, Grayhack J et al. (eds) Adult and pediatric urology, 2nd edn. Mosby, St. Louis, p 1831
Meyer R (1907) Zur Anatomie und Entwicklungsgeschichte der Ureterverdoppelung. Virchows Arch [A] 187:408
Nation EF (1944) Duplication of the kidney and ureter: a statistical study of 230 new cases. J Urol 51:456–465
O'Donnell B, Puri P (1986) Endoscopic correction of primary vesicoureteral reflux. Br J Urol 58:601–604
Olbing H (1987) Vesicoureteral reflux and the kidney. Pediatr Nephrol 1:638–646
Olbing H, Tamminen-Mobius T (1989) International Reflux Study in Children: development of new scars in children with reflux (abstract). Pediatr Nephrol 3C:62
Ortenberg J (1989) The quantitative renogram. Probl Urol 3:747
Politano V, Leadbetter W (1958) An operative technique for the correction of vesicoureteral reflux. J Urol 79:932–941
Polk H (1965) Notes on Galenic urology. Urol Surv 15:2
Pozzi A (1893) Ureteroverletzung bei Laparotomie. Zentralbl Gynakol 17:97
Ransley R, Risdon P (1974) Renal papillae and intrarenal reflux in the pig. Lancet II:1114
Ransley P, Risdon P (1975) Renal papillary morphology in infants and young children. Urol Res 3:105–109
Ransley P, Risdon P (1978) Reflux and renal scarring. Br J Radiol [Suppl 14]:1–34
Ransley P, Risdon P (1981) Reflux nephropathy: effect of antimicrobial therapy on the early pyelonephritic scar. Kidney Int 20:733–742
Rink R, Mitchell M (1990) Complications of reimplantation and ureterocele surgery. In: Marshall F (ed) Urologic complications, 2nd edn. Mosby, New York, p 409
Roberts JA (1990) Pathogenesis of non-obstructive urinary tract injections in children. J Urol 144:475–479

Ruston G, Majd M, Chandra R et al. (1988) Evaluation of ^{99m}Technetium-dimercaptosuicinic. Acid renal scans in experimental acute pyelonephritis in piglets. J Urol 140:1169–1174

Sampson J (1903) Ascending renal infection: with special reference to reflux of urine from the bladder into the ureters as an etiologic factor in its causation and maintenance. Johns Hopkins Hosp Bull 14:334

Shopfner C (1970) Vesicoureteral reflux. Radiology 95:637

Silver T, Kass E, Thornburg J et al. (1976) The radiologic spectrum of acute pyelonephritis in adults and adolescents. Radiology 118:65–71

Skoog S, Belman A (1991) Primary vesicoureteral reflux in the black child. Pediatrics 4:538–543

Skoog S, Belman A, Majd M (1987) A non-surgical approach to the management of primary vesicoureteral reflux. J Urol 138:941–946

Smellie J, Ransley P, Normand I (1985) Development of new scars: a collaborative study. Br Med J I:1957–1960

Stephens F, Lenaghan D (1962) The anatomic basis and dynamics of vesicoureteral reflux. J Urol 87:669–680

Tamminen-Mobius T (1990) Disappearance of vesicoureteral reflux during medical treatment after five years follow-up of randomly allocated children. Abstract No. 93. Presented at the American Academy of Pediatrics Urology Section, Boston, Mass.

Troell S, Berg U, Johansson B et al. (1988) Comparison between renal parenchymal sonographic volume, renal parenchymal urographic area, glomerular filtration rate and renal plasma flow in children. Scand J Urol Nephrol 22:207

Uson A, Lattimer J, Melicow M (1961) Ureteroceles in infants and children: a report based on 44 cases. Pediatrics 27:971–983

Van den Abbeele, Treves S, Lebowitz R (1987) Vesicoureteral reflux in asymptomatic siblings of patients with known reflux: radionuclide cystography. Pediatrics 79: 147–153

Walker R (1990) Renal functional changes associated with vesicoureteral reflux. Urol Clin North Am 17:307–316

Walker R (1991) Vesicoureteral reflux. In: Gillenwater J, Grayhack J et al. (eds) Adult and pediatric urology, 2nd edn. Mosby, St. Louis, p 1889

Walker R, Duckett J, Bastone F et al. (1977) Screening school children for urologic disease. Pediatrics 50: 239–243

Weigert C (1877) Ueber einige Bildungsfehler der Ureteren. Virchows Arch [A] 70:490

White R (1989) Vesicoureteral reflux and renal scarring. Arch Dis Child 64:407–412

Winsberg J, Claesson J, Jacobsson B et al. (1979) Renal growth after acute pyelonephritis in childhood. An epidemiological approach. In: Hodson J, Kincaid-Smith P (eds) Reflux nephropathy. Masson, New York, p 309

Woodard J, Filardi G (1976) The demonstration of vesicoureteral reflux under general anethesia. J Urol 116: 501–502

Yip C, Leach G, Rosenfield S et al. (1985) Delayed diagnosis of voiding dysfunction. Occult spinal dysraphism. J Urol 134:694–698

Zhang G, Day D, Loken M et al. (1987) Grading of reflux by radionuclide cystography. Clin Nucl Med 12:106–109

8 Anatomy and Physiology of the Prostate

E. STEPHEN AMIS, Jr.

CONTENTS

8.1 Anatomy

The adult prostate is a firm, elastic gland having the shape of an inverted pyramid and located at the base of the bladder (Fig. 8.1). It is traversed by the prostatic urethra and the paired ejaculatory ducts, the latter emptying distally on the verumontanum. The verumontanum is a small mound of tissue posteriorly situated in the distal prostatic urethra. It contains a small central cavity communicating with the urethra, the utricle. The average measurements for the prostate are 3.4 cm in length, 4.4 cm in width, and 2.6 cm in thickness. The weight of the normal gland is between 15 and 20 g.

A venous plexus surrounds the prostate, being somewhat more prominent anteriorly between the prostate and pubic symphysis (VAN ENGLESHOVEN and KREEL 1979). Surrounding this plexus there is a fascial layer which is an extension of the visceral layer of endopelvic fascia. Posteriorly, the rectum is separated from the prostate by a dense layer of connective tissue, the rectovesical or Denonvilliers' fascia. Anterolaterally, the prostate is fixed by the puboprostatic ligaments. The inferior apex of the prostate rests on the urogenital diaphragm, through which passes the membranous urethra.

Classical descriptions of prostate anatomy define five lobes which confluently compose the gross gland. These lobes include the two lateral lobes, the anterior lobe, the posterior lobe, and

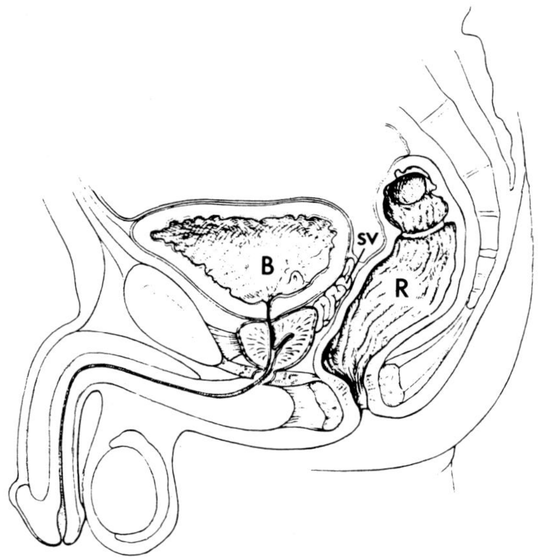

Fig. 8.1. Diagram of the gross anatomic relationship of the prostate to other pelvic structures. *B*, bladder; *SV*, seminal vesicle; *R*, rectum

the median lobe. However, vestigial prostatic tissue can occur superiorly to the gland itself, and when hypertrophied can result in further lobes. If this occurs in the region behind the bladder neck, the result is the subcervical lobe of Albarran (the sixth lobe), and if behind the trigone, the subtrigonal lobe of Home (the seventh lobe) (LICH et al. 1978). Gross dissections of the prostate do not reveal clear demarcations of the gland along lobar divisions.

More recent work by McNEAL (1981) indicates that the anatomy of the prostate is zonal, rather than lobar (Fig. 8.2). A small transitional zone, accounting for about 5% of the volume of the prostate, surrounds the proximal prostatic urethra. This zone appears to be the site of origin of benign prostatic hyperplasia. The remaining bulk of the glandular prostate lies posterior to the urethra and is divided into central and peripheral zones. The central zone comprises the smaller,

E. STEPHEN AMIS, Jr., M.D., Professor and Chairman, Department of Radiology, Albert Einstein College of Medicine and Montefiore Medical Center, 111 East 210th Street, Bronx, NY 10467, USA

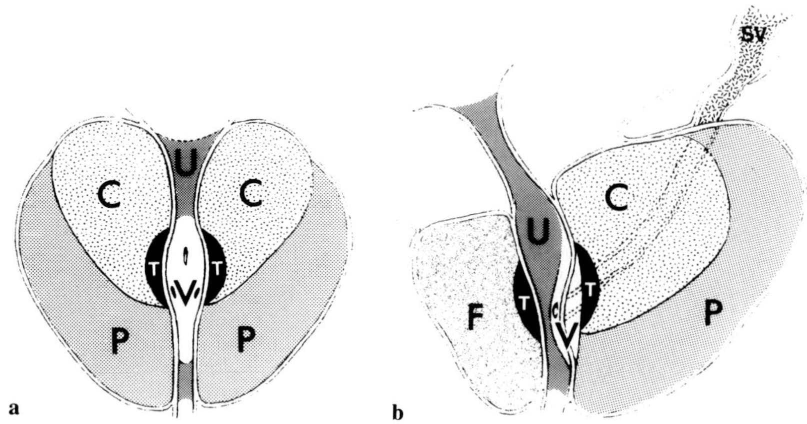

Fig. 8.2. **a** Coronal and **b** sagittal diagrams of the prostate showing zonal anatomy. Note the significant anterolateral extent of the peripheral zone. *T*, transitional zone; *V*, verumontanum; *P*, peripheral zone; *C*, central zone; *U*, urethra; *F*, anterior fibrous zone

proximal sector of the glandular prostate, while the peripheral zone occupies almost the entire posterolateral portion of the prostate and the bulk of the prostatic apex, cupping the central prostate as a baseball glove would cup a baseball. Prostatic carcinoma and prostatitis generally are found originating in this peripheral zone. Tissue anterior to the prostatic urethra is primarily fibrous in nature. The zonal division has been reported to be relatively constant from infancy through adulthood (Hiraoka and Akimoto 1987).

In composition, the prostate is a heterogeneous organ composed of fibromuscular and glandular tissues, each contributing approximately 50% of prostatic weight (Fornage 1986). Histologically, the functional, or glandular, prostate comprises 20–40 tubuloalveolar glands with their excretory ducts emptying into the floor of the prostatic urethra around the base of the verumontanum.

Intimately related to the prostate are the seminal vesicles. These are paired saccular organs extending superolaterally above the prostate between the lower bladder segment and the anterior rectal wall. The ducts from these glands join the convoluted portion of the vasa deferentia in the pelvis just above the superior margin of the prostate to form the ejaculatory ducts. The close contiguity of the seminal vesicles to the prostate is an important anatomic point in the not uncommon spread of prostatic carcinoma to these organs.

The primary arterial supply to the prostate is a branch of the inferior vesical artery, which derives from the anterior division of the internal iliac (hypogastric) artery. The veins of the prostate drain into the previously mentioned periprostatic plexus (the plexus of Santorini), which in turn drains into the hypogastric veins. There are also anastomoses between the prostatic veins and the venous plexus of Batson, which invests the lumbar spine, the sacrum, and the iliac wings (Lich et al. 1978). This venous communication is of paramount importance in understanding the frequency of bony metastases from prostate cancer in these regions. The lymph drainage of the prostate originates in the glandular acini, forming an intraprostatic network that drains peripherally to a periprostatic subcapsular lymphatic network (Johnson and von Eschenbach 1981). This network gives rise to lymphatic trunks which drain to the obturator, external iliac, hypogastric, and presacral lymph nodes. Again, this anatomy is important, as it clarifies the nodal metastatic pattern most commonly seen with prostate cancer. Since tumor tends to spread sequentially along the pattern noted above, metastases in the para-aortic area are almost never seen unless the primary pelvic nodes have first become involved.

8.2 Physiology

Functionally, the prostate is an accessory sex organ, contributing to the total seminal ejaculate at the time of orgasm. Secretion is stimulated by parasympathetic nerves during the plateau phase of ejaculation (deGroat and Booth 1980), and the prostate is thus caused to contribute approximately 0.5 cc to the average ejaculate volume of 3.5 cc. Emission of semen into the urethra depends on sympathetic nerves that cause contractions of smooth muscles in the vasa deferentia, the seminal vesicles, and the prostate. From this point, antegrade (normal) ejaculation requires continued contraction of the bladder neck. The primary function of the prostatic portion of semen appears to be that of liquefaction of the semen, which initially coagulates into a gelatinous clot.

The growth of the prostate, both normal and abnormal, is mediated by circulating androgens (Wilson 1980). This functional relationship may be permissive rather than active, but both benign and malignant change occur only in patients with intact testes or in whom exogenous androgens are being administered. This relationship is also species specific, occurring only in humans and dogs. The gonads produce 95% of all circulating androgen in the form of testosterone (Grayhack et al. 1987). The remaining androgens are secreted by the adrenal glands in the forms of dihydroepiandosterone and androstenedione. Extremely important in the management of advanced prostate cancer, orchiectomy is the penultimate procedure for elimination of the large part of circulating androgens, serum testosterone reaching castrate levels in an average of 3 h following removal of the testes. Indirect suppression of testicular androgen can be accomplished by the administration of estrogens, progestational agents, and luteinizing hormone.

Yet another important physiologic aspect of the prostate is the secretion of so-called tumor markers. Prostatic acid phosphatase (PAP) is a monoester phosphohydrolase present in large amounts as an exocrine secretion of the normal prostate (Huben and Murphy 1986). Not normally found in serum, its presence there usually parallels the extent or stage of prostatic carcinoma. Prostate-specific antigen (PSA), a protein that is immunologically distinct from acid phosphatase, is another potentially useful serum marker. PSA has been found elevated in 122 of 127 patients with newly diagnosed, untreated prostate cancer, including seven of 12 patients with early disease and all of 115 with more advanced disease (Stamey et al. 1987). However, PSA was increased in 86% and PAP in 14% of patients with benign prostatic hyperplasia, thus somewhat limiting their diagnostic usefulness. Further, both were increased following prostate massage and biopsy or surgery of the prostate. Their major usefulness may lie in the follow-up of patients being treated for carcinoma of the prostate.

References

deGroat WC, Booth AM (1980) Physiology of male sexual function. Ann Intern Med 92:329–331

Fornage BD (1986) Normal US anatomy of the prostate. Ultrasound Med Biol 12:1011–1021

Grayhack JT, Keeler TC, Kozlowski JM (1987) Carcinoma of the prostate. Cancer 60:589–601

Hiraoka Y, Akimoto M (1987) Anatomy of the prostate from fetus to adult–origin of benign prostatic hyperplasia. Urol Res 15:177–180

Huben RP, Murphy GP (1986) Prostate cancer: an update. CA 36:274–292

Johnson DE, von Eschenbach AC (1981) Roles of lymphangiography and pelvic lymphadenectomy in staging prostate cancer. Urology [Suppl] 17:66–71

Lich R Jr, Howerton LW, Amin M (1978) Anatomy and surgical approach to the urogenital tract in the male. In: Harrison JH, Gittes RF, Perlmutter AD, Stamey TA, Walsh PC (eds) Campbell's urology, 4th edn. W.B. Saunders, Philadelphia, 1:3–33

McNeal JE (1981) Normal and pathologic anatomy of prostate. Urology [Suppl] 17:11–16

Stamey TA, Yang N, Hay AR, McNeal JE, Freiha FS, Redwine E (1987) Prostate-specific antigen as a serum marker for adenocarcinoma of the prostate. N Engl J Med 317:909–916

van Engelshoven JMA, Kreel L (1979) Computed tomography of the prostate. J Comput Assist Tomogr 3:45–51

Wilson JD (1980) The pathogenesis of benign prostatic hyperplasia. Am J Med 68:745–756

9 Diseases of the Prostate

E. STEPHEN AMIS, Jr.

CONTENTS

9.1 Introduction

The prostate is an inhomogeneous organ. This is true in both normal and diseased states, and it results in a great deal of complexity when the prostate is imaged. Further, though the prostate is affected by a limited number of disease processes, it is not at all uncommon to find these diseases occurring concurrently, especially in the aging male. Generally speaking, three diseases occur in the prostate. These are prostatitis, beign prostatic hypertrophy (BPH), and adenocarcinoma. Of course, within these broad categories there are classifications and degrees of disease, and there are other quite rare entities that can occur in the gland such as transitional cell carcinoma arising in the prostatic urethra, endometrioid tumors in the utricle, and sarcomas in the connective tissue elements, including the rhabdomyosarcomas occurring in young boys. Further, metastases from primary tumors elsewhere, most commonly lung or malignant melanoma, are occasionally found. However, this discussion will concern itself with the triad of infection, BPH, and prostatic cancer. Trauma to the prostate usually involves the prostatomembranous urethral junction, and will be covered in the chapter on the urethra.

Despite the limited number of specific pathologic processes, the prostate is the most frequently diseased internal organ (PHILLIPS and KRESSEL 1987). The incidence of cancer of the prostate (CAP) is equalled only by that of pulmonary malignancy according to 1988 statistical estimates, and it accounts for approximately 20% of all neoplasms occurring in the male (SILVERBERG and LUBERA 1988). BPH has been found to be the most frequently occurring proliferative disease found in any male internal organ, and is so common in the aged male that it is almost considered a normal condition. Finally, prostatitis, usually of the chronic variety, is a frequent resident of the prostate, even in younger men. Because of the frequency of these diseases, it is rather common to find the triad of prostatitis, BPH, and CAP coexisting in the same gland. This does not simplify the clinical or radiographic evaluation of symptomatology related to the prostate.

E. STEPHEN AMIS, Jr., M.D., Professor and Chairman, Department of Radiology, Albert Einstein College of Medicine and Montefiore Medical Center, 111 East 210th Street, Bronx, NY 10467, USA

9.2 Prostatitis

In the past there has been confusion regarding the classification of inflammatory disease of the prostate, and uniform terminology was lacking. However, it is now generally accepted that the prostatitis syndromes can be classified as acute bacterial prostatitis, chronic bacterial prostatitis, nonbacterial prostatitis, and prostatodynia (MEARES et al. 1978). The acute form supposes recovery of bacteria from prostatic fluid expressed by digital rectal examination, purulence of the fluid on microscopic examination, and clinical symptoms consistent with an infectious disease process. The chronic variety exists when pathogens are found in significant numbers from expressed prostatic fluid in the absence of systemic signs of acute infection. Nonbacterial prostatitis is defined as the syndrome of chronic lower tract irritative symptoms accompanied by the finding of white blood cells in the expressed prostatic fluid. In such cases, significant numbers of bacteria cannot be cultured from the prostatic fluid. There remains a group of patients with lower tract symptoms suggestive of infection, but in whom the prostatic fluid contains no bacteria or inflammatory cells. These patients are classified as having prostatodynia, or pain in the prostate. They do not have a true infection, and psychological factors may be important in the pathogenesis of the syndrome.

In addition to the above, occasional patients develop granulomatous prostatitis, a characteristic histologic reaction of the prostate to a variety of insults (KRIEGER 1984). Low grade fever, dysuria, and urinary frequency are in keeping with an infectious disease. It has been reported that only about 3% of all cases diagnosed as prostatitis have a granulomatous etiology (O'DEA et al. 1977). In some cases, granulomatous prostatitis follows a bout of acute bacterial prostatitis. However, it must be remembered that there are a number of specific causes of this granulomatous reaction in the prostate, including tuberculosis, *Treponema pallidum*, fungi, metazoa, and brucella (NEY et al. 1983). Despite its rarity, granulomatous disease of the prostate is important because of its ability to mimic CAP.

The frequency of prostatitis (all varieties) is attested to by the autopsy findings of the disease in 40 of 91 adult prostates (MCNEAL 1968). Clinically, it has been estimated that some 50% of men will experience symptoms related to prostate infection during their lifetimes.

The causative agents in true bacterial prostatitis are similar in type and prevalence to those causing urinary tract infection (MEARES 1980). It is felt that reflux of infected urine into the prostatic ducts emptying into the prostatic urethra may play an important etiologic role in the disease. This theory is supported by the fact that crystallographic analysis shows many prostatic calculi to contain elements common to urine but foreign to prostatic secretions. It is therefore clear that urine must enter the prostatic ducts, probably by reflux, and participate in the formation of such stones.

Yet another inflammatory condition occurring in the prostate is true abscess formation. While the exact etiology of this condition is unknown, it has been postulated that it may result from progression of prostatitis, or be associated with infarction of the gland or BPH (DAJANI and O'FLYNN 1968). Certainly, as is the case with abscesses elsewhere, diabetes mellitus seems to be a major predisposing factor (PAI and BHAT 1972). It is usually a disease found in men older than 50 years, but can be seen in much younger patients.

As mentioned above, prostatic calculi may be found in association with prostatitis. However, in most cases these calculi are incidental findings and are not associated with symptoms or clinically evident disease (MEARES 1974). In either case, they are felt to form in response to reflux of urine into the prostatic ducts. Their average age of occurrence is 56 years (FOX 1963) and MEARES (1974) has reported their incidence on plain film of the abdomen as 13.8%. However, this incidence is probably significantly low, as CT is capable of detecting calculi not seen by routine radiography and stones are a frequent finding. Just as their presence does not necessarily denote current or prior infection of the prostate, they are not predictors of other diseases, such as CAP or BPH. Their incidence in patients with CAP is reported as 6.37% and with BPH as 7.9% (FOX 1963), probably not a statistically significant difference.

9.3 Benign Prostatic Hypertrophy

Benign prostatic hypertrophy is the most common pathologic entity involving the prostate. Both normal and abnormal growth of the prostate appears to be mediated by circulating androgens, 95% of which are secreted by the testes as testosterone (see Chap. 8). The development of BPH is a common manifestation of the aging process, with 50% of the male population having pathologic BPH when they are between the ages of 51 and 60 years (BERRY et al. 1984). This is contrasted with an incidence of only 8% in the fourth decade. As noted in the section on anatomy, the normal prostate reaches about 20 g in adult weight. This occurs in the third decade, and remains stable with increasing age unless, or until, BPH develops. The average weight of a prostate that is recognized at autopsy to contain BPH is 33 g. Only 4% prostates attain a weight of 100 g or more (BERRY et al. 1984), only 1% reach 200 g (SPRING et al. 1980), and the largest recorded prostate reached a giant 820 g (OCKERBLAD 1946).

In cases of obstruction secondary to BPH, there is a general direct agreement between the severity of symptoms and the size of the gland. It has been reported that, in spite of the prevalence of the disease, only 10% or so of men with BPH will require surgical intervention to relieve lower urinary tract symptoms or upper tract compromise (BLANDY 1971). It is not known why this selective obstruction occurs, though perhaps there is something about the gland, perhaps its stiffness or its bulk, which disturbs the normal mechanism of the bladder neck (BLANDY 1978). Currently, more than a decade after BLANDY's initial estimation that only one man in ten with BPH will need surgery, some urologists estimate a need for surgery to relieve symptomatology in up to 50% of cases (KIRBY 1992).

9.4 Cancer of the Prostate

Cancer of the prostate is a common neoplasm in the aging man. Ninety-five percent of prostatic malignancies are adenocarcinomas arising from the epithelium of the active prostatic acini. This group will form the subject of this discussion. As with BPH, it has been reported that cancerous cells in the prostate may develop in response to high circulating levels of androgen (PASQUALINI 1982). The mean glandular activity of prostates with CAP has also been shown to be higher than that of benign glands (McNEAL 1969). CAP does not occur in eunuchs, and rapidly regresses in response to androgen reduction, both facts supporting the androgen stimulation theory. Environmental and hereditary factors have also been postulated as etiologic factors.

As previously noted, the incidence of CAP is quite high, being estimated as 20% of all male malignancies in 1988. Men under the age of 50 are rarely afflicted, accounting for less than 1% of all reported cases of CAP (HUBEN et al. 1982). The average age at the time of diagnosis is 73 years (HUBEN and MURPHY 1986). The diagnosis is usually made on the basis of needle biopsy (transrectal or transperineal) of abnormalities in the prostate detected by the examining finger on rectal examination, or upon microscopic examination of tissue removed at the time or transurethral or open prostatectomy for presumed benign disease. In 386 patients undergoing transurethral resection of the prostate for BPH, MURPHY et al. (1986) found a 17.2% incidence of occult CAP. Similarly, of 847 patients who underwent open prostatectomy for disease initially felt to be benign, 6.5% were reported to have CAP (BAUER et al. 1960). Autopsy figures are even more dramatic for men not dying from CAP. FRANKS (1954), in summarizing ten such studies, reports a 20.4% incidence of CAP in 2716 males. It is well known that the incidence increases with age, as evidenced by one study showing CAP in 57% of men over the age of 80 undergoing autopsy (SCOTT et al. 1969).

It should be obvious from the above that in many instances CAP can occur in the prostate and lie dormant for many years. This could give rise to speculation that there might be two varieties of CAP, one that remains latent and one that progressively grows, locally at first, then with invasion of adjacent tissues and subsequently metastasis. Current thinking, however, is that there is only a single form of CAP, having an initial slow growth rate that eventually exhibits a logarithmic growth curve. If this concept is to be better understood, then predictors of growth must be defined, as indeed they have been. These include the size of the primary tumor, stage of the disease, and histologic differentiation (grade of the tumor) (DE LA MONTE et al. 1986).

These predictive factors are closely interrelated. For example, size and stage are usually closely dependent on the grade of the neoplasm. Poorly differentiated tumors have been reported to be three times more likely to spread through the capsule than are well-differentiated tumors (SCOTT et al. 1969). Also, size is important in assigning a stage to tumors localized to the prostate. McNEAL et al. (1986) feel that CAP undergoes a gradual increase in malignant potential which is closely linked to tumor size, as evidenced by metastases being found only in association with primary tumors larger than 4 ml in 138 cases of CAP. He and his co-workers concluded that the capacity to metastasize probably develops only in tumors significantly larger than 1 ml in volume.

The degree of histologic differentiation (grade) of CAP is also a significant predictor of further aggressive potential, regardless of the stage or size at the time of initial diagnosis. The Gleason system is currently widely employed (GLEASON et al. 1974). This system is based on the microscopic study of tumors at low magnification to identify predominant (primary) and lesser (secondary) growth patterns. Five patterns of growth are numbered from 1 to 5. The primary and secondary pattern scores are then added to obtain the final Gleason grade, which can range from 2 to 10. For example, a tumor which is predominantly of low grade (primary pattern score = 2), but

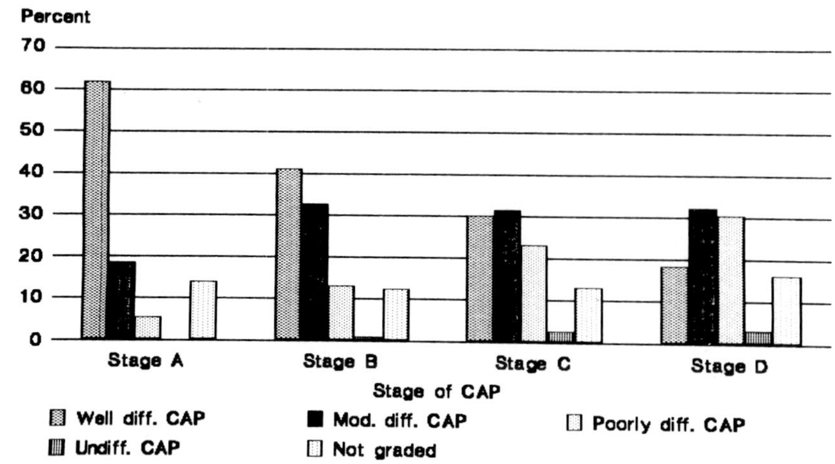

△

Fig. 9.1. Bar graph showing the varying degrees of differentiation of CAP for each stage of tumor. Note the increasing lack of differentiation for increasing stage of CAP

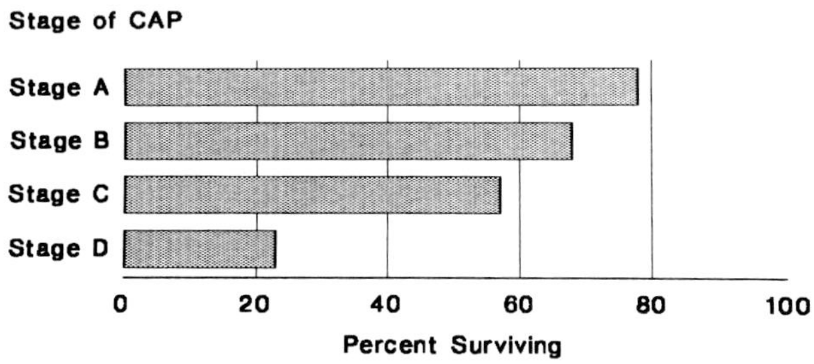

◁

Fig. 9.2. Bar graph showing the overall 5-year survival for patients with CAP by clinical stage

which has a focus of rather malignant cells (secondary pattern score = 4), would have a Gleason grade of 6 (2 + 4). This diversity of patterns is not unusual (Mostofi 1976). Clinical experience with the Gleason grading system has found it to be reliable and reproducible. Kramer et al. (1980) found that patients with Gleason grades 8, 9, or 10 had regional nodal metastases in 93% of cases, while patients with grades 4 or lower had no nodal spread. Figure 9.1 shows the relationship between grade and stage of CAP (Murphy et al. 1982).

Staging of CAP is based on the extent of involvement of the prostate, local invasion of the capsule into adjacent tissues, and distant spread. The importance of accurate staging can be seen in the dramatic decrease in 5-year survival with increasing stages of CAP (Fig. 9.2) (Murphy et al. 1982). While the TNM system can be applied, an alphabetical system is the current choice in the United States, and is felt to avoid confusion between tumor stage and grade. Staging is initially performed clinically, and then confirmed or altered based on radiographic evaluation. The gold standard remains histopathologic examination of the removed tissues. Unfortunately, discrepancies exist between clinical, radiographic, and pathologic staging. One comparison study between tumor size estimated on rectal examination and actual tumor size found a close correlation in only one of 17 cases (Siegelman et al. 1986). Further, seven patients had actual tumor areas that were more than twice as large as the estimate from palpation. Sensitivity and specificity of various imaging modalities in staging CAP will be discussed in subsequent sections.

Stage A CAP is divided into two categories, A1 and A2. Neither is palpable on rectal examination. A recently proposed definition of A1 disease is tumor involving 5% or less of tissue removed at prostatectomy (Epstein et al. 1986). This stage would also include small tumors initially diagnosed by transrectal ultrasound or magnetic resonance imaging (MRI), and subsequently confirmed by biopsy. High grade tumor, regardless of its size, should be considered as stage A2. Generally, however, A2 disease involves tumors diffusely infiltrating the prostate, though not resulting in a palpable nodule. While A2 tumors have been shown to exhibit more malignant potential than A1 lesions, patients with A1 disease are not entirely free from risk. An 8-year follow-up of 94 patients with A1 tumors showed a 16% incidence of progression of the disease (EPSTEIN et al. 1986). On the other hand, A2 disease is often very poorly differentiated, and has a worse prognosis than do B1 tumors, which usually have a more benign histology (DE VERE WHITE et al. 1977).

Stage B CAP is also divided into two categories. B1 tumors are palpable nodules less than 1.5 cm in diameter which are confined within the prostatic capsule. B2 lesions are larger than 1.5 cm in diameter, more diffuse, and also palpable; they, too, are confined to the limits of the prostate. Understaging can easily occur in this stage, as it is frequently difficult to separate lesions that are confined to the gland from those that have penetrated the capsule or that have microscopic spread to the seminal vesicles by either clinical or radiographic means. It was recently reported that mapping of excised prostates found small stage A lesions to be located more anteromedially in the peripheral zone than small stage B tumors (MCNEAL et al. 1988). This helps to explain the difference in palpability of the two stages. However, both types of lesion showed progressive regression in differentiation with increasing volume.

Stage C tumors have invaded the prostatic capsule or involved the seminal vesicles. Gross involvement locally is usually easily detectable by either rectal examination or various imaging modalities, notably computed tomography, magnetic resonance imaging, or transrectal ultrasound (MULHOLLAND 1988). After progressing to stage C, the tumor is no longer amenable to cure by radical prostatectomy and is usually treated with radiation therapy. Therein can be seen the importance of staging, especially between localized lesions (stage A or B) and those that have breached the capsule but have not spread distally (stage C). However, studies have shown that up to 66% of patients with presumed stage A or B disease have microscopic spread into adjacent tissues at the time of prostatectomy (SPIRNAK and RESNICK 1984). One can therefore see the difficulty in patient selection for radical surgical cure, especially since slightly over 50% of patients are initially staged clinically as having A or B tumors (Fig. 9.3) (MURPHY et al. 1982).

Stage D1 tumors are lesions exhibiting regional nodal spread. D2 lesions have widespread metastases. Both substages can occur regardless of the size or local extent of the primary tumor. Treatment in these advanced cases is usually limited to hormonal manipulations, often accompanied by radiation of bone metastases for symptomatic relief. CAP most commonly metastasizes to lymph nodes, with bone being the next most common site (JACOBS 1983). When nodal spread occurs, there is a predictable order of node involvement. First involved are the obturator nodes, then the external and internal iliac nodes (FRIEDLAND 1987). Bony metastases are found in approximately 70% of patients with advanced disease (SPIRNAK and RESNICK 1984). Sites involved, in decreasing order of frequency, are the spine, femur, pelvis, ribs, sternum, skull, and humerus (JACOBS 1983). Early metastases to the lower spine and pelvis occur through communications of the prostatic veins directly with the plexus of Batson, which invests these bony areas. Visceral metastases are most commonly found in the lung, liver, and adrenal, but any organ can be affected (CATALONA and SCOTT 1978).

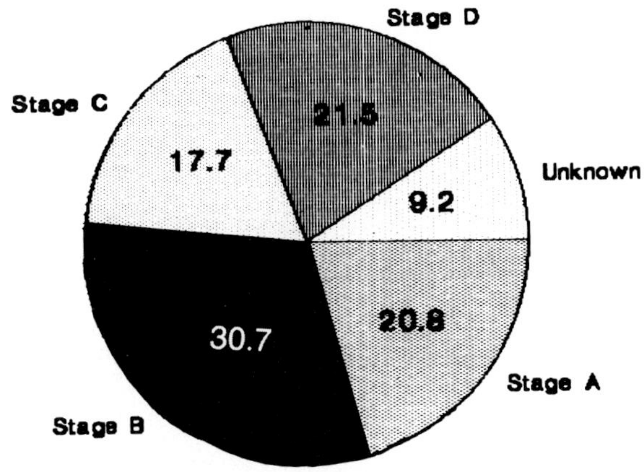

Fig. 9.3. Pie graph showing the incidence (in %) of the stages of CAP on initial clinical diagnosis (American College of Surgeons' survey). Note that stages A and B, which are potentially curable by radical surgery, constitute more than half of the cases

Given the weaknesses in both clinical and radiographic staging which currently exist, patients considered candidates for radical prostatectomy usually undergo a staging pelvic lymphadenectomy. This is considered a diagnostic rather than therapeutic modality by many urologists (FAIR and KADMON 1983; MCLAUGHLIN and SALTZSTEIN 1976; WALSH and LEPOR 1987). The patient who is then found to be free of spread becomes the beneficiary of radical surgery, and rightly so, as there is no current evidence that other treatments provide better control of the

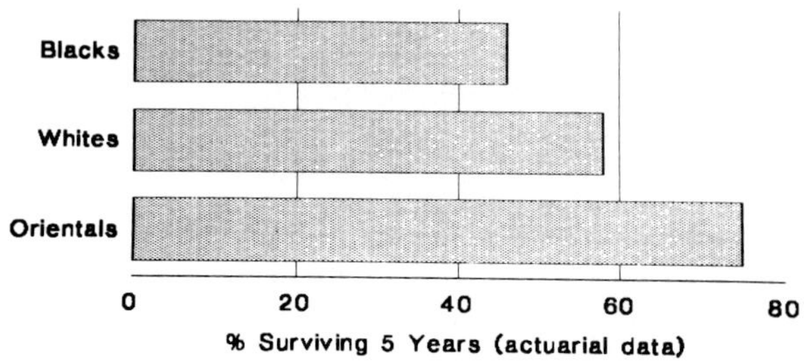

Fig. 9.4. Bar graph showing actuarial 5-year survival for three races of patients with CAP (American College of Surgeons' survey)

tumor. Fortunately, the surgical technique has been recently modified by WALSH (1987) to allow intraoperative identification and preservation of the branches of the pelvic plexus that innervate the corpora cavernosa, thus preserving erectile function in 70% of patients (WALSH 1992).

While approximately 60000 new cases of CAP were identified each year in the United States during the mid-1970s, estimates for 1988 indicated that 99000 new cases would be diagnosed (METTLIN and NATARAJAN 1987; SILVERBERG and LUBERA 1988). This increase ex-cedes that which would have been expected given the rise in population during that time frame. However, during this same period the death rate for CAP has remained about the same. The increased incidence, coupled with the stable death rate, resulted in an increase in the overall 5-year survivial to the 1982 level of 71.3% (METTLIN and NATARAJAN 1987). It should be noted, however, that the survival for black men is significantly lower than for whites, while that for Orientals is somewhat higher than for whites (Fig. 9.4) (MURPHY et al. 1982). However, regardless of race, the apparent improvement in survival may be skewed somewhat because many of the newly discovered lesions are early tumors with perhaps only minimal lethal potential (LEE et al. 1992). Since CAP is a disease of elderly men whose natural life expectancy is short and who may have other potentially fatal diseases, more than half of the patients will die from causes other than CAP (KIRK 1987). In the group who will die from other causes, treatment of their CAP will not increase their life span. On the other hand, the average age of the male population is increasing, and more men will consequently be at risk for CAP (MCCLENNAN 1988). Therefore, as the newer imaging modalities, notably transrectal ultrasound and magnetic resonance imaging, gain greater capabilites in detecting smaller and smaller lesions, the accurate prediction of the malignant potential of these early lesions becomes extremely important in determining which patients should be subjected to radical prostatectomy. Obviously, much work remains to be done in this regard.

References

Bauer WC, McGavran MH, Carlin MR (1960) Unsuspected carcinoma of the prostate in suprapubic prostatectomy specimens. Cancer 13:370–378
Berry SJ, Coffey DS, Walsh PC, Ewing LL (1984) The development of human benign prostatic hyperplasia with age. J Urol 132:474–479
Blandy JP (1971) Urinary tract diseases: benign prostatic enlargement. Br Med J 1:31–35
Blandy JP (1978) The indications for prostatectomy. Urol Int 33:159–170
Catalona WJ, Scott WW (1978) Carcinoma of the prostate: a review. J Urol 119:1–8
Dajani AM, O'Flynn JD (1968) Prostatic abscess. Br J Urol 40:736–739
de la Monte SM, Moore GW, Hutchins GM (1986) Metastatic behavior of prostate cancer: cluster analysis of patterns with respect to estrogen treatment. Cancer 58:985–993
de Vere White R, Paulson DF, Glenn JF (1977) The clinical spectrum of prostate cancer. J Urol 117: 323–327
Epstein JI, Paull G, Eggleston JC, Walsh PC (1986) Prognosis of untreated stage A1 prostatic carcinoma: a study of 94 cases with extended follow-up. J Urol 136:837–839
Fair WR, Kadmon D (1983) Carcinoma of the prostate: diagnosis and staging. World J Urol 1:3–11
Fox M (1963) The natural history and significance of stone formation in the prostate gland. J Urol 89:716–727
Franks LM (1954) Latent carcinoma of the prostate. J Pathol Bact 68:603–616
Friedland GW (1987) Staging of genitourinary cancers. Cancer 60:450–458
Gleason DF, Mellinger GT, The VA Cooperative Urological Research Group (1974) Prediction of prognosis for prostatic adenocarcinoma by combined histological grading and clinical staging. J Urol 111:58–64
Huben RP, Murphy GP (1986) Prostate cancer: an update. CA 35:274–292
Huben R, Nararahan N, Pontes E et al. (1982) Carcinoma of prostate in men less than fifty years old. Urology 20:585–588
Jacobs SC (1983) Spread of prostatic cancer to bone. Urology 21:337–344
Kirby RS (1992) Clinical assessment of benign prostatic hyperplasia. Cancer 70:284–290
Kirk D (1987) Trials and tribulations in prostatic cancer. Br J Urol 59:375–379
Kramer SA, Spahr J, Brendler CB, Glenn JF, Paulson BF (1980) Experience with Gleason's histopathologic grading in prostate cancer. J Urol 124:223–225
Krieger JN (1984) Prostatitis syndromes: pathophysiology, differential diagnosis, and treatment. Sex Transm Dis 11:100–112

Lee F, Torp-Pedersen S, Cooner W, Drago J, Holtgrewe L, Littrup P, Resnick M (1992) Detection and screening for prostate cancer. Cancer 70:355–356

McClennan BL (1988) Transrectal US of the prostate: is the technology leading the science? Radiology 168:571–575

McLaughlin AP, Saltzstein SL (1976) Prostatic carcinoma: incidence and location of unsuspected lymphatic metastases. J Urol 115:89–94

McNeal JE (1968) Regional morphology and pathology of the prostate. Am J Clin Pathol 49:347–357

McNeal JE (1969) Origin and development of carcinoma in the prostate. Cancer 23:24–34

McNeal JE, Kindrachuk RA, Freiha FS, Bostwick DG, Redwine EA, Stamey TA (1986) Patterns of progression in prostate cancer. Lancet I:60–63

McNeal JE, Price HM, Redwine EA, Freiha FS, Stamey TA (1988) Stage A versus stage B adenocarcinoma of the prostate: morphological comparison and biological significance. J Urol 139:61–65

Meares EM (1974) Infection stones of prostate gland. Urology 6:560–565

Meares EM (1980) Prostatitis syndromes: new perspectives about old woes. J Urol 123:141–147

Meares EM, Stamey TA, Drach GW, Fair WR (1978) Classification of benign diseases associated with prostatic pain: prostatitis or prostatodynia? J Urol 120:266

Mettlin C, Natarajan N (1987) End results for urologic cancers trends and interhospital differences. Cancer 60:474–479

Mostofi FK (1976) Problems of grading carcinoma of prostate. Semin Oncol 3:161–169

Mulholland SG (1988) Impact of radiology on the management of prostatic disease: a clinician's perspective. Semin US CT MR 9:335

Murphy GP, Natarajan N, Pontes JE, Schmitz RL, Smart CR, Schmidt JD, Mettlin C (1982) The national survey of prostate cancer in the United States by the American College of Surgeons. J Urol 127:928–934

Murphy WM, Dean PJ, Brasfield JA, Tatum L (1986) Incidental carcinoma of the prostate: how much sampling is adequate? Am J Surg Pathol 10:170–174

Ney C, Miller HL, Levy JL (1983) Granulomatous prostatis. Urology 21:320–323

Ockerblad NF (1946) Giant prostate: the largest recorded. J Urol 56:81–82

O'Dea MJ, Hunting DB, Greene LF (1977) Non-specific granulomatous prostatitis. J Urol 118:58–60

Pai MG, Bhat HS (1972) Prostatic abscess. J Urol 108:599–600

Pasqualini JR (1982) Hormonal regulation of the prostatic gland: physiology and pathology. Triangle 21:21–26

Phillips ME, Kressel HY (1987) Prostatic disorders: MR imaging at 1.5T. Radiology 164:386–392

Scott R, Mutchnik DL, Laskowski TZ, Schmalhorst WR (1969) Carcinoma of the prostate in elderly men: incidence, growth characteristics and clinical significance. J Urol 101:602–607

Siegelmann SS, McNeal JE, Freiha FS, Stamey TA (1986) Rectal examination in volume determination of carcinoma of the prostate: clinical and anatomical correlations. J Urol 22:1228–1230

Silverberg E, Lubera JA (1988) Cancer statistics, 1988. CA 38:5–22

Spirnak JP, Resnick MI (1984) Clinical staging of prostatic cancer: new modalities. Urol Clin North Am 11: 221–235

Spring DB, Schroeder DE, Watson RA, Agee RE (1980) Perivesical mass and vertical bladder caused by massive prostatic enlargement. Urology 15:207–208

Walsh PC, Lepor H (1987) The role of radical prostatectomy in the management of prostatic cancer. Cancer 60:526–537

Walsh PC (1992) Why make an early diagnosis of prostate cancer (editorial). J Urol 147:853–854

10 Urography and the Prostate

E. Stephen Amis, Jr.

CONTENTS

10.1 Consequences of Outlet Obstruction

To understand the urographic findings relating to diseases of the prostate, it is necessary to be aware of the response of the bladder and upper urinary tract to outlet obstruction. Whatever the etiology of obstruction of urine outflow from the bladder, the detrusor of the bladder compensates by hypertrophy. In the early stages, much as occurs with the heart, functionality of the bladder is manitained by increased contractility. As muscular hypertrophy progresses, there is resultant thickening of the bladder wall, including the trigonal region. With increasing intraluminal pressure, the bladder mucosa begins to herniate between the thickened muscle bands of the wall. Small mucosal herniations that do not protrude beyond the bounds of the bladder are known as cellules. With persistent obstruction these progress to frank bladder diverticula. Not being invested with a muscular coat, these diverticula do not empty well at voiding, and in fact may increase their volume. This results in stasis of urine, which can lead to infection and calculus formation. Long-term obstruction will eventually culminate in failure of the bladder, again similar to the failure seen in the heart pumping against increased resistance. With failure comes increasing residual urine and intravesical pressure and concomitant decreasing functional bladder capacity. The latter leads to the symptoms of frequency of urination and nocturia, as well as the feeling of incomplete emptying. These symptoms, coupled with hesitancy and a weak urinary stream, constitute the symptom complex known as prostatism.

In most cases of outlet obstruction, the valve mechanism at the ureterovesical junction retains its competence. However, even without reflux, increased pressure in the bladder lumen is relayed to the upper tracts by a decrease in the frequency and effectiveness of ureteral peristalsis. This results in poor delivery of the urine bolus from the renal pelvis to the bladder. In such a scenario, the end result is a functional obstruction of the upper tracts, though a catheter can easily be passed through the ureteral orifices. However, in some cases the valve mechanism preventing vesicoureteral reflux may fail in response to significant increases in lumen pressure, and reflux may then contribute to upper tract dilatation by direct transmission of pressure to the collecting systems. Beck (1970) reported on 2171 patients with a clinical diagnosis of benign prostatic hypertrophy (BPH). At the time of presentation, 14.5% of these patients were found to be azotemic, indicating some degree of functional compromise of the upper tract. The average age of this group was 78 years. The institution of bladder drainage resulted in an improvement in renal function in the majority of affected patients. The factors determining when surgical intervention should be undertaken in patients with prostatism due to benign disease include the severity of symptoms, the degree of decompensation of the bladder, and the presence or absence of upper urinary tract compromise. Intravenous urography remains the study of choice for initially evaluating bladder and upper tract changes.

10.2 Excretory Urography

Approximately four million excretory urograms are performed in the United States each year

E. Stephen Amis, Jr., M.D., Professor and Chairman, Department of Radiology, Albert Einstein College of Medicine and Montefiore Medical Center, 111 East 210th Street, Bronx, NY 10467, USA

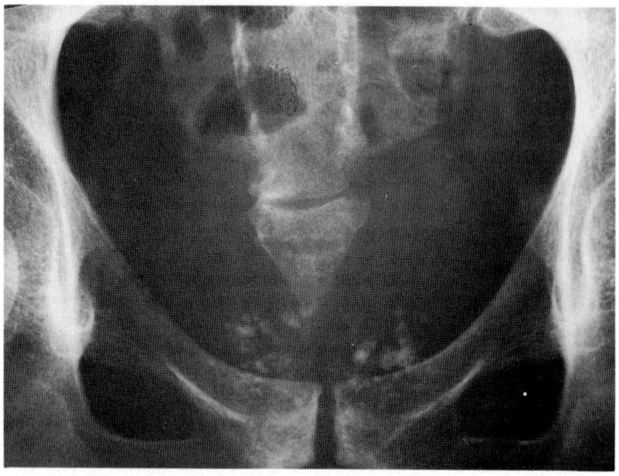

Fig. 10.1. Coned plain film of pelvis showing prostatic calcifications. The numerous stones in this patient are due to massive intraprostatic reflux secondary to bladder detrusor–external sphincter dyssynergia

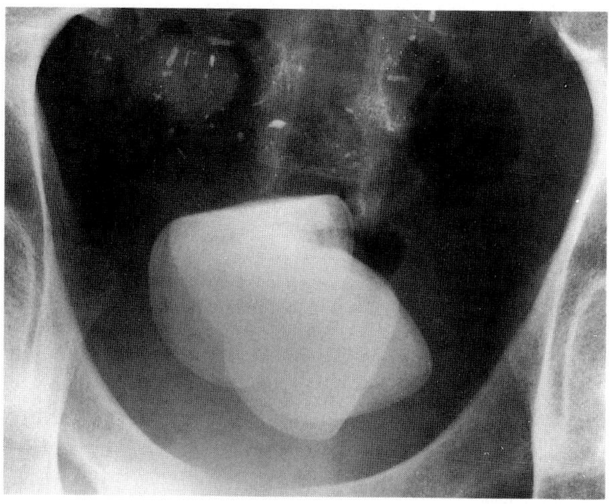

Fig. 10.2. Coned plain film of pelvis showing several large, faceted bladder calculi secondary to bladder outlet obstruction

(KUMAR and SCHREIBER 1985). With the increasing pressure to use the more expensive low osmolality contrast agents for more and more indications, the economic consequences can be easily deduced. Excretory urograms are somewhat routinely obtained in most men with prostatism, and certainly in the large majority of men in whom prostatic surgery is anticipated. There has been an ongoing debate in the radiologic and urologic literature as to the efficacy of this practice, with both pros and cons being pointed out (BAUER et al. 1980; BUTLER et al. 1978; MELLINS et al. 1979; PANG et al. 1979, 1980; WASSERMAN et al. 1987). Rather than delve into the dozen or so arguments in print, it is best to refer to the overall review of the arguments by TALNER (1986). The proponents of routine urography primarily base their recommendation on the anticipated discovery of renal lesions in patients in whom these are otherwise unsuspected. As previously mentioned, evaluation of the urinary tract proximal to the prostate remains a compelling reason for the study also. TALNER's review found that 15 renal tumors (either renal cell carcinoma or transitional cell carcinoma) were discovered in the 3828 patients reported in the literature. This would indicate a prevalence of renal tumors in this select group (patients with prostatism) of 0.4%. He concludes that, even were we to acknowledge a slight increase in prevalence of renal tumors in men with prostatism, it would not be sufficient to support routine urography in prostatism patients. Nevertheless, the practice continues on a somewhat routine basis in many institutions. Certainly, excretory urography is the most commonly employed radiographic study in the evaluation of urinary tract disease. Anatomic detail and gross renal function are assessed, as are the complications of bladder outlet obstruction.

Prior to the intravenous injection of contrast material for urography, a preliminary film of the abdomen is obtained. This is also referred to as a KUB (kidney, ureters, bladder) or scout film. This film yields information only indirectly regarding prostatic disease, since the prostate itself is not visualized. The only exception is that of prostatic calculi, and it must be realized that these do not delineate the actual size of the prostate, even when numerous. In BPH, distribution of these stones is frequently peripheral, though still beneath the compressed peripheral zone and surrounding the expanding adenoma arising from the central portion of the prostate (Fig. 10.1). In cancer of the prostate (CAP), calcifications are likely to be small and scattered when present, but this is a nonspecific pattern (FOX 1963). Further, in prostates where significant infection has occurred, calculi may be larger and coalescent due to previous destruction of intervening tissue by the inflammatory process. In rare instances, calcifications may occur on, or protrude through, the surface of an enlarged prostate. In such cases, if there is significant intravesical extension of the prostate, they may seem to originate within the bladder lumen or wall (POLLACK et al. 1981). If bladder outlet obstruction has been longstanding,

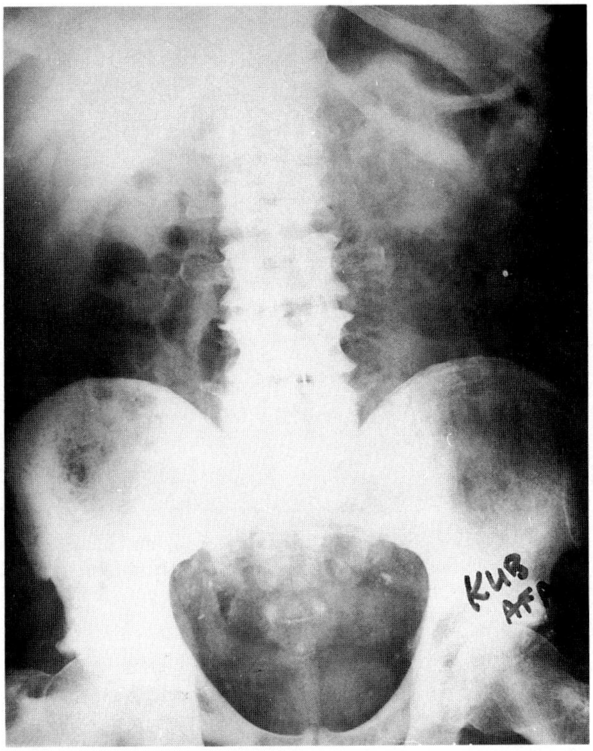

Fig. 10.3. Plain film of abdomen showing diffuse involvement of right pelvis by blastic metastases from CAP. Note the dense smudgy appearance of involved bone

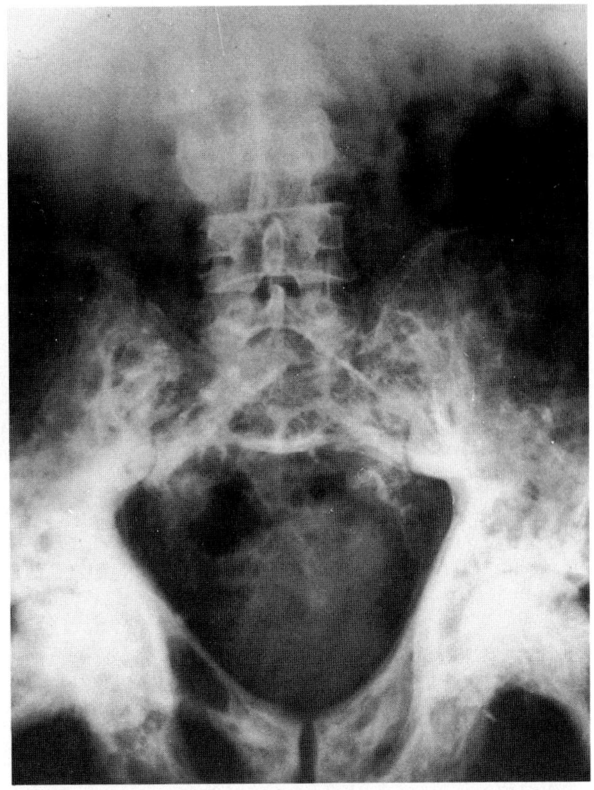

Fig. 10.4. Plain film of abdomen showing gross involvement of the bony pelvis by Paget's disease. The trabecular pattern is very prominent, and there is bilateral internal protrusion of the acetabuli due to softening of bone

bladder calculi may occur (Fig. 10.2), and in the case of upper tract dilatation, a search should be made for stones in that region since they have a higher incidence with urine stasis and infection.

In viewing any abdominal film, bony structures should be carefully scrutinized for metastatic lesions (Fig. 10.3). The frequency of bony metastases with CAP has been previously mentioned and is quite high. The majority of these are blastic, and have a homogeneously dense, rather smudgy appearance, though they can also be well defined. On occasion Paget's disease (Fig. 10.4) and degenerative joint disease may be difficult to differentiate from metastatic CAP.

When filled with contrast, the normal bladder base on the standard anteroposterior view parallels the superior margin of the pubis. Enlargement of the prostate results in an inferior intrusion into the bladder with elevation of the base (Fig. 10.5), but there is no direct correlation of the degree of elevation with the weights of resected prostatic tissue (MEYHOFF et al. 1981). On oblique views this extravesical encroachment can be seen to be somewhat posterior. With progressive enlargement, there can be significant elevation of the trigone and hence the ureteral orifices, resulting in "J-ing" or "hooking" of the distal ureters (Fig. 10.6). This abnormal ureteral course is among the more reliable signs of significant prostatic enlargement.

With hypertrophy of the subcervical or subtrigonal vestigial prostatic tissue, as previously discussed in Chap. 8, so-called intravesical protrusion of the prostate occurs. This has the appearance of a smooth, round filling defect within the lumen of the bladder (Fig. 10.7). Since the enlarged prostate is protruding into the bladder from a posterior rather than inferior direction, it can be entirely surrounded by contrast in the supine patient. In such cases, the differential diagnosis includes an inflated Foley balloon, a müllerian duct cyst invaginating the bladder posteriorly (YODER and PFISTER 1983), and a large bladder calculus, though the last-mentioned can usually be appreciated on the plain film. With the smooth margins that are characteristic for this

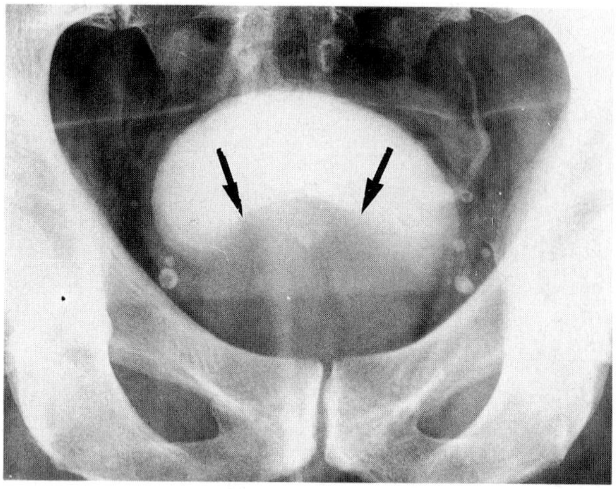

Fig. 10.5. Coned view of bladder from intravenous urogram showing smooth protrusion into the bladder base of a benignly enlarged prostate (*arrows*)

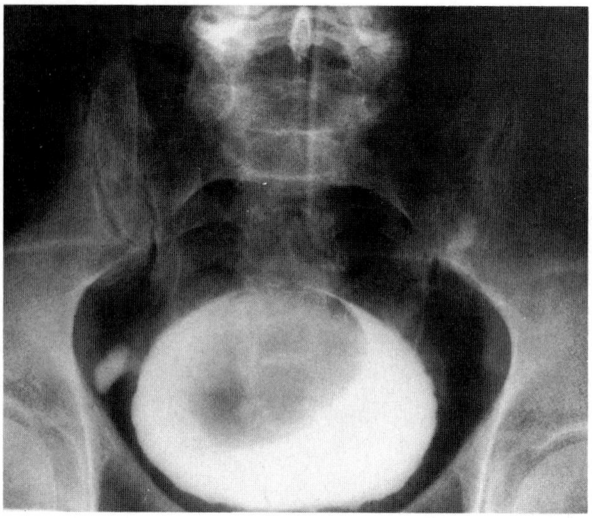

Fig. 10.7. Coned view of bladder from intravenous urogram showing a smooth filling defect in the central bladder due to hypertrophy of prostatic tissue behind bladder (lobe of Albarran)

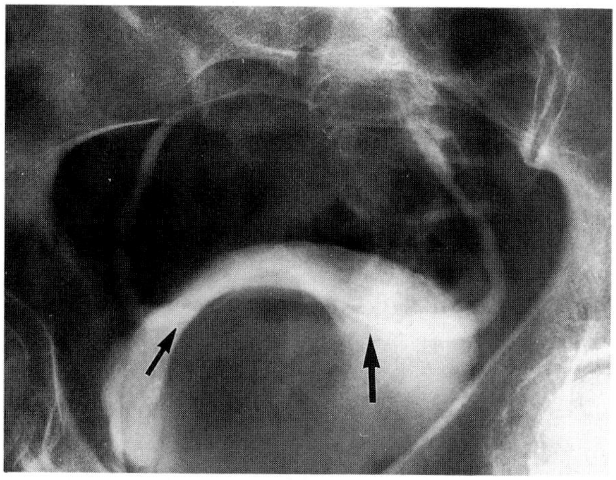

Fig. 10.6. Coned view of bladder from intravenous urogram showing "J-ing" of distal ureters (*arrows*) secondary to significant enlargement of the prostate (BPH)

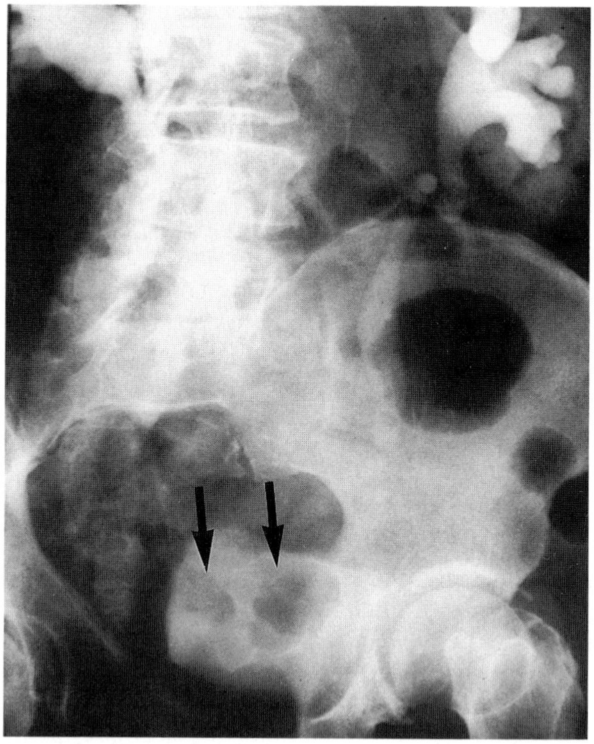

▷ **Fig. 10.8.** Fifteen-minute oblique film from intravenous urogram showing a grossly nodular enlargement of the prostate due to CAP (*arrows*)

lesion, clots in the bladder or bladder carcinoma are highly unlikely.

As opposed to the smooth impression on the bladder caused by the benignly enlarged prostate, gross irregularity or nodularity of the prostate should suggest the possibility of CAP (Fig. 10.8). It must be remembered, however, that transitional cell carcinoma arising from the bladder floor may have a similar appearance (Fig. 10.9). Further, on rare occasions, BPH may also exhibit a nodular appearance, though it does not usually have an irregular surface in such cases.

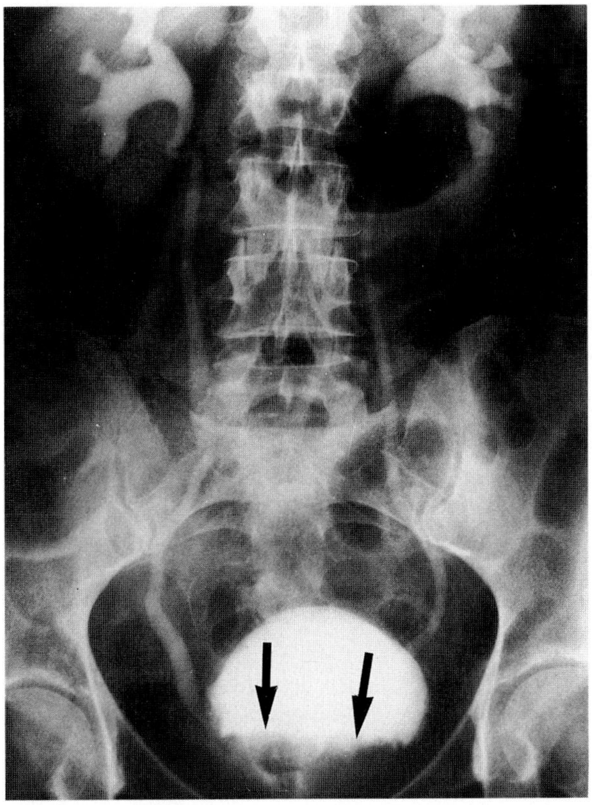

Fig. 10.9. Coned view of bladder from intravenous urogram showing an irregular mass in the bladder base which proved to be transitional cell carcinoma (*arrows*)

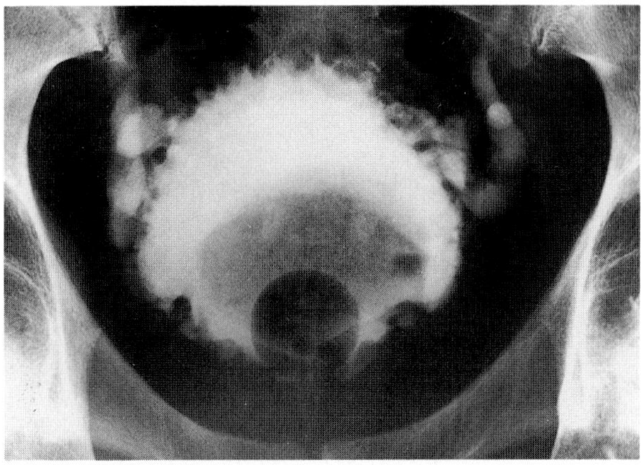

Fig. 10.10. Coned view of bladder from intravenous urogram showing an irregular bladder margin and multiple diverticula in this patient with BPH. Trabeculation can be confidently diagnosed with these gross findings

In the normal bladder following opacification, the detrusor measures only about 2 or 3 mm in thickness, and the wall is smooth. Increase in thickness may become radiographically apparent if muscle hypertrophy occurs in the face of bladder outlet obstruction. It is difficult to diagnose trabeculation on radiographs, but a diffusely feathery appearance of the bladder wall when the bladder is filled is suggestive of this entity. However, when cellules or frank diverticula are seen, the diagnosis can be made with confidence (Fig. 10.10). As the bladder fails, dilatation becomes prominent, with subsequent high levels of residual urine after voiding. In such cases, acute urinary retention may be imminent.

Estimation of residual urine from urographic studies is notoriously inaccurate. This is true for several reasons, including the environment of the study not being conducive to normal voiding and the introduction of an unknown time factor between the time of voiding and exposure of the postvoid film. The only clinically valid postvoid film is one which shows complete emptying of the bladder.

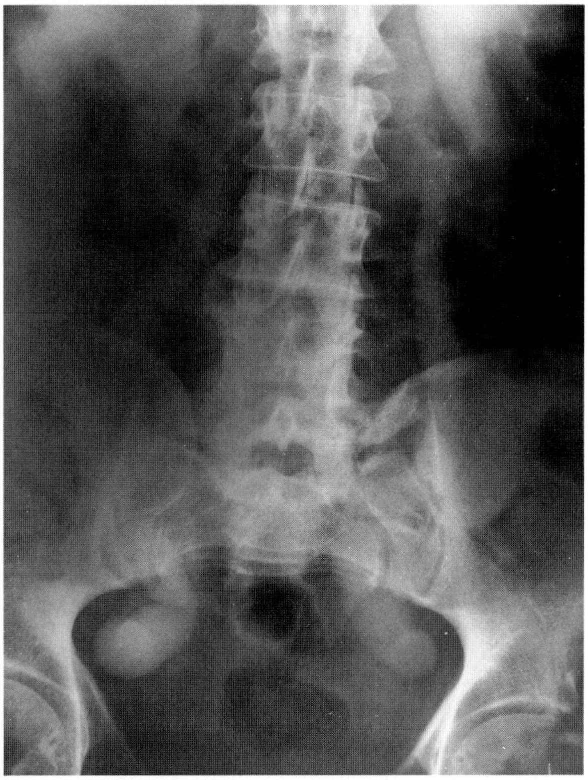

Fig. 10.11. Ten-minute urogram film showing bilateral, symmetric hydronephrosis in the patient with outlet obstruction secondary to BPH. Note that the bladder has not opacified on this film as it was full at the beginning of the study and there is delay in entry of contrast into the high pressure bladder

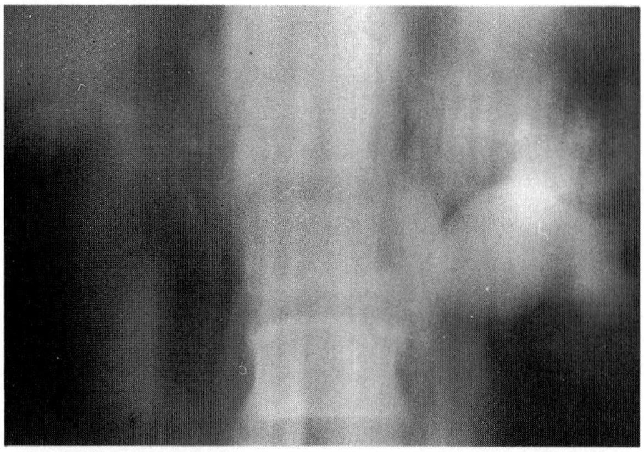

Fig. 10.12. Tomogram of the kidneys from intravenous urogram showing asymmetric hydronephrosis secondary to invasive CAP

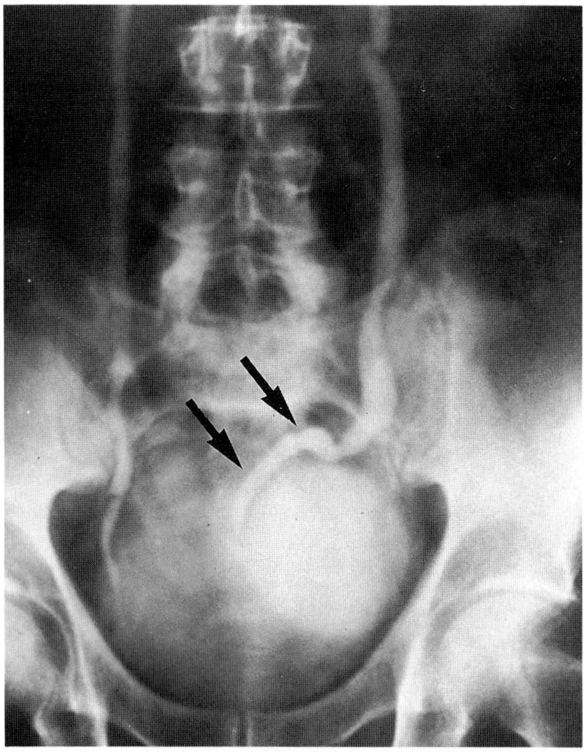

Fig. 10.13. Coned view of distal ureters and bladder from intravenous urogram showing abrupt medial deviation of distal left ureter (*arrows*) around a large bladder diverticulum

As previously noted, increased intravesical pressure and high levels of residual urine may result in functional obstruction of the upper tracts, or, on some occasions, in vesicoureteral reflux. In either case, the upper tracts eventually show signs of dilatation, usually bilateral and symmetric (Fig. 10.11). This is most commonly due to BPH and usually resolves after prostatectomy or following catheter drainage of the bladder. CAP, on the other hand, can invade the retrotrigonal area and involve one or both distal ureters. This may result in unilateral or asymmetric hydronephrosis, and CAP should be suspected when this pattern is seen (Fig. 10.12).

An acute medial deviation of either distal ureter is frequently seen in association with a bladder diverticulum, which on early films may be nonopacified. If such is the case, subsequent films, especially the postvoid film, will usually demonstrate the diverticulum because of mixing of contrast with the originally nonopacified urine (Fig. 10.13). Though less likely, one should consider the possibility of a pelvic mass or enlarged nodes when this pattern is encountered.

References

Bauer DL, Garrison RW, McRoberts JW (1980) The health and cost implications of routine excretory urography before transurethral prostatectomy. J Urol 123:386–389

Beck AD (1970) Benign prostatic hypertrophy and uraemia. Br J Surg 57:561–565

Bernstein RG, Siegelman SS, Tein AB, Bosniak MA (1969) Huge filling defect in the bladder caused by intravesical enlargement of the prostate. Radiology 92: 1447–1452

Butler MR, Donnelly B, Komaranchat A (1978) Intravenous urography in evaluation of acute retention. Urology 12:464–466

Fox M (1963) The natural history and significance of stone formation in the prostate gland. J Urol 89:716–727

Kumar R, Schreiber MH (1985) The changing indication for excretory urography. JAMA 254:403–405

Mellins HZ, McNeil BJ, Abrams HL, VanHouten FX, Murphy MA, Korngold E (1979) The selection of patents for excretory urography. Radiology 130:293–296

Meyhoff HH, Ingemann L, Nordling J, Hald T (1981) Accuracy in preoperative estimation of prostatic size. Scand J Urol Nephrol 15:45–51

Pang SMW, Keresteci AG, Rankin JT, Jewett MAS (1979) Role of preoperative urography in benign prostatic hyperplasia. Urology 16:292–294

Pinck BD, Corrigan MJ, Jasper P (1980) Pre-prostatectomy excretory urography: does it merit the expense? J Urol 123:390–391

Pollack HM, Banner MP, Martinez LO, Hodson CJ (1981) Diagnostic considerations in urinary bladder wall calcification. AJR 136:791–797

Talner LB (1986) Routine urography in men with prostatism. AJR 147:960–961

Wasserman NF, Lapointe S, Eckmann D, Rosel PR (1987) Assessment of prostatism: role of intravenous urography. Radiology 165:831–835

Yoder IC, Pfister RC (1983) Congenital anomalies of the adult bladder and urethra. Semin Roentgenol 18:267–275

11 Ultrasound of the Prostate

LINDA M. SANDERS

CONTENTS

11.1 Introduction

Both benign and malignant prostatic disease are common in the aging male and may result in significant morbidity and mortality. Assessment until recently has depended upon clinical methods such as the digital rectal examination and laboratory tests, coupled with biopsy results. However, data suggest that 50% of the hard nodules found during digital examination are benign (JEWETT 1956). In addition, transperineal and transrectal biopsies used to confirm a diagnosis have an accuracy of only between 50% and 90% (ABU-YOUSEF and NARAYANA 1985). Prostate imaging therefore has developed as a complementary diagnostic tool. Of all the modalities used in prostate evaluation, ultrasonography has probably received the most attention.

11.2 Methods of Examination and Instrumentation

Three different sonographic approaches to the prostate are currently used. The first, and oldest, is the transabdominal approach. Due to the retropubic location of the prostate, sagittal and transverse scans require a caudal tilt of the scanning plane of up to 30–40° (FORNAGE 1986). Visualization is best performed through a distended bladder, generally using a 3.5-MHz transducer for adequate depth penetration. As part of the transabdominal evaluation, the same probe may acquire coronal images if it is placed in a perineal location. Advantages of the transabdominal approach are high patient tolerance and ability to perform simultaneously digital rectal examination. Also, associated upper urinary tract and retroperitoneal pathology may be identified. In some patients, however, this technique proves limited because of abdominal wall thickness which results in sound beam attenuation and scatter with image degradation. Also, in some patients, the pubic symphysis is so prominent that the inferior aspect of the prostate cannot be seen. This is disadvantageous in that deep focal lesions may be missed, and measurements for prostatic volume may be inaccurate.

The use of transrectal sonography of the prostate has increased in parallel with technologic advances. Compared to transabdominal ultrasound, placement of the scanning head closer to the area of interest allows better resolution of detail within the prostate. WILD and REID (1957) were the first to develop a transrectal probe. However, WATANABE and associates (1968) are generally credited with obtaining the first clinically useful images of the prostate. The current examination is usually performed in the lithotomy, supine, or lateral decubitus positions. The rectal probe is inserted approximately 8–9 cm above the anal verge and a rubber condom covering the outer assembly of the probe is inflated with approximately 50–100 cc of water to ensure good contact with the rectal mucosa. The original transducers were radial and rotated in an axial plane. Serial transverse images are thus produced which allow a comparison between the left and right sides of the prostate. In almost every current

LINDA M. SANDERS, M.D., Department of Radiology, Saint Barnabas Medical Center, Old Short Hills Road, Livingston, NJ 07039, USA

system, separate transducers are required for longitudinal images, often using a small linear array attachment, with frequencies usually between 5 and 7.5 MHz. The ideal system is one in which both transverse and longitudinally oriented scans are obtainable from the same probe handle, eliminating the need for a second rectal insertion. Such transducers are becoming more readily available. Compared to transabdominal ultrasound, placement of the scanning head closer to the area of interest allows better resolution of detail within the prostate. The third approach, which is not widely used, employs a transurethral transducer. This mode of scanning is performed as a part of cystoscopy using a small rotating 4.5-MHz transducer inserted through the cystoscope. When the scanner is in place, the bladder is distended with fluid. Prostate scans are obtained by withdrawing the cystoscope until the transducer is within the prostatic urethra (Fornage 1986; Gammelgaard and Holm 1980). This type of imaging has been shown to be particularly useful in staging bladder carcinoma. The limited size of the transducer produces a reduced energy output and the peripheral regions of large prostate are not well imaged. Also, the rotating tip of the probe is not shielded and may cause urethral trauma (Fornage 1986).

11.3 Normal Appearance of the Prostate

11.3.1 Transabdominal and Transperineal Approaches

On suprapubic transverse scans caudally angled through the distended bladder, the prostate has a symmetric, roughly triangular, oval or semilunar shape. The echotexture is generally homogeneous. The rectum is identified posterior to the prostate. On sagittal scans, the prostate apex and inferior portion of the gland are less well seen. Transperineal images produce coronal slices of the prostate which appear triangular, limited by the bladder floor superiorly, the obturator internus muscles laterally, and the levator ani, ischio-, and bulbocavernosus muscles inferiorly. In theory, these views may better demonstrate the apex than the suprapubic approach since the transducer head is nearer to the apex in the perineal approach.

11.3.2 Transrectal Approach

The transrectal approach has proved better in obtaining detailed images of prostate architecture (Rickards 1992). On transverse views, the normal prostate appears triangular and symmetric. If the rectal balloon surrounding the probe is overinflated, this may indent the posterior margin of the gland. The transitional zone may be identified as a globular, sonolucent area occupying the anterior midportion of the cranial half of the prostate, adjacent to the bladder neck and surrounding the proximal segment of the prostatic urethra. This feature has been assumed to represent normal periurethral tissue (Rifkin 1987) and may have been an unrelated finding present in 100% of prostates with suspected inflammatory disease in one study (Griffiths et al. 1984). The peripheral zone extends along the posterior and posterolateral aspect of the prostate from apex to base and its echogenicity is the reference point by which lesions are classified. Superior to the prostate and posterior to the bladder are the seminal vesicles. Sometimes the demarcation between the peripheral zone and the seminal vesicles is difficult to identify unless the seminal vesicles are echopenic, as they occasionally are (Sanders et al. 1987). The central zone is usually isoechoic with the peripheral zone and thus is indistinguishable on ultrasound although occasionally may appear as a hypoechoic band of tissue along the anterior aspect of the prostate on sagittal views, extending from bladder neck to apex (Fornage 1986). Musculature is identified laterally and inferiorly. The rectal wall is depicted as an echogenic arcuate layer of tissue against the distended balloon. On midsagittal scans, the prostate is elongated, tapering from base to apex, and sometimes slightly concave anteriorly (Fig. 11.1). The longitudinal scans optimally show bladder neck and apex; however, the lateral borders of the prostate are poorly assessed due to the tangential orientation of the scan plane. The rectal wall is again identified as a linear, echogenic layer. The periprostatic venous plexus may be identified anteriorly as an anechoic oval structure (Fig. 11.2), unless phleboliths are present, in which case echogenic foci with or without shadowing are noted. Posterior to the apex of the prostate, perirectal fat is frequently seen as relatively hypoechoic. Infrequently, the collapsed urethra (Fig. 11.3) and ejaculatory ducts may be traced. Transurethral resection

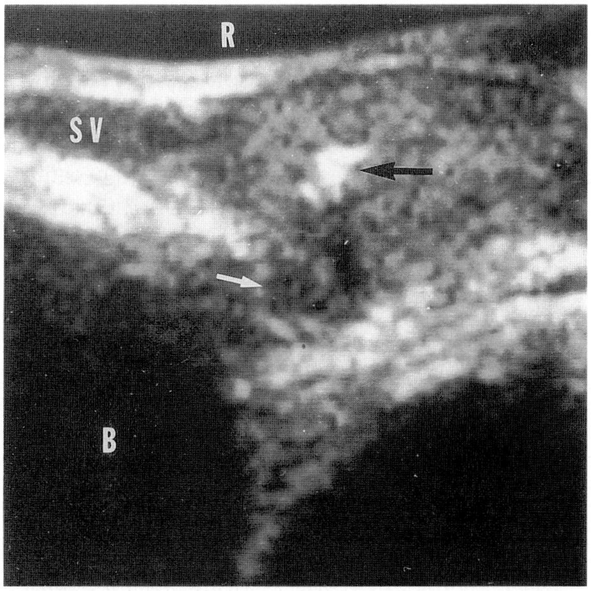

Fig. 11.1. Longitudinal transrectal image demonstrating normal hypoechoic transitional periurethral zone (*white arrow*). Incidental calcification is present, with shadowing (*black arrow*). *R*, rectum; *SV*, seminal vesicles; *B*, bladder

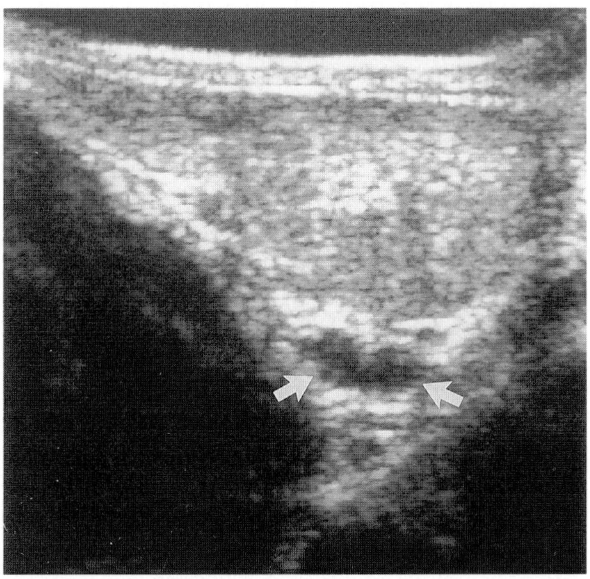

Fig. 11.2. Longitudinal transrectal image demonstrating normal hypoechoic structures anterior to the prostate which represent the prostatic venous plexus (*white arrows*)

of the prostate (TURP) may produce a defect identifiable as a cone-shaped expansion of the prostatic urethra at the bladder neck (Fig. 11.4).

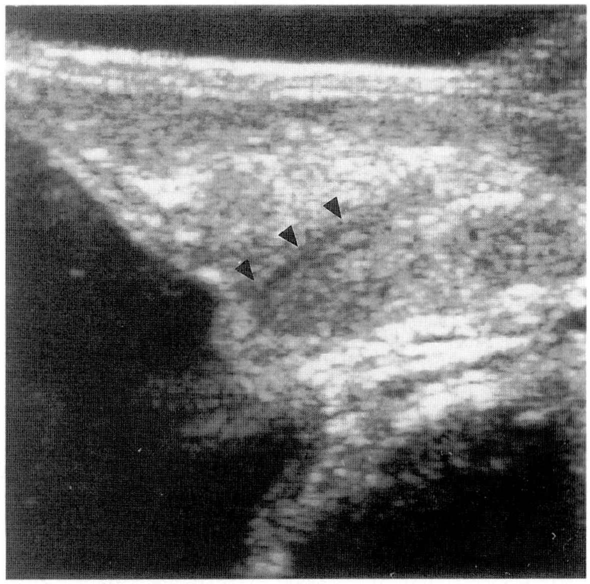

Fig. 11.3. Longitudinal midline image demonstrates the normal prostatic urethra (*black arrowheads*)

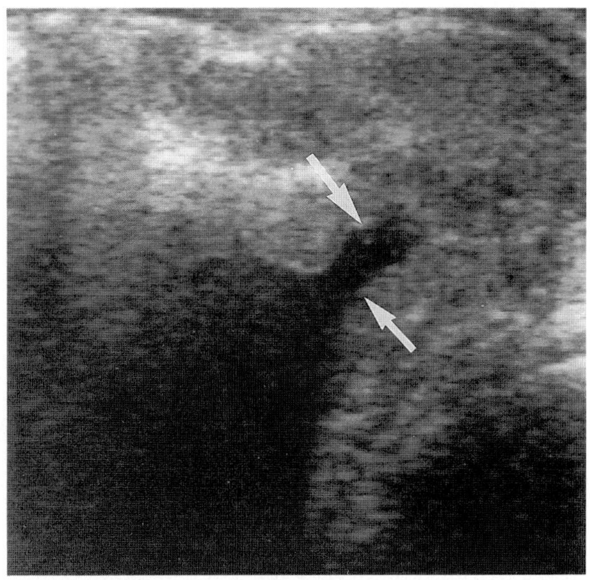

Fig. 11.4. Large transurethral resection (TUR) defect (*white arrows*)

11.3.3 Transurethral Approach

Images obtained with this method depict the prostate as an inverted heart, with a midline posterior cleft formed by the median sulcus. Because of beam orientation, this approach may best evaluate the prostatic capsule, which is normally higly echogenic (Fornage 1986).

11.4 Pathology

Interpretation of prostate images is confounded by age-related changes which occur naturally in the prostate. Corpora amylacea, present predominantly in the posterolateral gland, may calcify, or calculi of various sizes may develop in the transitional and central zones (Fox 1963). These result in bright sonographic reflectors which may or may not shadow (Dahnert et al. 1986b) and disrupt the normal homogeneous echotexture. Adenomyomatous changes of benign prostatic hypertrophy (BPH) are found almost without exception in the older patient as well. Transrectal ultrasound has been used extensively in evaluation of prostatic disease and attempts have been made to ascertain a characteristic appearance of each type of pathology, especially to distinguish carcinoma of the prostate (CAP) from BPH and prostatitis. Most investigators agree that there is considerable overlap in the sonographic appearances of these common disease processes (Rifkin et al. 1983a, 1990; Burks et al. 1986; Lee et al. 1986; Griffiths et al. 1990). Rare entities such as malacoplakia, likewise, have been known to mimic carcinoma sonographically (Chantelois et al. 1990).

11.4.1 Carcinoma of the Prostate

One of the difficulties in interpreting the literature is that assumptions regarding the location, size, and echotexture of CAP cannot be made on the basis of biopsies or TURP alone, since the smaller the tumor, the more easily it may be missed on biopsy (Lee et al. 1987). On the other hand, if a biopsy specimen contains carcinoma, it cannot be assumed that the sonographic features of that lesion represent cancer since a benign abnormality may and often does coexist with infiltrative tumor cells which cause no visible macroscopic and therefore sonographic alteration (Dahnert 1988). This is supported by data that tumor volume is underestimated by ultrasound (Lee et al. 1988; Dähnert 1992; Rathaus et al. 1991). A recent review by Dahnert (1988) dealt with the shortcomings of biopsy proof and analyzed the ultrasound appearance of CAP according to pathologic studies of entire resected prostates. Only seven such studies with pathologic–sonographic correlation are currently present within the literature (Hamper et al. 1990a). As the author points out, however, any retrospective analysis of sonographic images of prostates known to contain CAP suffers from interpreter bias. To date, no prospective study of a large series of autopsy specimens has been performed to obtain information on the true sensitivity and specificity of ultrasound in detecting CAP (Coffield et al. 1992).

If the results of the above-mentioned seven studies are combined, 61% of CAPs appear hypoechoic (Chang and Friedland 1990). Conversely, 39% are sonographically isoechoic or contain foci of hyperechogenicity (Hamper et al. 1990b). The most plausible explanation for the hypoechogenicity of most CAPs is that spongelike, glandular cystic spaces in normal prostatic tissue cause more sound reflections than tissue of uniformly solid character, such as carcinoma. Many authors report that they have detected no echogenic CAPs (Sanders et al. 1987; Lee et al. 1986; Dahnert et al. 1986a; Rifkin et al. 1989). Nevertheless, when a neoplasm invades the internal zone it may involve areas where calcification exists and therefore theoretically may have regions of hyperechogenicity (Sanders et al. 1987; Lee et al. 1985; Egawa et al. 1992). Based on work by Dähnert et al. (1986a), who correlated sonograms with xeroradiographs of resected prostates, these echogenic areas are felt to represent calcium even in the absence of shadowing. The work of Dähnert et al. supports the notion that tumors may contain calcium secondarily rather than as a result of dystrophic change. No correlation between the ultrasound appearance of cancer and its histologic grading has ever been established (Griffiths et al. 1987).

Location of a lesion within the prostate is an additional aspect which has been addressed. The site of origin of CAP has been analyzed in multiple studies. Recently, McNeal et al. (1988) reported that small stage A lesions were located more anteromedially in the peripheral zone than were small stage B lesions. However, overall, 70%–100% of cancers originate peripherally (McNeal 1969; Lee et al. 1985; McClennan 1988). This is fortunate for the sonographer since a hypoechoic tumor may be more easily identified within the homogeneous peripheral zone. On the other hand, it is extremely difficult to detect CAP within the

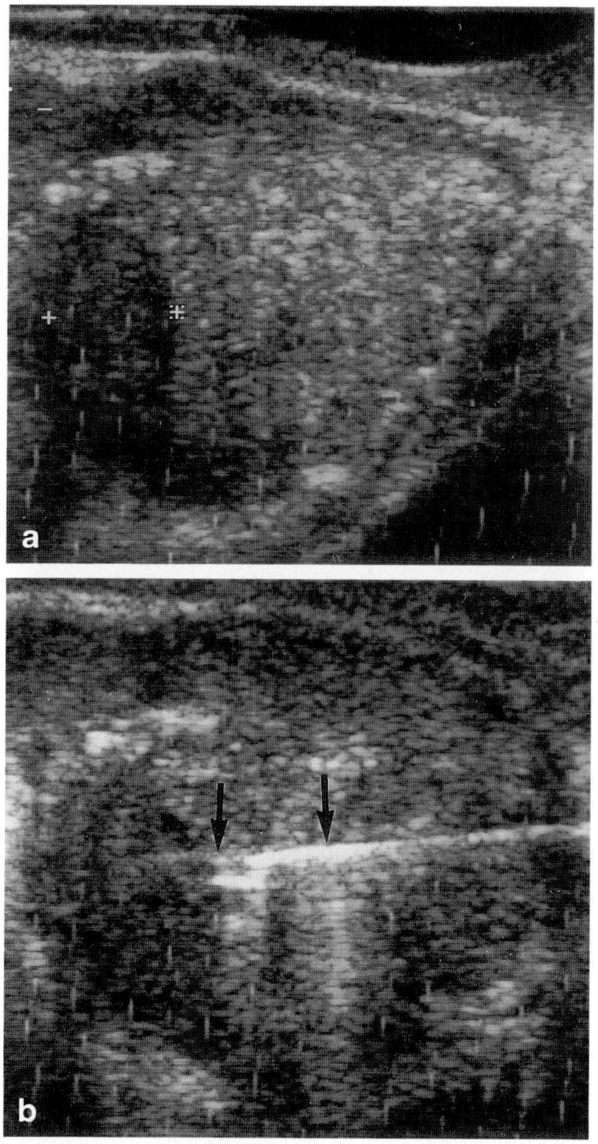

Fig. 11.5 a,b. Hypoechoic nodule. **a** Hypoechoic nodule in the base of the prostate involving the peripheral and central zones (*within cursors*). **b** Biopsy needle (*black arrows*) placed so that its tip is in contact with the edge of the nodule. Histology was adenocarcinoma. (*Vertical white lines* on both images are artifacts.)

central zone secondary to frequent concomitant BPH. Many authors have abandoned making a diagnosis of cancer in the central zone (SANDERS et al. 1987). These data suggest that the characteristic appearance of CAP is a peripherally located hypoechoic lesion (Fig. 11.5). However, in a recent series (RIFKIN and CHOI 1988), only 21% of peripheral hypoechoic lesions were malignant. BURKS et al. (1986) reported that of 55 peripheral hypoechoic lesions, approximately

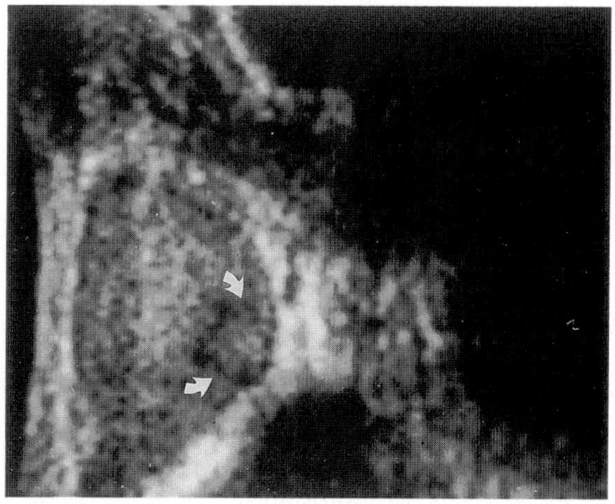

Fig. 11.6. Isoechoic nodule with surrounding halo (*white arrows*)

45% were malignant. However, LEE et al. (1986) reported that approximately 60% of peripheral hypoechoic lesions were cancerous.

Finally, mass effect may be helpful in establishing a lesion as real. CAP, when subcapsular, may cause a localized bulge in the contour of the capsule. If invasive, a peripheral carcinoma may also obliterate the echogenic line of the capsule. Further, a halo may be seen at the borders of a lesion and uninvolved gland, perhaps due to compressed parenchyma (Fig. 11.6). This finding has been helpful in identifying isoechoic lesions (DAHNERT 1988). However, these haloes may also be found surrounding benign nodules (BURKS et al. 1986).

To determine the true sensitivity and specificity of ultrasound in the detection of CAP, the true prevalence of the disease must be known. Even theoretically, this value is disputed. MONTIE et al. (1988) demonstrated a surprising 46% incidence of unsuspected CAP in prostatectomy specimens removed for bladder cancer. Other authors assume a lower prevalence in their calculations of between 2.8% and 15% in men aged over age 60 (LEE et al. 1988).

In studies performed in vivo, calculated sensitivities and specificities are affected by not knowing the true incidence of CAP in the study group because of less than perfectly accurate biopy results. This error is compounded by the fact that not all patients in every study undergo biopsies. For example, patients with abnormal sonograms but impalpable abnormalities were not biopsied in one series (CHODAK et al. 1986), and in another, healthy patients with no palpable or ultrasonographic abnormalites were not biopsied (LEE et al. 1988). Despite an imperfect gold standard for the diagnosis of the disease, the reported sensitivity and specificity of ultrasound in the detection of CAP range between 80% and 90% and 40% and 60% respectively (CHODAK et al. 1986; FRITZSCHE et al. 1983). Positive predictive values are uniformly low, generally falling in the 30% range (CHODAK et al. 1986; LEE et al. 1988; TERRIS et al. 1992). SALO et al. (1987b) and RIFKIN and CHOI (1988) assert that these numbers preclude the use of ultrasound as a screening method. Overall, there appears to be no characteristic sonographic features which allow reproducibly accurate differentiation between benign and malignant lesions (RIFKIN et al. 1986, 1990).

Although adequate information on true false-negative rates for transrectal ultrasound of CAP is not available, ultrasound can provide important staging information to complement findings on digital examination (MCCLENNAN 1988). Ultrasound may be useful for patients with known, clinically localized CAP being considered for radical prostatectomy. Reports dealing with staging are somewhat contradictory. In one series using transabdominal ultrasound, capsule invasion could not be reliably predicted (GREENBERG et al. 1982); in another, using transrectal ultrasound, extracapsular extension could be accurately assessed, with a sensitivity of 86% and a specificity of 94% (SALO et al. 1987a; LORENTZEN et al. 1992). One series reported an equally high sensitivity of 89%, but claimed a specificity of only 50% (PONTES et al. 1985). Invasion into seminal vesicles, manifested by loss of the normal fat plane between prostate and seminal vesicle, has been demonstrated with ultrasound (SPIRNAK and RESNICK 1984). PONTES et al. (1985) reported a sensitivity of 100%; however, a more recent study indicates that transrectal ultrasound is less reliable in revealing seminal vesicle invasion (SANDERS et al. 1987). One series reported a sensitivity of 29% and a specificity of 100% (SALO et al. 1987a). This accuracy may improve with further refinements of diagnostic criteria (MCCLENNAN 1988).

The multitude of controversial issues regarding transrectal ultrasound of the prostate notwithstanding, many authors agree on certain indications for this procedure. Ultrasound-guided biopsies may allow a more adequate tissue sampling (MCCLENNAN 1988) or may be used to guide or document actual needle placement into a palpable or impalpable lesion (RIFKIN et al. 1983b; ABE et al. 1987; HOLM and GAMMELGAARD 1981; LIDDELL et al. 1986), thus increasing the yield of biopsy (TORP-PEDERSON et al. 1989; DYKE et al. 1990) (Fig. 13.5b). Recently, however, RESNICK (1988) stressed that transrectal ultrasound guidance may not be routinely necessary in the biopsy of a palpable nodule. Transrectal ultrasound may also demonstrate impalpable CAP in patients with positive laboratory tests, such as elevated acid phosphatase or prostate specific antigen, or bone scintigraphy (COONER et al. 1988; TORP-PEDERSON et al. 1990).

In terms of therapeutic alternatives, transrectal ultrasound provides a method for effective radioactive seed placement (LOENING and ROSENBERG 1987) or may be useful in determination of port size for radiotherapy (LEE et al. 1980). It may be useful as well in following patients with known CAP to assess response to treatment, either hormonal or radiation. Tumor response may be reflected as changes in tumor volume or overall gland size, or as changes in tumor echogenicity, or both (RESNICK et al. 1980). Although tumor volume may be underestimated by ultrasound (LEE et al. 1988), volumetric assessments of the entire prostate may indicate local recurrence or systemic progression (CARPENTIER et al. 1982; FUJINO and SCARDINO 1986). In the former series, both hormonal and radiation therapy resulted in loss of prostatic volume, although an early increase in prostatic size in some radiated patients was thought to reflect prostatic edema. Volume increases were not observed in many patients who did have systemic progression. In the latter study, positive response to radiotherapy included a reconstitution of the integrity of the capsule and a normalization of the size and shape of the prostate and seminal vesicles.

Ultrasound may also be of use in the follow-up of patients who have undergone radical prostatectomy, since tumor recurrence may be inaccessible to palpation by rectal examination (SPIRNAK and RESNICK 1984; ABI-AAD 1992; WASSERMANN et al. 1992). Finally, both transrectal and transabdominal ultrasound have proven useful for identification of enlarged regional nodes, particularly the internal iliac chain, and transabdominal ultrasound may also detect more distant metastases (LANG 1983).

11.4.2 Benign Prostatic Hypertrophy

The role of ultrasound in the evaluation of this common disorder is somewhat limited in comparison to its role in CAP. Sonography is effective in determining accurate prostatic dimensions for volumetric assessment, which correlates closely with prostatic weight and thus the degree of hypertrophy (WATANABE et al. 1974; KADOW et al. 1985). Some urologists use the sonographically derived volumetric measurements in determining whether prostate resection should be performed via a transabdominal or a transurethral approach (SANDERS et al. 1987). OKAFOR et al. (1983) used transrectal ultrasound to assess volume changes in

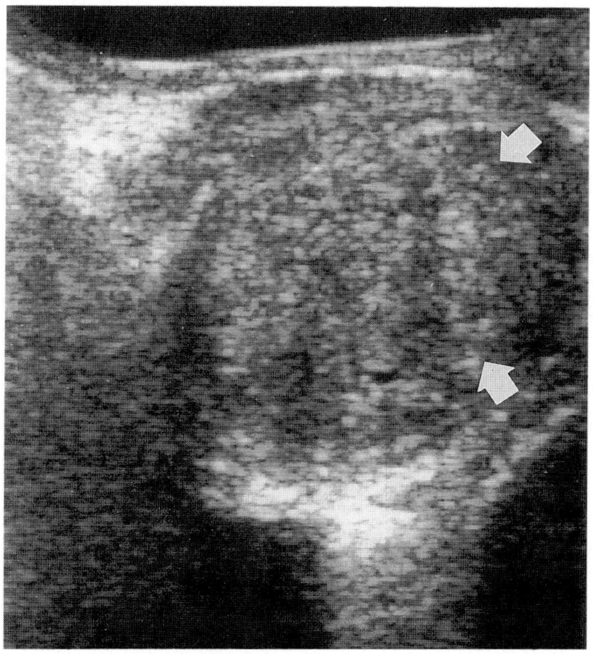

Fig. 11.7 Enlarged prostate with coarsened echotexture and a dominant nodule (*white arrows*) typical of BPH

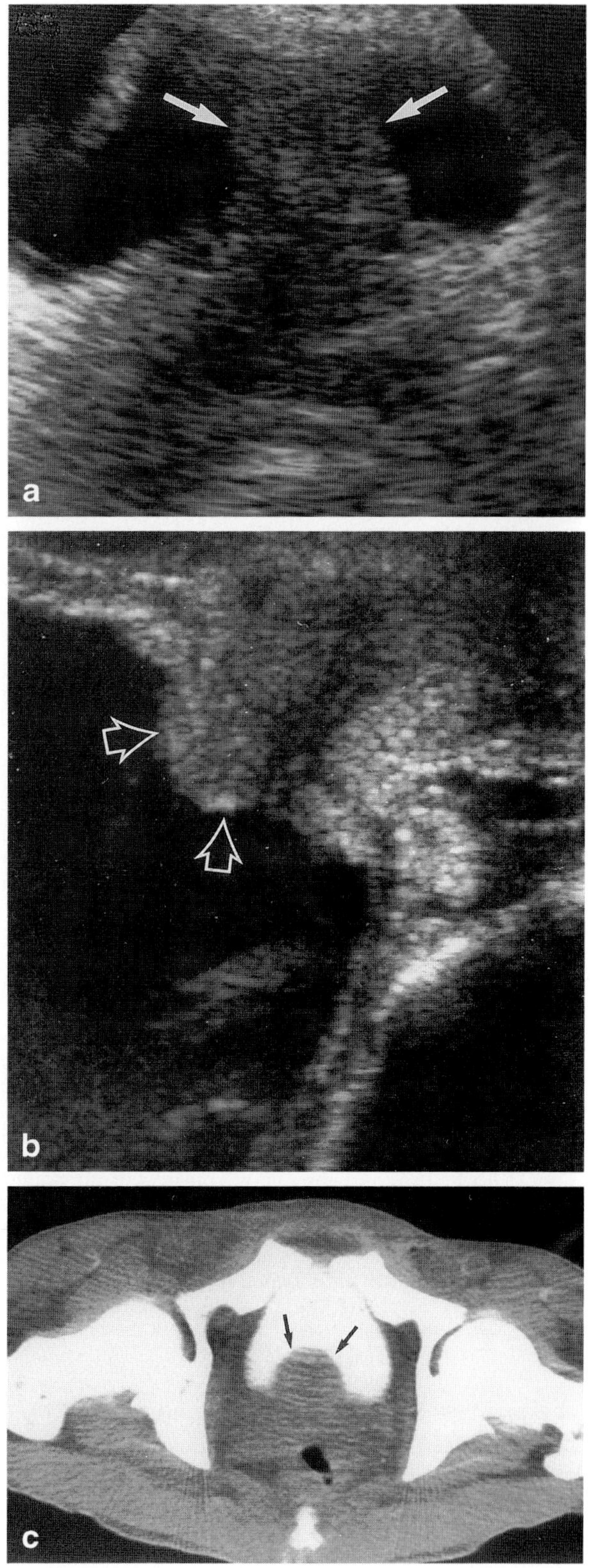

▷

Fig. 11.8a–c. Lobe of Albarran. **a** Transabdominal ultrasound demonstrates a large soft tissue mass protruding into the bladder from the prostate (*white arrows*). **b** Transrectal ultrasound demonstrates the protruding mass (*white arrows*). **c** CT image shows posterior protrusion of the mass into the contrast – filled bladder (*black arrows*)

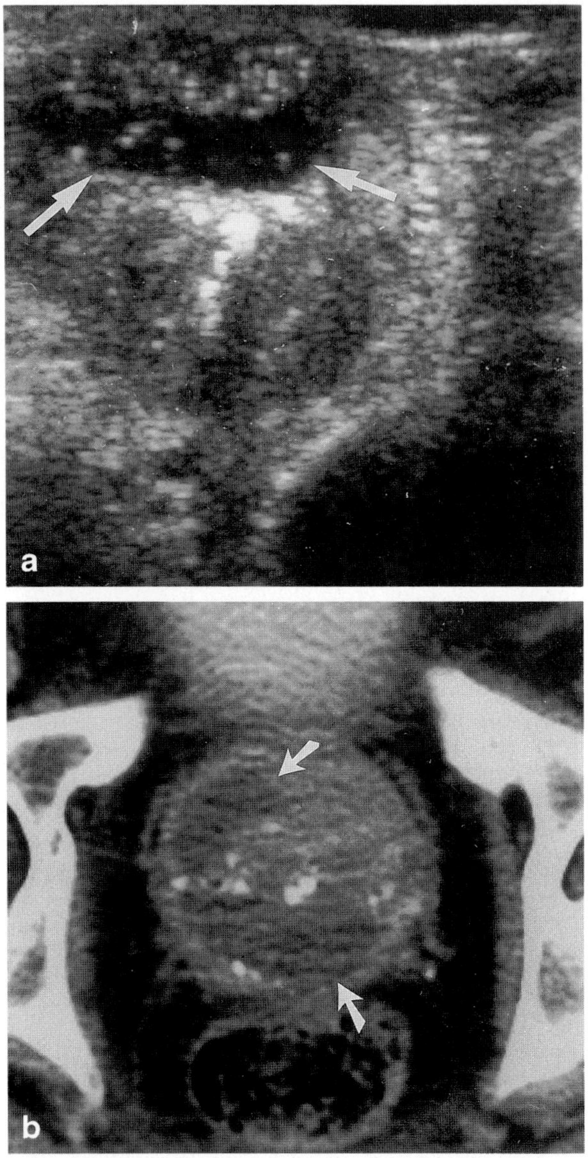

Fig. 11.9 a,b. Prostatic abscess. **a** Transrectal ultrasound demonstrating cystic mass involving the right seminal vesicle and prostate (*white arrows*). Calcifications with posterior shadowing are incidentally present. **b** CT showing low density prostatic mass (*white arrows*). At surgery, a large abscess involving the prostate and right seminal vesicle was unroofed

the prostate after TURP and demonstrated high correlation.

An increase in the anteroposterior dimension is reported to be the earliest finding in BPH, followed by rounding of the contour of the gland (PEELING and GRIFFITHS 1984; CLEMENTS et al. 1992). In addition, an increase in coarseness of the echotexture (Fig. 11.7) as well as focal enlargement of one segment of the prostate may be seen (SANDERS et al. 1987) (Fig. 11.8). In one particular series, a majority of prostates with BPH demonstrated discrete central nodules of varying echogenicity, though rarely purely hypoechoic (BURKS et al. 1986; LEE et al. 1992).

Calcifications are found in glands with BPH as frequently as in glands with CAP (HASSLER 1968). In one study (DAHNERT et al. 1986b), calcifications were never identified in the external gland where 98% of the identified carcinomas were located, but only in the central gland. They are not commonly present in adenomatous tissue (HASSLER 1968). Thus, calcifications are considered incidental findings. The sonographic appearance of calicifications has been elucidated by DAHNERT et al. (1986) and has been discussed in a prior section. Sonourethrography has been described as a useful technique to detect the presence of adenomatous nodules impinging upon the prostatic urethra. This method, not widely used, relies upon patient voiding with the transrectal probe in place (RIFKIN 1984).

11.4.3 Inflammatory Disease

Although the sonographic appearance of CAP has received the bulk of attention, several studies have attempted to define the sonographic features of prostatic inflammation (DE LA ROSETTE et al. 1992). Hypoechoic areas may be noted as well as poor definition of the prostatic capsule, both nonspecific findings (GRIFFITHS et al. 1984). However, if frankly cystic areas with thick walls or septations are identified in the prostate in the clinical setting of frequency, urgency, and pyuria, a diagnosis of abscess may be suggested (PAPANICOLAOU et al. 1987) (Fig. 11.9). Prostatic abscesses may be easily differentiated on ultrasound from a müllerian duct cyst or seminal vesicle cyst or abscess, based on the location of these latter conditions outside the prostate (NGHIEM et al. 1990). In one case report, sonography was found useful in demonstrating resolution of a prostatic abscess during antibiotic therapy (THORNHILL et al. 1987). Some authors have advocated transrectal ultrasound for the investigation of the cause of hemospermia (ETHERINGTON et al. 1990).

References

Abe M, Hashimoto T, Matsuda T, Saitoh M, Watanabe H (1987) Prostatic biopsy guided by transrectal ultrasonography using real-time linear scanner. Urology 24:567–569

Abid-Aad AS, Macfarlane MT, Stein A, DeKernion JB (1992) Detection of local recurrence after radical prostatectomy by prostate specific antigen and transrectal ultrasound. J Urol 147:952–955

Abu-Yousef MM, Narayana AS (1985) Prostatic carcinoma: detection and staging using suprapubic US. Radiology 156:175–180

Burks DD, Drolshagen LF, Fleischer AC, Liddell HT, McDougal WS, Karl EM, James AE (1986) Transrectal sonography of benign and malignant prostatic lesions. AJR 146:1187–1191

Carpentier PJ, Schroeder FH, Blom JHM (1982) Transrectal ultrasonography in the followup of prostatic carcinoma patients. J Urol 128:742–746

Chang P, Friedland GW (1990) Hypoechoic lesions of the prostate: clinical relevance of tumor size, digital rectal examination prostate specific antigen. Radiology, 175:581–582

Chantelois AE, Parker SH, Sims JE, Horne DW (1990) Malacoplakia of the prostate sonographically mimicking carcinoma. Radiology 177:193–195

Chodak GW, Wald V, Parmer E, Watanabe H, Ohe H, Saitoh M (1986) Comparison of digital examination and transrectal ultrasonography for the diagnosis of prostatic cancer. J Urol 135:951–954

Coffield KS, Speighs VO, Brawn PN, Riggs MW (1992) Ultrasound detection of prostate cancer in postmortem specimens with histological correlation. J Urol 147: 822–826

Cooner WH, Mosley BR, Rutherford CL (1988) Clinical applications of transrectal ultrasound and prostatic specific antigen in the search for prostate carcinoma. J Urol 139:758–761

Clements R, Penney MD, Etherington RJ, Griffiths GJ, Hughes H, Peeling WB (1992) Volume of normal prostate, of prostate cancer, and of benign prostatic hyperplasia: are correlations with prostate specific antigen clinically useful? Prostate 4:51–57

Dähnert WF (1988) Ultrasonography of carcinoma of the prostate: a critical review. Appl Radiol XX:39–44

Dähnert WF (1992) Determination of prostate volume with transrectal US for cancer screening. Radiology 183:625–626

Dähnert WF, Hamper UM, Eggleston JC, Walsh PC, Sanders RC (1986a) Prostatic evaluation by transrectal sonography with histopathologic correlation: the echopenic appearance of early carcinoma. Radiology 158:97–102

Dähnert WF, Hamper UM, Walsh PC, Eggleston JC, Sanders RC (1986b) The echogenic focus in prostatic sonograms, with xeroradiographic and histopathologic correlation. Radiology 159:95–100

De la Rosette JJ, Karthaus HF, Debruyne FM (1992) Ultrasonographic findings in patients with nonbacterial prostatitis. Urol Int 48:323–326

Dyke CH, Toi A, Sweet JM (1990) Value of random US-guided transrectal prostate biopsy. Radiology 176:345–349

Etherington RJ, Clements R, Griffiths GJ et al. (1990) Transrectal ultrasound in the investigation of hemospermia. Clin Radiol 41:175–177

Egawa S, Wheeler TM, Greene DR, Scardino PT (1992) Unusual hyperechoic appearance of prostate cancer on transrectal ultrasonography. Br J Urol 69:169–174

Fornage BD (1986) Normal US anatomy of the prostate. Ultrasound Med Biol 12:1011–1021

Fox M (1963) The natural history and significance of stone formation in the prostate gland. J Urol 89: 716–727

Fritzsche PJ, Axford PD, Ching VC, Rosenquist RW, Moore RJ (1983) Correlation of transrectal sonographic findings in patients with suspected and unsuspected prostatic disease. J Urol 130:272–274

Fujino A, Scardino PT (1986) Transrectal ultrasonography for prostatic cancer – the response of the prostate to definitive radiotherapy. Cancer 57:935–940

Gammelgaard J, Holm HH (1980) Transurethral and transrectal ultrasonic scanning in urology. J Urol 124:863–868

Greenberg M, Neimen HL, Vogelzang R, Falkowski W (1982) Ultrasonographic features of prostatic carcinoma. J Clin Ultrasound 10:307–312

Griffiths GJ, Crooks AJR, Roberts EE, Evans KT, Buck AC, Thomas PJ, Peeling WB (1984) Ultrasonic appearances associated with prostatic inflammation: a preliminary study. Clin Radiol 35:343–345

Griffiths GJ, Clements R, Jones DR, Roberts EE, Peeling WB, Evans KT (1987) The ultrasound appearances of prostatic cancer with histologic correlation. Clin Radiol 38:219–227

Griffiths GH, Clements R, Peeling WB (1990) Current status of transrectal ultrasonography in the diagnosis and management of prostatic cancer. Clin Radiol 40: 337

Hamper UM, Epstein JI, Sheth S et al. (1990a) Cystic lesions of the prostate gland: a sonographic-pathologic correlation. J Ultrasound Med 9:395–402

Hamper UM, Sheth A, Walsh PC, Epstein JI (1990b) Bright echogenic foci in early prostatic carcinoma: sonographic and pathologic correlation. Radiology 176:339–343

Hassler O (1968) Calcifications in the prostate gland and adjacent tissues: a combined biophysical and histological study. Pathol Microbiol 31:97–107

Holm HH, Gammelgaard J (1981) Ultrasonically guided precise needle placement in the prostate and seminal vesicles. J Urol 125:385–387

Jewett HJ (1956) Significance of the palpable prostatic nodule. JAMA 160:838–839

Kadow C, Gingell JC, Penry JB (1985) Prostatic ultrasonography: a useful technique? Br J Urol 57:440–443

Lang EK (1983) Neoplasms of the bladder, prostate and urethra. Semin Roentgeno 28:288–298

Lee DJ, Leibel S, Shiels R, Sanders R, Siegelman S, Order S (1980) The value of ultrasonic imaging and CT scanning planning the radiotherapy for prostatic carcinoma. Cancer 45:724–727

Lee F, Gray JM, McLeary RD et al. (1985) Transrectal ultrasound in the diagnosis of prostate cancer: location, echogenicity, histopathology, and staging. Prostate 7:117–129

Lee F, Gray JM, McLeary RD et al. (1986) Prostatic evaluation by transrectal sonography: criteria for diagnosis of early carcinoma. Radiology 158:91–95

Lee F, Littrup PJ, McLeary RD et al. (1987) Needle aspiration and core biopsy of prostate cancer: comparative evaluation with biplanar transrectal US guidance. Radiology 163:515–520

Lee F, Littrup PJ, Torp-Pederson ST et al. (1988) Prostate cancer: comparison of transrectal US and digital rectal examination for screening. Radiology 168:389–394

Lee F, Littrup PJ, Loft-Christensen L, Kelly BS Jr, McHugh TA, Siders DB, Mitchell AE, Newby JE (1992) Predicted prostate specific antigen results using transrectal ultrasound gland volume. Differentiation of benigne prostatic hyperplasia and prostatic cancer. Cancer 70:211–220

Liddell HT, McDougal WS, Burks DD, Fleischer AC (1986) Ultrasound versus digitally directed prostatic needle biopsy. J Urol 135:716–718

Loening SA, Rosenberg SJ (1987) Percutaneous placement of radioactive gold seeds in localized prostatic carcinoma. Urology 29:250–252

Lorentzen P, Nerstrom H, Iversen P, Torp-Pedersen ST (1992) Local staging of prostate cancer with transrectal ultrasound: a literature review. Prostate 4:11–16

McClennan BL (1988) Transrectal US of the prostate: Is the technology leading the science? Radiology 168:571–575

McNeal JE (1969) Origin and development of carcinoma of the prostate. Cancer 23:24–34

McNeal JE, Price HM, Redwine EA, Freiha FS, Stamey TA (1988) Stage A versus stage B adenocarcinoma of the prostate: morphological comparison and biological significance. J Urol 139:61–65

Montie JE, Wood DP, Pontes JE, Boyett JM, Levin HS (1988) Adenocarcinoma of the prostate in cystoprostatectomy specimens removed for bladder cancer. Presented at the 83rd Annual Meeting of the American Urologic Association, Boston, June 3–7, 1988

Nghiem HT, Kellman GM, Sandberg SA, Craig BM (1990) Cystic lesions of the prostate. Radiographics 10: 635–650

Okafor PIS, Wild SR, Beynon LL, Chisholm GD (1983) Progress in transrectal ultrasonography for prostatic disease. Br J Urol 55:721–725

Papanicolaou N, Pfister RC, Stafford SA, Parkhurst EC (1987) Prostatic abscess: imaging with transrectal sonography and MR. AJR 149:981–982

Peeling WB, Griffiths GJ (1984) Imaging of the prostate by ultrasound. J Urol 132:217–224

Pontes JE, Eisenkraft S, Watanabe H, Ohe H, Saitoh, Murphy GP (1985) Preoperative evaluation of localized prostatic carcinoma by transrectal ultrasonography. J Urol 134:289–291

Rathaus V, Richter S, Nissenkorn I, Goldberg E (1991) Transperineal ultrasound examination in evaluation of prostatic size. Clin Radiol 44:383–385

Resnick MI (1988) Transrectal ultrasound guided versus digitally directed prostatic biopsy: a comparative study. J Urol 139:754–757

Resnick MI, Willard JW, Boyce WH (1980) Transrectal ultrasonography in the evaluation of patients with prostatic carcinoma. J Urol 124:482–484

Rifkin MD (1984) Sonourethrography: technique for evaluation of prostatic urethra. Radiology 153:791–792

Rifkin MD (1987) Endorectal sonography of the prostate: clinical implications. AJR 148:1137–1142

Rifkin MD, Choi H (1988) Implications of small, peripheral hypoechoic lesions in endorectal US of the prostate. Radiology 166:619–622

Rifkind MD, Kurtz AB, Choi HY, Goldberg BB (1983a) Endoscopic ultrasonic evaluation of the prostate using a transrectal probe: prospective evaluation and acoustic characterization. Radiology 149:265–271

Rifkin MD, Kurtz AB, Goldberg BB (1983b) Sonographically guided transperineal prostatic biopsy: preliminary experience with a longitudinal linear-array transducer. AJR 140:745–747

Rifkin MD, Friedland GW, Shortliffe L (1986) Prostatic evaluation by transrectal endosonography: detection of carcinoma. Radiology 158:85–90

Rifkin MD, McGlynn ET, Choi H (1989) Echogenicity of prostate cancer correlated with histologic grade and stromal fibrosis: endorectal US studies. Radiology 170:549

Rifkin MD, Dahnnert W, Kurtz AB (1990) State-of-the-art: endorectal sonography of the prostate gland. AJR 154:691–700

Salo JO, Kivisaari L, Rannikko S (1987a) Computerized tomography and transrectal ultrasound in the assessment of local extension of prostate cancer. J Urol 137:435–438

Salo JO, Rannikko S, Makinen J, Lehtonent T (1987b) Echogenic structure of prostatic cancer imaged on radical prostatectomy specimens. Prostate 10:1–9

Sanders RC, Hamper UM, Dahnert WF (1987) Update on prostatic ultrasound. Urol Radiol 9:110–118

Spirnak JP, Resnick MI (1984) Transrectal ultrasonography. Urology 23:461–467

Terris MK, McNeal JE, Stamey TA (1992) Transrectal ultrasound imaging and ultrasound guided prostate biopsies in the detection of residual carcinoma in clinical stage A carcinoma of the prostate. J Urol 147:864–869

Thornhill BA, Morehouse HT, Coleman P, Hoffman-Tretin JC (1987) Prostatic abscess: CT and sonographic findings. AJR 148:899–900

Torp-Pederson ST, Lee F (1990) Hypoechoic lesions of the prostate: clinical relevance of tumor size, digital rectal examination, and prostate specific antigen: reply. Radiology 175:583

Torp-Pederson ST, Lee F, Littrup PJ, Siders DB, Kumasaka GH, Solomon MH, McLeary RD (1989) Transrectal biopsy of the prostate guided with transrectal US: longitudinal and multiplanar scanning. Radiology 170:23–27

Wassermann NF, Kapoor DA, Hildebrandt WC, Zhang G, Bohn MN, Eppel SN, Reddy PK (1992) Transrectal ultrasound in evaluation of patients after prostatectomy; part 2 ultrasound and biopsy findings in the presence of residual and early recurrent prostatic cancer. Radiology 185:367–372

Watanabe H, Kato H, Kato T, Morita M (1968) Diagnostic application of ultrasonotomography to the prostate. Jpn J Urol 59:273–279

Watanabe H, Igari D, Tanahashi Y, Harada K, Saitoh M (1974) Measurements of size and weight of prostates by means of transrectal ultrasonography. Tohoku J Exp Med 114:277–285

Wild JJ, Reid JM (1957) Progress in techniques of soft tissue examination by 15 MC ultrasound. In: Kelly E (ed) Ultrasound in biology and medicine. American Institute of Biological Sciences, Washington, p 30

12 Computed Tomography of the Prostate

HOWARD M. LEVY

CONTENTS

12.1 Introduction

The prostate and surrounding structures can be clearly depicted by computed tomography (CT). The prostate is optimally evaluated by contiguous thin sections with the patient in the supine position. The upper extent of the gland lies at the inferior margin of the seminal vesicles while the most inferior border lies just above the bulb of the penis. The anterior, posterior, and lateral borders are delineated by the periprostatic fat. Neither the specific lobes nor zones of the prostate can be distinguished by CT.

12.2 The Normal Prostate

The normal prostate generally has a smooth contour and is of homogeneous density. On unenhanced scans it has an attenuation value of approximately 50 Hounsfield units. The morphology of the normal prostate changes with age. In a retrospective study of 55 males who had CT scans for reasons other than suspected prostate disease, the prostate was measured and found to increase in size with age (VAN ENGELSHOVEN and KREEL 1979). The average measurements in the 6–30 year age group were in craniocaudad, anterior-posterior, and transverse dimensions

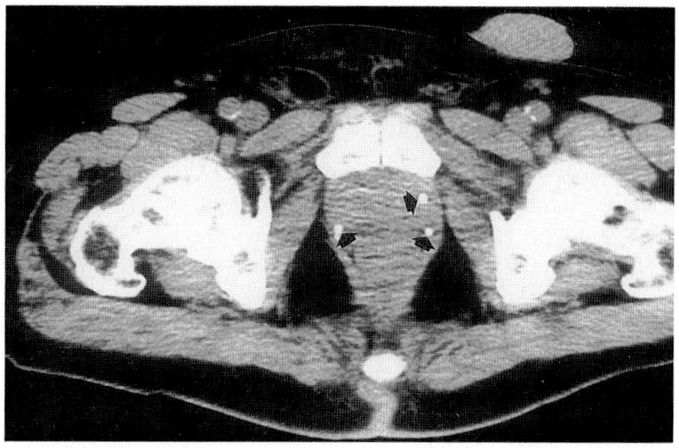

Fig. 12.1. Multiple punctate calcifications (*arrows*) are present at the periphery of the prostate

3.0 cm, 2.3 cm, and 3.1 cm. respectively, while in the 70-year-old age group the corresponding measurements were 5.0 cm, 4.4 cm, and 5.3 cm. The majority of patients greater than 50 years of age had calcifications within the prostate (Fig. 12.1), while in the under 30 age group, none were found to have calcifications.

12.3 Carcinoma of the Prostate

Computed tomography has essentially no role in screening for carcinoma of the prostate (CAP). CAP generally has attenuation values similar to normal prostatic tissue and thus cannot be detected. Focal contour abnormalities, however, can signify carcinoma. In one study the authors found that CAP could produce a nodular contour of the gland (PRICE and DAVIDSON 1979). This was not observed in patients with benign disease. Alternatively though, the prostate can be normal in contour and still be involved by cancer.

The principal role of CT in patients with CAP is to define the extent of disease. Specifically this involves distinguishing disease localized to the prostate from disease which has spread outside

HOWARD M. LEVY, M.D., Christina Hospital, Medical Center of Delaware, 4755 Ogletown-Stanton Road, Newark, DE 19718, USA

Table 12.1. CT criteria for staging CAP

Stage	CT findings
A or B	No evidence of tumor extension outside prostate capsule
C	Local extension (periprostatic fat, bladder, seminal vesicles, levator ani)
D1	Pelvic adenopathy
D2	Distant metastases

the gland. By accurately assessing the extent of disease, CT can aid the clinician in planning appropriate treatment.

The CT criteria for staging CAP are given in Table 12.1. There are some general problems which have been encountered in the staging process. Stage A and B disease cannot be distinguished from one another and generally show no evidence of abnormality on CT. In stage C and D1 disease, microscopic tumor involvement cannot be detected, while on the contrary, benign etiologies can result in findings indistinguishable from malignancy. As scanning done for the purpose of staging is generally confined to the abdomen and pelvis, D2 disease outside this area will not be detected.

Problems also arise in drawing conclusions from the different published studies. There has been a wide discrepancy in reported results with regard to certain staging parameters. The investigators have utilized different models and generations of CT scanners as well as various scanning techniques. The stage of disease at the time of CT scanning varied widely among the studies and in some investigations the study populations were very small (as few as 15 patients). All of these factors have led to wide statistical variations.

While the primary role of CT is to identify local invasion and lymph node metastases, it has been only moderately successful in staging CAP. The overall accuracy, sensitivity, and specificity have been reported to be 67%–77%, 33%–50%, and 75%–100% respectively (Emory et al. 1983; Platt et al. 1987; Price and Davidson 1979; Morgan et al. 1981).

The presence of local invasion classifies CAP as stage C. The common sites of involvement include the seminal vesicles, bladder, levator ani muscle, and periprostatic fat. The accuracy, sensitivity, and specificity for determining local invasion range from 47% to 73%, from 18% to 64%, and from 60% to 100% respectively (Emory et al. 1983; Golimbu et al. 1981; Hricak et al. 1987; Platt et al. 1987).

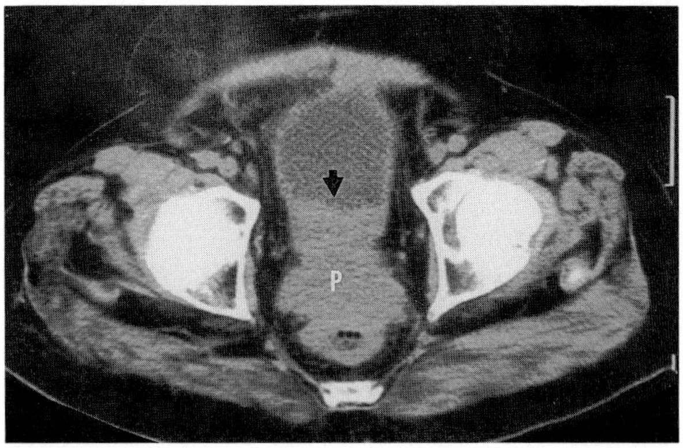

Fig. 12.2. CAP invading the bladder with resulting marked thickening of the posterior bladder wall (*arrow*). *P*, prostate

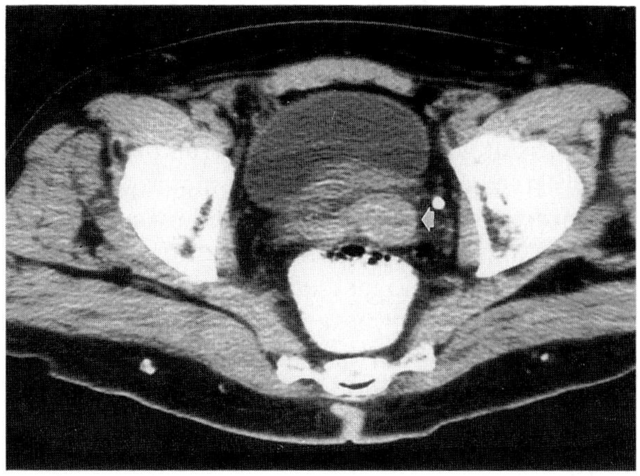

Fig. 12.3. Seminal vesicle involvement. An asymmetrically enlarged seminal vesicle on the left (*arrow*) in a patient with stage C CAP

The criteria for ascertaining bladder involvement are asymmetric thickening of the bladder wall or a mass extending into the bladder (Fig. 12.2). Involvement of the bladder is via direct extension. Due to its proximity to the prostate, the base of the bladder is the most common region involved. As this interface between the prostate and bladder is transverse in nature, it is very difficult to evaluate in the transaxial plane. Thus, accurately assessing tumor involvement in this area can present a very real dilemma.

Seminal vesicle involvement can also be difficult to determine. The criteria for involvement are either asymmetry of the seminal vesicles

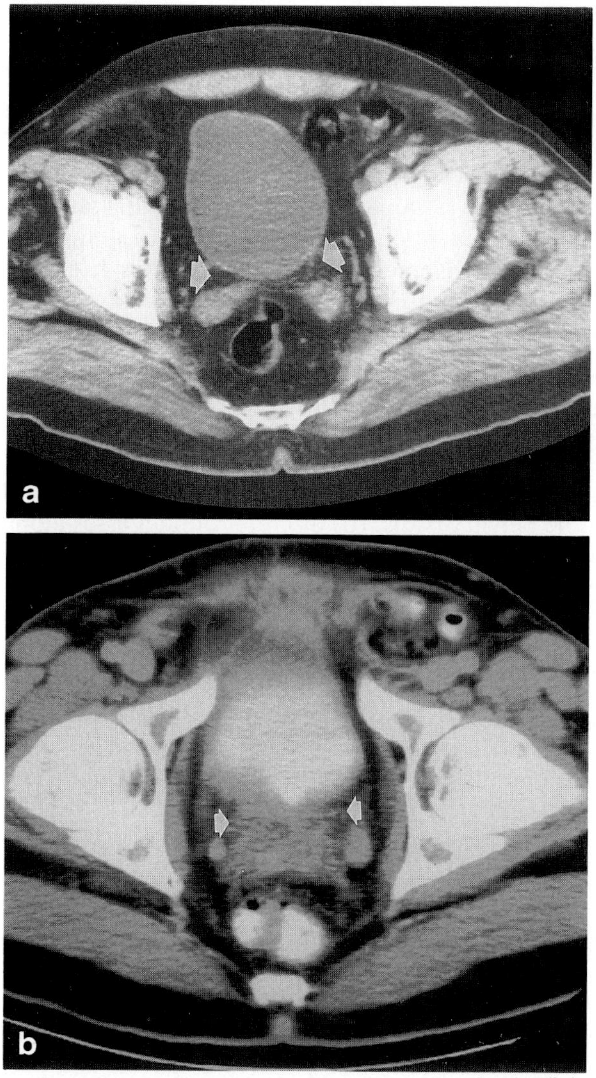

Fig. 12.4a,b. Seminal vesicle angle. **a** The acute angles between the seminal vesicles and posterior bladder wall (*arrows*) are preserved in a patient with CAP. **b** There is loss of both the right and left seminal vesicle angles (*arrows*) in a patient with stage C CAP

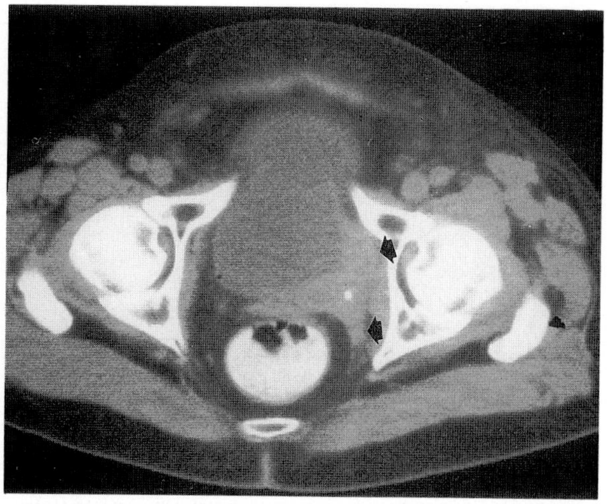

Fig. 12.5. Periprostatic invasion. Extraprostatic tumor extending towards the left pelvic side wall (*arrows*)

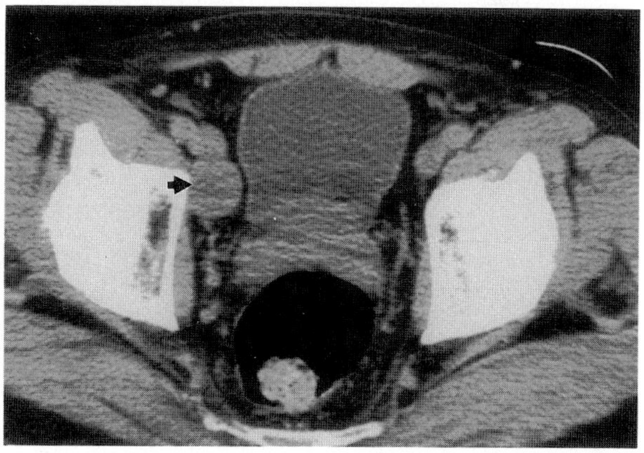

Fig. 12.6. Stage D1 disease. An enlarged obturator node is present on the right (*arrow*)

(Fig. 12.3) or loss of the seminal vesicle angle (Seidelman et al. 1977). The seminal vesicle angle refers to the region between the seminal vesicle and posterior wall of the bladder. This angle is typically acute and is occupied by fat (Fig. 12.4a). Obliteration of this angle (Fig. 12.4b) is a nonspecific sign and can result from a number of causes other than malignancy such as benign disease and prior surgery (Price and Davidson 1979). The degree of bladder distention can also affect the appearance of the interface between bladder and seminal vesicle (Golimbo et al. 1981).

The periprostatic fat is another common area of local invasion (Fig. 12.5). CT appears to be slightly more sensitive for determining involvement in this area as opposed to invasion of the seminal vesicles (Platt et al. 1987). However, benign disease as well as prior biopsies can produce changes in the periprostatic fat that are indistinguishable from malignancy. Further, microscopic extracapsular disease can lead to a false-negative diagnosis.

The levator ani muscle is yet another area that can be involved via direct extension of CAP. However, in addition to malignancy, enlargement

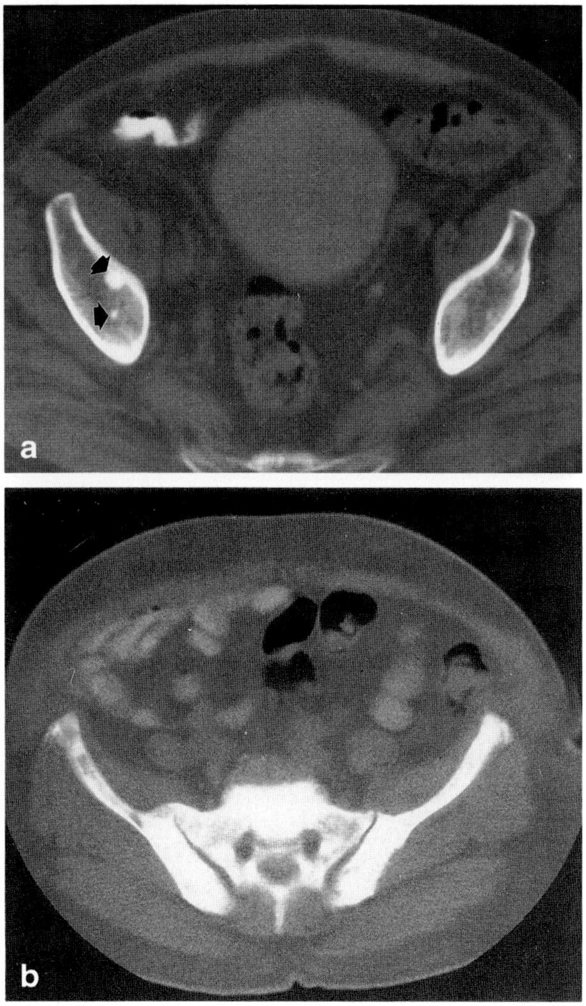

Fig. 12.7a,b. Metastatic CAP (stage D2). **a** Two well-defined osteoblastic metastases (*arrows*) in the right ilium. **b** Diffuse sclerosis of the iliac wings and sacrum

can result from prior interventional procedures or inflammatory processes.

The nodes of the pelvis include the common, internal, and external iliac chains. The nodes are named for the corresponding vessel. The external iliac nodes are the ones most commonly involved with CAP. This nodal group comprises three chains: the external, middle, and internal chains. The node most commonly involved with CAP is the obturator node, which is in the internal chain (Flocks et al. 1959) (Fig. 12.6). The obturator nodes lie just below the external iliac vein near the pelvic side wall.

The reported accuracy, sensitivity, and specificity for determining pelvic lymph node metastases from CAP (stage D1) range from 67% to 93%, from 0% to 100%, and from 78% to 100% respectively (Emory et al. 1983; Giri et al. 1982; Platt et al. 1987; Morgan et al. 1981; Levine et al. 1981; Weinerman et al. 1983; Salo et al. 1986). There are numerous reasons for these wide discrepancies in values. Most importantly, CT cannot specifically identify architectural abnormalities within nodes. Thus individual authors have relied upon different criteria to determine nodal involvement. Generally size has been the major criteria. While most authors report nodes of 1.2–1.5 cm or larger as abnormal, some consider nodes over 1 cm abnormal while others report nodes up to 2 cm as normal. Other authors have relied solely upon anatomic features to determine nodal metastases (Giri et al. 1982). These features include (a) asymmetry around the pelvic vessels, (b) discrete round masses along the pelvic side wall, and (c) separation of these masses from the primary tumor.

Most investigators, but not all, have relied upon histopathologic correlation to confirm lymphadenopathy. Finally, in reporting abnormal nodes, some have calculated their statistics based upon pelvic node involvement solely. However, others have included retroperitoneal node involvement in their analyses.

The presence of adenopathy plays a major role in determining treatment. In most centers, the presence of D1 disease will exclude the patient from a radical prostatectomy. In addition to malignancy, enlargement of nodes can be secondary to fibrosis, hyperplasia, fatty replacement, or inflammation (Hricak 1987; Harell 1983). In order to avoid a false-positive diagnosis and preclude potentially curative surgery, a staging lymphadenectomy or percutaneous fine needle biopsy may be necessary to confirm the diagnosis (Klein 1979).

After lymph nodes, bone is the most common site of metastatic disease in CAP. These metastases are typically osteoblastic and appear as sclerotic regions which are either focal or diffuse (Fig. 12.7). They can be associated with a soft tissue mass. Metastasis confined to the bones of the abdomen and pelvis can usually be detected by CT, particularly if bone windows are utilized. However, in the staging process, radionuclide bone scan is considered the modality of choice for evaluation of the bones.

Computed tomography can be helpful in monitoring the response of CAP to all types of treatment. Currently parameters such as weight loss, bone pain, acid phosphatase levels, and hemoglobin are monitored in order to determine response. However, these indicators have on occasion been shown to improve in patients with documented progression of disease (SCHMIDT et al. 1976). By assessing change in tumor bulk, CT offers a more direct method of determining response to therapy. This can be particularly helpful in the evaluation of experimental protocols.

Computed tomography can also aid the radiation therapist with treatment planning. As the prostate is located between two relatively radiosensitive structures, the bladder and rectum, it is important that the radiation port be accurate to avoid unnecessary complications. Further, since clinical staging underestimates the extent of the tumor in as many as 20%–50% of patients (WHITMORE and MACKENZIE 1959; KLEIN 1979; BYAR and MOSTOFI 1972; FRANKS 1975; JEWETT 1975), CT can provide additional information regarding the local extent of disease which can alter the size of the radiation treatment field. In one study (MUNZENRIDER et al. 1977), CT findings resulted in a change of field size in 47% of patients.

Computed tomography has been reported to be useful in patients being treated with ^{125}I seeds. Not only can it be helpful in determining tumor response, but it can aid in determining the distribution of the seeds. GORE and MOSS (1983) found that CT demonstrated errors in seed implantation in up to 85% of patients.

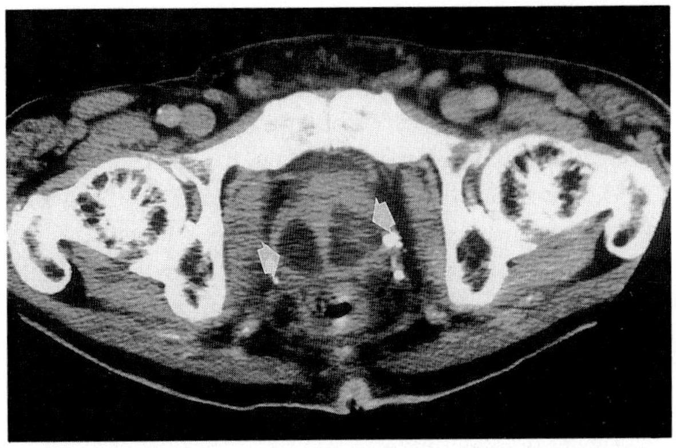

Fig. 12.8. Prostatic abscess. Two low attenuation fluid collections (*arrows*) involving separate lobes of the prostate

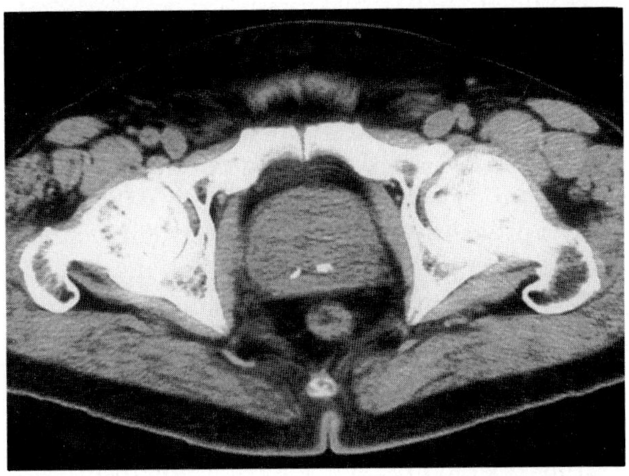

Fig. 12.9. BPH. A markedly enlarged prostate with calcifications

12.4 Other Diseases of the Prostate

While CT finds its greatest use in imaging the prostate by staging CAP or monitoring its response to therapy, other disease processes can also be studied with this modality. These include prostatic abscesses, benign prostatic hypertrophy (BPH), some uncommon tumors, and even congenital conditions such as müllerian duct cysts (HIGASHI et al. 1990).

12.4.1 Abscesses

Abscesses of the prostate are uncommon. The largest reported CT series included only five patients (THORNHILL et al. 1987). Predisposing factors include diabetes mellitus, intravenous drug abuse, and prior genitourinary instrumentation. These abscesses can be difficult to diagnose clinically as the presenting symptoms can be similar to those of acute prostatitis and/or acute cystitis. As many as one-third of patients with prostatic abscesses have been found to have concurrent CAP (JAMESON 1968).

As with any abscess, an abscess in the prostate can be life threatening. Thus it is important that it be promptly diagnosed and adequately treated. In contrast to CAP, intraprostatic abscesses can be identified with CT. Typically these appear as low attenuation lesions which can easily be distinguished from adjacent prostatic tissue (Fig. 12.8). They usually enlarge the gland and can be uni- or multiloculated. In later stages they can extend outside the prostatic capsule and invade adjacent pelvic soft tissues.

12.4.2 Benign Prostatic Hypertrophy

The typical appearance of BPH on CT is that of an enlarged, smoothly contoured gland of homogeneous density (PRICE and DAVIDSON 1979) (Fig. 12.9). On rare occasions lesions cause obliteration of the seminal vesicle angle or periprostatic fat planes or have an associated extraprostatic soft tissue component which make them indistinguishable from CAP (PRICE and DAVIDSON 1979).

12.4.3 Uncommon Tumors

There have been reports of some uncommon tumors of the prostate studied by CT. These include rhabdomyosarcoma, mucinous adenocarcinoma, and leiomyoma.

Rhabdomyosarcomas are predominantly malignancies of children but can occur in adults. Although the prostate is not a common site, this tumor can originate there. In contrast to CAP, these are typically large bulky masses. They have a propensity for local invasion. These malignancies are treated with chemotherapy and radiation to reduce the tumor bulk, followed by surgery. CT has completely modified the diagnostic approach and follow-up of these lesions. It serves an essential role in determining the extent of tumor, assessing the response to therapy, predicting operability, and screening for recurrence (GEOFFRAY et al. 1987). More recently MRI has been advocated for the same purpose (BARTOLOZZI et al. 1988).

There has been one reported case in the CT literature of mucinous adenocarcinoma (DUNNICK et al. 1982) and one of leiomyoma of the prostate (REGAN et al. 1987). Mucinous adenocarcinoma is a rare malignancy of the prostate which usually arises from the central portion of the gland (CHICA et al. 1977). Due to the mucin production, this lesion measured 12 Hounsfield units and was easily identified on CT. An abscess can have a similar appearance and thus clinical history is necessary to make the correct diagnosis. Leiomyomas are rare lesions of the prostate. They are benign but can cause obstructive symptoms. The one case described was very large (approximately 12 cm), well circumscribed, and inhomogeneous in appearance.

References

Bartolozzi C, Selli C, Olmastroni M, Di Candio G (1988) Rhabdomyosarcoma of the prostate: MR findings. AJR 150:1333–1334

Byar DP, Mostofi FK (1972) Carcinoma of the prostate: prognostic evaluation of certain pathologic features in 208 radical prostatectomies: examined by the step-section technique. Cancer 30:5–13

Chica G, Johnson DE, Ayala AG (1977) Mucinous adenocarcinoma of the prostate. J Urol 118:124–125

Dunnick NR, Walther PJ, Ford KK, Korobkin M, Paulson DF (1982) Mucinous adenocarcinoma of the prostate. J Comput Assist Tomogr 6:1198–1199

Emory TH, Reinke DB, Hill AL, Lange PH (1983) Use of CT to reduce understaging in prostatic cancer: comparison with conventional staging techniques. AJR 141:351–354

Flocks RH, Culp D, Porto R (1959) Lymphatic spread from prostatic cancer. J Urol 81:194–196

Franks LM (1975) Etiology, epidemiology and pathology of prostatic cancer. Cancer 32:1092–1095

Geoffray A, Couanet D, Montagne JP, Leclere J, Flamant F (1987) Ultrasonography and computed tomography for diagnosis and follow-up of pelvic rhabdomyosarcomas in children. Pediatr Radiol 17:132–136

Giri PGS, Walsh JW, Hazra TA, Texter JH, Koontz WW (1982) Role of computed tomography in the evaluation and management of carcinoma of the prostate. Int J Radiat Oncol Biol Phys 8:283–287

Golimbu M, Morales P, Al-Askari S, Shulman Y (1981) CAT scanning in staging of prostatic cancer. Urology 18:305–308

Gore RM, Moss AA (1983) Value of computed tomography in interstitial ^{125}I brachytherapy of prostatic carcinoma. Radiology 146:453–458

Harell GS (1983) The retroperitoneum. In: Haaga JR, Alfidi RJ (eds) Computed tomography of the whole body. C.V. Mosby, St. Louis, p 753

Higashi TS, Takizawa K, Suzuki S et al. (1990) Muellerian duct cyst: ultrasonographic and computed tomographic spectrum. Urol Radiol 12:39

Hricak H (1987) Urologic cancer: methods of early detection and future developments. Cancer 60:677–685

Hricak H, Dooms GC, Jeffrey RB et al. (1987) Prostatic carcinoma: staging by clinical assessment, CT, and MR imaging. Radiology 162:331–336

Jameson RM (1968) Prostatic abscess and carcinoma of the prostate. Br J Urol 40:288–292

Jewett HJ (1975) The present status of radical prostatectomy for stages A and B prostatic cancer. Urol Clin North Am 1:105–123

Klein LA (1979) Medical progress: prostatic carcinoma. N Engl J Med 300:824–833

Levine MS, Arger PH, Coleman BG, Mulhern CB Jr, Pollack HM, Wein AJ (1981) Detecting lymphatic metastases from prostatic carcinoma: superiority of CT. AJR 137:207–211

Morgan CL, Calkins RF, Cavalcanti EJ (1981) Computed tomography in the evaluation, staging, and therapy of carcinoma of the bladder and prostate. Radiology 140: 751–761

Munzenrider JE, Pilepich MD, Rene-Ferrero JB, Tchakaroua I, Carter BL (1977) Use of body scanner in radiotherapy treatment planning. Cancer 40:170–179

Platt JF, Bree RL, Schwab RE (1987) The accuracy of CT in the staging of carcinoma of the prostate. AJR 149: 315–318

Price JM, Davidson AJ (1979) Computed tomography in the evaluation of the suspected carcinomatous prostate. Urology Radiol 1:39–42

Regan JB, Barrett DM, Wold LE (1987) Giant leiomyoma of the prostate. Arch Pathol Lab Med 111:381–382

Salo JO, Kivisaari L, Rannikko S, Lehtonen T (1986) The value of CT in detecting pelvic lymph node metastases in cases of bladder and prostate carcinoma. Scand J Urol Nephrol 20:261–265

Schmidt JD, Johnson DE, Scott WW, Gibbons RP, Prout GR, Murphy GP (1976) The national prostatic cancer project: chemotherapy of advanced prostatic cancer: evaluation of response parameters. Urology 7:602–610

Seidelman FE, Reich NE, Cohen WN, Bryan PJ, Havrilla TR (1977) Computed tomography of the seminal vesicles and seminal vesicle angle. Comput Axial Tomogr 1:281–284

Thornhill BA, Morehouse HT, Coleman P, Hoffman-Tretin JC (1987) Prostatic abscess: CT and sonographic findings. AJR 148:899–900

Van Engelshoven JMA, Kreel L (1979) Computed tomography of the prostate. J Comput Assist Tomogr 3: 45–51

Weinerman PM, Arger PH, Coleman BG, Pollack HM, Banner MP, Wein AJ (1983) Pelvic adenopathy from bladder and prostate carcinoma: detection by rapid-sequence computed tomography. AJR 140:95–99

Whitmore WF, Mackenzie AR (1959) Experience with various operative procedures for the total excision of prostatic carcinoma. Cancer 12:396–405

13 Magnetic Resonance Imaging of the Prostate

David S. Moss

CONTENTS

13.1 MRI of the Normal Prostate

Magnetic resonance imaging (MRI) provides the best inherent soft tissue contrast of any imaging modality and has provided unprecedented details of prostate anatomy in vivo. The normal prostate has an intermediate intensity, homogeneous signal on T1-weighted images which provides no information about internal prostatic architecture. However, prostatic zonal anatomy is well-delineated with T2 weighting. The relatively low signal anterior fibromuscular zone, the intermediate signal central zone (CZ), and the high signal peripheral zone (PZ) are consistently identified (Hricak et al. 1987a; Phillips et al. 1987a; Gevenois et al. 1990) (Fig. 13.1). With T2 weighting the urethra and the periurethral glands are often inseparable, appearing as a bright linear band (Koslin et al. 1987); occasionally details of urethral anatomy such as the verumontanum can be visualized (Hricak et al. 1987a).

The fibromuscular zone is seen anterior to the urethra and has a signal intensity similar to that of muscle. It is composed of the preprostatic sphincter (smooth muscle) at the prostatic base and the prostatic sphincter (striated muscle) located at the apex. Authors differ on whether the two sphincters can be distinguished by MRI, with some claiming the preprostatic sphincter signal approximates that from the bladder wall while the prostatic sphincter signal appears similar

David S. Moss, M.D., Assistant Professor of Radiology, Department of Radiology, Columbia-Presbyterian Medical Center, 622 West 168th Street, New York, NY 10032, USA

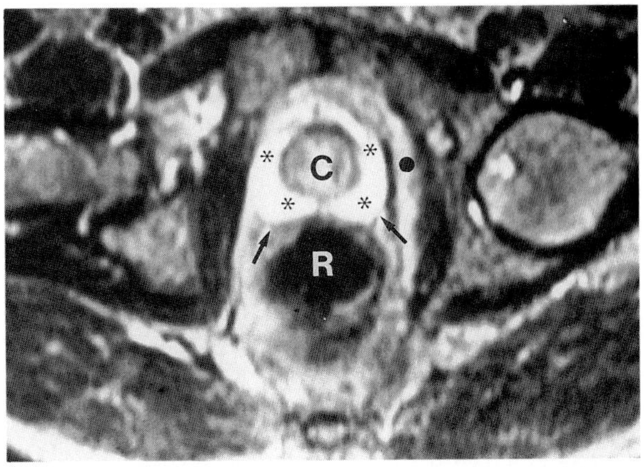

Fig. 13.1. MR image of normal prostate gland. Axial view; spin echo; TR 2500 ms/TE 80 ms; field strength 1.5 T. On this T2-weighted image the zonal architecture of the prostate is displayed. The periphery of the prostate is outlined by the prostatic capsule on either side of the gland (*arrows*). Within the substance of the prostate both the high signal intensity peripheral zone (*) and the lower, mixed signal intensity central gland (*C*) can be delineated. On the *left*, periprostatic fat is seen (●). The median raphe of the prostate is seen as a low signal intensity linear structure at 6 o'clock between the right and the left portions of the peripheral zone. *R*, rectum. (Courtesy of Dr. Howard Pollack)

to that of other striated muscle (Sommer et al. 1986; Koslin et al. 1987). The low intensity of the signal from this zone is attributed to the relative lack of free water in fibrous and muscular tissue (Phillips et al. 1987a).

The CZ lies posterolateral to the cephalic half of the prostatic urethra; it extends caudally as far as the verumontanum. The PZ, the most frequent site of origin of carcinomas and prostatitis, is a bright, symmetric crescent lying posterolateral and caudal to the CZ. Some degree of CZ heterogeneity, once considered pathologic, is now seen routinely in normal subjects examined with heavily T2-weighted sequences on mid or high field strength machines (Koslin et al. 1987; Carrol et al. 1987).

The intermediate intensity of the CZ is usually separable from the peripheral bright crescent of the PZ (on T2-weighted images). The relatively lower signal of the CZ may be explained by its relative abundance of smooth muscle within its stroma (PHILLIPS et al. 1987a). In addition, HRUBAN et al. (1987) have shown that the ducts of the PZ have relatively larger lumens which probably contribute to a relative increase in free water and, therefore, in signal intensity on T2-weighted images.

McNeal described a transitional zone (TZ) which blends with the periurethral glands and with the preprostatic sphincter and which is the most frequent site of origin of benign prostatic hypertrophy (BPH). With normal aging the CZ atrophies and is replaced by an expanded and increasingly heterogeneous TZ. Authors have been unable to visualize a discrete TZ separate from the neighboring CZ and periurethral glands despite scanning with a wide variety of pulse sequences (HRICAK et al. 1987a; KOSLIN et al. 1987).

The CZ and PZ are distinguishable in nearly all young adults; however, authors dispute the ability of MRI to make this distinction in older normal subjects (ALLEN et al. 1989). HRICAK et al. (1987a) could separate these zones in only 8 of 23 normal subjects over 40 years of age. PHILLIPS et al. (1987b), however, could separate these zones in 30 of 31 patients with various prostatic pathology (mean age 65 years). KOSLIN et al. (1987) also were able to separate these zones in his aging normal volunteers. Technical parameters were similar and there is presently no obvious explanation for these discordant findings.

The periprostatic venous plexus (PVP) is seen immediately adjacent to the prostate and, with T2 weighting, has a signal equal to or slightly greater than the neighboring PZ (POON et al. 1985, 1988). Such a bright signal is commonly seen in small vessels with relatively slow flow. The veins approach the prostate through the posterolateral aspect of its base and flow anteriorly to join the venous plexus of Santorini directly anterior to the prostate. These anterior veins are the most consistently identified portion of the PVP as the lateral veins are frequently not appreciated in older patients. This may be because they are compressed by increasing prostate size and, for unknown reasons, they often appear isointense with and therefore inseparable from the PZ in older patients (PHILLIPS et al. 1987b). The region directly posterior to the prostate is the avascular Denovilliers' fascia, which appears dark on T2-weighted images (HRICAK et al. 1987a).

A thin dark line, presumed to represent the prostatic capsule, is often seen around the periphery of the PZ, separating it from the PVP. This structure is usually incompletely visualized and may not be seen at all (PHILLIPS et al. 1987a; ALLEN et al. 1989).

The seminal vesicles are routinely visualized with an intermediate signal on T1-weighted sequences and a very bright signal on T2-weighted images. On these latter images they usually appear as bright as the bladder. However, in some normal patients the signal may be only slightly brighter than that of muscle (PHILLIPS et al. 1987a; HRICAK 1988).

The recently advocated use of endorectal surface coils promises to further enhance definition of lesions in the peripheral zone, but also in the central and transitional zones (MARTIN et al. 1988; SCHNALL et al. 1989).

13.2 MRI of Benign Prostatic Hypertrophy

T1-weighted images of patients with BPH usually show a heterogeneous prostate, often with discrete nodules. However, the gland may appear completely homogeneous and still harbor clinically significant BPH (Fig. 13.2).

Several authors have described the appearance of BPH on T2-weighted images (CARROL et al. 1987; HRUBAN et al. 1987; PHILLIPS et al. 1987b; LING et al. 1986). One sees central nodules varying from very low to very high in signal intensity, presumably corresponding to the wide range in their histologic makeup (SCHIEBLER et al. 1989; KAHU et al. 1989). Most nodules are of moderate signal intensity. Presumably this reflects the usual mix of fibrous tissue, glandular lumen, and epithelium. Increased fibrosis has been shown to accompany infarction of nodules and probably accounts for the lesions with lower signal. Those with a smaller than average percentage of fibrous tissue and some of those having undergone recent hemorrhage would be expected to appear brighter on T2-weighted images (the hemorrhagic ones may also appear bright on T1-weighted images).

Nodules of BPH are typically discrete and well defined, and are often surrounded by a dark rim which has been shown by HRUBAN et al. (1987) to represent a fibrous capsule. As they grow they can compress and obliterate the PZ and the anterior fibromuscular zone as well as the lateral portion of the PVP.

While these nodules are typical they are by no means invariably seen in patients with BPH. LING et al. (1986) found nodules in 7 of 12 patients with biopsy-proven BPH. LARKIN et al. (1986), using a 0.15-T magnet, could not identify any discrete nodules in his 12 patients with BPH. CARROL et al. (1987) used pathologic mapping techniques of resected specimens to closely correlate regional pathology with findings on each MRI slice. The central regions of most of their specimens (with and without BPH) were heterogeneous, containing many tiny bright foci, but none of these bright foci corresponded to the location of any hyperplastic nodules. They detected one nodule, while pathology-proven nodules up to 20 mm in eight other patients were not seen. Thus, although a typical appearance has been described, current techniques can frequently miss hyperplastic nodules within a heterogeneous or even within a completely homogeneous appearing prostate.

13.3 MRI of Carcinoma of the Prostate

The signal from intraprostatic carcinoma (CAP) has been said to vary from hypo- to iso- to hyperintense on T2-weighted images (LING et al. 1986; BRYAN et al. 1986; THICKMAN et al. 1990; SCHIEBLER et al. 1989; POLLACK and SCHNALL 1992; SCHIEBLER et al. 1992). Current MRI techniques have not been able to distinguish hyperplastic nodules from neoplastic foci solely on the basis of the type of signal generated by each entity. In fact, in vivo quantification of T1 and T2 values showed no significant difference between BPH and CAP (KJAER et al. 1987). Because of the propensity for CAP to arise from the PZ it is hoped that by pinpointing the exact location of small lesions one will be able to distinguish a peripheral carcinoma from a central hyperplastic nodule (of course, larger lesions may grow centrally, confusing the issue) (CARROL et al. 1987).

Recent investigators have carefully examined the PZ in patients with CAP and have found hypointense defects in the otherwise bright PZ in many patients (SCHIEBLER et al. 1989) (Fig. 13.3). CARROL et al. (1987) found such a defect in 8 of 12 patients with carcinoma. This defect was proven by pathologic analysis to correspond to foci of tumor in these eight patients. Whether or not a

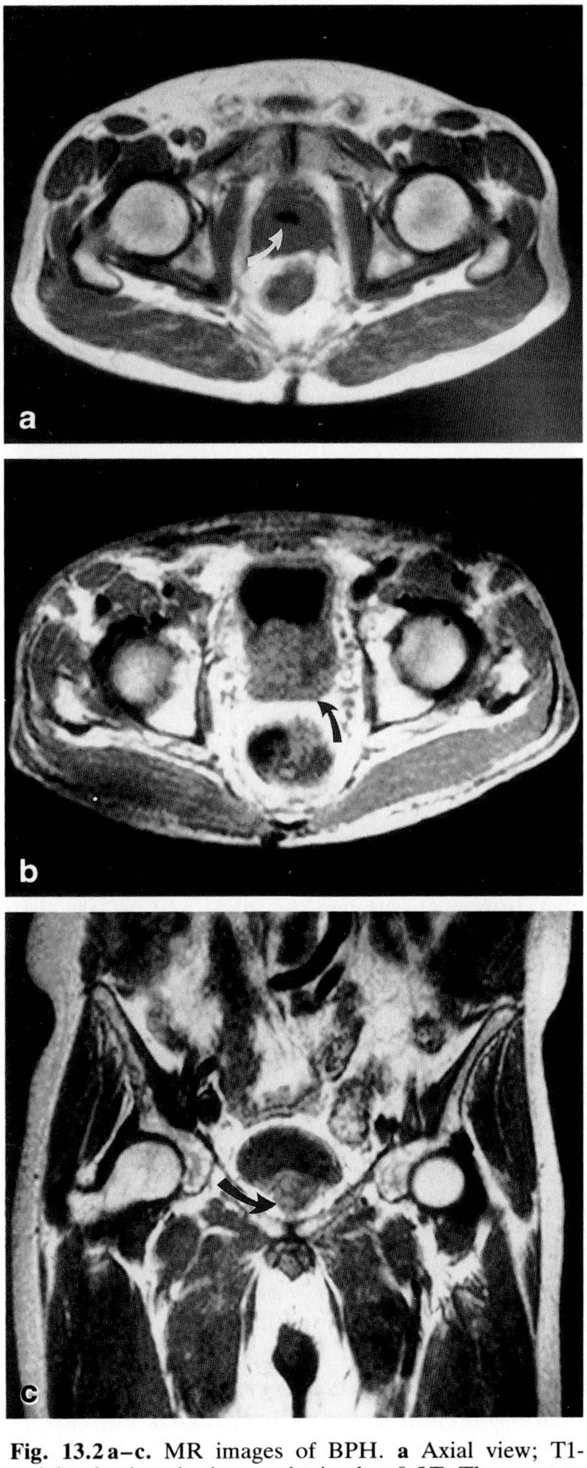

Fig. 13.2a–c. MR images of BPH. **a** Axial view; T1-weighted spin-echo image obtained at 0.5 T. The prostate appears homogeneous; the central low intensity structure (*arrow*) represents the urethra with a post-TURP defect. **b,c** Axial and coronal T1-weighted images show the prostate (*arrow*) to be inhomogeneous with discrete hyperplastic nodules indenting the bladder base

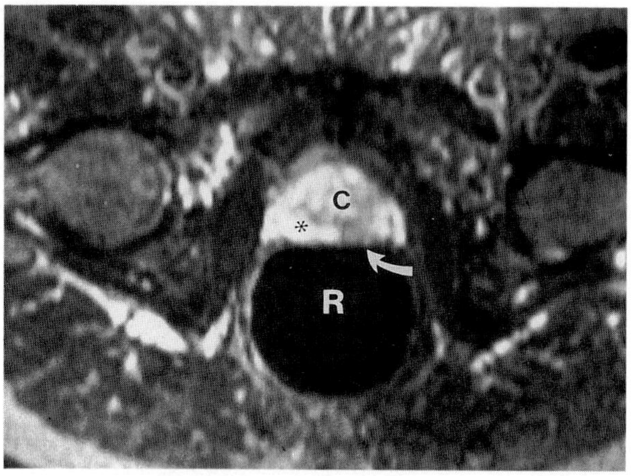

Fig. 13.3. MR image of adenocarcinoma of the prostate. Stage C. Spin-echo; TR 2500 ms/TE 80 ms; field strength 1.5 T. A low signal intensity lesion replaces a part of the left half of the peripheral zone of the prostate at 4, 5, and 6 o'clock. The right half of the peripheral zone (*) is intact and demonstrates its normal high signal intensity. The lesion extended to the capsular surface as suggested by the MR image, but microscopically invasion of the capsule was present, which was not detectable by MR. Note the heterogeneous signal central gland (*C*), attributable to a combination of glandular hyperplasia (high signal) and fibromuscular hyperplasia (low signal). (Courtesy of Dr. HOWARD POLLACK)

PZ defect was visible in this small series was unrelated to tumor size and to histologic grade of the tumor. Furthermore, the tumor size was grossly underestimated in five of the eight patients in whom it was seen, and in four patients no focal inhomogeneity to suggest tumor was appreciated even in retrospect.

BEZZI and co-workers (1988) found a hypointense PZ defect in 34 of 37 patients with CAP who subsequently underwent a radical prostatectomy. These defects were inferred to represent carcinoma because they all corresponded to the location of tumor palpated on physical examination and documented by biopsy. An earlier study at the same institution showed this to be a nonspecific finding as an identical PZ defect was seen in five of ten BPH patients with no known malignancy. Moreover, it is known that prostatitis has a marked predilection for the PZ. Acute or chronic prostatitis could produce a PZ lesion mimicking that seen with CAP, thereby further limiting the specificity of this finding.

Even though current MRI techniques are not able to definitively diagnose intraprostatic foci of tumor, they could prove useful in assessing tumor volume. McNeal has suggested that aggressive behavior is correlated with tumor volume and that tumors >4 cm are the ones most likely to metastasize.

BEZZI and co-workers did find a correlation between estimated volume and invasiveness; however, they did not have detailed pathologic analysis of resected prostates available for a gold standard of actual tumor volume. They discussed two important obstacles to estimating tumor size: (a) invasion into the CZ is difficult to separate from the heterogeneity normally seen in this zone, and (b) subacute hemorrhage (which can appear hypo- or hyperintense) is frequently seen as almost all patients are imaged following biopsy. BEZZI et al. found 40% of patients had bright intraprostatic foci on T1-weighted images, which they attributed to subacute postbiopsy hemorrhage. Others have found few or no patients with changes they attributed to biopsy (MIROWITZ 1992).

In its most promising current application, investigators have been using MRI to predict local extracapsular spread of CAP, thereby helping the urologists to decide which patients should undergo radical prostatectomy (AISEN 1990; KAHN et al. 1989; SCHIEBLER et al. 1989; SCHIEBLER and SCHNALL 1992; POLLACK and SCHNALL 1992).

Transverse T1-weighted images have been generally regarded as the best for detecting adenopathy as the dark lymph nodes are easily discernible against the bright fat. Several studies have shown that MRI is at least as effective as computed tomography (CT) in detecting enlarged pelvic lymph nodes (BEZZI et al. 1988; AISEN 1990). Current techniques do not permit MRI identification of small foci of tumor within normal-sized lymph nodes. T1- and T2-weighted images are used to evaluate the periprostatic fat, which is usually homogeneous and has a sharp interface with the gland. Linear streaking as well as focal masses in the fat are suspicious for extracapsular spread. The levator ani muscles are examined for symmetry in size and signal. Bright foci within the levator muscles on T2-weighted images have been correlated with tumor invasion (HRICAK et al. 1987b). An important caveat in evaluating the levator ani is the frequent presence of the chemical shift artifact (HRICAK et al. 1987a). This phenomenon, which occurs at the interface between fat and other tissues, can cause asymmetric signal from the levator which can be confused with neoplastic involvement. It usually manifests as a low signal rim at one margin and a high signal rim at the opposite margin of the contralateral levator muscle. This artifact can also cause the levator to appear indistinct and therefore difficult to evaluate. While it most frequently involves the levator, this artifact has been seen to affect the bladder wall as well. Often the chemical shift artifact can be confidently recognized and disregarded. However, if doubt persists, coronal views are usually helpful. Alternatively, the transverse view can be repeated after changing the direction of the frequency-encoding gradient.

Tumor involvement in the seminal vesicles usually appears as a dark focus within these otherwise bright structures on T2-weighted images. Despite reported sensitivities ranging from 50% to 83%, even macroscopic involvement has been missed with current MRI techniques.

Carcinoma of the prostate extending to the bladder base and rectum has been documented with MRI. Sagittal or coronal views are often helpful supplements to transverse views in this regard. Nevertheless, asymmetric thickening of the bladder base can sometimes be seen in patients with BPH and following transurethral resection of the prostate (TURP), making the diagnosis of tumor invasion difficult.

In the largest correlative series of CAP to date, HRICAK et al. (1987b) compared the surgical/pathologic findings in 46 patients who underwent radical prostatectomy with their preoperative CT and MRI studies. CT was 61% accurate in differentiating intra- from extracapsular tumor. Using transverse T1- and T2-weighted images the reported accuracy of MRI was 74%; this jumped to 83% when either coronal or sagittal T2-weighted images were used to supplement the transverse views. There were ten cases where the findings on MRI differed from CT, and MRI was proven to be correct in nine of these. The addition of a coronal or sagittal view was helpful in overcoming chemical shift artifact and in imaging the bladder neck. Limitations of MRI included missing microscopic local invasion and mistaking periprostatic fibrosis for tumor, both of which are well-known pitfalls in CT interpretation.

BIONDETTI and co-workers (1987) correlated surgical findings in 18 patients with their preoperative MRI scans obtained at either 0.35 T or 0.5 T, utilizing contiguous 1 cm thick slices. In this series each of four parameters was evaluated independently and the conclusion was that, overall, MRI correctly separated stage B from stages C and D in 16 of the 18 patients. Alterations of the periprostatic fat was an insensitive but 100% specific parameter. Preoperative MRI detected three of six infiltrated seminal vesicles, again with a high specificity (29 of 30 normal seminal vesicles appeared normal on MRI).

BIONDETTI et al.'s most controversial parameter related to the integrity of the PVP. Every patient whose PVP appeared abnormal did indeed have extracapsular disease, although the capsular invasion was often contralateral to the side of the PVP abnormality. Thus, combining these parameters (plus adenopathy), BIONDETTI et al. claimed an 87% MRI sensitivity and a 90% specificity in staging CAP.

PHILLIPS and co-workers (1987), however, found the PVP prohibitively difficult to evaluate in 31 patients with various prostatic diseases (the PVP in younger, normal controls was much easier to see). There was very poor interobserver agreement, and this parameter was not felt to be useful. HRICAK et al. (1987b) also could identify the anterior and lateral PVP in almost all younger patients but could do so in only 10 of 23 older normal subjects. Thus, although PHILLIPS et al.'s series lacked the extensive surgical correlation of that of BIONDETTI et al., it does call into question the significance of not finding a normal PVP: Is this simply a result of BPH and/or normal aging, or is it a specific indication of extracapsular disease?

BEZZI and co-workers (1988) used a 1.5-T magnet and 5-mm slices to study 37 CAP patients who underwent radical prostatectomy. Their results were similar to those of BIONDETTI et al.: irregular gland margins, foci of decreased signal from adjacent fat, and an abnormal PVP all combined for a 44% sensitivity and an 81% specificity. With the addition of lymph node and seminal vesicle parameters BEZZI et al. achieved an overall accuracy of 78% in separating intra- from extracapsular involvement.

BEZZI et al. also found that all five cases of extracapsular disease which were mistakenly classified as stage B by MRI involved only microscopic capsular invasion. In a few centers those with only microscopic capsular invasion are considered for radical prostatectomy; therefore, at these centers MRI would have been 100% sensitive in determining who is a surgical candidate.

In this same study all three cases of stage B disease mistakenly labeled as stage C demonstrated either unilateral or bilateral decreased signal from biopsy-proven normal seminal vesicles. HRICAK (1988) has recently pointed out that a diffuse decrease in seminal vesicle signal can be seen in a variety of nonmalignant conditions and has suggested that localized foci of decreased signal should raise the greatest suspicion of tumor invasion.

Published data are based on so few cases that any conclusions can only be considered tentative. Regarding technique, most current investigators obtain transverse T1- and T2-weighted images, usually supplemented by coronal T2-weighted images. If there is clinical concern about bladder or rectal involvement, sagittal views may be more helpful than coronal views. Most acquire a T1-weighted image with the TR in the range of 500–800 ms and the TE in the range of 20–50 ms. For T2-weighted images the TR should be in the range of 2000–2500 ms, with a TE in the range of 50–100 ms. Recent reports have shown excellent anatomic detail when the slice thickness is reduced to 5 or 7 mm (with two excitations). Most of these studies have been performed on machines with a strength of 0.5 T or higher.

Using current techniques MRI cannot reliably distinguish BPH from CAP. Furthermore, it has not been accurate in determining the size of the carcinomas which have been visualized. It is possible that different pulse sequences, for example, gradient-recalled echoes, may prove helpful. MRI is similar to CT in detecting pelvic adenopathy and is probably more accurate in detecting local extracapsular spread of tumor, especially seminal vesicle involvement. It is not yet known whether it is sensitive or specific enough to be clinically useful in this latter regard.

The role of position emission Tomography in identifying prostatic cancer with Tagged androgen receptors is as yet not established but shows promise (Liu et al. 1992).

References

Aisen AM (1990) Body MR imaging in the local staging of neoplasms. Radiology 176:617

Allen KS, Kressel HY, Arger PH, Pollack HM (1989) Age-related changes of the prostate: evaluation by MR imaging. AJR 152:77–81

Bezzi M, Kressel HY, Allen KS, Schiebler ML, Altman HG, Wein AJ, Pollack HM (1988) Prostatic carcinoma: staging at 1.5T. Radiology 169:339–346

Biondetti PR, Lee JKT, Lind D, Catalona WJ (1987) Clinical stage B prostate carcinoma: staging with MR imaging. Radiology 162:325–329

Bryan PJ, Butler HE, Nelson AD et al. (1986) Magnetic resonance imaging of the prostate. AJR 146:543–548

Carrol CL, Sommer FG, McNeal JE, Stamey TA (1987) The abnormal prostate: MR imaging at 1.5T with histopathological correlation. Radiology 163:521–525

Gevenois PA, Salmon I, Stallenberg B et al. (1990) Magnetic resonance imaging of the normal prostate at 1.5T. Br J Radiol 63:101

Hricak H (1987) Urologic cancer: methods of early detection and future developments. Cancer 60:677–685

Hricak H (1988) Imaging prostate carcinoma (editorial). Radiology 169:569–571

Hricak H, Dooms G, McNeal JE et al. (1987a) MR imaging of the prostate: normal anatomy. AJR 148:51–58

Hricak H, Dooms GC, Jeffrey RB et al. (1987b) Prostatic carcinoma: staging by clinical assessment, CT, and MR imaging. Radiology 162:331–336

Hruban RH, Zerhouni EA, Dagher AP, Pessar ML, Hutchins GM (1987) Morphologic basis of MR imaging of benign prostatic hypertrophy. J Comput Assist Tomogr 11:1035–1041

Kahn T, Burrig K, Schmitz-Drager B, Furst G, Modder U (1989) Prostatic carcinoma and benign prostatic hyperplasia: MR imaging with histopathologic correlation. Radiology 173:847–851

Kjaer L, Thomsen C, Iverson P, Henriksen O (1987) In vivo estimation of relaxation processes in benign hyperplasia and carcinoma of the prostate gland by magnetic resonance imaging. Magn Reson Imaging 5:23–30

Koslin DB, Kenney PJ, Koehler RE, Van Dyke JA (1987) Magnetic resonance imaging of the internal anatomy of the prostate gland. Invest Radiol 22:947–953

Larkin BT, Berquist TH, Vtz DC (1986) Evaluation of the prostate by magnetic resonance imaging. Magn Reson Imaging 4:53–58

Ling D, Lee JKT, Heiken JP, Balfe DM, Glazer HS, McClennan BL (1986) Prostatic carcinoma and benign prostatic. Hyperplasia: inability of MR imaging to distinguish between the two diseases. Radiology 158:103–107

Liu A, Carlson KE, Katzenellenbogen JA (1992) Synthesis of high affinity fluorine-substituted ligands for androgen receptor. Potential agents for imaging prostatic cancer by position emission tomography. J Med Chem 35: 2113–2129

Martin JF, Hajek P, Baker L, Gylys-Morin D, Fitzmorris-Glass R, Mattrey RR (1988) Inflatable surface coil for MR imaging of the prostate. Radiology 167:268

Mirowitz SA (1992) Seminal vesicals biopsy related hemorrhage simulating tumor invasion at endorectal MR imaging. Radiology 185:373–376

Phillips ME, Kressel HY, Spritzer CE et al. (1987a) Normal prostate and adjacent structures: MR imaging at 1.5T. Radiology 164:381–385

Phillips ME, Kressel HY, Spritzer CE et al. (1987b) Prostatic disorders: MR imaging at 1.5T. Radiology 164: 386–392

Pollack HM, Schnall MD (1992) Magnetic resonance imaging of carcinoma the prostate. Prostate 4:17–31

Poon PY, McCallum RW, Henkelman MM et al. (1985) Magnetic resonance imaging of the prostate. Radiology 154:143–149

Poon PY, McCallum RW, Henkelman MM et al. (1988) MRI of periprostatic venous plexus in staging of prostatic carcinoma. J Can Assoc Radiol 39:111

Schiebler ML, Tomaszewski JE, Bezzi M et al. (1989) Prostatic carcinoma and benign prostatic hyperplasia: correlation of high-resolution MR and histopathologic findings. Radiology 172:131–137

Schiebler ML, Schnall MD, Altwater E (1992) Magnetic resonance imaging of the prostate. JCAT 16:493–494

Schiebler ML, Yankankas BC, Tempany C, Spritzer CE, Rifkin MD, Pollack HM, Zerhouni EA (1992) MR imaging in carcinoma of the prostate: interobserver variation and efficacy for determining stage C disease. AJR 158:559–562

Schnall MD, Lenkinski RE, Pollack HM, Imai Y, Kressel HY (1989) Prostate: MR imaging with an endorectal surface coil. Radiology 172:570–574

Sommer FG, McNeal JE, Carrol CL (1986) MR depiction of zonal anatomy of the prostate at 1.5T. J Comput Assist Tomogr 10:983–989

Thickman D, Miller GJ, Hopper KD et al. (1990) Prostate cancer comparison of preoperative 0.35T MRI with whole mount histopathology. MRI 8:205

14 Interventional Radiology of the Prostate

E. STEPHEN AMIS, Jr.

CONTENTS

Interventional techniques involving the prostate may be utilized for either diagnostic or therapeutic purposes. The most important of these techniques are pedal lymphangiography with needle aspiration biopsy of visualized nodes, embolization of postprostatectomy or postbiopsy prostatic bleeding, and balloon dilation of obstructing benign prostatic hypertrophy (BPH). These will be individually addressed. Needle biopsy of the prostate under sonographic guidance has been previously discussed.

14.1 Lymphangiography and Percutaneous Node Biopsy

Lymphangiography and combined needle aspiration biopsy is a diagnostic technique used in some institutions for staging of carcinoma of the prostate (CAP). The pedal lymphangiogram, using an oily contrast medium, results in opacification of pelvic and retroperitoneal lymph nodes. This occurs by trapping of the contrast within the lymph node, thereby displaying not only the lymph node size and contour, but also internal architectural details (CASTELLINO et al. 1980). This trapping is within the intranodal sinusoidal network, with very little contrast, if any, entering into the denser aggregates of cells composing the follicles and medullary cords. Therefore, the normal lymphangiogram is characterized by a diffuse, homogeneous stippled appearance of the nodes, representing the opacified sinuses and the nonopacified follicular tissue. Metastatic lesions in the node alter this appearance, producing well-demarcated negative defects and perhaps an associated focal bulging of the node contour (Fig. 14.1).

Unfortunately, benign processes can mimic this appearance. These include fatty and fibrous tissues replacing normal nodal tissue, and inflammatory or infectious involvement of the nodes. The defects seen with these benign lesions frequently occur in the aging population, precisely the age group at risk for CAP, thus causing problems with arriving at the correct diagnosis of metastatic disease (CASTELLINO and MARGLIN 1982). One differentiating factor is that the benign defects are not usually associated with local expansion of the node. Yet another source of error in lymphangiography is that of microscopic metastatic lesions in nodes which are too small to produce radiographic defects. Thus, as can be seen from the above discussion, a lymphangiogram interpreted as positive should carry a high level of correlation with the clinical presentation of the patient (e.g., defects in nodes in a patient with highly undifferentiated CAP are highly likely to represent metastases). A negative lymphangiogram, on the other hand, indicates only the absence of radiographically detectable lesions.

As noted previously, CAP metastasizes first to the nodes in the region of the obturator nerve. Whether these nodes are opacified on lymphangiography has been the subject of some debate in the literature. However, MERRIN et al. (1977), in studying 50 samples of excised obturator nodes from patients with pelvic malignancy that had undergone preoperative lymphangiography, found that all nodes contained radiopaque contrast.

To overcome the weaknesses of lymphangiography in staging CAP, as enumerated above,

E. STEPHEN AMIS, Jr., M.D., Professor and Chairman, Department of Radiology, Albert Einstein College of Medicine and Montefiore Medical Center, 111 East 210th Street, Bronx, NY 10467, USA

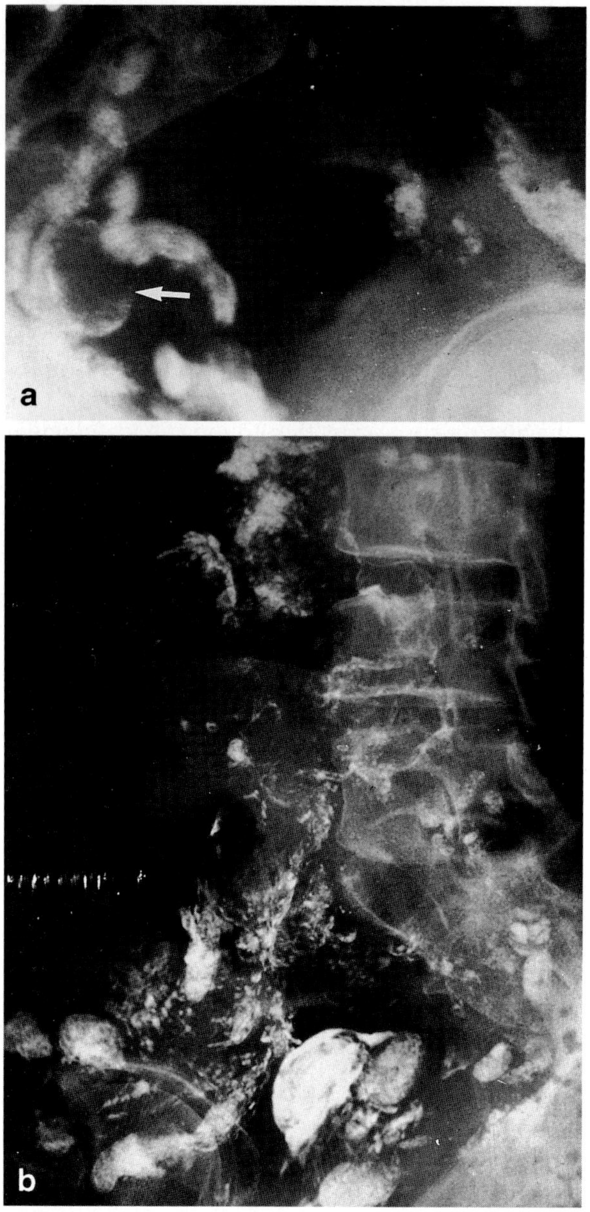

Fig. 14.1. **a** Coned view of lymphangiogram in patient with CAP. The filling defect seen (*arrow*) was proven to be a metastatic focus. Note that the node bulges in response to this focus. **b** Grossly abnormal lymphangiogram in patient with widespread CAP. Note the almost total replacement of many nodes with metastatic tumor

biopsies of both normal-appearing and abnormal nodes as imaged during the study have been advocated. This technique involves the use of a skinny needle (22 gauge) passed percutaneously into an opacified node, or a filling defect within an otherwise opacified node, under fluoroscopic control (Amis et al. 1983). The efficacy of this technique, like the visualization of obturator nodes, has also been subject to debate in recent years. In one study, 66 suspect nodes were biopsied, and positive cytology for CAP was obtained in 29 (Efremidis et al. 1981). The authors felt this sufficient to recommend the technique highly. Carrying the process one step further, Gothlin and Hoiem (1981) biopsied six to ten normal appearing nodes in each of 24 patients with low-grade CAP, and found metastases in six patients. However, this success could not be confirmed in another study in which normal-appearing nodes were biopsied in 49 patients with carcinoma of the prostate or bladder without finding a single metastasis (Kidd and Correa 1984).

Perhaps the best studies for determining the accuracy of lymphangiography are those in which the histopathology and radiographic appearance of excised nodes are compared. One such study yielded high false-negative rates for the lymphangiogram as a staging tool, detecting only 40% of patients with involved nodes (low sensitivity) (Sherwood and O'Donoghue 1981). In the same study, however, the specificity was found to be fairly high, allowing recognition of 80% of those patients who were free of node deposits by a normal lymphangiogram. A recent study evaluated 587 excised nodes from 23 patients with CAP 5 to 10 days after pedal lymphangiography (Komatsu et al. 1987). Each node was radiographed, and the radiograph compared to the histologic findings. A total of 17 nodes were positive for CAP. Of these, only five showed a defect on the radiography, one was suspicious, nine were negative, and two showed nonfilling of the positive node by contrast. False-negative calls occurred chiefly because metastatic foci were microscopic. As can be easily seen, the lymphangiogram, with or without needle biopsy of nodes, cannot equal the accuracy of staging pelvic lymphadenectomy.

14.2 Embolization for Control of Prostatic Hemorrhage

Significant bleeding from the prostate, whether after prostatectomy or needle biopsy, is fortunately a rare occurrence. In the past such cases would have been treated with bladder irrigation, packing of the bladder, or, as a last resort, surgical ligation of both hypogastric arteries. More recently, reports have indicated the efficacy of percutaneous transfemoral embolization of branches of the hypogastric arteries. Success with this technique has been reported in an animal study (DAREWICZ et al. 1980) as well as in several human series (BENSON et al. 1980: GALLOWAY 1982; MITCHELL et al. 1976; NADALINI et al. 1981; SMITH et al. 1975; LANG 1981). Failures were generally due to hemorrhage that was diffuse or secondary to multiple vessel inflow.

Because of the extensive collateral blood flow to the prostate, preembolization studies should include injection of both hypogastric arteries (Fig. 14.2a). Similarly, embolization should usually be carried out bilaterally, with repeated injections to document the sites of emboli and the cessation of bleeding (Fig. 16.2b,c). Once small test doses of contrast material reveal marked stasis of flow, or backflow into the common iliac artery, embolization should cease (GALLOWAY 1982). A rich collateralization from the external iliac and femoral, as well as from the inferior mesenteric arteries, allows maintenance of viability of the bladder despite bilateral occlusion of the branches of the hypogastric arteries (SMITH et al. 1975).

Although a number of embolic agents have proven effective in control of hemorrhage, autologous clot, Amicar-enforced autologous clot, and Gelfoam are favored (GALLOWAY 1982; SMITH et al. 1975; LANG 1981). The propensity of autologous clot to embolize at the level of muscular branch arteries maintains perfusion via the precapillary plexus. Moreover, lysis of such clots results in reconstitution of flow and thereby minimizes the risk of tissue necrosis particularly of necrosis of the bladder.

Apart from necrosis of the bladder, complications have included pain, fever, and rebleeding (HIETALA 1978).

14.3 Balloon Dilation of Benign Prostatic Hypertrophy

Benign prostatic hypertrophy has been discussed in detail in a previous chapter. Suffice it to say that a majority of the adult male population over the age of 50 are afflicted, with a not insignificant number of this group suffering bothersome symptoms. Classic treatment for this condition continues to be open or transurethral prostatectomy. However, recent work on balloon dilation of the benignly enlarged prostate seems to indicate that this simple procedure may provide long-term

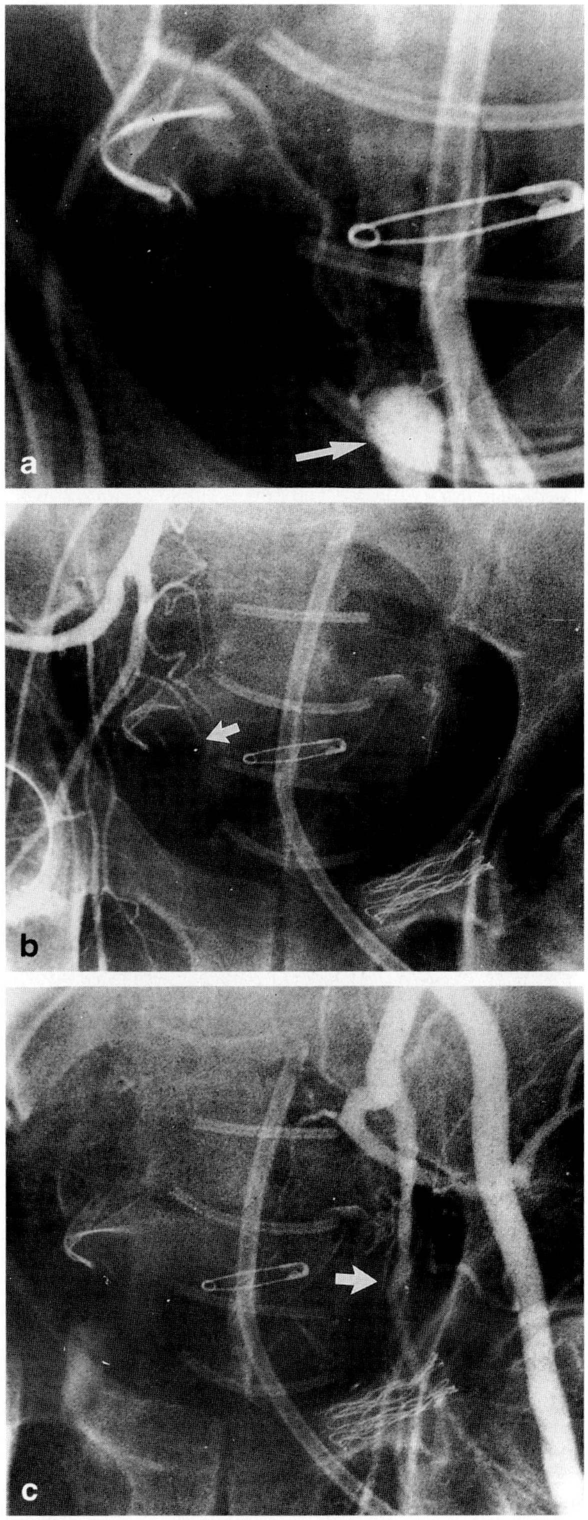

Fig. 14.2a–c. Angiographic embolization of prostatic hemorrhage in a patient who has undergone recent biopsy. **a** Subselective injection of the right hypogastric artery showing extravasation of contrast in the region of the prostate. **b,c** Postembolization hypogastric injections showing occlusion of branches feeding the prostate bilaterally

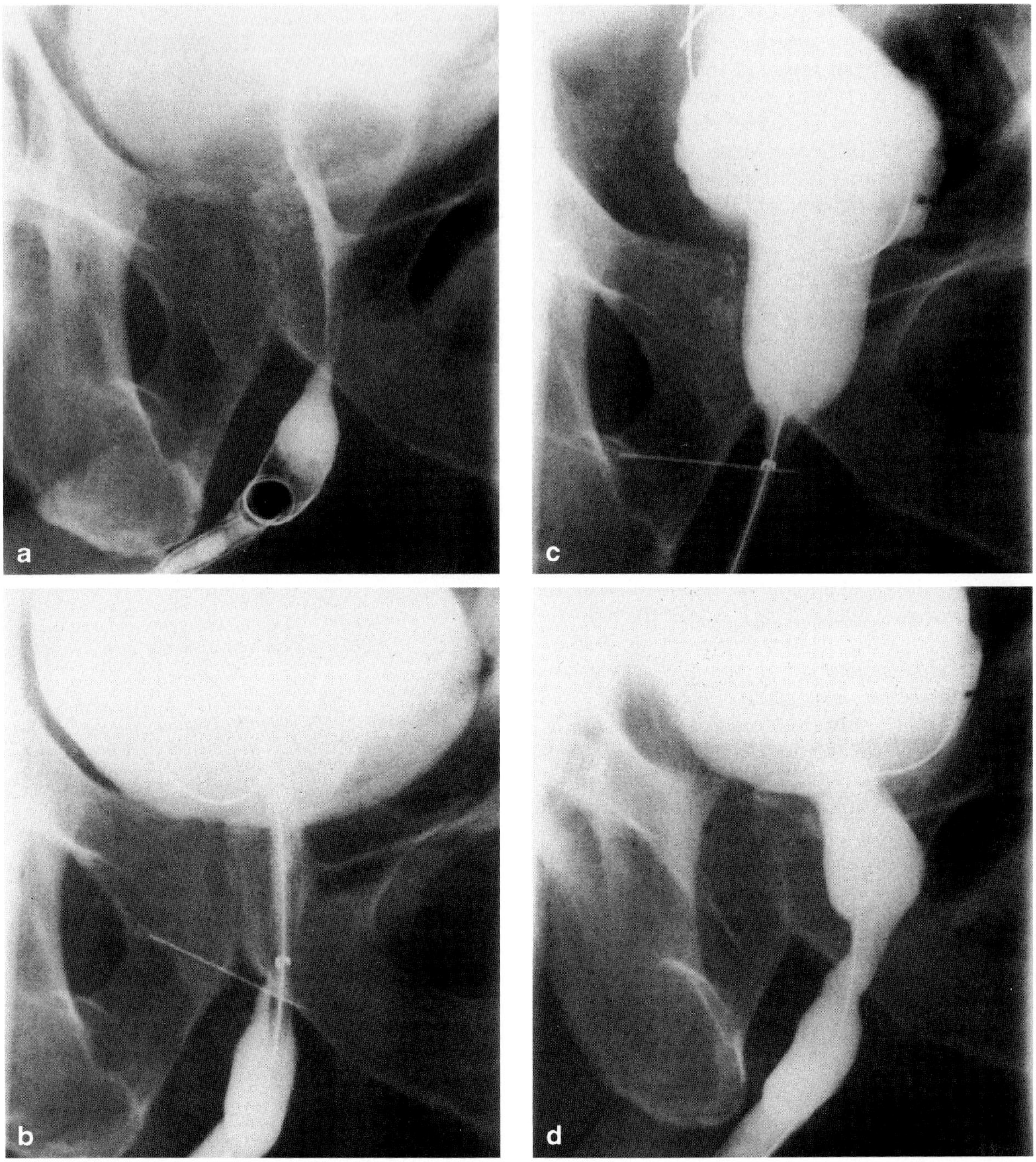

Fig. 14.3 a–d. Balloon dilation of BPH. **a** Councill catheter within the mid-anterior urethra with balloon partially inflated to occlude urethral lumen. Retrograde urethrogram performed via this catheter shows a significant degree of prostatic urethral narrowing due to BPH. **b** The external sphincter has been marked by a needle placed over the drapes. The dilating catheter is in proper position with the proximal marker just above the sphincter. Contrast has been injected retrograde through a small pediatric feeding tube to double check the position of the balloon with respect to the external sphincter. **c** The balloon is fully inflated, with the bladder neck included in the dilation. **d** Retrograde study performed immediately after the dilation via the Councill catheter. The guide wire is still in place. Significant dilation of the bladder neck and prostatic urethra can be appreciated. (Case courtesy of Dr. Wilfrido Castaneda)

symptomatic relief. BURHENNE et al. (1984) reported performing the technique on cadavers. More recently, CASTANEDA et al. (1987) experimentally dilated the prostatic urethra in a group of dogs, finding good results in follow-up over a period of 14 months. They then progressed to dilation of the prostatic urethra in human males with BPH (CASTANEDA and REDDY 1987). Of five subjects, four experienced significant resolution of obstructive symptoms over follow-up periods of up to 8 months. Under topical anesthesia and mild sedation, dilation was performed with a 25-mm urethroplasty balloon catheter inflated at 3–6 atm for 10 min (Fig. 14.3). Great care was taken not to dilate the external sphincter. In the failed patient, dilation was felt to be ineffectual due to predominantly middle lobe hypertrophy, which allowed the enlarged segment of the prostate, extending into the bladder, simply to be pushed away by the inflated balloon. This condition is now considered to be a contraindication to dilation.

Placement of a metallic stent into the prostatic urethra has been another modification recently advocated for the management of obstructive prostatic hypertrophy. The initial reported results are better than those for mere balloon dilation (RICKARDS et al. 1989). Improvement of objective parameters such as flow rate and residual urine are cited as major advantages of this latter technique. Self-retaining intraurethral stents have also been advocated as a viable alternative to long-term indwelling catheters in the treatment of prostatism (YACHIA et al. 1990).

References

Amis ES Jr, Pfister RC, Yoder IC (1983) Interventional radiology of the adult bladder and urethra. Semin Roentgenol 18:322–330

Benson RC, Marquis WE, Crummy AB, Uehling DT (1980) Embolization for genitourinary disorders. Urology 16:587–591

Burhenne HJ, Chisholm RJ, Quenville NF (1984) Prostatic hyperplasia: radiological intervention. Radiology 152:655–657

Castaneda F, Lund G, Larson BW (1987) Prostatic urethra: experimental dilation in dogs. Radiology 163:645–648

Castaneda F, Reddy R (1987) Benign prostatic hypertrophy: retrograde transurethral dilation of the prostatic urethra in humans. Radiology 163:649–653

Castellino RA, Marglin SI, Carroll BA, Young SW, Harell GS, Blank N (1980) The radiographic evaluation of abdominal and pelvic lymph nodes in oncologic practice. Cancer Treat Rev 7:153–160

Castellino RA, Marglin SI (1982) Imaging of abdominal and pelvic lymph nodes: Lymphography or computed tomography? Invest Radiol 17:433–443

Darewicz J, Cylwik B, Musierowicz A, Boczon S (1980) The effect of internal iliac artery embolization on the prostatic gland in the dog. Int Urol Nephrol 12:37–41

Efremidis SC, Dan SJ, Nieburgs H, Mitty HA (1981) Carcinoma of the prostate: lymph node aspiration for staging. AJR 136:489–492

Galloway DC (1982) Transcatheter embolization for control of bleeding after prostatic biopsy. South Med J 75:1128–1130

Hietala SO (1978) Urinary bladder necrosis following selective embolization of the internal iliac artery. Acta Radiol [Diagn] (Stockh) 19:316–320

Gothlin JH, Hoiem L (1981) Percutaneous fine-needle biopsy for radiographically normal lymph nodes in the staging of prostatic carcinoma. Radiology 141:351–354

Kidd R, Correa R (1984) Fine-needle aspiration biopsy of lymphangiographically normal lymph nodes: a negative view. AJR 141:1005–1006

Komatsu H, Hayashi S, Tanabe N, Shirasu N (1987) Evaluation of early metastatic lesion of pelvic lymph nodes from carcinoma of the bladder or prostate. J Urol 138:341–343

Lang EK (1981) Transcatheter embolization of pelvic vessels for control of intractable hemorrhage. Radiology 140:331–339

Merrin C, Wajsman Z, Baumgartner G, Jennings E (1977) The clinical value of lymphangiography: Are the nodes surrounding the obturator nerve visualized? J Urol 117:762–764

Mitchell ME, Waltman A, Athanasoulis CA, Kerr WS Jr, Dretler SA (1976) Control of massive bleeding with angiographic techniques. J Urol 115:692–695

Nadalini VF, Positano N, Bruttini GP, Medica M, Fasce L (1981) Occlusione arteriosa terapeutica delle arterie ipogastriche con isobutil-2-cianoacrilato nelle neoplasie vescicali e prostatiche. Radiol Med (Torino) 67:61–66

Rickards D, Milroy E, Chapple C, Edlin A, Wallstein H (1989) New noninvasive treatment for prostate outflow obstruction; transrectal guided insertion of Wallstent endoprosthesis. RSNA, paper 276, Chicago, Ill.

Sherwood T, O'Donoghue EPN (1981) Lymphograms in prostatic carcinoma: false-positive and false-negative assessments in radiology. Br J Radiol 54:15–17

Smith JC, Kerr WS Jr, Athanasoulis CA, Waltman AC, Ring EJ, Baum S (1975) Angiographic management of bleeding secondary to genitourinary tract surgery. J Urol 113:89–92

Yachia D, Lask D, Rabinson S (1990) Self-retaining intraurethral stent: an alternative to long-term indwelling catheters or surgery in the treatment of prostatism. AJR 154:111–113

15 Screening Examinations for Carcinoma of the Prostate

Reid M. Morse and Martin I. Resnick

CONTENTS

15.1 Definition of Problem

Carcinoma of the prostate (CAP) was the cause of 24000 deaths in the United States in 1983 (Catalona and Scott 1986). According to the American Cancer Society, approximately 30000 men will die of this disease in 1990, which makes it second only to carcinoma of the lung as a cause of cancer-related death in American men (American Cancer Society 1990). It has also been predicted that approximately 99000 new cases of CAP will be diagnosed during this period.

Digital rectal examination (DRE) and incidental findings of cancer on histologic examination of tissue following transurethral or open prostatectomy are the most common ways that CAP is detected. Unfortunately, many cancers discovered in this manner are not confined to the prostate. More than 75% of patients have metastatic or locally invasive disease at the time of diagnosis and between 12% and 66% of patients undergoing radical prostatectomy for presumed localized disease have direct extension into the seminal vesicles or periprostatic tissue (Elder et al. 1982; Jewett et al. 1972; Walsh and Jewett 1980). These patients may or may not have symptoms referable to their disease.

Much effort has been dedicated to the development of diagnostic modalities that can aid in the early detection of CAP. When such modalities are employed prior to the appearance of symptoms this is called screening. Most of the present research related to this problem has been directed towards imaging and biochemical studies. This chapter will begin with a review of statistical models used for screening and a discussion of the ideal screening test. Following this, specific screening techniques including DRE, biochemical markers, and transrectal ultrasonography will be addressed.

15.2 Principles of Screening

The detection of a disease process in an asymptomatic individual or population requires the use of some type of test or study. Results of these tests are often reported or compared using statistical terms which relate to the effectiveness of that study in obtaining an early and accurate diagnosis. In order to appreciate fully the concept of screening, the following terms will be defined: sensitivity, specificity, positive predictive value, and negative predictive value.

Sensitivity refers to the number of patients who actually have a disease and test positive divided by the total number of patients with the disease. As it relates to CAP, sensitivity can be mathematically expressed as:

$$\frac{\text{\# of patients with true positive study}}{\text{\# of patients with positive histology}} \times 100$$

Specificity is a term that refers to the number of patients who actually do not have the disease and test negative divided by the total number of patients without the disease. Again relating this

Reid M. Morse, M.D., Resident in Urology, Case Western Reserve University, School of Medicine, Cleveland, OH 44106, USA

Martin I. Resnick, M.D., Lester Persky Professor of Urology, Chairman, Department of Urology, University Hospitals of Cleveland, 2074 Abington Road, Cleveland, OH 44106, USA

to prostate cancer, specificity can be expressed mathematically as:

$$\frac{\text{\# of patients with true negative study}}{\text{\# of patients with negative histology}} \times 100$$

Positive predictive value and negative predictive value are important terms to use as they relate the particular study to disease prevalence. The prevalence of a disease refers to the number of individuals in a specified population who have that disease at one point in time. *Positive predictive value* is the probability that the disease is in fact present given a positive test result. It can be expressed using the data on sensitivity (*Se*), specificity (*Sp*), and prevalence (*P*) as (WATSON and TANG 1980; VECCHIO 1966):

$$\frac{(Se) \times (P)}{(Sp)(P) + (1 - Sp)(1 - P)} \times 100$$

Negative predictive value is the probability that a disease is absent given a negative test result. It can be expressed using similar terms as:

$$\frac{(S)(1 - P)}{(Sp)(1 - P) + (P)(1 - Se)} \times 100$$

With the terminology defined, various issues regarding screening should be addressed. First, it is important to consider the indications for screening and who should be evaluated. For a disease to be suitable for screening the consequences to the health of a population should be serious (LOVE 1985). One way to quantify this is to measure the impact of a disease in terms of mortality or in person and work years of life lost in that population. CAP fits this criterion, being the second most common cause of cancer-related death in American men, although some might claim that its higher incidence among older men makes it less important to productivity than a disease affecting younger men.

Another issue to consider is that of the age of individuals to be included in a screening program. Certainly it is advisable to choose an age range high enough to include a significant number of individuals who might have the disease but not so high as to detect the disease after it has become disseminated. Additionally, the upper limit should not be so high that successful therapy will be negated by a poor general state of health in an individual. Utilizing these principles, the age range for the screening of CAP should probably be from 40 to 75 years, although others may have various reasons to expand or contract this group.

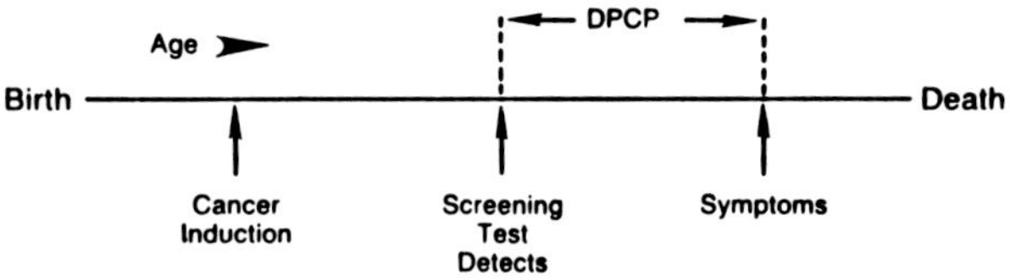

Fig. 15.1. Natural history of a cancer. *DPCP*, detectable preclinical phase

The ability to reduce mortality from CAP through screening is based on the premise that finding the disease in advance of the usual time of detection will permit an alteration in its lethal course. For this concept to be effective, a detectable preclinical phase (DPCP) must exist such that at some point during the natural history of the disease a specific property such as the production of an enzyme or the shedding of cells is recognizable by an available test before the onset of symptoms (Fig. 15.1) (LOVE 1985). Additionally, once the disease is discovered, treatment during the DPCP (also referred to as lead time) must alter the prognosis in a favorable direction (American Cancer Society 1990). Although the natural history of CAP is variable and unpredictable, several limited studies indicate that screening programs potentially improve the cure rates of this malignancy (VIHKO et al. 1985; CHODEK and SCHOENBERG 1984; GUINAN et al. 1980).

The frequent claim that early treatment of cancer prolongs survival is sometimes difficult to prove because the starting point from which survival is measured is nearly always the time when treatment was initiated (SMITH 1985). For this reason the term "length-time bias" has been used and refers to the bias of detecting a disproportionate number of slower growing tumors which take longer to surface. In order to avoid fundamental errors in interpreting true survival benefit, survival needs to be measured from the time of diagnosis and not simply from the start of therapy.

Lastly, it is important to determine the optimal interval at which a screening test should be utilized. This decision should not only reflect the concept of length-time bias but also take into consideration economic factors. Models which show the relationship between cost of the screening program and lives saved per patient screened are shown in Fig. 15.2. The purpose of this illustration is to describe how to achieve the goal of lowering mortality from a cancer with the greatest return per unit of monetary investment (LOVE 1985).

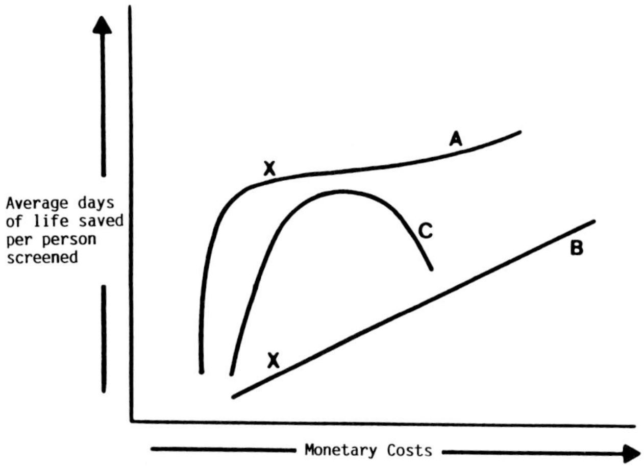

Fig. 15.2. Cost-effectiveness curves for hypothetical screening program

Three hypothetical cancer screening programs are shown. It is apparent that for the same financial investment per person the average number of days of life saved by screening for cancer A is greater than the average saved by screening for cancer B. For cancer A, a point (X) is reached beyond which increased frequency (and cost) of screening results in only a minimal increase in days of life saved. This would be a cost-effective position to operate a screening program for cancer A. Further input into this program would obviously be nonproductive. This curve might fit CAP because if more and more patients were to be detected and subsequently treated, a point would eventually be reached at which many patients whose lives would not be affected by the disease would undergo therapy. For cancer B increasing cost continues to show increased days of life saved. The third model demonstrates how increasing costs and test frequency can have a negative effect and actually result in decreased days of life saved. This might be seen in a program where the submission of greater numbers of cytologic specimens to detect bladder or cervical cancer would result in increased misreading and improper diagnosis. Additionally, if the morbidity and mortality of evaluation and treatment exceed those associated with the natural course of the untreated disease, this type of curve would be seen. This curve theoretically could also represent CAP. Although it may sound callous to judge screening programs in terms of cost- and risk-benefits, these are real considerations and their estimation should be required when programs are being assessed. For CAP a yearly examination in men aged 40–75 years does not seem unreasonable.

15.3 The Ideal Screening Test

The ideal test for screening a population to detect potentially curable disease would have several features. Most would agree that such a test should be noninvasive, inexpensive, rapid, objective, reproducible, reliable, and well accepted by patients. For example, an especially desirable test would be one which utilizes an easily obtainable body fluid such as serum, urine, or prostatic secretions. Ideally, the test should have both a high sensitivity and a high specificity and also be reliable in predicting either the presence or absence of the disease in a specific population. In general, a test with a higher specificity is preferable to one with a higher sensitivity, as small decrements in specificity may cause large numbers of false-positive results and lead to unnecessary and more invasive testing (Thompson 1987). It has been suggested by some authors that to be acceptable a cancer screening test should have a sensitivity of at least 95% and a specificity of 100% (Galen and Galimbo 1975).

Another concern has to do with the ability to determine the biologic potential of a discovered cancer. In the case of CAP a spectrum of disease exists, ranging from a malignant potential so great that metastases are present prior to the onset of local signs or symptoms, to cases so indolent that they remain dormant for the duration of the patient's life. Those patients in the former category require further evaluation and therapy while those in the latter would neither benefit from nor require other therapeutic approaches. McNeal and associates (1986) have shown in a recent autopsy study that 1 cm of tumor volume was associated with the capacity to metastasize and that tumors of smaller volume did not appear to have acquired this ability. They suggest that further growth and the development of poor differentiation by the tumor affect the ability to metastasize and believe that a tumor volume of 1 cm is the critical size that must be detected by a screening program if it is to be of value. Others have not quantified this volume as accurately but agree that there appears to be an increased propensity for local and distant spread as tumor volume increases (Cantrell et al. 1981).

Regarding the high incidence of CAP with advancing age, it has been stated that more people die *with* the disease than *of* the disease. Because the biologic potential of small tumors is not known, it is not clear who will benefit from treatment and who should be left alone. It is certainly possible that the morbidity of treatment (radical prostatectomy, radiation therapy) may be greater than the morbidity of the disease and this is especially important in the older population.

To date there is no consensus as to the one ideal screening test for CAP nor is it entirely clear as to what is needed (GRAYHACK and BOCKRATH 1981). The remainder of this chapter will be devoted to the discussion of specific screening studies dealing with physical findings, laboratory determinations, and imaging.

15.4 Rectal Examination

Digital rectal examination (DRE) provides information regarding the size, consistency, symmetry, and heterogeneity of the prostate. It is well recognized that routine use of this examination is associated with the early detection of CAP, and for these reasons DRE remains the single most important step in the physical examination for detecting CAP (VAN BUSKIRK and KIMBROUGH 1954; KIMBROUGH and ROWE 1951). With this in mind, however, it is interesting that DRE is not universally accepted as a screening modality for CAP and that the value and frequency of the examination have yet to be clearly established (VIHKO et al. 1985; CHODAK and SCHOENBERG 1984; LEE et al. 1992; SCHHIDT 1992).

The actions of many clinicians are guided by the observation that a hard prostate or prostatic nodule often represents cancer and that biopsy is the next step in establishing a diagnosis. The shortcoming of this approach is that the physical findings of many benign conditions such as benign prostatic hyperplasia, acute and chronic prostatitis, calculi, granulomatous disease, prostatic infarcts, periprostatic venous thrombosis, and hormonal influences leading to squamous metaplasia can mimic those found in cancer (GRABSTALD 1965). Prostatic nodules that are found to be malignant may be adenocarcinoma, squamous cell carcinoma, transitional cell carcinoma, sarcoma, lymphoma, or metastatic tumors.

Studies performed several decades ago showed that approximately one-half of patients with prostatic nodules or indurated areas of the prostate have cancer and that there is little or no correlation between the clinical impression as determined by rectal palpation and the results of the pathologic report from biopsy (JEWETT 1956; EMMETT et al. 1962; GOLDSTEIN and WEINBERG 1954; BARNES and OKAMATO 1961). More recently, investigators have stated that the specificity of DRE is 29% (CHODAK and SCHOENBERG 1984). However, what is presented as the specificity of the test is actually the positive predictive value of rectal examination in the detection of CAP in asymptomatic men (Letters to the editor 1984). Utilization of the formulas presented earlier in this chapter reveals that the 11 cancers found among the 38 men with positive rectal examinations represent a positive predictive value of 29%.

An additional problem with DRE is related to the location of malignancies within the prostate. For many years it was taught that carcinoma arose from the posterior lobe of the gland, which is adjacent to the rectum. It is now readily accepted that most carcinomas (70%) arise in the peripheral zone of the gland but that 30% have their origin in the anterior portion of the prostate, which is not as accessible to the examining finger and may be missed by this method (ANSELL 1982; STAMEY TA, personal communication).

The positive predictive values and negative predictive values of DRE range from 11% to 29% and from 85% to 95% respectively, based on varying prevalence rates. These data refer to the unlikely chance of having CAP with a negative rectal examination while only one to three men out of ten with a positive rectal examination will be found to have CAP. Despite these problems a carefully performed annual DRE remains an efficient and cost-effective approach when attempting to detect CAP at an early and curable stage.

15.5 Tumor Markers: Prostatic Acid Phosphatase and Prostatic Specific Antigen

Recognized chemical markers for CAP exist in serum, urine, and prostatic fluid and are routinely measured by means of biochemical and immunologic methods (BAN et al. 1984; SCHACHT et al. 1984). Though many of these substances contribute to the diagnosis, staging, and assessment of treatment and follow-up evaluations of patients with CAP, their role in screening has been limited due to high false-positive rates inherent to the study. The two most popular markers in use, prostatic acid phosphatase and prostatic specific antigen, will be discussed.

Acid phosphatase enzymes are found in erythrocytes, platelets, osteoclasts, bile, and prostate in high concentrations and can manifest elevations in Gaucher's and Paget's disease, hyperthyroidism, CAP, and benign prostatic hypertrophy. Prostatic acid phosphatase is produced in the acinar cells of the gland and is secreted into the seminal fluid by the ductal system. The small amount that is absorbed into the circulation can be detected by a relatively simple enzymatic assay as well as a more recently used immunoassay known as a radioimmunoassay (RIA). Each type of assay is fraught with unique problems as the RIA has a high false-positive rate and a minor elevation or high normal level measured by the enzymatic assay may indicate metastatic disease (Bahnson and Catalona 1987; Whitesel et al. 1984).

Prostatic acid phosphatase has been used in the evaluation and follow-up of patients with metastatic CAP since the 1940s. It was later suggested that this marker might be valuable in the detection of cancer confined to the prostate but studies have shown that this test does not predict all patients with stage A disease and that 6% of men with benign prostatic hyperplasia test positive (Foti et al. 1978; Fleischmann et al. 1983; Carroll 1978). Assuming CAP to have a disease prevalence rate of 30%, the reported values of sensitivity and specificity of prostatic acid phosphatase in the literature can be used to calculate a positive predictive value approaching 63% and a negative predictive value of 94%. Watson and Tang (1980) have calculated that the positive predictive value of the test in the absence of a prostatic nodule falls within the range of approximately 30%. These data argue against the use of prostatic acid phosphatase as a screening test for the early detection of CAP (Flam et al. 1992; Littrup et al. 1992).

A prostatic specific antigen (PSA) was isolated in 1979 by injecting crude extracts of human prostatic tissue into rabbits. Like prostatic acid phosphatase, this antigen has been extensively studied as a marker for CAP. Although it has been shown to be useful in detecting recurrent and residual disease following radical prostatectomy, radiation therapy, or bilateral orchiectomy, PSA has not been universally accepted as a marker for the selection of men with cancer confined to the prostate (Stamey et al. 1987; Oesterling et al. 1988; Perimenis 1992). It has been shown by both the Yang and Hybritech assays that PSA can be elevated in patients who have benign prostatic hyperplasia, thereby limiting the role of this test as a useful screening modality (Marden and Williams 1987).

Recently Catalona and associates (1991) reexamined the issue of using PSA to detect occult CAP. PSA levels were drawn from 1653 healthy men and compared to a control group of 300 individuals. Their results indicated that rectal examination and transrectal ultrasonography yielded increases in the ability to predict cancer but that PSA level as an independent predictor of cancer provided the highest positive predictive value of the three tests.

15.6 Transrectal Ultrasonography

Early success in transrectal ultrasonography of the prostate was achieved by Watanabe and Katoh in 1968. As technology in this area improved, other investigators began working with transabdominal and transurethral ultrasonography to visualize the prostate but it was determined that transrectal ultrasonography was superior to these modalities in providing the most consistent and reproducible images of the prostate (Henneberry et al. 1979; Holm and Northeved 1974). Recently, transrectal ultrasonography of the prostate has proven to be useful in the preoperative staging of patients with localized CAP although microscopic invasion of the capsule cannot be delineated (Cohen and Resnick 1983; Pontes et al. 1985; Hamper et al. 1991; Egender et al. 1986). Even impalpable cancers may be identified by transrectal ultrasonography (Lee et al. 1991; Sheth et al. 1991). This technique has also been credited as being useful in the documentation of the response of CAP to orchiectomy, radiation therapy, and the administration of estrogens (Carpenter et al. 1986; Fujimo and Scardino 1985, 1986).

The major controversy regarding transrectal ultrasonography of the prostate has to do with its application as a screening technique for carcinoma (Chang and Friedland 1990). Several investigators, including Watanabe and Lee, have been proponents of its use in this manner but others have not advocated its use in this regard (FUJIMO and SCARDINO 1986; WATANABE et al. 1984; LEE et al. 1985; RESNICK 1985). The problem with the application of this study in the early detection of CAP is related to the low sensitivity and specificity of the examination. Benign and malignant disorders of the prostate are often difficult if not impossible to differentiate and may occur simultaneously.

Early studies with this technique characterized carcinomas as areas of increased echogenicity (WATANABE and KATOH 1968; KING et al. 1973; RESNICK et al. 1977, 1980). With the advent of newer instrumentation and higher frequency transducers, many investigators have shown that CAP appears only as hypoechoic areas while others have shown that these tumors are hyperechoic, hypoechoic, isoechoic, or of mixed echogenicity (LEE et al. 1985; RIFKIN et al. 1986; DANHERT et al. 1986).

The observation that many benign conditions such as nodules of benign prostatic hyperplasia, prostatitis, prostatic cysts, and blood vessels perforating the prostatic capsule will mimic the echo changes seen with carcinoma adds to the difficulty in interpretation (DANHERT et al. 1986; RESNICK 1980). It is also important to recognize that stage A2 carcinomas cannot be visualized with reliability (SHETH et al. 1991). This problem was made evident by the finding of diffuse carcinoma in patients having undergone simple prostatectomy for presumed benign disease in the presence of normal preoperative ultrasonographic examinations (RESNICK 1980; RESNICK et al. 1980). Because up to one-third of CAPs arise anteriorly, a region not well visualized by transrectal ultrasonography, these cancers may not be discovered by this modality while at a small and potentially curable stage (MCNEAL et al. 1988).

Utilizing data from various studies, the sensitivity and specificity of transrectal ultrasonography have been reported to average 71% and 85% respectively. Assuming a disease prevalence of 30%, this yields a positive predictive value of approximately 36% and a negative predictive value of 93%. These figures are not significantly different from those for DRE. For this reason it appears that the added gain from screening a population with transrectal ultrasonography is not worth the time and expense because the additional useful information is minimal to nonexistent (CHANG and FRIEDLAND 1990). A recent report by CHANCELLOR and associates (1987) addressed this problem utilizing state of the art transrectal ultrasonography. Of the 53 men found to have benign prostatic hyperplasia, 23 (43.4%) had preoperative ultrasonograms which were suggestive of carcinoma. Ultrasonographic findings were consistent with malignancy in only one patient who had histologic evidence of cancer. Utilizing these data, the sensitivity and specificity can be calculated as 8.3% and 56.6% respectively and the positive predictive value is below 5%. In another study only 29% of men with ultrasonographically suspicious prostatic examinations were found to have cancer (COONER et al. 1988). Again, it is the high rate of false-positive and false-negative examinations obtained with current ultrasonographic instrumentation that negates the application of this study in the screening for CAP.

In an effort to compare the clinical usefulness of transrectal ultrasonography and DRE in a screening program for CAP, LEE and associates (1988) examined 784 self-referred men over 60 years of age. Biopsy was performed on the basis of the findings on ultrasonography and/or digital examinations. The overall detection rate for CAP was found to be two times higher with ultrasonography than with DRE and the sensitivity of the former was reported as two times higher than that of the latter. In reality, sensitivity cannot be determined because healthy patients did not undergo biopsy. Also the reported positive predictive values for transrectal ultrasonography and DRE of 31% and 34% respectively are not statistically significant and are in fact in line with those reported by other authors (SEIDMAN et al. 1987). Furthermore, because one out of every ten blind biopsies in this age group would be positive by chance alone, the transrectal ultrasonography group would be expected to yield more positive biopsies simply on the basis that twice as many biopsies were performed compared to the other group.

COONER and associates (1990) have demonstrated that the combination of DRE, PSA, and transrectal ultrasonography could increase the success of screening from 1.7% to 14.6%. They did not, however, conclude that routine ultrasonography should be utilized for screening in men less than 64 years of age if the DRE and PSA level were normal. The reason for this is the very low rate of cancer detected in this group.

15.7 Magnetic Resonance Imaging

The role of magnetic resonance imaging in the diagnosis and screening of CAP is as yet not well defined. However, the modality adds additional parameters to staging of the disease (THICKMAN et al. 1990). The recently introduced innovation of an endorectal surface coil for magnetic resonance imaging of the prostate promises to improve further our ability for finite assessment of tumor extension and hence staging (SCHNALL et al. 1989, 1991; TEMPANY et al. 1991).

15.8 Conclusion

The ability to detect CAP in an asymptomatic population at an early and curable stage is an appealing prospect. At the present time noninvasive imaging modalities and biochemical markers are not useful for this purpose due to the poor sensitivity, specificity, and predictive values of these techniques. Falsely positive tests are often followed by anxiety on the part of the patient and family and the use of extensive and invasive investigations by the physician. Falsely negative values result in a delay in diagnosis.

More carefully designed clinical studies are needed to evaluate the future of transrectal ultrasonography of the prostate as well as any test deemed useful in the screening for CAP. If a lesson can be learned from colleagues studying the value of routine mammography as a means of detecting breast cancer in women, it is that large numbers of patients should be investigated and with good follow-up in order to make sound recommendations. The American Cancer Society has recently reported data relating to this issue in which 280000 women were studied and followed up to 11 (LEE et al. 1988). These concerns regarding CAP are recognized and three cooperative studies are currently either in progress or are being planned that will hopefully provide answers regarding which test is most beneficial, the optimal screening frequency (e.g., semiannually, annually, biannually), and which population should be studied (e.g., age, race).

At the present time screening for early detection of CAP is best done with yearly digital rectal examinations on all men greater than 40 years of age. This represents the most efficient and cost-effective approach when attempting to diagnose the disease at an early and curable stage. It does not seem unreasonable to screen a population of men between the ages of 40 and 75 on a yearly basis. Such a practice should yield a significant group of men who would be cured of their disease by either radiotherapy or radical prostatectomy.

References

American Cancer Society (1990) Cancer Statistics for 1990. 40:9

Ansell ID (1982) Histopathology of prostatic cancer. In: Chisholm GD, Williams DI (eds) Scientific foundations of urology. Year Book Medical, New York, pp 737–752

Bahnson RR, Catalona WJ (1987) Adverse implications of acid phosphatase levels in the upper range of normal. J Urol 137:427–430

Ban Y, Wang MC, Chu TM (1984) Immunologic markers and the diagnosis of prostate cancer. Urol Clin North Am 11:269

Barnes RW, Okamato S (1961) Diagnosis of prostatic carcinoma: a statistical study. West J Surg 9:362

Cantrell BB, Deklerk DP, Eggleston JC (1981) Pathological factors that influence prognosis in stage A prostatic cancer. J Urol 125:516

Carpentier PJ, Schroeder FH, Schmitz PIM (1986) Transrectal ultrasonography of the prostate: the prognostic relevance of volume changes under endocrine management. WJ Urol 4:159

Carroll BJ (1978) Radioimmunoassay of prostatic acid phosphatase in carcinoma of the prostate. N Engl J Med 298:912

Catalona WJ, Scott WW (1986) Carcinoma of the prostate. In: Walsh PC, Gittes RE, Perlmutter AD, Stamey TA (eds) Campbell's urology. W.B. Saunders, Philadelphia, pp 1463–1534

Catalona WJ, Smith DS, Ratliff TL et al. (1991) Measurement of prostatic specific antigen in serum as a screening test for prostate cancer. N Engl J Med 324:1156–1161

Chancellor MB, McHugh TA, Dorr RP, VanAppledorn CA (1987) Transrectal prostate ultrasonography before transurethral prostatectomy, its value for screening stage A cancer (abstr). J Urol 137:241A

Chang P, Friedland GW (1990) The role of imaging in screening for prostate cancer: a decision analysis perspective. Invest Radiol 25:591–595

Chodak GW, Schoenberg HW (1984) Early detection of prostatic cancer by routine screening. JAMA 252: 3261–3264

Cohen JM, Resnick MI (1983) The use of transrectal ultrasonography in the diagnosis of stage A prostatic carcinoma. West J Urol 1:12

Cooner WH, Mosley BR, Rutherford CL Jr, Beard JH, Pond HS, Bass RB Jr, Terry WJ (1988) Clinical application of transrectal ultrasonography and prostate specific antigen in the search for prostate cancer. J Urol 139:758–761

Cooner WH, Mosely BR, Rutherford CL et al. (1990) Prostate cancer detection in a clinical urological practice by ultrasonography, digital rectal examination and prostate specific antigen. J Urol 143:1146

Danhert WF, Hamper UM, Eggleston JC, Walsh PC, Sanders PC (1986) Prostatic evaluation by transrectal sonography with histopathologic correlation: carcinoma. Radiology 158:97

Egender G, Furtschegger A, Schachtner W, Parker E, Bartsch G (1986) Transrectal ultrasonography in diagnosis and staging of prostatic cancer. W J Urol 4:163

Elder JS, Jewett HJ, Walsh PC (1982) Radical perineal prostatectomy for clinical stage B2 carcinoma of the prostate. J Urol 127:704–706

Emmett JL, Barber KW Jr, Jackman RJ (1962) Transrectal biopsy to detect prostatic carcinoma: a review and report of 203 cases. J Urol 87:460

Fleischmann J, Catalona WJ, Fair WR, Heston WDW, Menon M (1983) Lack of value of radioimmunoassay for prostatic acid phosphatase as a screening test for prostatic cancer in patients with obstructive prostatic hyperplasia. J Urol 129:312–314

Flam TA, Brawer MK, Cooper EH, Javadpour N (1992) Diagnosis and markers in prostatic cancer. Cancer 70:357–358

Foti AG, Cooper JF, Herschman H, Malvaez RR (1978) Detection of prostatic cancer by solid-phase radioimmunoassay of serum prostatic acid phosphatase. N Engl J Med 289:912

Fujimo A, Scardino PT (1985) Transrectal ultrasonography for prostatic cancer: its value in staging and monitoring the response to radiotherapy and chemotherapy. J Urol 133:806

Fujimo A, Scardino PT (1986) Transrectal ultrasonography for prostatic cancer. II. The response of the prostate to definitive radiotherapy. Cancer 57:935

Galen RS, Galimbo SR (1975) Beyond normality: the predictive value and efficiency of medical diagnosis. John Wiley, New York, p 80

Goldstein AE, Weinberg T (1954) The importance of correct diagnosis of carcinoma of prostate: clinical application. Am Surg 20:971

Grabstald H (1965) The clinical and laboratory diagnosis of cancer of the prostate. Cancer 15:76

Grayhack JT, Bockrath JM (1981) Diagnosis of carcinoma of prostate. Urology 27:54–60 [Suppl, March]

Guinan P, Bush I, Ray V, Vieth R, Rao R, Bhatti R (1980) The accuracy of the rectal examination in the differential diagnosis of prostate carcinoma. N Engl J Med 303:499–503

Hamper UM, Sheth S, Walsh PC, Holtz PM, Epstein JI (1991) Capsular transgression of prostatic carcinoma: evaluation with transrectal ultrasound with pathologic correlation. Radiology 178:791–796

Henneberry M, Carter MF, Neiman HL (1979) Estimation of prostatic size by suprapubic ultrasonography. J Urol 121:615

Holm NH, Northeved A (1974) A transurethral ultrasonic scanner. J Urol 111:238

Jewett HJ (1956) Significance of the palpable nodule. JAMA 160:838

Jewett JH, Eggleston JC, Yawn DH (1972) Radical prostatectomy in the management of cancer of the prostate: probable causes of some therapeutic failures. J Urol 107:1034–1040

Kimbrough JC, Rowe RB (1951) Carcinoma of the prostate. J Urol 66:373

King WW, Wilkiemeyer RM, Boyce WH, McKinney WM (1973) Current status of prostatic echography. JAMA 266:444

Lee F, Gray JM, McLeary RD et al. (1985) Transrectal ultrasound in the diagnosis of prostate cancer: location, echogenicity, histopathology and staging. Prostate 7: 117–129

Lee F, Littrup PJ, Torp-Pederson ST et al. (1988) Prostate cancer: comparison of transrectal US and digital rectal examination for screening. Radiology 168:389–394

Lee F Jr, Bronson JP, Lee F, Torp-Pedersen S, Siders DB, Thornbury JR, McHugn TA (1991) Nonpalpable cancer of the prostate: assessment by transrectal ultrasound. Radiology 178:197–200

Lee F, Torp-Pedersan S, Cooner W, Drago J, Holtgrewel, Littrup P, Resnick H (1992) Detection and screening for prostate carcinoma. Cancer 70:355–356

Lee F, Littrup PJ, Loft-Christensen L, Kelly BS Jr, McHugh TA (1992) Predicted prostate specific antigen: Results using transrectal ultrasound gland volume. Differentiation of benign prostatic hyperplasia and prostatic carcinoma. Cancer 70:211–220

Schmidt JD (1992) Clinical diagnosis of prostatic cancer. Cancer 70:221–224

Letters to the editor (1984) Problematic prostatic prediction. JAMA 254:1171–1173

Littrup PJ, Lee F, Mettlin C (1992) Prostate cancer screening: current trends and future implication. Ca Cancer J Clin 42:198–211.

Love RL (1985) Principles of cancer screening. In: Stoll BA (ed) Screening and monitoring of cancer. John Wiley, Chichester, pp 3–17

Marden A, Williams RD (1987) Comparison of two commercially available immunoassays for serum prostatic specific antigen (abstr). Presented at North Central Section, American Urological Association, Detroit, Michigan

McNeal JE, Kindrachuk RA, Freiha FS, Bostwick DG, Redwine EA, Stamey TA (1986) Patterns of progression in prostate cancer. Lancet I:60–63

McNeal JE, Price HM, Redwine EA, Freiha FS, Stamey TA (1988) Stage A versus stage B adenocarcinoma of the prostate: morphological comparison and biological significance. J Urol 139:61–65

Oesterling JE, Chan DW, Epstein JI et al. (1988) Prostatic specific antigen in the preoperative and postoperative evaluation of localized prostatic cancer treated with radical prostatectomy. J Urol 139:766–772

Pontes JE, Eisenkraft S, Watanabe H, Ohe H, Saitoh M, Murphy GP (1985) Preoperative evaluation of localized prostatic carcinoma by transrectal ultrasonography. J Urol 134:289

Resnick MI (1980) Evaluation of prostatic carcinoma: non-invasive and reoperative techniques. Prostate 1: 311–320

Resnick MI (1985) Use of transrectal ultrasound in evaluating prostatic cancer. J Urol 134:314

Resnick MI, Willard JW, Boyce WH (1977) Recent progress in ultrasonography of the bladder and prostate. J Urol 117:444

Resnick MI, Willard JW, Boyce WH (1980) Transrectal ultrasonography in the evaluation of patients with prostatic carcinoma. J Urol 124:482–484

Perimenis P, Markou SA, Barbalias G (1992) Prostate-specific antigen test: operating characteristics and assessment criteria in the diagnosis of prostatic cancer. Urol Int 48(2):171–174

Rifkin MD, Friedland GW, Shortliffe L (1986) Prostatic evaluation by transrectal endosonography: detection of carcinoma. Radiology 158:85

Schacht MJ, Garnett JE, Grayhack JT (1984) Biochemical markers in prostatic cancer. Urol Clin North Am 11:253

Schnall MD, Lenkinski RE, Pollack HM, Imai Y, Kressel HY (1989) Prostate: MR imaging with an endorectal surface coil. Radiology 172:570–574

Schnall MD, Imai Y, Tomaszewski J, Pollack HM, Lenkinski RE, Kressel HY (1991) Prostate cancer: local staging with endorectal surface coil MR imaging. Radiology 178:797–802

Seidman H, Gelb SK, Silverberg E, LaVerda N, Lubera JA (1987) The breast clinic detection demonstration project end results. CA 37:258–290

Sheth S, Hamper UM, Walsh PC, Holtz PM, Epstein JI (1991) Stage A adenocarcinoma of the prostate: transrectal ultrasound and pathologic correlation. Radiology 179:35–40

Smith IE (1985) Assessing effect of treatment on survival. In: Stoll BA (ed) Screening and monitoring of cancer. John Wiley, Chichester, pp 335–353

Stamey TA, Yang M, Hay AR, McNeal JE, Freiha FS, Redwine E (1987) Prostatic specific antigen as a serum marker for adenocarcinoma of the prostate. N Engl J Med 317:909–915

Tempany CM, Rahmouni AD, Epstein JI, Walsh PC, Cerhouni EA (1991) Invasion of the neurovascular bundle by prostatic carcinoma: evaluation with MR imaging. Radiology 181:17–112

Thickman D, Miller GJ, Hopper KD, Raife M (1990) Prostate cancer: comparison of preoperative 0.35 T MRI with whole-mount histopathology. Magn Reson Imaging 8:205–211

Thompson IM (1987) The early detection of genitourinary neoplasms. AUA Update Series. Lesson 26, vol 6

vanBuskirk KE, Kimbrough JC (1954) Carcinoma of the prostate. J Urol 71:742

Vecchio TJ (1966) Predictive value of a single diagnostic test in unselected populations. NEJM 274:1171–1173

Vihko P, Kontturi M, Lukkarinen O, Ervasti J, Vihko R (1985) Screening for carcinoma of the prostate. Rectal examination and enzymatic and radioimmunologic measurements of serum acid phosphatase compared. Cancer 56:173–177

Walsh PC, Jewett HJ (1980) Radical surgery for prostate cancer. Cancer 45:1906–1911

Watanabe H, Katoh H (1968) Diagnostic application of the ultrasonography of the prostate. J Urol 59:279

Watanabe H, Ohe H, Inabe T, Itakura Y, Saitoh M, Nakao M (1984) A mobile mass screening unit for prostatic disease. Prostate 5:559–565

Watson RA, Tang DB (1980) The predictive value of prostatic acid phosphatase as a screening test for prostatic cancer. N Engl J Med 303:497–499

Whitesel JA, Donohue RE, Mani JH et al. (1984) Acid phosphatase: its influence on the management of carcinoma of the prostate. J Urol 131:70–72

16 Neurogenic Disease and Incontinence: Physiology, Pathophysiology, Diagnostic Imaging, and Urodynamic Studies

GERALD W. FRIEDLAND, INDER PERKASH, and GEORGE M. SEGALL

CONTENTS

Neuromuscular dysfunction of the bladder and urethra is common; it has been estimated that the prevalence in adults of various forms of dysfunction may be as high as 10% (FRIEDLAND and PERKASH 1983). The principal reason for this relatively high figure is that neuromuscular bladder dysfunction can be caused by common diseases, including, for example, diabetes mellitus, cerebrovascular disease, Alzheimer's disease, and Parkinson's disease (DENNIS et al. 1991; LOSE and COLSTRUP 1991; O'DONNELL and BECK 1991; LOSE 1991; VAN GOOL et al. 1992). It is not sufficiently realized, however, how frequent this problem has become with drug therapy. Figure 16.1 illustrates commonly used drugs that can contract or relax the detrusor and urethra. It should be noted that this list includes common drugs like antidepressants and those used for cardiovascular disease, such as β-blockers and calcium channel blockers. As these drugs are now used very widely, it is not surprising that side-effects in the urinary tract occur more often. Unfortunately, such side-effects are frequently not immediately recognized.

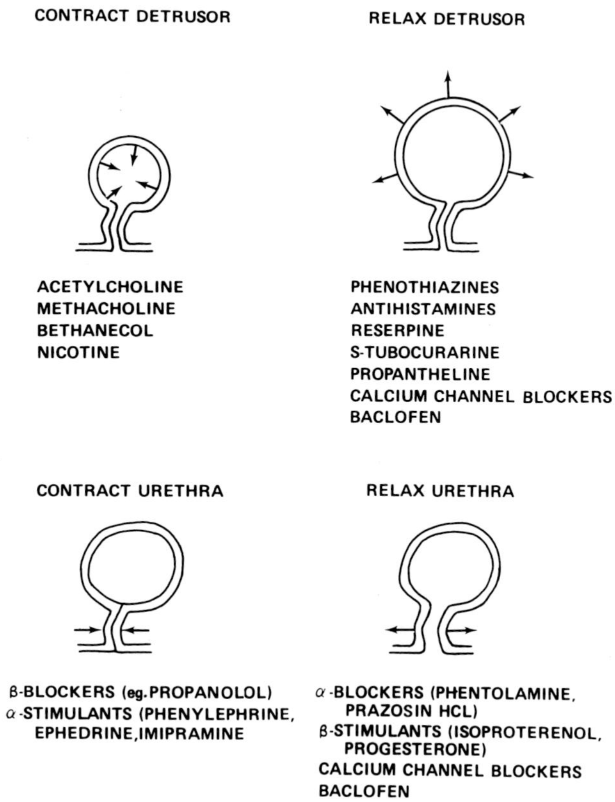

Fig. 16.1. Effect of drugs on the detrusor and urethra

GERALD W. FRIEDLAND, M.D., Chief, Radiology Service; INDER PERKASH, M.D., Chief, Spinal Cord Injury Service; GEORGE M. SEGALL, M.D., Assistant Chief, Nuclear Medicine Service; Veterans Administration Medical Center, 3801 Miranda Avenue, Palo Alto, CA 94304, USA

In discussing neurogenic disease and incontinence it is important to bear in mind the relevant anatomy of the lower urinary tract.

16.1 Anatomy

16.1.1 Muscles

Normally, the wall of the entire bladder, the bladder neck, and the upper half of the prostatic urethra in the male and the upper half of the urethra in the female contains smooth muscle, whereas the wall of the lower half of the urethra in the female and the lower half of the prostatic urethra in the male also contains striated muscle (Fig. 16.2). There may be significant normal variations in this ratio, however; in some individuals, the muscular wall of the entire urethra is striated, for example.

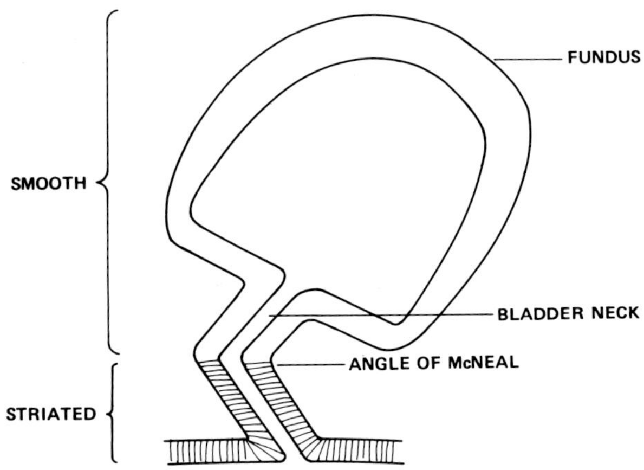

Fig. 16.2. Distribution of smooth and striated muscle

16.1.2 Neural Control

Neural control involves both the central nervous system and the peripheral nerves.

16.1.2.1 Central Control

The pathways in the central nervous system are complex, and controversial with regard to which central pathways control the bladder and urethra. As illustrated in Fig. 16.3, however, there is some agreement as to the basics, namely that there is a frontal cortical center, a pontine center, and a sacral cord or conal center, with afferent and efferent pathways between each center.

16.1.2.2 Peripheral Control

The peripheral control involves three different groups of nerves:

1. The *parasympathetic nerve supply* arises from the anterior columns at S3 (Tanagho and Schmidt 1982); the nerve endings secrete acetylcholine, which contracts the detrusor during voiding (Fig. 16.4).

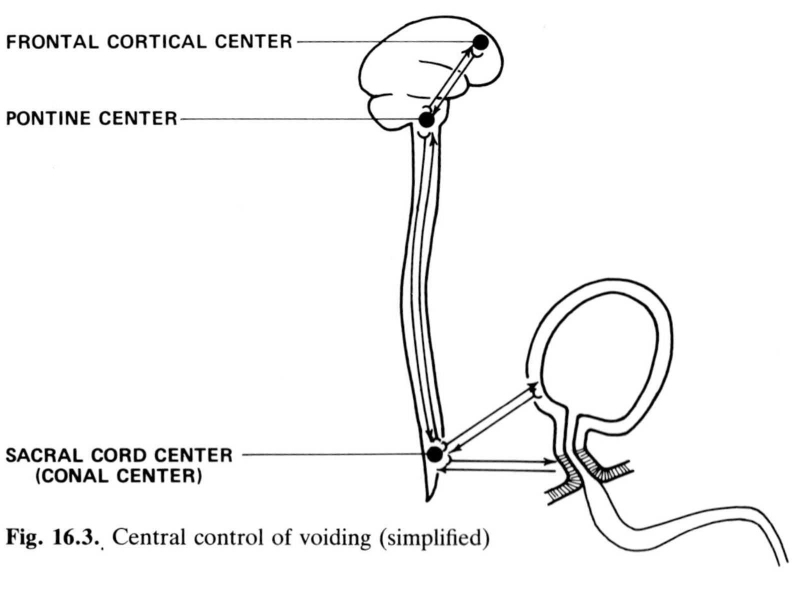

Fig. 16.3. Central control of voiding (simplified)

2. *The pudendal nerves* arise from the anterior columns of S2 and supply the periurethral striated sphincter and the urogenital diaphragm (Fig. 16.5) (AMIS and BLAIVAS 1990).
3. *The sympathetic nerve supply* arise from the anterior gray columns of T11-L2 (FRIEDLAND and PERKASH 1983). The nerve endings produce norepinephrine during bladder filling, the effect of which is different in different parts of the bladder (Fig. 16.6). The fundus, for example, has β-adrenergic receptors, so norepinephrine relaxes the fundus as the bladder fills. The bladder neck, on the other hand, has α-adrenergic receptors, so norepinephrine contracts the bladder neck during bladder filling.

Relative Distribution of the Peripheral Nerve Supply. The above description of the peripheral nerve supply to the bladder is somewhat oversimplified. The detrusor has β-adrenergic receptors and a cholinergic nerve supply, whereas the bladder neck has primarily α-adrenergic receptors, although it does have some β-adrenergic receptors and a cholinergic nerve supply as well. The urethra has both α- and β-adrenergic receptors and a cholinergic nerve supply (Fig. 16.7) (FRIEDLAND and PERKASH 1983). This multiple supply may explain why, during voiding, there is perfect synergy in the lower urinary tract, as first the periurethral striated sphincter relaxes, then the detrusor contracts and the bladder neck opens (Fig. 16.8) (FRIEDLAND and PERKASH 1983). Any disturbance in this perfect synergy is called dyssynergia.

16.2 Investigation

Neuromuscular dysfunction of the lower urinary tract can be investigated using plain radiography, an intravenous urogram, a cystogram, the voiding cystourethrogram, the dynamic retrograde urethrogram, ultrasound, computed tomography, magnetic resonance imaging, urodynamic studies, and scintigraphy. Currently, the most widely used studies are urodynamic studies, ultrasonography,

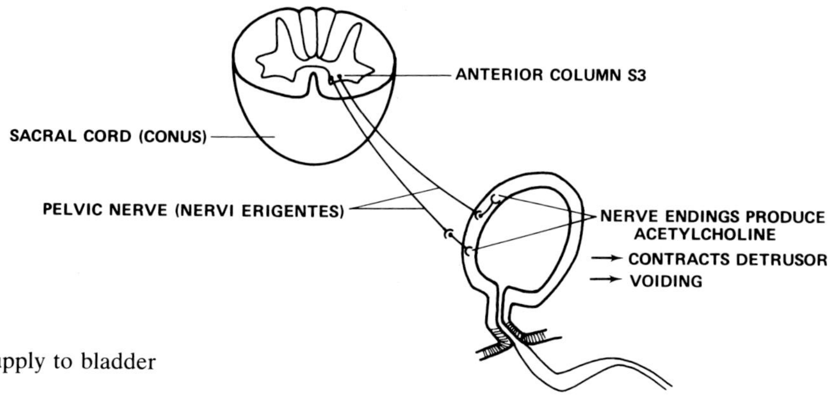

Fig. 16.4. Parasympathetic nerve supply to bladder

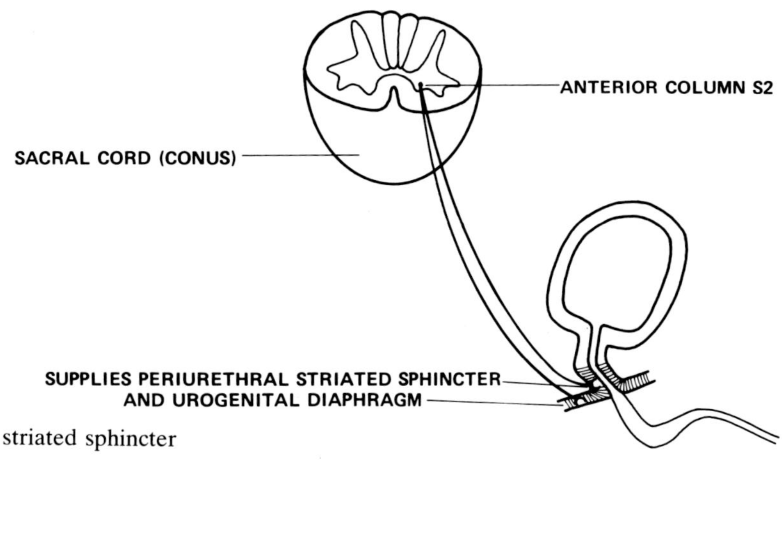

Fig. 16.5. Nerve supply of periurethral striated sphincter and urogenital diaphragm

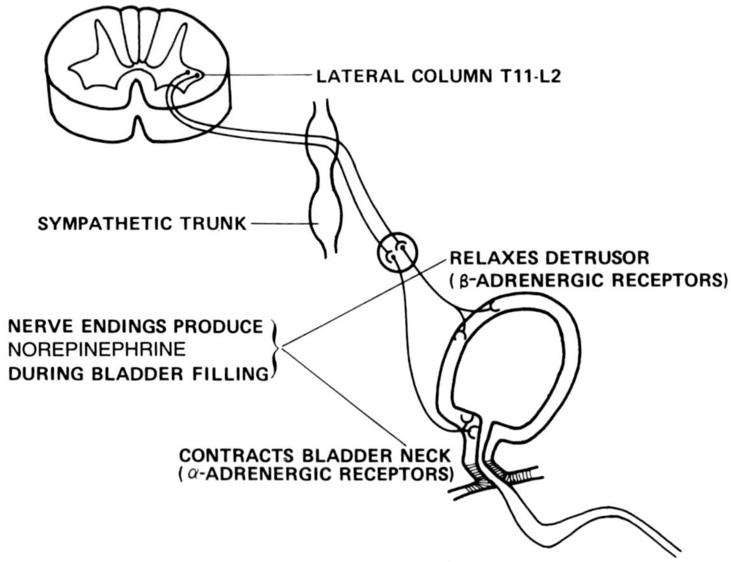

Fig. 16.6. Sympathetic nerve supply to the bladder

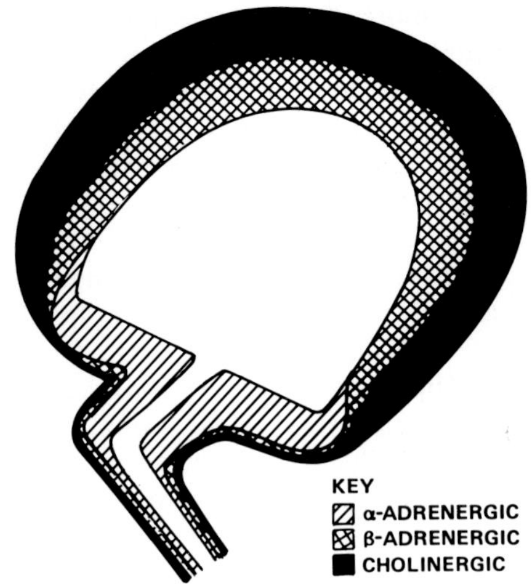

Fig. 16.7. Relative distribution of the peripheral nerve supply

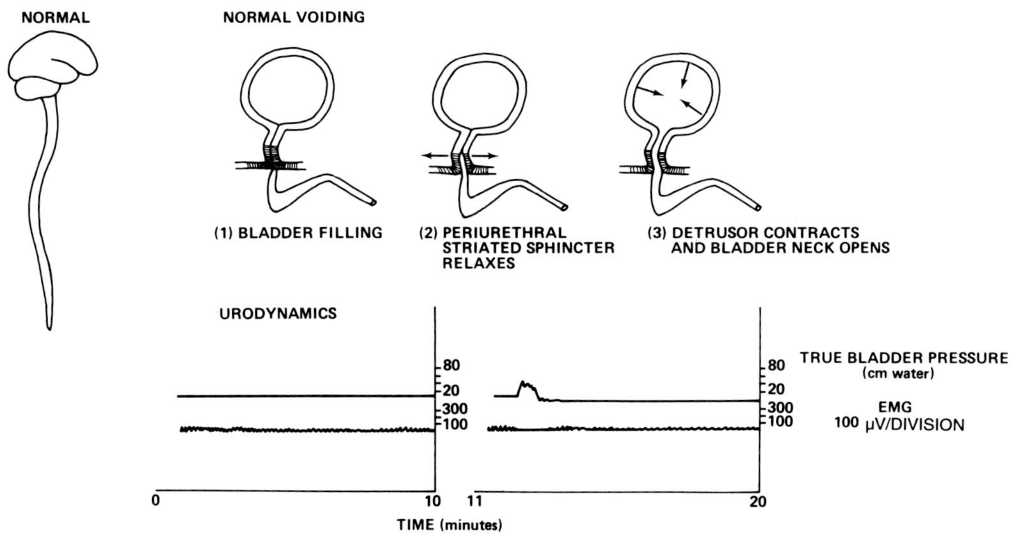

Fig. 16.8. Normal voiding: physiologic events and urodynamic findings

the voiding cystourethrogram, the intravenous urogram, and scintigraphy (AMIS and BLAIVAS 1990). For the purposes of the current discussion, we will concentrate on these widely used studies.

16.3 Urodynamic Studies

16.3.1 Voiding Speed

The simplest urodynamic study is the voiding speed, which is an examination performed particularly in patients with no *obvious* neurologic lesion or in whom bladder outlet obstruction is possible (DEMUYLDER et al. 1992).

The two parameters of most interest are the time in seconds to empty the bladder and the peak voiding flow rate in milliliters per second. To do the examination, the patient simply voids into a container to which is attached an electronic flowmeter (DRACH and BINARD 1976). The normal time to empty the bladder is 20–30 s; the normal peak voiding flow rate in women under age 50 years is at least 25 ml/s, whereas in women over 50 it is at least 18 ml/s (DRACH and BINARD 1976). In men under 60 the rate is at least 22 ml/s; in men aged 40–60 it is at least 18 ml/s, whereas in men over 60 it is at least 13 ml/s (DRACH and BINARD 1976).

16.3.2 The Formal Urodynamic Study

16.3.2.1 Urodynamics Equipment

A four-channel machine is completely adequate for modern urodynamic studies (PERKASH and FRIEDLAND 1987a), provided it can measure: (a) bladder pressure (the cystometrogram); (b) the urethral pressure, (c) the electromyogram of the periurethal striated sphincter, and (d) the rectal pressure.

The machine should also have a coaxial cable capable of attachment to the monitor either of fluoroscopic equipment or transrectal ultrasonographic equipment, in order to obtain simultaneous images on the same monitor upon which are displayed urodynamics data (PERKASH and FRIEDLAND 1987a).

16.3.2.2 Urodynamics Catheters

Three types of urodynamics catheter are available (PERKASH and FRIEDLAND 1987a): (a) the triple lumen catheter, which we use; (b) the membrane catheter, in which the side hole in the urethra is covered by a membrane – this catheter is, however, prohibitively expensive; and (c) a catheter with a strain gauge at the tip, which unfortunately tends to injure the urethra.

16.3.2.3 Transrectal Ultrasonographic Urodynamics

Transrectal ultrasonographic urodynamics is a method still used in only a few institutions, although its use is becoming more widespread (NISHIZAWA et al. 1982; SHAPEERO et al. 1983; PORENA et al. 1987; SHABSIGN et al. 1987). It involves a linear array transducer introduced intrarectally, which produces sagittal images of the bladder and urethra. A coaxial cable from the ultrasonographic equipment is attached to the urodynamics monitor, so that both ultrasonographic and urodynamic images can be seen simultaneously on the same monitor, which can then be videotaped or photographed.

Transrectal ultrasonography has the following advantages: (a) it involves no radiation; (b) there are no bones overlapping the bladder neck or the urethra; (c) no contrast material is used, which, for centers with a large volume of cases, can amount to a significant annual saving; and (d) catheterization is not required. If urodynamic studies are performed using a catheter, however, it is possible to follow the course of the catheter as it is introduced into the urethra, which can be important for showing certain kinds of pathology (ledges, false passages), as discussed below. Transrectal ultrasonography can be a great help in preventing precipitous bladder contractions during introduction of the urodynamics catheter, as is also discussed below. Transrectal ultrasonography can also show the surrounding soft tissue, especially the prostate and seminal vesicles.

The disadvantage of transrectal ultrasonography is that it does not show vesicoureteral reflux or the pendulous urethra.

16.3.2.4 Methods of Urodynamic Study

First the patient voids. The electromyogram needle is then inserted into the periurethral striated sphincter. If ultrasonographic equipment is available, the ultrasonographic probe is then inserted intrarectally. The urodynamics catheter is inserted under ultrasonographic control, so that it does not touch the wall of the bladder, inducing precipitous bladder contraction; two strain gauges are then attached to the catheter, and the bladder and urethral pressures are measured. Water is infused into the bladder at 40 ml/min, and into the urethra at 4 ml/min. When the bladder is full, the patient voids.

If the patient is being tested for incontinence, this examination is done with the patient in the upright position, and the patient is asked to stop voiding and to hold. To measure the urethral pressure profile, the catheter is pulled out of the bladder under ultrasonographic control.

If the examination is being performed under ultrasonographic control, the ultrasonographic probe is then removed, a rectal balloon is inserted, and the urodynamic studies are repeated.

16.3.2.5 Normal Urodynamics

As fluid is dripped into the bladder, the normal person will feel full at about 150 ml water, and a strong urge to void at 400 ml water. The normal bladder pressure in cmH_2O varies between 10 and 20 during bladder filling; there may be sudden rises in this pressure, but no such rise should exceed 15 cmH_2O. During voiding, there is a sudden rise in pressure, which should be less than 50 cmH_2O, followed by a plateau lasting 20–30 s and then a sudden fall in bladder pressure as voiding ends (Fig. 16.8).

The electromyogram (EMG) of the periurethral striated sphincter in a normal person varies between 10 and 50 μv. When the patient is instructed to hold urine, however, electrical activity increases to between 100 and 150 μv. During voiding, there is no electrical activity in the periurethral striated sphincter (Fig. 16.8).

Two kinds of urethral pressure are relevant, the urethral pressure reading and the urethral pressure profile (Schmidt 1991).

The urethral pressure reading is obtained through the side hole of the catheter, which measures the pressure in the region of the periurethral striated sphincter during voiding.

To obtain the urethral pressure profile, the catheter is pulled out through the urethra when the patient is not voiding. The hole near the tip of the catheter measures pressure continuously at every point within the urethra. This can be useful for measuring the pressure gradient between the bladder and the bladder neck, in order to discover whether there are bladder neck problems; the normal pressure gradient is less than 3 cmH_2O. This examination can also be used as follow-up before and after surgery for the rest of the urethra, but, outside of these contexts, the examination is not particularly useful.

Thus, the normal voiding process (Fig. 16.8) would begin with a slow rise in bladder pressure during filling, not to exceed 20 cmH_2O, with electrical activity in the periurethral striated sphincter at normal levels (10–50 μV). As voiding begins, the periurethral striated sphincter relaxes, so that the EMG activity falls to zero, the detrusor contracts, and, simultaneously, the bladder neck opens. The bladder pressure rises suddenly to a value that may be as high as 50 cmH_2O, at which level it remains during the time necessary to complete voiding, some 20–30 s. As voiding continues, there is no electrical activity at the periurethral striated sphincter. As voiding ends, there is a precipitous drop in bladder pressure to the baseline, and electrical activity again appears, at normal levels, in the periurethral striated sphincter.

16.4 The Voiding Cystourethrogram

A number of factors can affect the success of the voiding cystourethrogram in spinal cord injury patients. The catheter can irritate the bladder, causing precipitous bladder contractions, but the contrast material itself may also do so; if it is too cold, it is run in too quickly, and if it is too concentrated, or if the bladder is infected, precipitous bladder contractions may result (Perkash and Friedland 1986c). The ideal, therefore, is to control all these variables in order to assure a successful examination.

We try, for example, to use as dilute a contrast material as possible, and have found sodium diatrizoate 12.5% to be quite adequate. We heat the contrast material to body temperature conveniently, by placing the drip bottle inside the X-omat well away from film, rollers, and other moving parts, 30 min before the examination. This brings the contrast material up to the body temperature in good time. Further, we never elevate the height of the dripset more than 50 cm above the bladder, and administer the contrast material at a rate of about 40 ml/min. All infection is controlled before the examination is done; if the patient has a history of autonomic dysreflexia there would be a serious problem, so all such patients should be treated ahead of time with an appropriate oral α-adrenergic blocker.

Thus the major problems associated with a voiding cystourethrogram in spinal cord injury patients usually can be circumvented.

Apart from detrusor–sphincter or detrusor–bladder neck dyssynergia, other pathologic conditions occurring in spinal cord injury patients (false passages or posterior ledges, as discussed below) are seen posteriorly in the urethra. Thus if the patient is examined in the frontal or oblique position, the pathology can be missed (Shapeero et al. 1983). The true lateral position is more favorable, although it involves increased radiation exposure and there is a problem with overlapping bones. Some compromises must be made, which is one reason why the radiologic voiding cystourethrogram has disadvantages where these patients are concerned.

The main advantage of the voiding cystourethrogram in patients with neuromuscular bladder dysfunction is that it is excellent at demonstrating vesicoureteral reflux; indeed, where transrectal ultrasonography is available, this is the main use for the voiding cystourethrogram, although, as is discussed below, it is also possible to demonstrate vesicoureteral reflux by means of scintigraphy.

16.5 The Intravenous Urogram

It has often been recommended that intravenous urography be done early to establish a baseline, and on an annual basis thereafter. We have found, however, that with modern care this is far too frequent. We obtain baseline studies at 3 months after the onset of the neuromuscular bladder dysfunction and then perform a repeat study only if there are signs and symptoms indicating that something has gone wrong which can usefully be studied by intravenous urography.

Thus the intravenous urogram is now commonly used to show anatomic problems, such as stones, well illustrated by a combination of plain film tomography and intravenous urography, or scars of chronic reflux pyelonephritis, or other unrelated pathology like cysts or neoplasms. As a function study, the intravenous urogram is extremely poor, and it is now clear that scintigraphy has major advantages over intravenous urography for determining the state of renal function.

In addition, patients with neuromuscular dysfunction of the bladder and urethra frequently are on a number of medications, including α-adrenergic blockers, and it has been our impression that if contrast material reactions occur in such patients, they are more difficult to treat and control than would usually be the case. We have no absolute data to support this feeling, but it does make us more wary in using intravenous urography in these patients than we might otherwise be.

16.6 Scintigraphy

Scintigraphy will be discussed in some detail, as it is now the most important method for examining the upper urinary tract in patients with neuromuscular dysfunction of the bladder and urethra. The two important studies for this purpose are radionuclide cystography for the detection of vesicoureteral reflux, and radioisotope renography for examining disturbances in renal perfusion. The latter may also reveal parenchymal abnormalities and obstruction.

16.6.1 Radionuclide Cystography in Patients with Neuromuscular Bladder Dysfunction

There are two methods of doing radionuclide cystography, direct and indirect (Conway 1985). The direct method is the same as the radiologic voiding cystourethrogram: the patient is catheterized, the bladder emptied, and the radionuclide is instilled directly into the bladder (Bower et al. 1985). This examination can be done simultaneously with urodynamic studies (Sfakianakis et al. 1984).

The indirect method is somewhat analogous to the intravenous urogram (Nielsen et al. 1985) and is the only method of radionuclide cystography we have used on patients with neuromuscular dysfunction of the bladder and urethra. The patient is given an intravenous injection of a radiopharmaceutical, which is then excreted by the kidneys into the bladder.

The advantage of this method is that it is a more physiologic test: the patient need not be catheterized, which means that there is no problem with the catheter-induced precipitous bladder contractions (see below). The disadvantage is that since the radiopharmaceutical is administered intravenously, there is a high background activity which can obscure low grades of reflux (Conway 1985; Bower et al. 1985). The literature further states that if the examiner waits for the bladder to fill, has the patient void, and images only at that point, the examiner may miss reflux at lower bladder volumes (Conway 1985; Bower et al. 1985). At our institution, however, we image throughout the excretory phase of the renogram, before the patient voids, and have managed to show reflux at low bladder volumes very nicely. A further disadvantage is that there is a slightly higher radiation dosage to the patient with the indirect method, since the radiopharmaceutical is administered intravenously, goes throughout the body, and is excreted by the kidney. Further, the bladder fills slowly, meaning that the radiopharmaceutical is in the bladder longer than if the direct method were used, which yields a more localized and time-limited radiation dosage.

The advantage of either direct or indirect radionuclide cystography over the conventional radiologic voiding cystourethrogram is that the radiation dosage to the patient is much lower. The disadvantage is that the anatomy of the urethra is not well seen; radionuclide cystography shows function, not structure. To diagnose detrusor–bladder neck dyssynergia or detrusor–sphincter dyssynergia, or to detect ledges or false passages, the radiologic or ultrasonographic voiding cystourethrogram is still much to be preferred.

The radiopharmaceuticals used for the indirect method of radionuclide cystography are ^{123}I- or ^{131}I-hippuran or ^{99m}Tc-diethylenetriamine pentaacetic acid (DTPA). The advantage of hippuran is that it is both filtered and secreted, and is therefore cleared much faster from the kidneys than DTPA, which is filtered. It consequently yields a much lower background activity, making low grades of reflux much easier to detect.

The direct method requires $^{99m}TcO_4$, or nonabsorbable sulfur colloid.

Patients with neuromuscular dysfunction of the bladder and urethra are examined in the supine position, and a sequence of posterior images is collected before and after voiding. The residual bladder volume is easily calculated using the following simple formula:

$$\text{Residual bladder volume} = \frac{\text{voided urine volume} \times \text{postvoid counts in bladder}}{\text{prevoid counts in bladder} - \text{postvoid counts}}$$

In our series at the Palo Alto Veterans Administration Medical Center, using the indirect method of radionuclide cystography, one-third of all patients studied have shown reflux. One-fourth had unilateral reflux, and the rest had bilateral reflux.

Indirect scintigraphy is a screening test only. If the results are positive for vesicoureteral reflux, and if the decision to perform a sphincterotomy depends on a positive result, it will be important to follow up either with direct scintigraphy or a radiologic voiding cystourethrogram. This is because a significant number of patients with positive results on indirect scintigraphy do not show reflux on a radiologic voiding cystourethrogram.

There are several possible reasons why the results of indirect scintigraphy and a radiologic voiding cystourethrogram may differ.

The first, and most likely, possibility is the so-called ureteroureteral reflux (the yo-yo phenomenon) (Peters et al. 1990). This occurs when a peristaltic wave, having traveled down toward the distal ureter, stops, and the ureteral muscles relax. If there is still urine left in the distal end of the ureter, retrograde flow is possible, given the relaxed state of the muscles of that ureter. This phenomenon is even more likely if the bladder wall has hypertrophied, because the hypertrophied bladder wall can partially obstruct the distal ureter. As the peristaltic wave distends the distal ureter, the partial obstruction prevents some proportion of the urine from entering the bladder, which then can flow back up the ureter toward the kidney when the peristaltic wave relaxes. This would mean that, while no vesicoureteral reflux is occurring, ureteroureteral reflux is, leading to a false positive result for vesicoureteral reflux.

Another possibility is that the radiologic voiding cystourethrogram is simply a less sensitive test than indirect scintigraphy.

The least likely possibility is that the vesicoureteral reflux is intermittent. This is relatively unlikely because, if the reflux is intermittent, statistically it should appear equally intermittent on indirect scintigraphy and a radiologic voiding cystourethrogram.

According to the principles of bayesian and decision analysis, if the prior probability is high and the consequences of missing the diagnosis are serious, a very sensitive test is required; specificity is less important (Chang 1989; Friedland et al. 1989; Friedland 1990). Certainly those criteria exist in this situation.

Thus, while indirect scintigraphy is fine as a screening examination, it will require the additional specificity of a radiologic voiding cystourethrogram or direct scintigraphy, both of which are still regarded as the "gold standard," to confirm the diagnosis.

To show reflux using the indirect method, we generate an image of each kidney, beginning 1 min after the intravenous injection of the radiopharmaceutical, and continuing at 1-min intervals for 27 min.

The resulting data can be analyzed in two ways. The first is simply to look at the images, to see if the activity in the ureter and kidney suddenly increases during the excretory phase, which would indicate that this increased activity must come from the bladder up to the ureter or the kidney. Because these levels are low, however, the images can be difficult to distinguish from the background radio activity. For this reason we use the time-activity curve, as follows. As images of the kidneys become available, we define regions of interest simply by drawing the renal outlines, and the computer can generate counts of radioactivity per minute within the designated region of interest. On the excretory phase, we would normally expect that each subsequent minute will show less activity than the preceding minute, as the kidney is constantly losing radiopharmaceutical. If there is an increase of 10% or more in any one minute compared with the preceding minute, reflux is indicated (Fig. 16.9).

Using this method, reflux must reach the kidney in order to be detected, which means that we are measuring grade II reflux and above, but not grade I reflux. Grade 1 reflux, however, is probably not significant.

16.6.2 Radioisotope Renography in Patients with Neuromuscular Bladder Dysfunction

Radioisotope renography is done in patients with neuromuscular dysfunction of the bladder and urethra to show disturbances in perfusion of the kidneys, gross renal parenchymal abnormalities, obstruction, and reflux.

The study is done in two phases. The first phase shows the renal parenchyma. It enables us to see the size and shape of each kidney and any anatomic defects in the renal parenchyma; it also allows us to compare the perfusion of one kidney with that of the opposite kidney. The latter is done by counting the activity in each kidney, which is proportional to the perfusion.

To do the examination, 1–5 mCi dimercaptosuccinate (DMSA) is administered intravenously. Between 85% and 90% of the compound binds to the sulfhydryl groups in the collecting tubules, thus showing the renal parenchyma; the remaining 10%–15% is excreted in the urine.

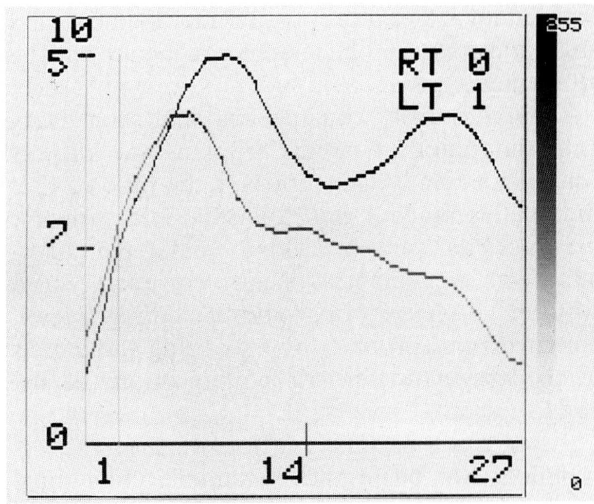

Fig. 16.9. Time-activity curve showing a sudden increase in activity during the excretory phase, indicating reflux

If the examiner is looking specifically for anatomic defects, tomography of the kidneys is much better at defining such defects than conventional planar views. For example, planar views cannot differentiate the renal pelvis from the renal parenchyma, but tomography does this very well. The resolution using this technique is not comparable to the intravenous urogram, however,

If anatomic defects are not a concern, then planar images in both the posterior and the anterior projection are required.

The reasons that both projections are required is that the two kidneys may not lie at the same depth within the body (Cosgriff and Brown 1990). In fact, in about 80% of the population, the lower pole of the right kidney is tilted more anteriorly than the lower pole of the left. This explains why the right kidney usually appears shorter on an intravenous urogram, although anatomically they are the same length; the right kidney is being foreshortened.

In addition, because the posterior abdominal wall and the retroperitoneum tilt anteriorly as the observer progresses inferiorly, the lower the kidney, the more anterior it will be. If the patient has a scoliosis, the kidney on the side of the convexity will also be more anterior than the opposite kidney.

This means that the further anteriorly the kidney is located, the lower the activity that will be recorded on a posterior view. Body tissues attenuate gamma rays, and the more anterior the kidney, the more tissue the gamma rays must traverse, and the more the beam will be attenuated.

Observationally, this means that, for every 1 cm difference in depth between two kidneys whose true relative function is in the ratio of 1:1, the relative function appears to be 1.25:1 if only the posterior view is used to make the determination. A geometric mean, however, which requires both anterior and posterior views, minimizes this problem by equalizing the effects of the attenuation across both portions of the body.

After the anatomic portion of the study is complete, we begin the dynamic or functional portion of the examination. For this purpose some institutions use technetium-labeled DTPA, which is filtered but not secreted; others, including our own, use orthoiodohippurate (hippuran). Hippuran is virtually identical to *p*-aminohippuric acid, which has been the classical drug of choice for this purpose for years. It is both filtered and excreted, and is therefore rapidly cleared from the kidneys; more than 70% of the renal activity will have washed out in the first 30 min after the beginning of the intravenous injection. The hippuran is labeled with either ^{131}I (dose: 300 μCi) or ^{123}I (dose: 1 mCi); ^{131}I is usually used at our institution because it is less expensive, although ^{123}I gives a lower radiation dosage to the patient, enabling us to use a larger amount and as a consequence to obtain better images.

Regardless of the isotope used, the patient is hydrated with 1 liter of water prior to the examination. No medications are discontinued, since the effects on the renogram are insignificant, except that if we are investigating a patient for hypertension, all diuretics are withheld.

All patients are examined in the supine position. The bladder is drained continuously via a Foley catheter in all patients, although we consider the latter to be optional.

The imaging sequence is one posterior view every minute for 27 min after the injection of the radiopharmaceutical. Regions of interest are marked around each kidney, and the computer measures the total radiocativity in each area of interest and then subtracts the background radioactivity, yielding true activity in each kidney, which is then plotted against time, yielding a time-activity curve for each kidney.

The normal scan in spinal cord injury patients will show symmetric uptake and excretion of the radiopharmaceutical by both kidneys, with peak activity at 3–5 min. The radioactivity in spinal cord injury patients should fall to at least 33% of peak activity, although in many patients it will fall to 25% or less.

The total effective renal plasma flow (ERPF) is calculated from the concentration of hippuran remaining in the plasma at 44 min. We use the method developed at the University of Alabama by Tauxe and Dubovsky (Tauxe et al. 1982) for obtaining this figure, which is both well tested and standardized, and is now widely available from commercial software vendors.

Normal values for the total ERPF depend on the size and age of the patient; thus males usually have higher values than females and younger patients tend to have higher values than older patients. A graph is available which relates total ERPF to the patient's size and age, but a useful rule of thumb is that the normal total ERPF is above 450 ml/min. Thus, if clinicians see a value below that figure they may regard the examination as abnormal.

To find the ERPF of each kidney, the total ERPF as derived above is multiplied by the relative uptake of hippuran by each kidney 1–2 min after injection, which is proportional to perfusion. (After 2 min, uptake of hippuran will reflect both perfusion and washout, which is the reason for choosing the 1–2 min time frame.)

Regions of interest are drawn around each kidney and, for example, if the right kidney is found to contribute 45% of the total renal activity and the left kidney 55%, then the ERPF of the right kidney is 0.45 × total ERPF, and that of the left 0.55 × total ERPF. In no case should the values for each kidney vary more than 10%; if they do, one or both kidneys is abnormal.

In a series at the Palo Alto Veterans Administration Medical Center, 28% of patients in the Spinal Cord Injury Center had a total ERPF of less than 450 ml/min, and 59% had more than a 10% difference in split function studies (Fig. 16.10).

The reason this 10% difference may exist is that the calculation of the ERPF uses only the posterior view. As discussed above, the two kidneys may be at a different level in the body, one more anterior than the other; this may yield a different apparent result for each kidney if only a posterior view is used (Cosgriff and Brown 1990).

Since ^{131}I has a higher energy than ^{99m}Tc, attenuation can be less of a problem with ^{131}I, but

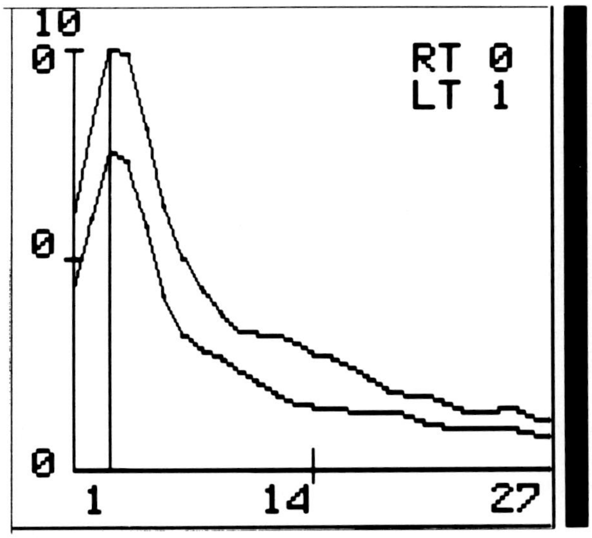

Fig. 16.10. Time-activity curve showing asymmetric ERPF with otherwise parallel curves

the problem is not eliminated. Asymmetries of more than 10% on ^{131}I hippuran studies should be confirmed by calculating the relative activity using the geometric mean on a ^{99m}Tc study, as discussed above.

In another series at the Palo Alto Veterans Administration Medical Center, the ERPF was shown to be significantly lower 1 year after the spinal cord injury than earlier (Tempkin et al. 1985). There was commonly a delay in the transit of the radiopharmaceutical through the renal parenchyma, and also a delay in emptying the renal pelvis.

In patients examined before and after the administration of the anticholinergic agent oxybutinin, the peak activity was delayed in patients prior to the administration of oxybutinin, but was normal in patients after its administration. In addition, at the end of the curve, at 27 min, residual activity in the kidneys was less after the administration of oxybutinin than before hand. Oxybutinin relaxes the bladder and as there is some evidence of cholinergic supply to the distal ureter, it may relax the distal ureter as well.

Another study (Kulemeier et al. 1985) involving a 10-year follow-up in spinal cord injury patients showed that the decrease in total ERPF was 4.5 ml per year. Factors affecting this decline significantly were found to be age (activity normally decreases as the patient ages), sex (males have a higher ERPF than females), and whether the patient was quadriplegic or paraplegic (quadriplegics lose function faster). The presence of kidney stones or episodes of acute pyelonephritis were found to lead to greater declines as well. Factors not affecting the total ERPF were found to be the number of years since the injury, whether the injury was complete or incomplete, the presence of bladder stones, bacteriuria without clinical pyelonephritis, and severe pressure sores (Galloway et al. 1991).

16.6.3 The Diuretic Renogram

The diuretic renogram is useful for showing obstruction, although it will not be worth doing it if the serum creatinine is above 2.0 mg/dl.

The procedure is to do the basic hippuran renogram, followed by the administration of 60–80 mg furosemide intravenously 10 min after the start of examination. The literature states that the dose should be 40 mg, but our experience has shown this to be inadequate.

The examination is interpreted by examining the renogram. There will be a normal steep slope after the administration of furosemide; if there is a patulous renal pelvis which is not obstructed, there will be a plateau before the administration of furosemide and a steep curve afterwards. If obstruction exists, there will be a plateau before and after the administration of furosemide.

One method of checking the adequacy of the dose is that, if only one kidney is believed to be obstructed, the other kidney should have a normal furosemide renogram; if it does not appear normal, the patient has not received enough furosemide.

16.7 Bladder Dysfunction

When there is neuromuscular dysfunction of the bladder and urethra, the bladder is either able to contract (reflex bladder) or unable to contract (areflexic bladder) (Friedland and Perkash 1983; Kaplan et al. 1991). If the bladder can contract, the patient has an upper motor neuron lesion; if the bladder cannot contract, the patient could have (a) a lower motor neuron lesion, (b) an upper motor neuron lesion leading to a chronically overdistended bladder due to improper or nonexistent treatment, or (c) a loss of sensory nerve roots, the most common cause of which is currently diabetes mellitis (Friedland and Perkash 1983).

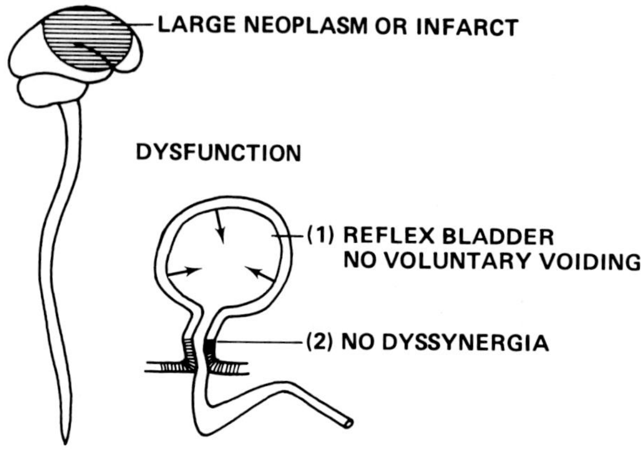

Fig. 16.11. Bladder dysfunction with a large suprapontine lesion

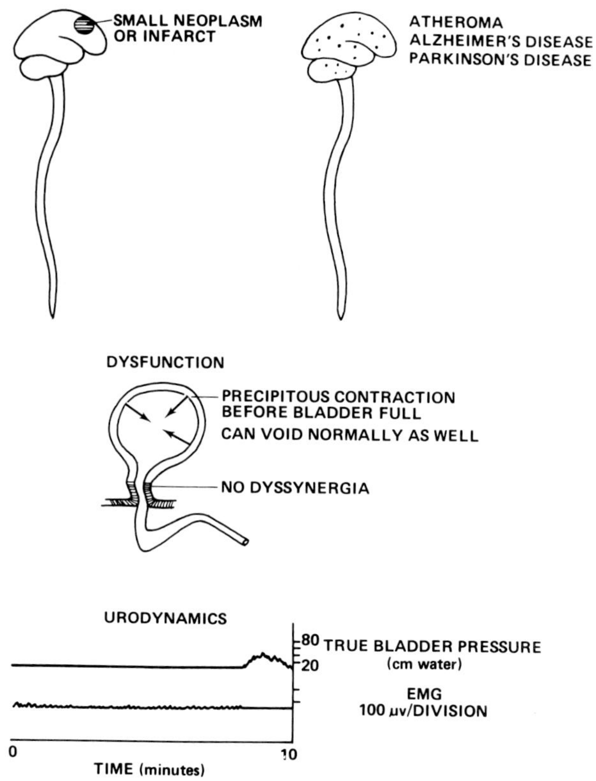

Fig. 16.12. Bladder dysfunction with small suprapontine lesion(s)

A reflex bladder contracts when less than 300 ml of urine is present. Such patients void involuntarily via a spinal cord reflex (Friedland and Perkash 1983).

16.7.1 Upper Motor Neuron Lesions

16.7.1.1 Supraportine Lesions

Large Suprapontine Lesions. Examples of large suprapontine lesions would include a large neoplasm or infarct. There is bladder dysfunction in these patients, involving a reflex bladder with no voluntary voiding (Resnick and Yalla 1985, 1987). There is no detrusor–bladder neck or detrusor–sphincter dyssynergia (Resnick and Yalla 1985, 1987) (Fig. 16.11).

Small Suprapontine Lesion(s). Common causes of a small single suprapontine lesion include a small neoplasm or a small infarct (Resnick and Yalla 1985, 1987). Multiple small lesions may be caused by atheroma, Alzheimer's disease, or Parkinson's disease (Resnick and Yalla 1985, 1987). Patients with a small suprapontine lesion or multiple small lesions usually have precipitous bladder contractions before the bladder is full, but they may also void normally, if they can reach the toilet in time. There is no detrusor–bladder neck or detrusor–sphincter dyssynergia (Resnick and Yalla 1985, 1987) (Figs. 16.12, 16.13).

The dysfunction we have just described is called detrusor hyperreflexia (Resnick and Yalla 1985; Hald et al. 1984) and it is now the most common cause of incontinence in the elderly (Resnick and

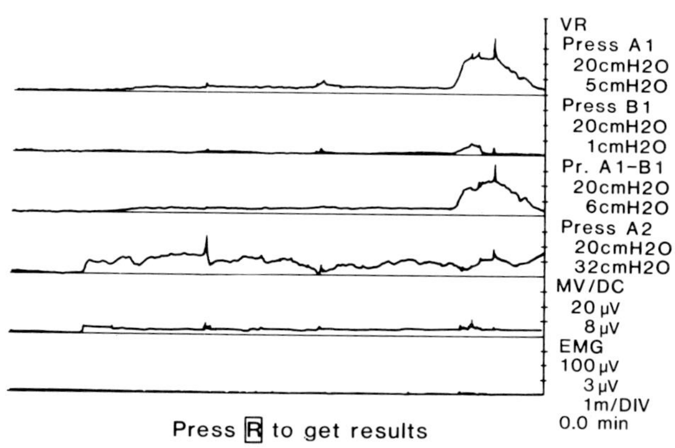

Fig. 16.13. Urodynamic study in a patient with a suprapontine lesion. *Press A1*, total bladder pressure; *Press B1*, intrarectal pressure; *Press A1 – B1*, true bladder pressure; *Press A2*, urethral pressure reading; in all the above, each small division = 20 cmH_2O pressure. *EMG*, electromyogram; each small division = 100 µV. (Perkash and Friedland 1987a)

YALLA 1985, 1987). It is an extremely expensive form of neuromuscular dysfunction of the bladder; indeed, the most common reason the elderly are placed in nursing homes is incontinence (RESNICK and YALLA 1985, 1987; BROCKLEHURST 1986) and the Office of the Surgeon General of the United States has estimated that 8 billion dollars is spent in that country alone in 1 year simply for incontinence pads for the elderly (BRASDA 1983). Of that figure, almost 3 billion dollars would be spent on elderly patients with detrusor hyperreflexia (RESNICK and YALLA 1987).

Common causes of detrusor hyperreflexia include stroke, Alzheimer's disease, and Parkinson's disease (RESNICK and YALLA 1985, 1987). Such patients have normal peak voiding flow rates, no postvoid residual urine, and voluntary control over their anal sphincters (RESNICK and YALLA 1985, 1987).

A significant subgroup of these patients are those with detrusor hyperactivity with impaired contractile function (RESNICK and YALLA 1987). Patients in this group have uninhibited contractions and no obstruction at the bladder neck. Their residual urine levels are often over 50% of capacity. There is marked bladder trabeculation, and possible episodes of acute retention.

This form of neuromuscular dysfunction is highly significant, as such patients are often misdiagnosed as having benign prostatic hyperplasia, which means that the patient's incontinence becomes much worse after prostatic surgery (RESNICK and YALLA 1987). They may also be correctly diagnosed as having detrusor hyperactivity, but the impaired contractile function is missed, so that when the patient is given medications to suppress bladder contractions, the incontinence gets much worse, and the patient may even go into acute retention following medications to suppress bladder contractions (RESNICK and YALLA 1987).

16.7.1.2 Subpontine Upper Motor Neuron Lesions

Subpontine upper motor neuron lesions have a number of causes, common ones being trauma, degenerative disease of the vertebrae and intervertebral disks, neoplasms (which may be primary or secondary), and infections.

Upper motor neuron spinal cord lesions can lead to four specific syndromes:

1. Detrusor–sphincter dyssynergia
2. Detrusor–bladder neck dyssynergia
3. The cauda equina syndrome
4. The central cord syndrome

1. *Detrusor–Sphincter Dyssynergia.* Detrusor–sphincter dyssynergia is caused by a lesion between the pons and the conus (sacral cord) (FRIEDLAND and PERKASH 1983). When the detrusor contracts, the periurethral striated sphincter does not relax; thus, on urodynamic studies it will be possible to observe that when the detrusor contracts the electromyogram of the periurethral striated sphincter increases, and the true bladder pressure during voiding becomes very high (PERKASH and FRIEDLAND 1987a) (Figs. 16.14, 16.15).

A voiding cystourethrogram in such patients will show a narrowing of the distal half of the prostatic urethra, due to the contraction of the periurethral striated sphincter (FRIEDLAND and PERKASH 1983; SHAPEERO et al. 1983). This contraction forces the verumontanum into the lumen of the urethra, so that the verumontanum looks prominent (FRIEDLAND and PERKASH 1983; SHAPEERO et al. 1983) (Fig. 16.16).

If untreated, the bladder neck in patients with detrusor–sphincter dyssynergia can become wide, since it is above the area of obstruction (FRIEDLAND and PERKASH 1983; SHAPEERO et al. 1983). The bladder itself may become thickened and trabeculated, and, if the pressure in the bladder is continuously above 70 mmH_2O, vesicoureteral reflux may develop, as well as reflux into the prostatic ducts, the vas, and the seminal vesicles (FRIEDLAND and PERKASH 1983; SHAPEERO et al. 1983).

The ultrasonographic voiding cystourethrogram will demonstrate the narrowing of the distal half of the prostatic urethra due to the contraction of the periurethral striated sphincter, the prominent verumontanum, and the wide bladder neck (SHAPEERO et al. 1983) (Fig. 16.16).

It is important to distinguish patients with detrusor–sphincter dyssynergia from those with urethral stricture without dyssynergia (Fig. 16.17). The major differences are: (a) an electromyogram of the periurethral striated sphincter will show increased activity during voiding if the patient has detrusor–sphincter dyssynergia, whereas there will be no activity in the striated muscle if the patient has stricture; (b) with suprapubic tapping, the periurethral striated sphinc-

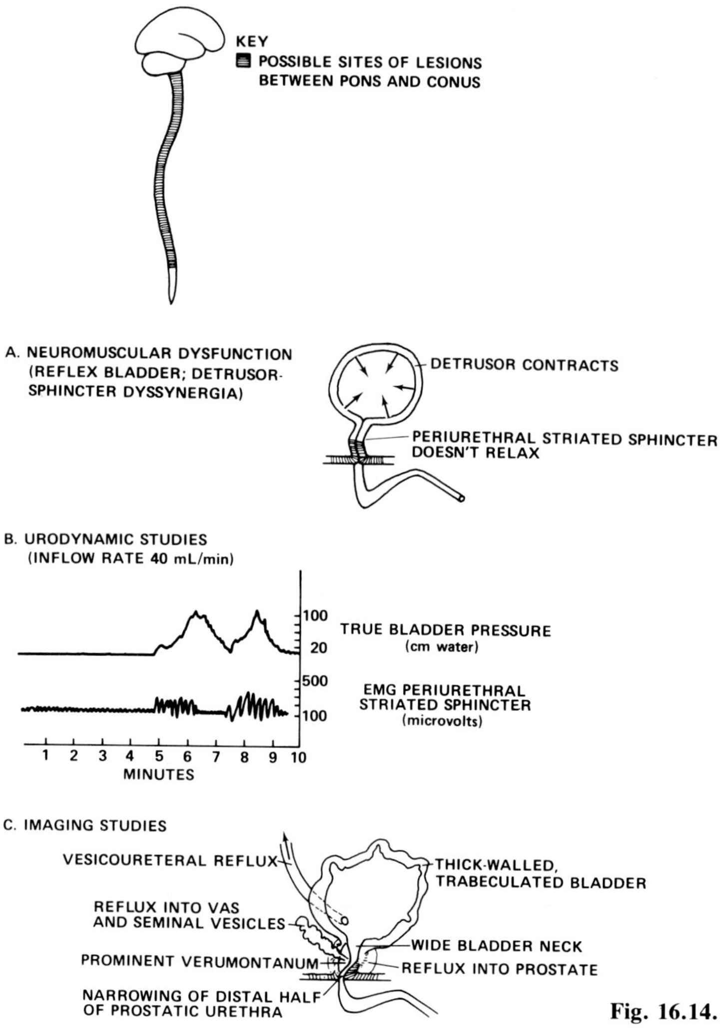

Fig. 16.14. Detrusor–sphincter dyssynergia

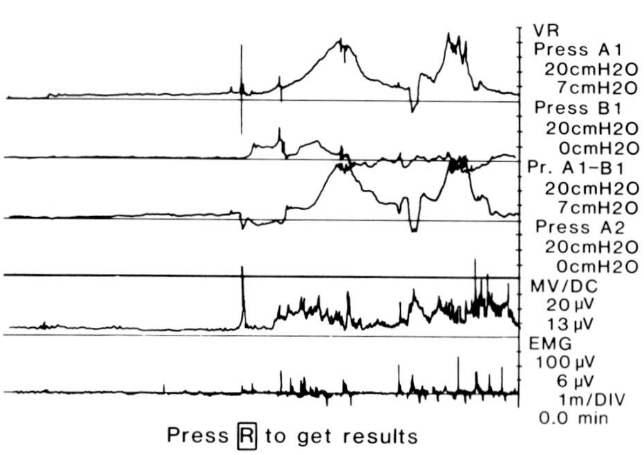

Fig. 16.15. Urodynamic studies in a patient with detrusor–sphincter dyssynergia. (PERKASH and FRIEDLAND 1987a)

ter eventually relaxes, so that the distal half of the prostatic urethra opens, whereas with stricture the urethra remains narrow; and (c) a dilator passes easily through the distal half of the prostatic urethra in a patient with dyssynergia whereas it meets resistance in a patient with stricture.

Failure of relaxation of the periurethral striated sphincter can also occur in a patient with the Hinman syndrome (HINMAN 1986), the spastic periurethral striated sphincter syndrome (RAZ and SMITH 1976), and psychogenic retention.

The Hinman syndrome occurs in children, whereas the spastic periurethral striated sphincter syndrome tends to occur in adult women. In all such cases, however, the person, for psychological reasons, keeps the periurethral striated sphincter contracted while voiding. The diagnostic feature in such cases is the electromyogram of the periurethral striated sphincter. In all such cases the periurethral striated sphincter relaxes briefly just before the detrusor contracts, and then contracts again as voiding continues (Blaivas 1984). In patients with detrusor–sphincter dyssynergia, however, this brief relaxation does not occur (Blaivas 1984).

2. *Detrusor–Bladder Neck Dyssynergia.* Detrusor-bladder neck dyssynergia occurs when there is a lesion of the cord between the pons and T5 (Friedland and Perkash 1983; Shapeero et al. 1983). In this functional abnormality, when the detrusor contracts, the bladder neck does not relax (Friedland and Perkash 1983; Shapeero et al. 1983). Most of these patients also have detrusor–sphincter dyssynergia, so that the periurethral striated sphincter also does not relax (Fig. 16.18) (Ganzer et al. 1991).

When combined urodynamic and imaging studies are performed, the bladder pressure is elevated, the neck either will not open or opens only slightly, and the patient either is unable to void or dribbles; over time, the detrusor hypertrophies.

If the patient is given α-adrenergic blockers, or if a sphincterotomy through the bladder neck as well as the periurethral striated sphincter is performed, the bladder neck will be open, the periurethral striated sphincter can open with suprapubic tapping, and the patient will be able to void (Fig. 16.19).

Autonomic dysreflexia is a complication in patients with detrusor–bladder neck dyssynergia (Friedland and Perkash 1983) (Fig. 16.20). When the detrusor contracts during attempted voiding, the contracted bladder neck is stretched, which results in excess secretion of norepinephrine. This excess causes sweating and peripheral arteriolar constriction, and the peripheral arteriolar constriction causes the blood pressure to rise.

Normally this rise in blood pressure is compensated for by reflex portal vasodilatation, but in patients with lesions above the greater splanchnic nerve there is no reflex portal vasodilatation, and the blood pressure will continue to rise. As a result, the baroreceptors are activated in the carotid sinus and the aortic arch, causing reflex bradycardia. This slowing of the pulse, however, is insufficient to lower the blood pressure, as a result of which the patient gets a headache. Thus the signs of autonomic dysreflexia are:

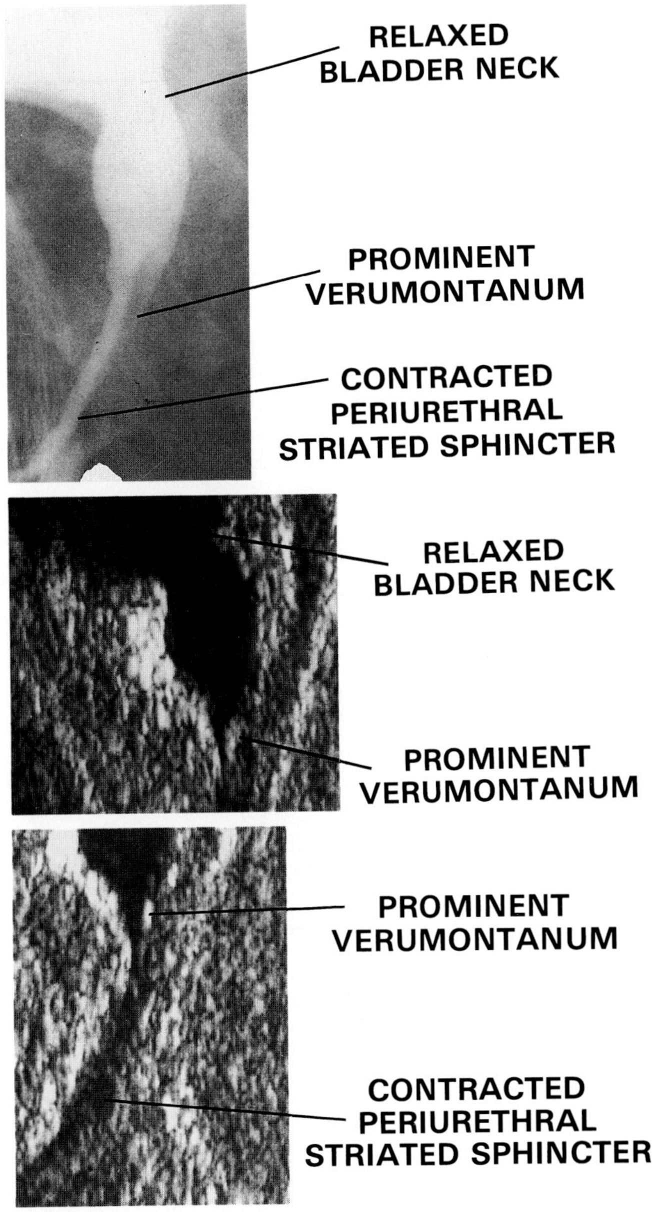

Fig. 16.16. Radiographic (*top*) and ultrasonographic (*middle* and *bottom*) voiding cystourethrograms in a patient with detrusor–sphincter dyssynergia, showing the characteristic appearance of the urethra. (Shapeero et al. 1983)

(a) hypertension, (b) sweating, (c) slow pulse, and (d) headache.

If the blood pressure remains high, there are two possible dangers to the patient: cerebral hemorrhage, or if the patient is to have an interventional procedure, e.g., percutaneous nephrostomy, he or she may bleed severely, so severely that the bleeding is difficult or impossible to control.

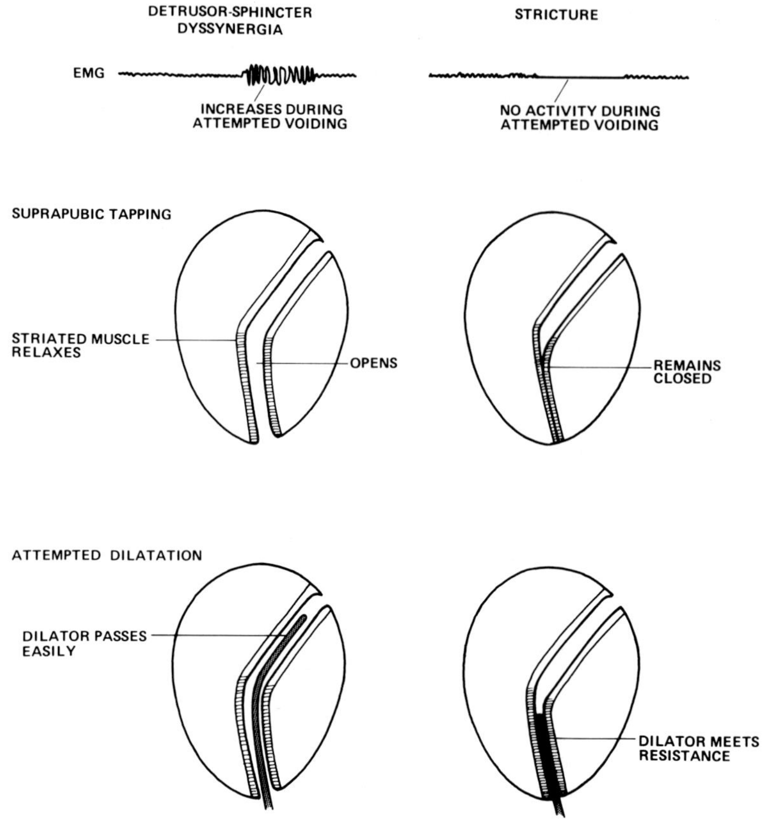

Fig. 16.17. Detrusor–sphincter dyssynergia versus urethral stricture. (FRIEDLAND and PERKASH 1989)

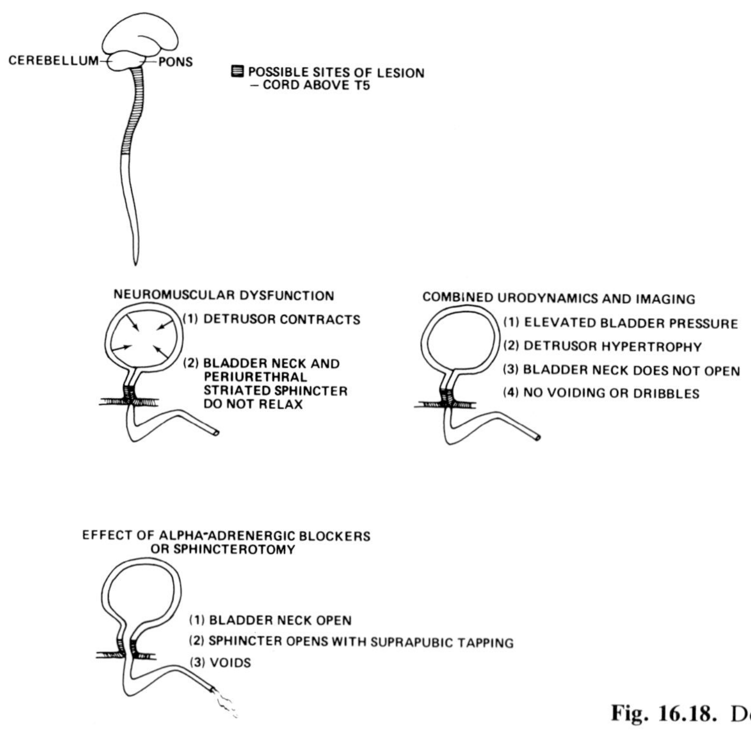

Fig. 16.18. Detrusor–bladder neck dyssynergia

Thus it is always important to be certain that the patient is receiving α-blockers and has a systolic pressure below 100 mmHg before performing any interventional or surgical procedure in a patient with detrusor–sphincter dyssynergia.

3. *The Cauda Equina Syndrome.* The cauda equina syndrome occurs in patients with lesions of the conus (sacral cord) (Fig. 16.21). The neuromuscular dysfunction in such patients is an areflexic bladder, because they have a lower motor neuron lesion. However, because the sympathetic nerve supply is unopposed, these patients also get detrusor–bladder neck dyssynergia. Thus, on a conventional or ultrasonographic voiding cystourethrogram, unlike other patients with a lower motor neuron lesion, patients with the cauda equina syndrome do not void when the Credé maneuver is performed, since the bladder neck will not open.

If these patients are given an α-adrenergic blocker, however, and if the Credé maneuver is subsequently performed, the bladder neck opens

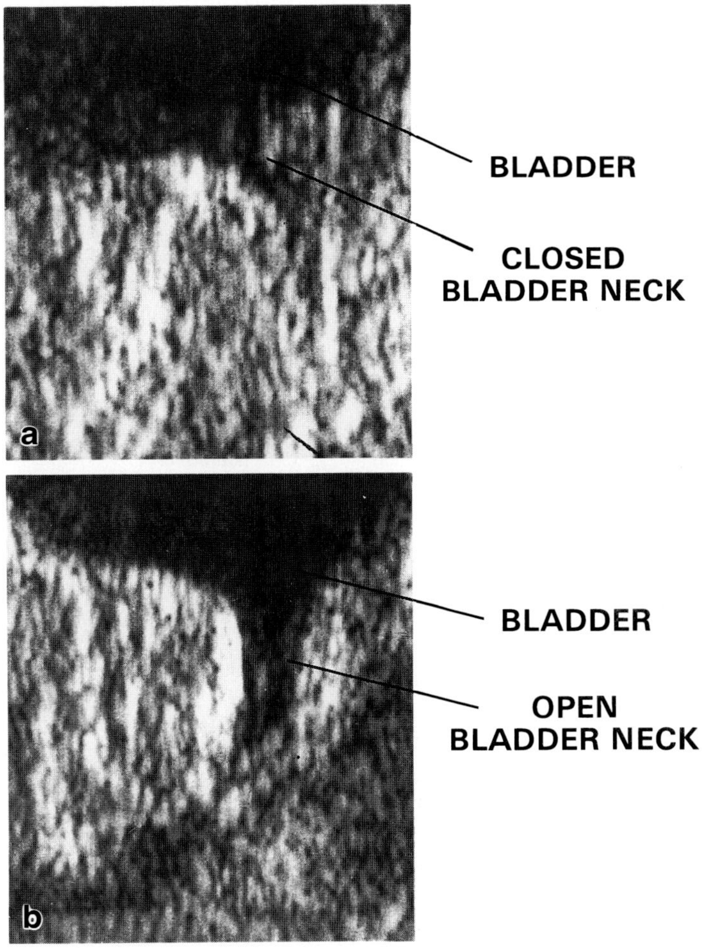

▷

Fig. 16.19 a,b. Ultrasonographic voiding cystourethrogram in a patient with detrusor–bladder neck dyssynergia. **a** Attempted voiding; the bladder neck is closed. **b** Five minutes after the patient had received 10 mg phentolamine intravenously, the bladder neck has opened

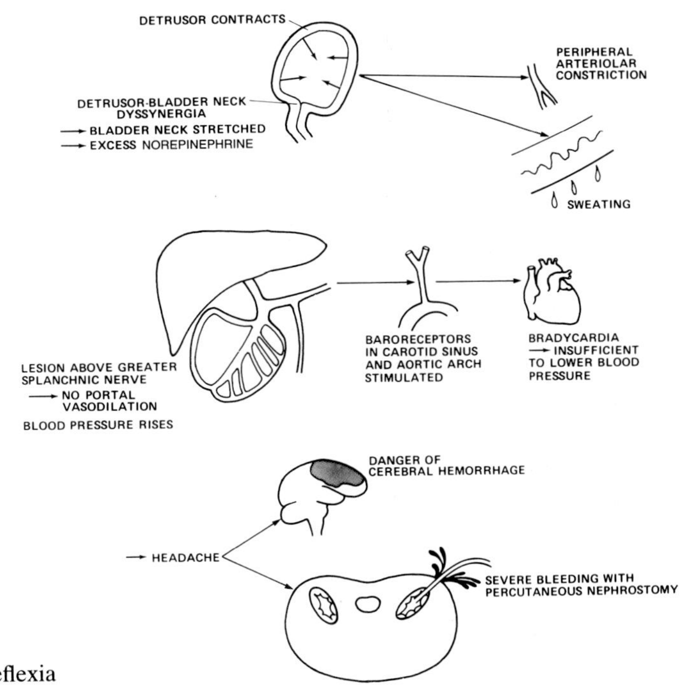

Fig. 16.20. Autonomic dysreflexia

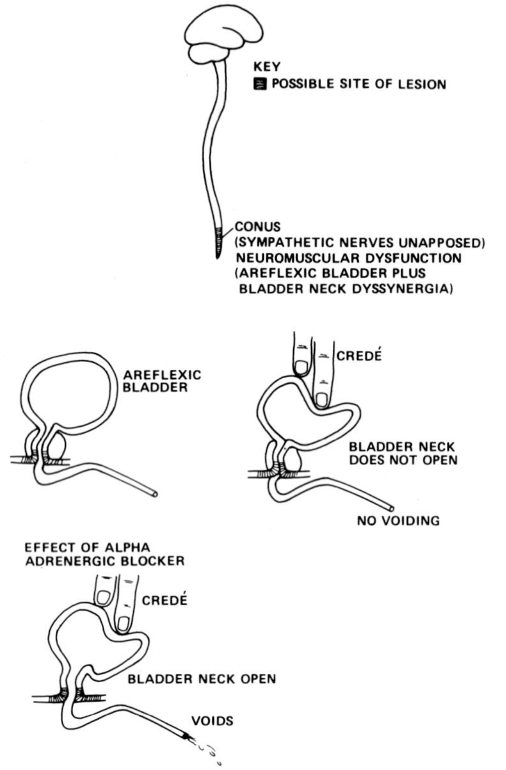

Fig. 16.21. The cauda equina syndrome

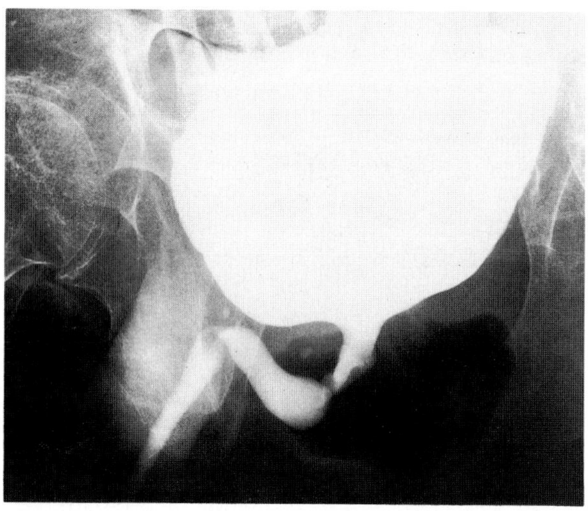

Fig. 16.22. Lower motor neuron lesion. The bladder has descended below the symphysis pubis. Note the narrow membranous urethra and the S-shaped urethra. (FRIEDLAND and PERKASH 1983)

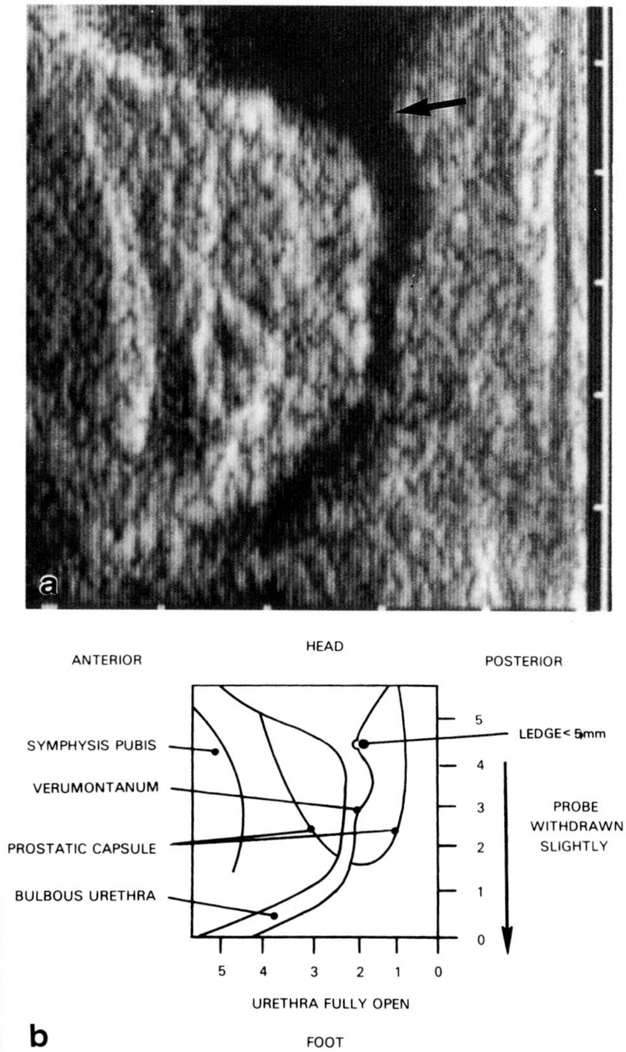

Fig. 16.23. a Normal ultrasonographic voiding cystourethrogram, showing a normal posterior ledge (*arrow*). **b** Diagrammatic illustration of **a**. (PERKASH and FRIEDLAND 1985)

and the patient is able to void. This is an example of a patient with an areflexic bladder due to a lower motor neuron lesion, who may have bladder trabeculation if appropriate treatment is not supplied.

Detrusor–bladder neck dyssynergia must be differentiated from primary bladder neck obstruction, originally described in young men (BLAIVAS and NORLEN 1984) but now shown to occur with equal frequency in older men and young women.

Patients with primary bladder neck obstruction show α-adrenergic overactivity at the bladder neck, which results in a narrowing of the bladder neck which can closely resemble detrusor–sphincter dyssynergia. These patients have

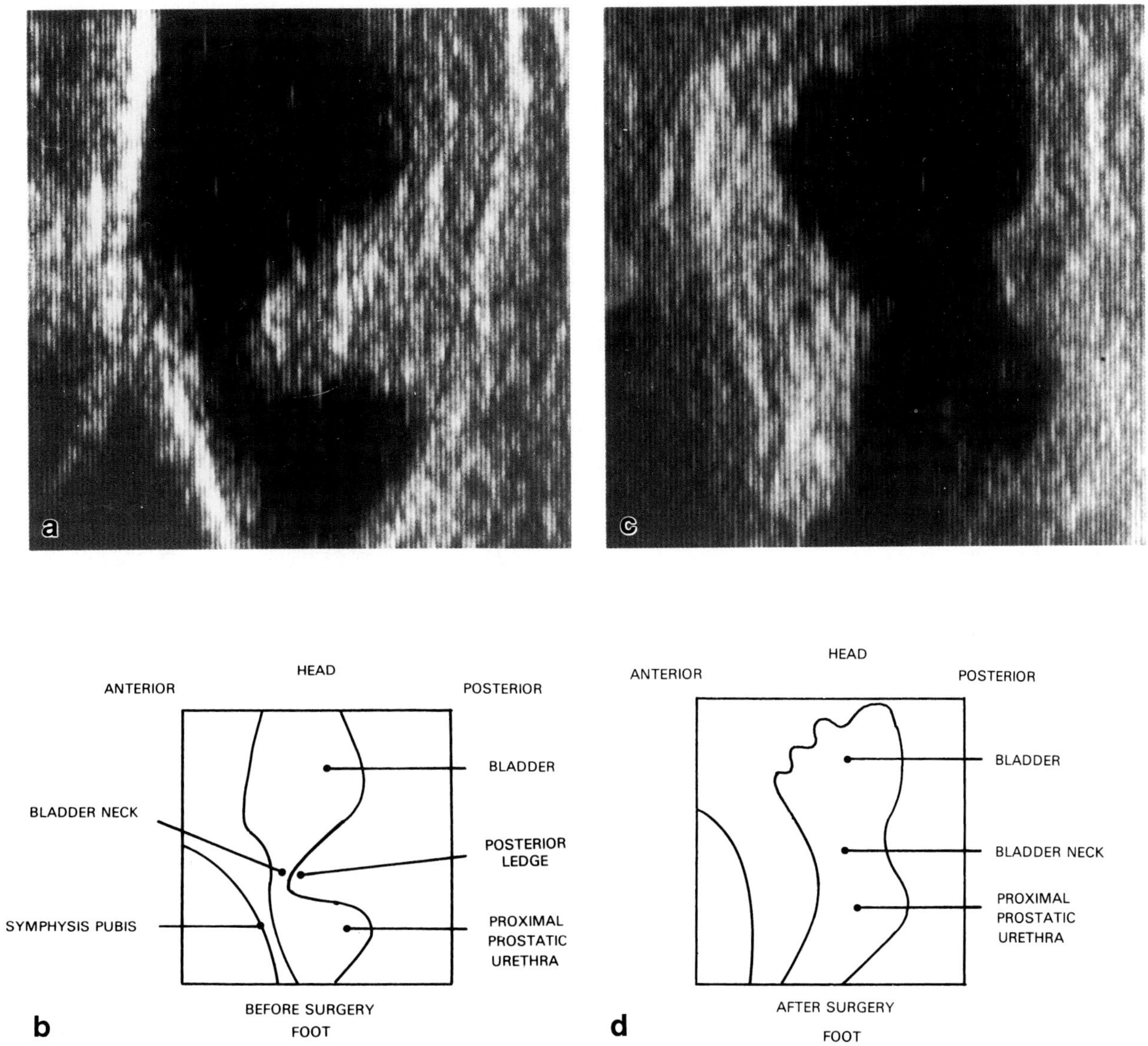

Fig. 16.24a–d. Pathologic posterior ledge. **a** Ultrasonographic voiding cystourethrogram, showing prominent posterior ledge. **b** Diagrammatic illustration of **a**. **c** Following a Perkash sphincterotomy, the ledge has receded. **d** Diagrammatic illustration of **c**. (PERKASH and FRIEDLAND 1985)

decreased urine flow, and may go into acute retention. There is no evidence of neuromuscular dysfunction.

Recently, the diameter of the bladder neck has been determined (MANOLIN 1987): the normal diameter is 6 mm or greater, the indeterminate range is 4–6 mm, whereas definite narrowing can be said to occur when the bladder neck measures less than 4 mm.

16.7.2 Lower Motor Neuron Lesions

In patients with a lower motor lesion, the bladder neck is usually widely patent and the urethra is open (FRIEDLAND and PERKASH 1983). The membranous urethra is usually narrow, which is said to be due to elastic recoil; presumably the pressure generated in the prostatic urethra is insufficient to distend the membranous urethra. Performing the Credé maneuver in such patients causes the bladder to descend, sometimes even below the symphysis pubis; because of this descent, the urethra may have a characteristic S-shaped configuration (FRIEDLAND and PERKASH 1983) (Fig. 16.22).

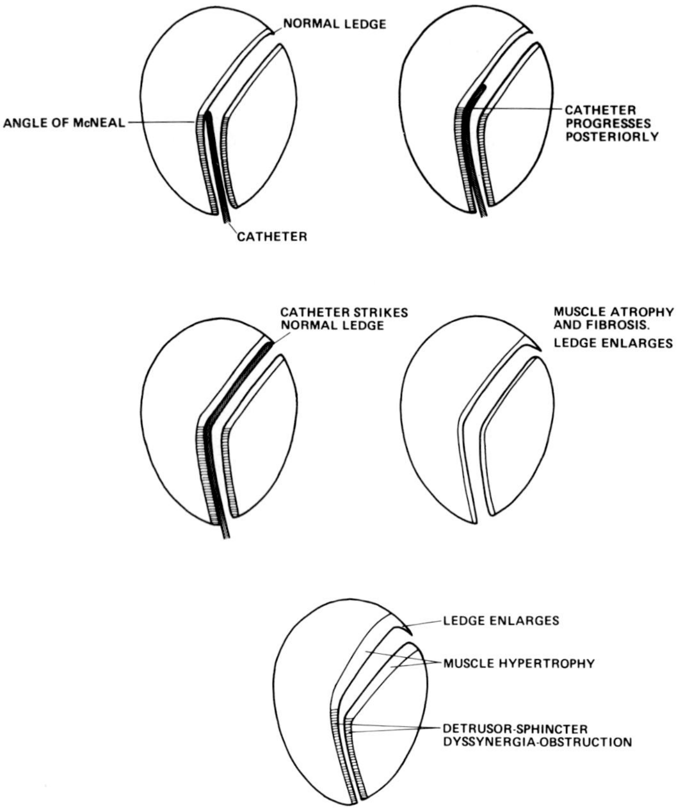

Fig. 16.25. Etiology of the posterior ledge. (FRIEDLAND and PERKASH 1989)

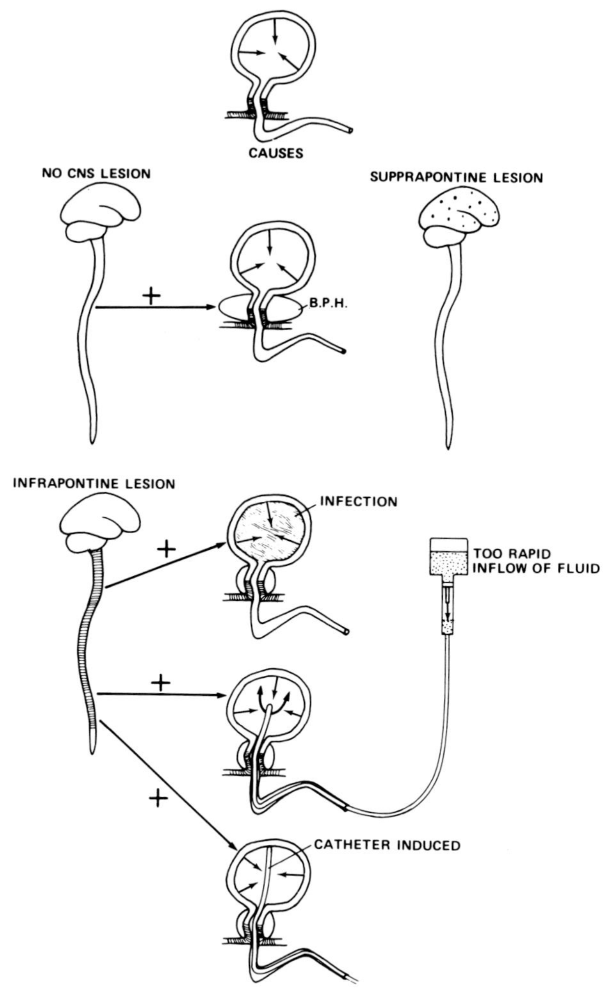

Fig. 16.26. Etiology of precipitous bladder contractions with less than 125 ml of urine in the bladder

16.8 Iatrogenic Bladder and Urethral Abnormalities

16.8.1 Ledges

We owe the discovery of posterior ledges of the bladder neck to transrectal ultrasonography (PERKASH and FRIEDLAND 1986a). Normally, there is a small posterior ledge 0–0.5 cm in length at the bladder neck (PERKASH and FRIEDLAND 1986a) (Fig. 16.23). This ledge can become pathologic when it reaches a size greater than 0.5 cm in length (PERKASH and FRIEDLAND 1986a) (Fig. 16.24).

The etiology is long-term intermittent catheterization and chronic detrusor–sphincter dyssynergia (Fig. 16.25). Intermittent catheterization can cause a ledge of increased length because, as the catheter is passed in the prostatic urethra, it is bent at the angle of McNeal and, because of its slight rigidity, progresses posteriorly through the urethra. Thus it strikes the normal ledge, and, should this occur repeatedly, it may cause muscle atrophy and fibrosis. In patients with chronic detrusor–sphincter dyssynergia, however, there is muscle hypertrophy at the bladder neck. As expected, histologic examination of these ledges has shown a mixture of muscle atrophy, muscle hypertrophy, and fibrosis.

The physiologic effect of an elongated ledge is a high pressure gradient between the bladder and the bladder neck. There may also be difficulty with catheterization, including bleeding. The treatment is the Perkash sphincterotomy, the success rate of which is about 98% (PERKASH and FRIEDLAND 1986a). This procedure involves incisions at 10 o'clock and at 2 o'clock, through both the periurethral striated sphincter and the bladder neck (PERKASH and FRIEDLAND 1986a).

The differential diagnosis includes bladder neck stricture, which causes a circumferential

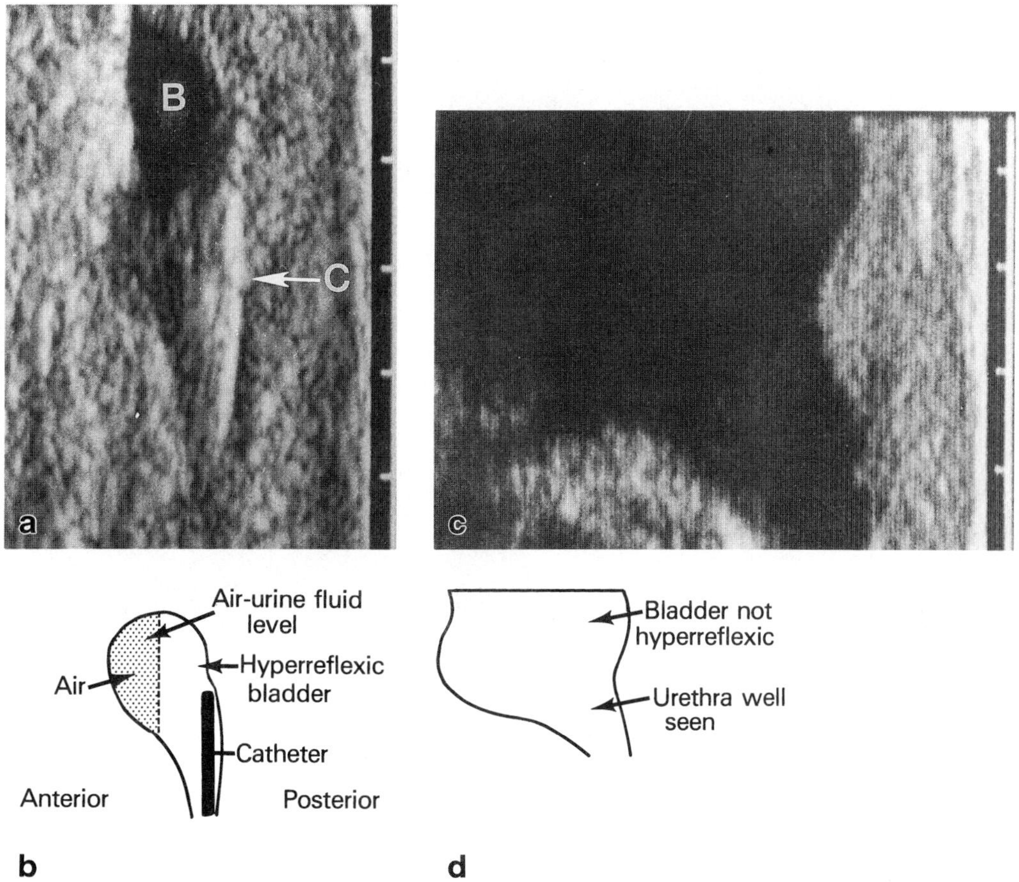

Fig. 16.27a–d. Catheter-induced precipitous bladder contractions. **a** Catheter (*C*) strikes the wall of the bladder (*B*), causing a precipitous bladder contraction with less than 125 ml of fluid in the bladder. **b** Diagrammatic illustration of **a**. **c** Examination repeated the next day without the catheter. No precipitous contractions. **d** Diagrammatic illustration of **c**. (PERKASH and FRIEDLAND 1986c)

narrowing of the bladder neck, and hyperplasia of the periurethral glands, which causes a rounded (not ledge-like) mass projecting into the bladder neck and bladder base posteriorly (PERKASH and FRIEDLAND 1986b).

16.8.2 Precipitous Bladder Contractions

Precipitous bladder contractions with less than 125 ml of urine in the bladder can occur in patients with no lesions of the brain or spinal cord, but who have benign prostatic hyperplasia (RESNICK and YALLA 1985, 1987). They are, however, very common in patients with suprapontine lesions, and may also occur in patients with infrapontine lesions, in patients with acute bladder infections, in patients in whom fluid has been introduced too rapidly into the bladder (as during urodynamic studies or a voiding cystourethrogram), or if the catheter touches the bladder wall and irritates it (PERKASH and FRIEDLAND 1986c; RESNICK and YALLA 1985, 1987) (Fig. 16.26).

Precipitous bladder contractions with less than 125 ml of urine in the bladder occur in 20% of patients with spinal cord injuries who have upper motor neuron lesions, but about 50% of these are catheter-induced precipitous bladder contractions (Fig. 16.27) and can be prevented entirely by introducing the catheter under ultrasonographic control (PERKASH and FRIEDLAND 1986c).

If the precipitous bladder contraction in a spinal cord injury patient is not catheter induced, the patient should receive an anticholinergic drug because it can prevent autonomic dysreflexia (Figs. 16.20, 16.28) if the lesion is above T5 (PERKASH and FRIEDLAND 1986c). If the precipitous bladder contraction is catheter-induced, no anticholinergic drug should be given, because it causes severe constipation, which is already a problem with spinal cord injury patients (PERKASH and FRIEDLAND 1986c).

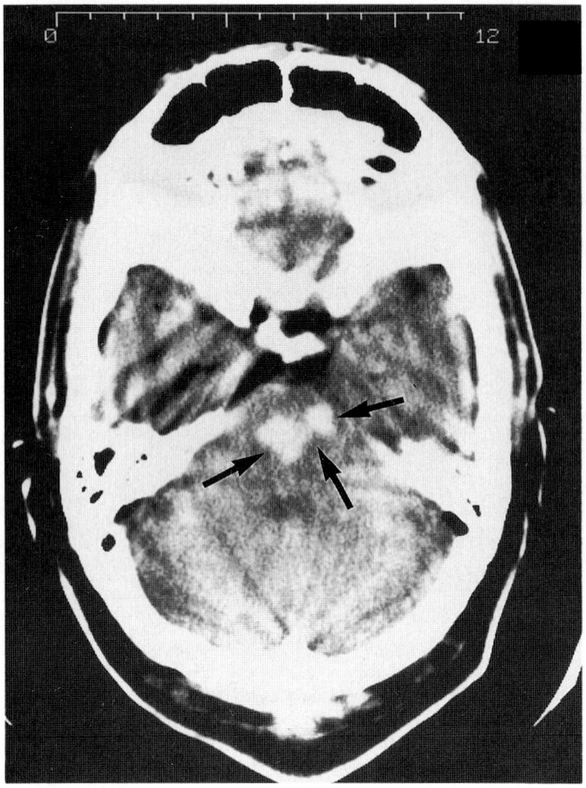

Fig. 16.28. CT scan showing a pontine hemorrhage (*arrows*) due to autonomic dysreflexia. This 32-year-old patient died as a result of the hemorrhage

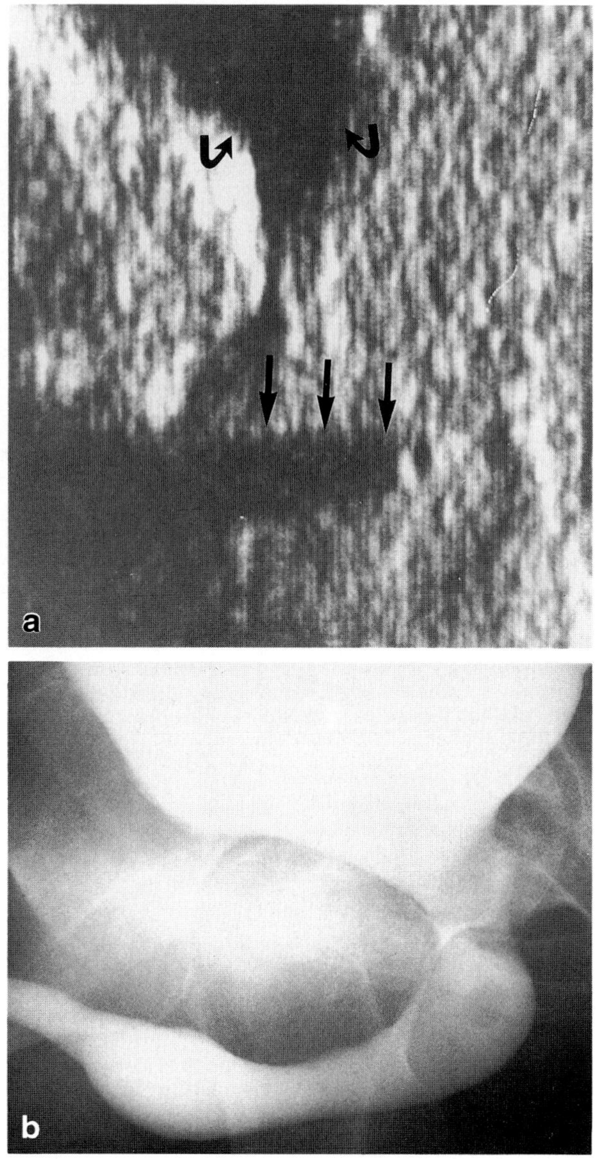

▷

Fig. 16.29 a,b. False passage in the prostatic urethra, well shown by introducing a catheter into the prostatic urethra under ultrasonographic control (*arrows*, **a**), but invisible on a radiographic voiding cystourethrogram (**b**). (Perkash and Friedland 1987b)

16.8.3 False Passages

False passages in the prostatic urethra can obstruct a catheter should it happen to go in that direction (Perkash and Friedland 1987b). A radiologic voiding cystourethrogram or retrograde urethrogram is usually negative in such cases, which must be diagnosed by introducing the catheter under ultrasonographic control and observing the catheter entering the false passage (Perkash and Friedland 1987b) (Fig. 16.29).

Such false passages have superior mucosal flaps, but during voiding, as, for example, during a voiding cystourethrogram, the urine stream forces the flap closed. When a catheter is pushed up the urethra, especially in the region of the angle of McNeal, its tip runs posteriorly because of its slight rigidity, elevates this flap, goes underneath it, and becomes impacted in the false passage (Perkash and Friedland 1987b) (Fig. 16.30).

Thus transrectal ultrasonography is an ideal method for diagnosing false passages (Perkash and Friedland 1987b). These false passages develop when the catheter repeatedly leaves the lumen in the same place, typically because it encounters an angle, typically at the junction of the bulbous and posterior urethra and in the midprostatic urethra (the angle of McNeal). Such repeated passages create a dead-ended

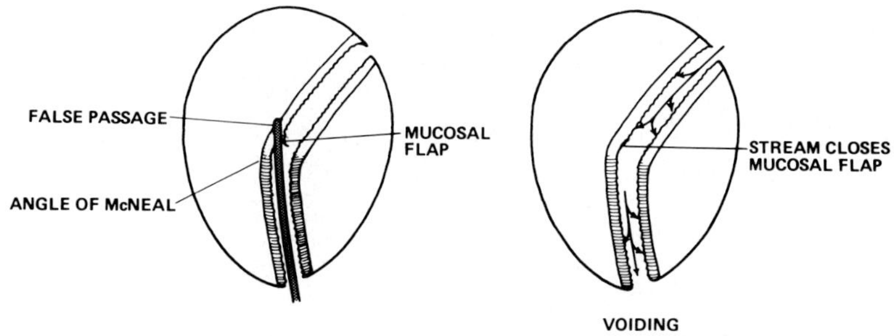

Fig. 16.30. Diagram illustrating how a catheter elevates the mucosal flap overlying a false passage, and how the urine stream forces the flap closed during voiding. (FRIEDLAND and PERKASH 1989)

false passage, which, on subsequent passes, the catheter may enter again.

16.9 The Angle of McNeal

McNEAL (1983) has described a 45° angle anteriorly at the midpoint of the prostatic urethra (Figs. 16.31, 16.32). We have described above how this may be a factor leading to a pathologic posterior ledge, and it probably contributes as well to the development of false passages in the prostatic urethra (McNEAL 1983).

A third problem, however, is that if a patient has some degree of detrusor–sphincter dyssynergia, and, as a result, some narrowing of the distal half of the prostatic urethra, the patient, attempting to void via the Credé maneuver, may actually close the bladder neck instead of opening it (PERKASH and FRIEDLAND 1984) (Fig. 16.33).

Thus, instead of the Credé maneuver, we instruct patients with detrusor–sphincter dyssynergia to undertake suprapubic tapping (PERKASH and FRIEDLAND 1984, 1985). If the patient has the use of his arms, he can do so himself, otherwise someone else must do it, but in either case 15–20 vigorous rapid taps with the ulnar side of the hand in the region of the bladder just above the symphysis pubis will help. Each tap does not elevate the bladder pressure much, but the periurethral striated sphincter contracts with each tap. Since this is striated muscle, after 15–20 such taps it tires, and suddenly relaxes, allowing the patient to void (Fig. 16.34). This is a very good method to initiate voiding in presphincterotomy patients, and the very best method of initiating voiding

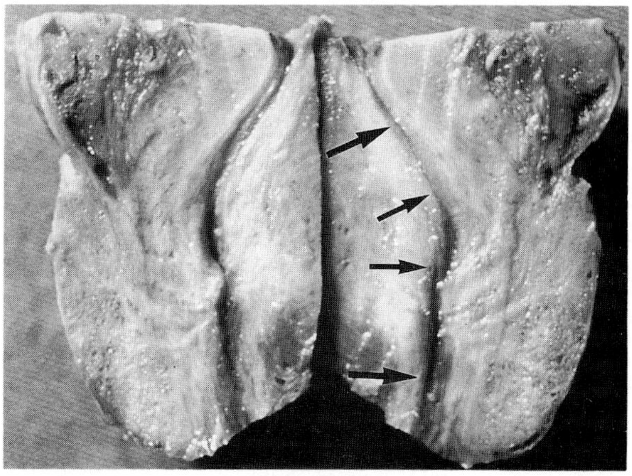

Fig. 16.31. Bivalved prostate, removed at autopsy from a 22-year-old man, showing how the urethra (*arrows*) angulates anteriorly at its midpoint. (PERKASH and FRIEDLAND 1986a)

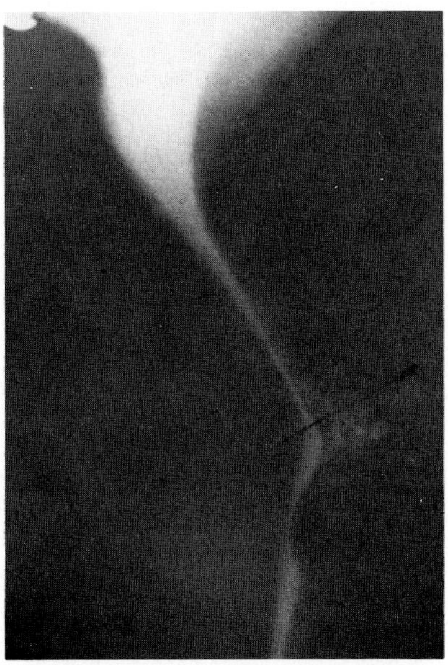

Fig. 16.32. Retrograde urethrogram performed at autopsy on the same patient shown in Fig. 18.31. Note the angle of McNeal. (PERKASH and FRIEDLAND 1986a)

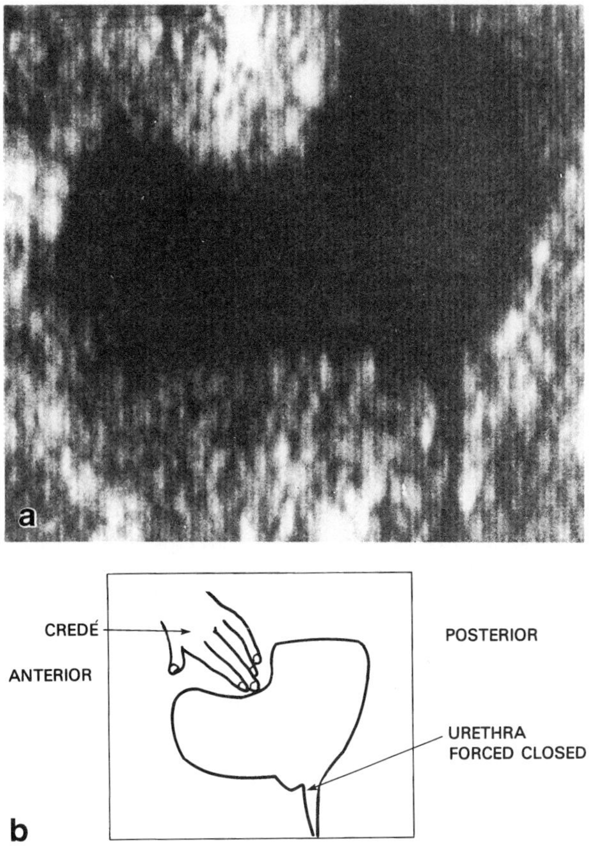

Fig. 16.33. **a** Ultrasonographic voiding cystourethrogram, showing how the Credé maneuver forces the urethra closed. **b** Lateral view: Diagrammatic illustration of **a**

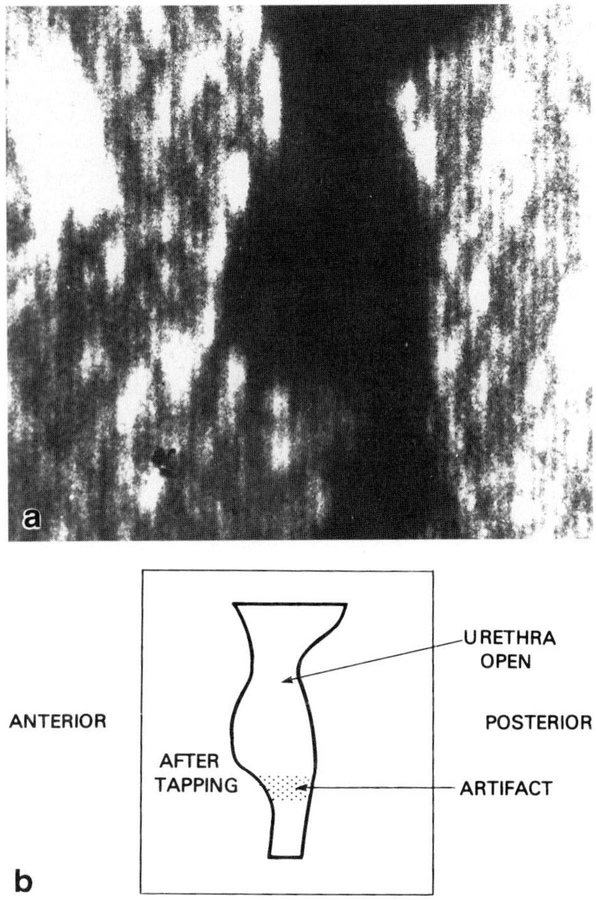

Fig. 16.34. **a** Ultrasonographic voiding cystourethrogram, showing that the urethra opens widely after suprapubic tapping (same patient as in Fig. 18.33). **b** Lateral view: Diagrammatic illustration of **a**. (Perkash and Friedland 1985)

after sphincterotomy, in order to be certain that the urethra relaxes completely.

16.8 Bladder Retraining

Transrectal ultrasonography is very useful in teaching patients the proper tapping maneuver in order to initiate voiding (Perkash and Friedland 1984). We ask them to observe the monitor during transrectal ultrasonography, and to teach themselves to tap in such a fashion as to open the urethra in a way that is correct for their own bodies (Perkash and Friedland 1984).

References

Amis SE Jr, Blaivas JG (1990) The role of the radiologist in evaluating voiding dysfunction. Radiology 175:317–318

Blaivas J (1984) Multichannel urodynamic studies. Urology 23:421–438

Blaivas JG, Norlen LJ (1984) Primary bladder neck obstruction. World J Urol 2:191–195

Bower GB, Lovegrove FT, Geysel H, Van der Schaff A, Guelfi G (1985) Comparison of "direct" and "indirect" radionuclide cystography. J Nucl Med 26:465–468

Brazda JF (1983) Washington Report. The Nation's Health 13:3

Brocklehurst JC (1986) The aging bladder. Br J Hosp Med 35:8–10

Chang PJ (1989) Bayesian analysis revisited: a radiologist's survival guide. AJR 152:721–727

Conway JJ (1985) Radionuclide cystography. In: Tauxe WN, Dubovsky EV (eds) Nuclear medicine in clinical urology and nephrology. Appleton-Century-Crofts, Norwalk, Connecticut, pp 305–320

Cosgriff P, Brown H (1990) Influence of kidney depth on the renographic estimation of relative renal function. J Nucl Med 31:1576–1577

Dennis PJ, Rohner TJ Jr, Hu TW, Igou JF, Yu LC, Kaltreider DL (1991) Simple urodynamic evaluation of incontinent elderly female nursing home patients. A descriptive analysis. Urology 37:173–179

Demuylder X, Claes H, Neven P, DeJaegher K (1992) Usefulness of urodynamic investigation in female incontinence. Eur J Obstet Gynecol Reproduct Biol 44: 205–208

Drach GW, Binard W (1976) Disposable peak urinary flow meter estimates lower urinary tract obstruction. J Urol 115:175–179

Friedland GW (1990) The urethra. Imaging and intervention in the 1990s. Clin Radiol 42:157–160

Friedland GW, Perkash I (1983) Neuromuscular dysfunction of the bladder and urethra. Semin Roentgenol 18:255–266

Friedland GW, Perkash I (1989) Imaging minzional nelle lesionic neurologiche. In: Pistolesi GF, Bergamo Andreis IA (eds) L'imaging del piccolo bacino funzionale. Libreria Cortina, Verona

Friedland GW, Chang P, Perkash I (1989) Imaging examinations in assessment of urethral disease. Prob Urol 3:820–860

Ganzer H, Madersbacher H, Rumpl E (1991) Cortico-evoked potential by stimulation vesicourethral junction: clinical value and neurophysiologic considerations. J Urol 146:118–123

Hald T, Bates P, Bradley WE (1984) The standardization of terminology of lower urinary tract function. International Continence Society, Glasgow, pp 1–34

Hinman F (1986) Nonneurogenic neurogenic bladder (the Hinman syndrome): 15 years later. J Urol 136:769–777

Kaplan SA, Chancellor MB, Blaivas JG (1991) Bladder and sphincter behavior in patients with spinal cord lesions. J Urol 146:113–117

Kulemeier KV, Lloyd LK, Stover SL (1985) Longterm followup of renal function after spinal cord injury. J Urol 134:8–11

Lose G (1991) Urethral pressure and power generation during coughing and voluntary contraction of the pelvic floor in healthy females. Br J Urol 67:580–585

Lose G, Colstrup H (1991) Mechanical properties of the urethra in healthy and in stress incontinent females: dynamic measurements in the resting urethra. J Urol 145:350–352

Manolin RA (1987) Voiding cystourethrography with synchronous measurements of pressures and flow in the diagnosis of subvesical obstruction in men: radiological view. J Urol 137:1196–1201

McNeal J (1983) The prostate gland: morphology and pathobiology. Monogr Urol 4:3–35

Nielsen JB, Jensen FT, Munch-Jorgensen T, Charles P, Djurhuus JC (1985) The diagnosis of vesico-ureteral reflux. Scand J Urol Nephrol 19:109–112

Nishizawa O, Moysiya I, Sato S, Harada T, Tsuchida S (1982) A new videourodynamics: combined ultrasonographic and urodynamic monitoring. Neurol Urodynam 1:295–301

O'Donnell PD, Beck C (1991) Urinar incontinence volume, patterns in elderly inpatient men. Urology 38:128–131

Perkash I, Friedland GW (1984) Using transrectal sonography to teach patients with spinal cord injuries to retrain their bladders. Radiology 152:228–229

Perkash I, Friedland GW (1985) Real-time gray-scale transrectal linear array ultrasonography in urodynamic evaluation. Semin Urol 3:49–59

Perkash I, Friedland GW (1986a) Posterior ledge of the bladder neck: the crucial diagnostic role of ultrasonography. Urol Radiol 8:175–183

Perkash I, Friedland GW (1986b) Transrectal ultrasonography of the lower urinary tract: evaluation of bladder neck problems. Neuroradiol Urodynam 5:299–306

Perkash I, Friedland GW (1986c) Catheter-induced hyperreflexia in spinal cord injury patients. Diagnosis by sonographic voiding cystourethrography. Radiology 159:453–455

Perkash I, Friedland GW (1987a) Principles of modern urodynamic studies. Invest Radiol 22:279–289

Perkash I, Friedland GW (1987b) Ultrasonographic detection of false passages arising from the posterior urethra in spinal cord injury patients. J Urol 137:701–702

Peters AM, Morony S, Gordon I (1990) Indirect radionuclide cystography demonstrates reflux under physiological conditions. Clin Radiol 41:44–47

Porena M, Vespaspiani G, Vergili G, Lombi R, Mearini E, Rosi P, Micali F (1987) Real-time transrectal sonographic voiding cystourethrography. Urology 30: 171–175

Raz S, Smith RB (1976) External sphincter spasticity syndrome in female patients. J Urol 115:443–446

Resnick M, Yalla SV (1985) Management of urinary incontinence in the elderly. N Engl J Med 313:800–805

Resnick NM, Yalla SV (1987) Detrusor hyperactivity with impaired contractile function. JAMA 257:3076–3081

Schmidt RA (1991) Urodynamics simplified. Urology 35: 449–454

Sfakianakis GN, Snuclovisky C, Strauss J, Hourani M, Lockhart G, Zilleruelo G, Freudlick M (1984) Improving the technique of nuclear cystography. Manometric approach. J Urol 131:1061–1064

Shabsign R, Fishman TJ, Krebs M (1987) The use of transrectal longitudinal real-time ultrasonography in urodynamics. J Urol 138:1416–1419

Shapeero G, Friedland GW, Perkash I (1983) Transrectal sonographic voiding cystourethrography. Studies in neuromuscular dysfunction. AJR 141:83–90

Tanagho AE, Schmidt RA (1982) Bladder pacemaker: scientific basis and clinical future. Urology 20:614–619

Tauxe WN, Dubovsky EV, Kidd T, Diaz F, Smith LR (1982) New formulas for the calculation of effective renal plasma flow. Eur J Nucl Med 7:51–54

Tempkin A, Sullivan G, Paldi J, Perkash I (1985) Radioisotope renography in spinal cord injury. J Urol 133: 228–230

VanGool JD, Vijverberg MA, Messer AP, Elzinger-Plomp A, VanJong TP (1992) Functional daytime incontinence: clinical and urodynamic assessment. Scan J Urol Nephrol Supplement 141:58–69

17 Testis and Scrotum

KYOUNG SIK CHO, BARBARA HSU, and ROBERT F. MATTREY

CONTENTS

17.1 Introduction

Cross-sectional imaging modalities have greatly improved the diagnosis of scrotal disease. In the clinical evaluation of scrotal abnormalities, physical examination may be difficult and inadequate because of severe pain, tenderness, swelling, and marked distortion of the inner contents of the scrotum. Currently, high-resolution ultrasonography is the imaging modality of choice because of its excellent depiction of scrotal anatomy, low cost, short examination time, and lack of ionizing radiation (LEOPOLD et al. 1979; CARROLL and GROSS 1983; HRICAK and FILLY 1983; KRONE and CARROLL 1985; BENSON et al. 1989; O'MARA and RIFKIN 1991). Color Doppler has added both anatomic and functional details relevant to the evaluation of the testis and its surrounding structures (MIDDLETON and MELSON 1989; BURKS et al. 1990; KRIEGER et al. 1990; LERNER et al. 1990; MIDDLETON et al. 1990; HORSTMAN et al. 1991a,b). Magnetic resonance imaging (MRI) is emerging as a powerful tool in the assessment of scrotal disease mostly because it has at least the sensitivity of ultrasonography but appears to have very high specificity. Like ultrasonography, it is capable of multiplanar imaging, displays flow, and is nonionizing. When compared to ultrasonography, the advantages of MRI are its wide field of view and its high contrast and spatial resolution. Its disadvantages are higher cost, limited patient access, and the necessity to sedate boys less than 8 years of age (BAKER et al. 1987a,b,c; RHOLL et al. 1987; THURNER et al. 1988; MATTREY and TRAMBERT 1990; FRITZSCHE et al. 1992).

The principal applications of scrotal imaging are to:

1. Localize a palpable mass as intratesticular or extratesticular
2. Detect occult neoplasm
3. Monitor the contralateral testis following unilateral orchiectomy for testicular carcinoma
4. Determine the cause of an acute scrotum
5. Evaluate the integrity of the testicle in cases of trauma or infection
6. Assess for complications when epididymitis does not respond to therapy
7. Determine the presence or absence of a varicocele in infertility
8. Assess testicular volume
9. Locate an undescended testis

Ultrasonography can resolve most of these problems; however, MRI becomes necessary when there is discrepancy between the clinical assessment and the ultrasonographic findings or when ultrasonography is equivocal or nonspecific (BAKER et al. 1987b; THURNER et al. 1988; MATTREY and TRAMBERT 1990).

KYOUNG SIK CHO, M.D., Associate Professor of Radiology, Asan Medical Center, University of Ulsan, 388-1 Poongnap-Dong, Songpa-Ku, Seoul 138-040, Korea
BARBARA HSU, M.D., Sharp Rees-Stealy Medical, 2001 Fourth Avenue, San Diego, CA 92101, USA
ROBERT F. MATTREY, M.D., Professor of Radiology, Magnetic Resonance Institute (8756), UCSD Medical Center, 200 West Arbor Drive, San Diego, CA 92103, USA

This chapter will describe the anatomy and embryology of the scrotum and the most useful imaging techniques for diagnosis. In addition we will demonstrate classical examples of scrotal pathology, providing background data to perform and interpret sonograms and MR scans of the scrotum.

17.2 Embryology

The testis and its efferent duct systems, the epididymis and vas deferens, develop from the gonadal ridges and mesonephric duct. Gonadal ridges develop by proliferation of the coelomic epithelium and condensation of the underlying mesenchyme during the fourth to fifth week of fetal life. Late in the fifth and early sixth week of embryologic development, the coelomic epithelium of the gonadal ridges proliferates and penetrates the underlying mesenchyme, where it forms a number of irregular shaped cords, named the primitive sex cords. During this time, both male and female gonads show the same morphology and are known as the indifferent gonads. Under the influence of the Y chromosome, the primitive sex cords continue to proliferate and penetrate deeper to form the testis or medullary cords. The cords split up into a network of tiny cell strands that point towards the hilus of the gland and give rise to the tubules of the rete testis. During the development the medullary cords are separated from the coelomic epithelium by a dense fibrous connective tissue, the tunica albuginea. During the fourth month of development, the testis cords become horseshoe shaped and their extremities continuous with those of the rete testis. At this point, the testis cords are composed of primitive germ cells and sustentacular cells of Sertoli derived from the surface epithelium gland. The testis cords remain solid until puberty, at which time they form the seminiferous tubules. At puberty they become canalized and join the rete testis tubules, which in turn enter the efferent ductules that are linked to the ductus deferens (MOORE 1988; SADLER 1990; O'MARA and RIFKIN 1991).

The interstitial cells of Leydig are derived from the mesenchyme of the gonadal ridge. In the eighth week of gestation, Leydig cells produce testosterone which affects sexual differentiation of the genital duct and external genitalia. Initially the embryo has two pairs of genital ducts, the mesonephric duct and the paramesonephric duct. In the male, as the mesonephros regresses, the mesonephric duct persists to form the main genital ducts, the ductus deferens and the epididymis. As the most cranial portion of the mesonephric duct regresses, it forms the appendix epididymis, and as the paramesonephric duct regresses, it forms the appendix testis. The caudal portion of the regressed mesonephros forms the paradidymis (ROLNICK et al. 1968; SADLER 1990).

The primitive testis is found in the posterior abdominal wall until the end of the second month. As the mesonephros degenerates, ligamentous bands (known as the caudal genital ligament and gubernaculum) descend to the inguinal region from the lower pole of the testes. Each gubernaculum then passes through the abdominal wall and attaches to the scrotal swelling. Independent from the descent of the testis, the peritoneal cavity evaginates following the course of the gubernaculum into the scrotal swelling to form the vaginal process. The vaginal process exits the fascial layers of the abdominal wall that form the inguinal canal accompanying the gubernaculum. By the 28th week of gestation, the testis descends to the level of the inguinal canal and by the 32nd week enters the scrotum. As the testis descends through the inguinal canal, it is covered by and becomes fused with reflected folds of the vaginal process to form the tunica vaginalis. At birth, 3% of male infants have undescended testes and this percentage decreases to 0.8% during the first year (MOORE 1988; SADLER 1990).

The mechanism of descent is not entirely clear. However, it has been shown that outgrowth of the extraabdominal gubernaculum produces intraabdominal migration of the testis, and that increasing intraabdominal pressure due to growth of intraabdominal organs causes the passage of the testis into the inguinal canal. Finally, regression of the gubernaculum produces testicular fixation to the scrotum. The process of descent is controlled by hormones, possibly androgens and müllerian inhibiting substances excreted by Sertoli cells (MOORE 1988; SADLER 1990).

17.3 Anatomy

The scrotum is a cutaneous pouch divided into two sacs by a partial median septum. Each sac contains the testis, epididymis, and lower portion of the spermatic cord. The tunica vaginalis invests the inner scrotal sac, partially covering all structures and forming an intravaginal space typically filled with 1–3 ml of fluid. In the order of outer to inner surface, scrotal wall consists of skin, subcutaneous fat, dartos muscle, external spermatic fascia, cremasteric muscle, inner spermatic fascia, and inner lining of parietal tunica vaginalis. Currently there are no imaging modalities that can differentiate these layers. However, swelling or scrotal wall hematoma in cases of inflammation or trauma can be recognized.

The normal adult testes are paired organs, ovoid in shape, measuring 4–5 cm in length, 2.5 cm in width, and 3 cm in anteroposterior diameter. They lie within the scrotal sac, suspended by the spermatic cord. The testis is covered by a visceral layer of the tunica vaginalis except for a strip that extends from the upper to lower pole leaving the region of the mediastinum testis uncovered. The mediastinum represents the invagination of the tunica albuginea. Inner components of the testis are divided into numerous lobules that contain the seminiferous tubules, the site of spermatogenesis. These lobules are separated from each other by fibrous septa that join at the mediastinum testis. The septa extend from the mediastinum to the tunica albuginea. The appendix testes measure 1–10 mm, are a remnant of the müllerian duct, and are present in 92% of males. They are attached to the tunica albuginea near the upper pole of the testis, are typically pedunculated, and are bilateral in 75% of males (Rolnick et al. 1968). Other testicular appendages are rarely identified, including the paradidymis (organ of Giraldés) and the superior and inferior vas aberrans of Haller.

The epididymis is the first part of the efferent route from the testis and lies along the superoposterolateral aspect of the testis. The epididymis is 6–7 cm in length, but it contains more than 6 m of a tortuous canal. It is divided into three parts: the head, body, and tail. The head of the epididymis (globus major, caput epididymis) is round or triangular and is situated at the upper pole of the testis. The epididymal head is approximately 6–15 mm in width.

The numerous straight seminiferous tubules within the testis enter the mediastinum testis to form a network named the rete testis. The upper end of the mediastinum testis forms 12–20 ducts termed the efferent ductules, which pass from the testis to the epididymal head. The efferent ductules become enlarged and exceedingly convoluted, forming a series of conical masses, which together form the epididymal head. All ductules in the head open into the one named the ductus epididymis, with complex convolution, forming the body of the epididymis. The body of the epididymis is approximately 2–4 mm in diameter. The epididymal duct is slightly enlarged and thickened at the lower pole of the testis, forming the tail of the epididymis (globus minor). The size of the epididymal tail is approximately 2–4 mm. From this point the epididymis ascends medially and superiorly to become the ductus deferens (Mattrey and Trambert 1990; O'Mara and Rifkin 1991; Tanagho 1992). A small protuberance may be identified adjacent to the epididymal head, named the appendix epididymis, which is a remnant of the mesonephric ducts. The epididymal appendix is present in 34% of males. One-third of these men have them bilaterally (Rolnick et al. 1968).

The ductus deferens (vas deferens) is a single muscular duct that connects the epididymis to the seminal vesicle duct to form the ejaculatory duct. The vas deferens is 2–3 mm in diameter and about 45 cm in length. It is part of the spermatic cord, which travels from the posterior border of the testis through the spermatic and inguinal canal to reach the deep inguinal region. In addition to the vas deferens, the spermatic cord consists of cremasteric muscle, vessels, nerve, and lymphatics.

When the testis descends into the scrotum, it is accompanied by the processus vaginalis, which originates from the peritoneum and becomes fused to the scrotal wall and a significant portion of the tunica albuginea of the testis to become the tunica vaginalis. There is typically 1–3 ml of fluid within the tunica vaginalis as lubricant. Since the epididymal head is also covered by the tunica vaginalis, it is also bathed in this fluid. In normal males, the tunica vaginalis leaves a bare area along the mediastinum testis that encompasses approximately one-third of the testicular equator and extends from the upper to the lower pole of the testis, providing a broad anchor.

The arterial supply of the scrotum is composed of three arteries, the testicular, cremasteric, and deferential arteries. The testicular artery is a branch of the aorta that arises just below the renal artery, descends within the retroperitoneum, and enters the deep inguinal ring. At that level, the testicular artery is joined by the vas deferens, the cremasteric artery, a branch of the inferior epigastric artery, and the deferential artery, a branch of the vesicular artery to form the spermatic cord.

Although there are anastomoses among these three arteries, the testis is mainly supplied by the testicular artery. After entering the scrotum, the testicular artery runs along the posterior aspect of the testis and penetrates the tunica albuginea, forming capsular arteries. These arteries run just beneath the tunica albuginea in a layer named the tunica vasculosa. The capsular arteries send centripetal branches that enter the testicular parenchyma and flow toward the mediastinum testis. When these branches reach the mediastinum, they turn back and travel in an opposite direction, forming the recurrent rami arteries (HARRISON and BARKELEY 1948; HORSTMAN et al. 1991a). In a significant number of males, a branch of the testicular artery enters the mediastinum testis and travels towards the tunica vasculosa to anastomose with the capsular arteries. The deferential and cremasteric arteries supply the epididymis, vas deferens, and peritesticular tissue. Venous outflow from the testis is through the mediastinum testis. The venous drainage then travels through the pampiniform plexus to exit from the scrotum along the spermatic cord.

17.4 Imaging Technique

17.4.1 Ultrasonography

The ultrasonographic examination of the testis is performed with a short-focused high-resolution real-time 7.5- to 10-MHz transducer. The patient is scanned in the supine position with the scrotum supported by towels draped beneath it or stabilized by the examiner's gloved hand. The latter instance has the advantage of allowing correlation between a palpable lesion and its ultrasonic findings, as the examiner's finger is readily identified as a highly echogenic band beyond the lesion (KRONE and CARROLL 1985). Examination is usually done with direct contact of the transducer coupled by acoustic gel applied evenly to the scrotal skin. On occasion a synthetic standoff is helpful when the testis is in the near-field of the transducer and proximal to the focal zone, as is encountered in prepubertal boys and when testes are atrophic (FORNAGE et al. 1984). The scrotal wall should be stretched and large amounts of acoustic gel used to avoid air entrapment in the hair or scrotal wall wrinkles. Imaging is done in the longitudinal and transverse planes as well as oblique sections if needed. In addition to the evaluation of the testis and epididymis in their entirety, an image of the epididymis and ipsilateral testis and an image of both testes across the septum should be obtained simultaneously to allow for the assessment of texture and echogenicity relationships. All gain settings are adjusted to provide uniform echogenicity of the testicle (KRONE and CARROLL 1985; BENSON et al. 1989; O'MARA and RIFKIN 1991).

After gray-scale examination of the scrotal contents, color Doppler ultrasonography may be used to evaluate blood flow. Scrotal color Doppler ultrasonography should be performed with a high-frequency transducer (equal to or greater than 5 MHz) to increase sensitivity to slow flow. This is important because on occasions, color Doppler performed at 5 MHz is unable to detect flow in normal adult males. It should be noted that although imaging on duplex systems is done at 7 MHz, the Doppler ultrasound wave may be operating at a lower frequency. Equipment manufacturers should be able to provide the transducer specification. The Doppler settings should be optimized for slow flow and should be able to detect flow as slow as 3 cm/s, particularly when imaging prepubertal boys. To achieve this high Doppler gain setting, low pulse repetition frequency, slow real-time frame rate, and a minimal wall filter may be required, which also increase the susceptibility to motion artifact and image noise (KRIEGER et al. 1990; HORSTMAN et al. 1991a; RALLS et al. 1991). Longitudinal, transverse, and oblique scanning should be performed to obtain the optimal display of testicular vascular anatomy. Color Doppler images of both testes should be comparable and symmetric.

17.4.2 Magnetic Resonance Imaging

The patient is placed supine on the scan table, feet first. The scrotum is elevated by means of a rolled towel or a specially designed triangular support placed between the thighs such that the testes lie in a horizontal plane. Another towel is draped over the thighs and scrotal region. To improve spatial and contrast resolution and signal homogeneity, a 12.5-cm circular surface coil is centered over the scrotum and placed horizontally on a 1-cm standoff. The coil is positioned such that the bottom of the coil is over the caudal tip of the scrotal sac. In infants and toddlers a diaper serves as the standoff. In infants and children, or when testes are very small, the use of the standard 9-cm circular coil should be considered, instead of the 12.5-cm coil. The entire area is then wrapped with the 14-in. strap, which is attached to the table to minimize patient motion. Ensure that the penis is left angled to the side in the patient's natural position. Do not angle the penis straight back against the anterior abdominal wall since the tight table strap could induce erection and cause motion. The isocenter is positioned at midscrotum (BAKER et al. 1987a; MATTREY and TRAMBERT 1990; MATTREY 1991).

A short TR and TE spin-echo sequence (400/12) is used in the sagittal plane to provide T1 contrast for tissue characterization and to serve as a localizer for further sequences. Note that the isocenter needs to be adjusted anteriorly since in most adults, the scrotum is approximately 3 cm anterior to isocenter. This adjustment may not be needed in smaller patients. A field of view of 20 cm is used to include the scrotum and inguinal region. This series is acquired with two acquisitions, 5-mm slice thickness and 1-mm interslice gap. No frequency or phase wrap should be used and no saturation pulses are needed. The sagittal plane defines the full anteroposterior dimension of the scrotum and ensures that the coronal plane covers the entire area of interest. Occasionally, the "bare area" of the testes and cord is best seen in this plane on T2-weighted sequences. However, sagittal images offer limited recognition of the epididymis, epididymis–scrotal wall interface, and epididymis–testis interface. They also do not allow for right and left comparison on the same image (BAKER et al. 1987a; MATTREY and TRAMBERT 1990; MATTREY 1991).

The next sequence is obtained in the coronal plane starting from the posterior aspect of the scrotum and proceeding anteriorly to include the anterior aspect of the external inguinal ring. This series is a double spin-echo sequence obtained with a long TR (2000/20/70). A fast spin-echo (FSE) sequence (3500/120) has yielded images analogous to the 2000/70 but with higher resolution and faster acquisition. Although we have adopted a T1 coronal (400/12) and an FSE sequence obtained in the coronal plane at the same plane levels as a replacement for the multiecho sequence, no data are available comparing these two techniques. Our preliminary data suggest that the two techniques are comparable. These series are obtained with a 16-cm field of view, 3-mm slice thickness, and 1.5-mm interslice gap as well as a 128 matrix and two acquisitions. A 192 matrix and an echo trail of 16 are used for the FSE technique. The T1 sequence obtained as a pair with the FSE technique is obtained with identical parameters as the FSE sequence except for a matrix size of 128 to speed imaging. The coronal plane is ideal for displaying scrotal anatomy (BAKER et al. 1987a; MATTREY and TRAMBERT 1990). It allows complete visualization of all the important anatomic structures and demonstrates the epididymis and the spermatic cord optimally. It also allows comparison of the right and left hemiscrotal and inguinal regions.

The sagittal T1 and coronal planes are sufficient in most individuals. At times when searching for a testicular lesion and the coronal series is normal or when the pathology is complex, an axial plane obtained as a multiecho or a combination T1 and FSE is of benefit (MATTREY and TRAMBERT 1990). Axial images allow right and left comparison and provide optimal visualization of the anterior and posterior aspects of the testis and scrotum, which are not well assessed on coronal sections.

Studies have not yet established whether the use of intravenous (IV) contrast agents is of benefit in MRI of the scrotum. We have shown that Gd-DTPA significantly enhances the normal testis and epididymis (CHO et al. 1991) and that the enhancement lasts for a significant length of time. Because the water-soluble agent is eliminated more rapidly from tumors than from normal testicular tissue, tumors that are typically invisible on T1-weighted images become more apparent following contrast administration (CHO et al. 1991; JUST et al. 1992). However, there is loss of specificity in that seminomatous and nonseminomatous lesions assume a similar appearance. A dose of 0.1 mmol/kg of body weight is usually used. Precontrast and postcontrast images should be obtained with otherwise identical imaging planes and techniques to allow for appropriate comparison. The use of IV contrast does aid in distinguishing cystic from solid lesions and allows the assessment of testicular vascularity. Although the enhancement is homogeneous and frequently highlights the rete testis in normal testes, inhomogeneous enhancement patterns have been observed, the reason for which remains unclear.

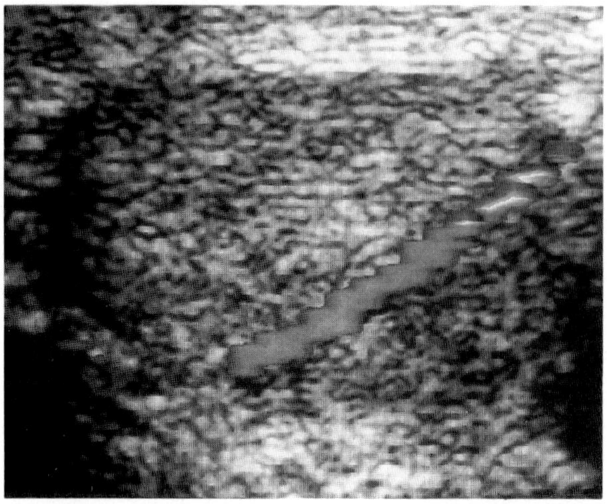

Fig. 17.1. Doppler ultrasonography of the normal testis demonstrating a major artery traversing the testis from the region of the mediastinum towards the tunica albuginea

17.5 Normal Appearance

17.5.1 Ultrasonography

The normal testis is homogeneous with low to medium level echotexture similar to that of other endocrine glands such as thyroid (Leopold et al. 1979; Hricak and Filly 1983; Krone and Carroll 1985; Benson et al. 1989; O'Mara and Rifkin 1991). Both testes should be symmetric and of equal echogenicity. Tunica albuginea and appendix testis are not generally identified unless a hydrocele is present (Krone and Carroll 1985). The mediastinum testis is frequently seen as an echogenic line along the long axis of the testicle paralleling the epididymis. The septa may be visualized as echogenic or hypoechoic strands radiating from the mediastinum testis into the parenchyma toward the tunica albuginea (Krone and Carroll 1985). On occasion a 2- to 3-mm-thick hypoechoic band is seen in the normal testicular parenchyma perpendicular to the mediastinum testis and oriented towards the upper pole (Fig. 17.1). This represents a normal variant of intratesticular vasculature (Fakhry et al. 1989). Although unusual, small (<2 mm) echogenic foci with or without shadowing may be seen scattered within both testes. Microlithiasis, as this condition has been called, is bilateral and is of no clinical significance. It is typically discovered as an incidental finding (Janzen et al. 1992). For further discussion see below.

The echogenicity of the globus major is similar to or slightly greater than that of the testis, although echotexture may be somewhat coarse. The echogenicity of the epididymal body and tail is similar to or slightly lower than that of the testis (Krone and Carroll 1985; O'Mara and Rifkin 1991). Although the tail is frequently visible, the body of the epididymis is difficult to identify and distinguish from peritesticular tissues. The reason for the greater echogenicity of head than body is presumed to be the numerous tubules that are present in the former. The pampiniform plexus at the base of the scrotum is typically hyerechoic and difficult to distinguish from adjacent fat. The spermatic cord is at times visible as a heterogeneous hyperechoic band with variable tubular hypoechoic structures. Flow within vessels in the pampiniform plexus and cord is easily depicted with color Doppler. The multiple layers of the scrotal wall cannot be distinguished. The normal wall is typically less than 3 mm in thickness and appears as a highly echogenic stripe. There is normally 1–3 ml of fluid bathing the testis that is visible as an anechoic space at the angles between the testis and epididymal head and tail (Krone and Carroll 1985; O'Mara and Rifkin 1991).

Color Doppler ultrasonography can display arterial flow in the normal spermatic cord and testis, but not in the normal epididymis. Venous flow within the normal scrotum is not usually seen. The main testicular artery is detected along the posterior superior aspect of the testis, where it penetrates the tunica albuginea to form the major capsular arteries. These arteries are well visualized along the outer margin of the testis in either longitudinal or transverse planes. The centripetal branches and the recurrent rami arteries are visible with flow towards the mediastinum in the former and towards the tunica in the latter. These intratesticular arteries are relatively straight and well visualized when imaged in a slightly oblique plane to the standard longitudinal and transverse planes. Although the capsular and centripetal arteries are visible in all normal adult testes, the recurrent rami are seen in only a few individuals. The Doppler wave form of the testicular artery and its branches exhibits a low-resistive pattern with high diastolic flow (Harrison and Barkeley 1948; Horstman et al. 1991a; Ralls et al. 1991).

17.5.2 Magnetic Resonance Imaging

The normal testis is a sharply demarcated oval structure with low to intermediate signal intensity on the T1- and intermediately weighted images and high signal intensity on the T2-weighted images (Fig. 17.2) (BAKER et al. 1987a; MATTREY and TRAMBERT 1990; FRITZSCHE et al. 1992). It is surrounded by the tunica albuginea, a thin layer of dense fibrous tissue, that has low signal intensity on T2-weighted images (Fig. 17.2). It can appear slightly brighter due to partial volume when the slice plane is nearly tangential to the testicular surface. The small amount of fluid present between the layers of the tunica vaginalis follows the expected signal behavior of water (slightly lower in signal than testis on T1-weighted images and slightly brighter than (testis on T2-weighted images) (BAKER et al. 1987a; MATTREY and TRAMBERT 1990).

The mediastinum testis yields a similar signal to testis on the T1-weighted sequence and becomes darker than testis on the T2-weighted sequence (Fig. 17.2). In some patients intrinsic testicular signal, while homogeneous, displays internal texture outlining lobules and rete testes that radiate from the mediastinum testis towards the tunical surface. Normal intratesticular vessels are infrequently seen in normal testes. In some men, however, a branch of the testicular artery can be seen emanating from the superior aspect of the mediastinum and coursing obliquely towards a diametrically opposed position in the upper aspect of the testis.

The epididymis is an inhomogeneous structure with signal intensity less than or equal to the normal testis on the T1- and intermediately weighted images but is moderately less intense than testis on T2-weighted images (MATTREY and TRAMBERT 1990; MATTREY 1991; FRITZSCHE et al. 1992). The head, body, and tail of the normal epididymis are easily delineated. The head of the epididymis is wedge shaped, lays lateral to the upper pole of the testis draping the tunical signal, and is frequently surrounded by a small amount of fluid. The normal tail, best seen when highlighted by fluid, is smaller than the epididymal head. The body of the epididymis lies alongside the mediastinum testis along the bare area of the testis. It can be easily distinguished from testis because it is darker than testis on the T2-weighted images and is separated from testicular tissue by the dark tunica albuginea.

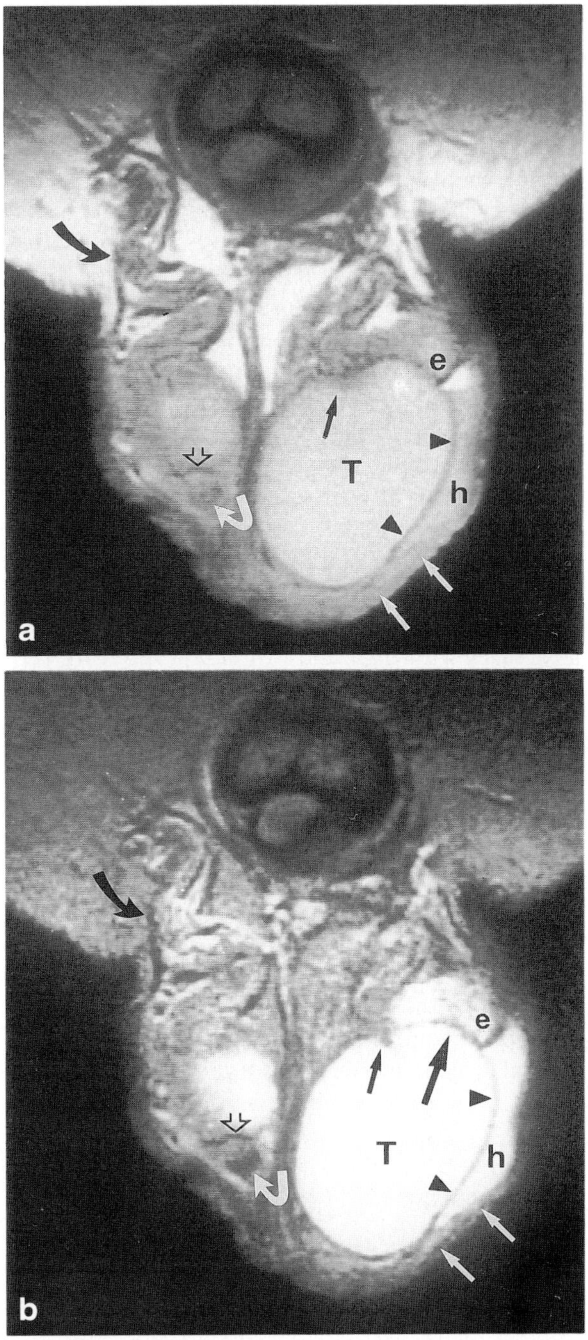

Fig. 17.2a,b. Normal testes (*T*), epididymis (*e*), tunica albuginea (*arrowheads*), and mediastinum testis (*small black arrow*), are shown in the coronal plane on **a** hydrogen density and **b** T2-weighted images. A small hydrocele (*h*) is shown best on the T2-weighted image; it is located within the tunical layers highlighting the lateral testis and epididymal head (*e*). Note the accordion-shaped spermatic cord (*curved black arrow*) entering the base of the right hemiscrotum. On the right, the tunica is not seen because the plane of section is too oblique to the testicular surface, thereby increasing partial volume. At the surface, a small superficial artery can be seen (*open arrow*). There is a focus of dark signal in the right epididymal tail (*curved white arrow*), probably representing chronic or old epididymitis. (BAKER et al. 1987a)

When the outer parietal and inner visceral layers of the tunica vaginalis are separated by a larger volume of fluid (hydrocele), the fluid surrounds the testes except posteromedially along the bare area where the testis is attached to the scrotal wall. The fluid volume is considered excessive when it surrounds the equator of the testis. The scrotal sac structures such as fat and dartos muscle are visualized on occasion.

The spermatic cord is easily imaged in all cases and is seen from the internal inguinal ring to the base of the scrotum. Serpiginous high signal intensity areas within the cord on intermediately and T2-weighted images are phase and chemical shift artifacts due to flow in the vascular structures, which are typically surrounded by fat. At times, the cremasteric reflex causes foreshortening of the cord that gives it a nodular appearance in cross-section. At the base of the scrotum, superior and lateral to the testis, the tortuous tubular structures with high and low signal intensity represent the pampiniform plexus, which can be followed into the inguinal canal. Since these vessels are intermixed with fat, both phase shift and chemical shift artifacts are frequently present. The deferent duct can be seen in some patients. When seen, it is a smooth undulating tubular structure similar in signal intensity to that of the testis. The deferent duct is not visualized in most patients. A more frequently encountered smooth undulating structure with signal similar to testis that follows the cords and epididymis and at times extends beyond the bare area of the testis to the scrotal wall is likely dilated veins with stagnant flow.

17.6 Pathology

17.6.1 Congenital Anomaly

17.6.1.1 Cryptorchidism

Cryptorchidism is the most common disorder of sexual differentiation in man. It occurs in 20%–33% of premature neonates and in 2.7%–6% of full-term infants. These testes will usually descend to their normal position during the first year of life. By 12 months of age, 0.8% of boys are considered as having undescended testes since spontaneous descent beyond the first year of life is unlikely (Scorer and Farrington 1972; Cour-Palar 1966; Hadziselimovic 1983; Fritzsche et al. 1987). Bilateral cryptorchidism occurs in about 10% of cases. Between 3% and 5% have total absence of testes at surgery (Krone and Carroll 1985; Friendland and Chang 1988; O'Mara and Rifkin 1991). An undescended testis may be intra-abdominal, intracanalicular, ectopic, atrophic, or absent. Undescended testes may be located anywhere from the renal hilum to the superior scrotum. However, 80% of cases are located near the inguinal canal (Krone and Carroll 1985). They may also be found in an ectopic location such as the perineum or superficial abdominal wall. Undescended testes located near the internal inguinal ring are not usually palpable. As a rule, undescended testes are smaller than the normal contralateral side and frequently have variable degrees of fibrosis that can give the testis a darker signal on T2-weighted images.

The etiologies of cryptorchidism are complex and unclear, including familial inheritance (prune belly syndrome), mechanical obstruction along the path of descent, congenital abnormality of the testicle, and abnormal hormonal effects (especially dihydrotestosterone) during embryogenesis (Friedland and Chang 1988). Cryptorchidism may be associated with other urogenital abnormalities including renal agenesis, renal ectopia, and prune belly syndrome. It is commonly associated with congenital inguinal hernia. Undescended testes located near the public rami can be easily injured in trauma. Further, because the spermatic cord may be attached to the undescended testis abnormally, torsion is more frequent in cryptorchidism (Krone and Carroll 1985; Friedland and Chang 1988; O'Mara and Rifkin 1991).

Impaired spermatogenesis occurs in cryptorchid testes. However, if the testis is brought to the scrotum by the age of 6, sterility may be avoided. Forty-four percent of men with repaired bilateral undescended testes maintain fertility (Krone and Carroll 1985). Undescended testes located near the inguinal ring have a four to five times greater risk of developing malignancy as compared to the general population. Intraabdominal testes have a yet higher incidence of malignancy. The malignant tumor is most frequently seminoma, and sarcomatous degeneration is the most ominous complication (Pinch et al. 1974; Batata et al. 1980; Rajfer 1992). It is currently accepted that the higher incidence of malignancy in cryptorchid testes is because they are intrinsically abnormal and surgical repair is necessary to allow the testis to be closely monitored or removed.

Ultrasonography. Various diagnostic modalities, such as ultrasonography (Wolveson et al. 1983; Weiss et al. 1986), computed tomography (Lee and Glazer 1982; Wolveson et al. 1983; Green 1985), spermatic venography (Glickman et al. 1977; Green 1985), arteriography, and MRI (Fritzsche et al. 1987; Landa et al. 1987; Kier et al. 1988; Friedland and Chang 1988) have been used to localize the cryptorchid testis. Reports on the accuracy of ultrasonography in detecting an undescended testis have been mixed, so that while some have claimed it to be extremely accurate (Wolveson et al. 1983), others have regarded it as unsatisfactory as a screening examination (Weiss et al. 1986). When testes are palpable, ultrasonography can recognize a normal undescended testis by visualizing the mediastinum testis and potential intrinsic flow on color Doppler (Zoeller and Ringert 1991). Using the proper gain setting, the echogenicity of the undescended testis is similar to the normal testis unless it is atrophic or neoplastic (Krone and Carroll 1985; O'Mara and Rifkin 1991). When testes are deep or intraabdominal they are difficult to detect (Weiss et al. 1986). Further, at times it is difficult to distinguish an inguinal testis from a lymph node on ultrasonography since the spermatic canal is difficult to identify. Although x-ray computed tomography can detect an intraabdominal testis with higher sensitivity and specificity than ultrasonography, it requires sedation of infants and young boys and delivers ionizing radiation (Lee and Glazer 1982; Wolveson et al. 1983). Further, the undescended testis assumes a soft tissue density similar to surrounding muscle or bowel. When the testis is surrounded by fat, it is easily recognized because of its ovoid shape and characteristic location along the course of testicular descent (Lee and Glazer 1982).

Magnetic Resonance Imaging. Magnetic resonance imaging has become the most accurate diagnostic modality for the detection of undescended testes. The first report of MRI in cryptorchidism showed that 15 of 16 undescended testes were correctly identified and only one intraabdominal testis was missed (Fritzsche et al. 1987). Other reports have had similar results (Landa et al. 1987; Kier et al. 1988; Friedland and Chang 1988). However, some authors reported difficulties identifying the intraabdominal testis (Fritzsche et al. 1987; Kier et al. 1988). As compared to the other imaging modalities, MRI allows the clear distinction of the undescended testis from its surrounding structures because of the multiplanar imaging capability as well as high tissue contrast . Further, it is nonionizing but does require sedation. MRI can clearly differentiate testis from adjacent hernia fluid, omental fat, and lymph nodes and can clearly delineate atrophic testes (Landa et al. 1987; Fritzsche et al. 1987; Kier et al. 1988; Friedland and Chang 1988).

The MRI technique to detect undescended testes is different from conventional scrotal MRI (Mattrey and Trambert 1990; Mattrey 1991). A high field system and surface coils are more adequate for this examination because of the ability to perform thin slices and a higher signal to noise ratio on T2-weighted images for adequate contrast resolution. A standard 5-in. circular surface coil is centered approximately over the symphysis pubis to ensure that the base of the scrotum and lower pelvis are included in the field of view. The coil is placed on a 1-cm standoff to decrease the high near-signal. In less than 20% of subjects, a body coil sequence, or head coil in infants, is used to image the pelvis and lower abdomen when testes are not found on the surface coil study. A small field of view (16–20 cm), high acquisition matrix, and thin slice thickness (usually 3 mm) are used to provide adequate spatial resolution. Axial T1-weighted scans are obtained in 5 mm thickness from the base of the scrotum to midbladder. This is followed by coronal T1- and T2-weighted scans that cover from the posterior aspect of the scrotum to the anterior surface of the abdominal wall. We now use a T1 and an FSE pair obtained at identical locations.

However, a variable echo sequence (2000/20/7) is also adequate. Since 80% of undescended testes are located near the inguinal canal, these sequences are sufficient. If the testes are near the internal inguinal ring or are intraabdominal, an axial T2-weighted scan over the testis is helpful to locate the testis relative to the iliac vessels and inguinal canal and ligament. If the testis or its cord structures are not seen, a T1-and T2-weighted axial series, using the body or head coil when appropriate, is acquired from the symphysis pubis to the renal hilum with a large field of view (20–34 cm) and a thicker slice (5–10 mm). The testis located above the inguinal ring is usually found along the path of the testicular artery, which courses along the anterior surface of the psoas muscle to the iliac vessels and then along the midpelvic sidewall to the bladder and finally

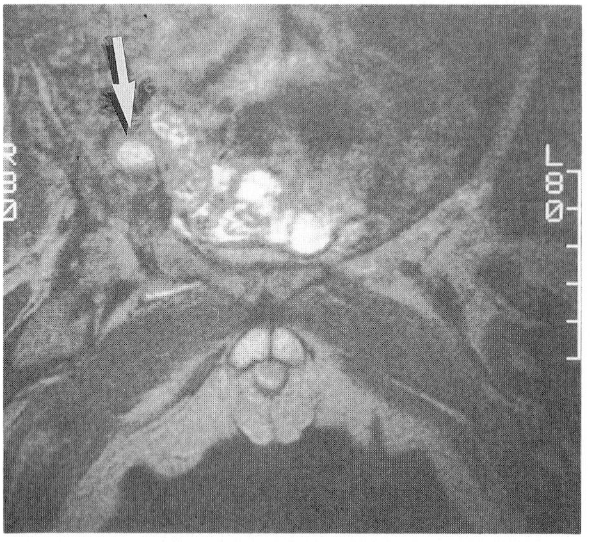

Fig. 17.3. T2-weighted image in a newborn with bilateral hernias and bilateral undescended testes. The right testis is located in a typical intraabdominal location (*arrow*), as was proven surgically. The left testis is not shown. (MATTREY and TRAMBERT 1990)

upwards lateral to the bladder towards the internal inguinal ring (Fig. 17.3).

The MR report should describe both the testis and the spermatic cord. If the testis is seen, its location, size, and signal intensity should be reported. If the testis is not visualized, the report should describe the spermatic cord. If the spermatic cord is seen, describe the location of its distal end, its thickness, and whether it enters the internal inguinal ring. These findings allow the surgeon to assess whether surgery is necessary, plan the surgical approach and treatment, and determine whether laparoscopy is required.

The task of locating intraabdominal testes is the most difficult in that confusion with lymph nodes and bowel is possible. In both published reports each missed a high intraabdominal testis (FRITZSCHE et al. 1987; KIER et al. 1987). With the advent of MR oral contrast and with increased experience, this problem could be partially overcome. Because testes enhance with IV contrast, the utility of fat-suppressed IV-enhanced studies has not been assessed to determine whether improvement can be achieved. However, there will always be a degree of uncertainty when testes are not clearly depicted. Whereas it is important to visualize these high intraabdominal testes (FRIEDLAND and CHANG 1988), it is the author's belief that there will always be a degree of uncertainty concerning whether laparoscopy should precede exploration. Therefore, the inability to visualize the high intraabdominal testis is less critical for patient management, since patients with absent cord and testis would have to undergo surgical exploration that would be preceded by laparoscopy. When the testis, cord, or both are well evaluated, laparoscopy is not necessary.

Assessment of the spermatic cord and testis together is essential for proper diagnosis. An empty spermatic canal is visible on MRI. It appears as a thin line extending from the inguinal canal to the base of the scrotum, most likely representing the gubernaculum, a thin fibrous strand. This should not be mistaken for an atrophic cord. The latter has significant width but is thinner than the normal contralateral cord. While an empty canal and an absent cord suggest the possibility of an intraabdominal testis, the presence of cord structures in the canal does not exclude this possibility. Cord structures may precede the testis, or if attached to a long mesentery the testis may flip-flop between an intracanalicular and an intraabdominal location. In fact, testicular venography performed to localize undescended testes have been known to show elements of the pampiniform plexus leading the testis by as much as 10–12 cm (Fig. 17.4).

The majority of intraabdominal testes will be found near the internal inguinal ring, where MRI should be reasonably accurate. Therefore, the goal of the imaging schemes should be to maximize the assessment of the internal inguinal ring. The technique described above would allow such assessment. The 5-in. surface coil should be centered over the pubic tubercle to place the testis at an optimal position in the field.

Magnetic resonance imaging is extremely accurate in its ability to locate inguinal testes because testes are contrasted with fat, and because they are depicted along with their epididymis and surrounding intravaginal fluid which is present in many cases (Fig. 17.5). The testis has a normal ovoid shape with clear demonstration of the tunica albuginea and mediastinum. These testes can assume three positions: the subcutaneous space anterior to the external inguinal ring; the spermatic canal; or the inguinal canal. When testes do not exit the inguinal canal, they frequently proceed laterally and insinuate themselves over the femoral vessels. In this location, they are frequently impalpable.

Intracanalicular testes are easily differentiated from lymph nodes, because their tunica albuginea

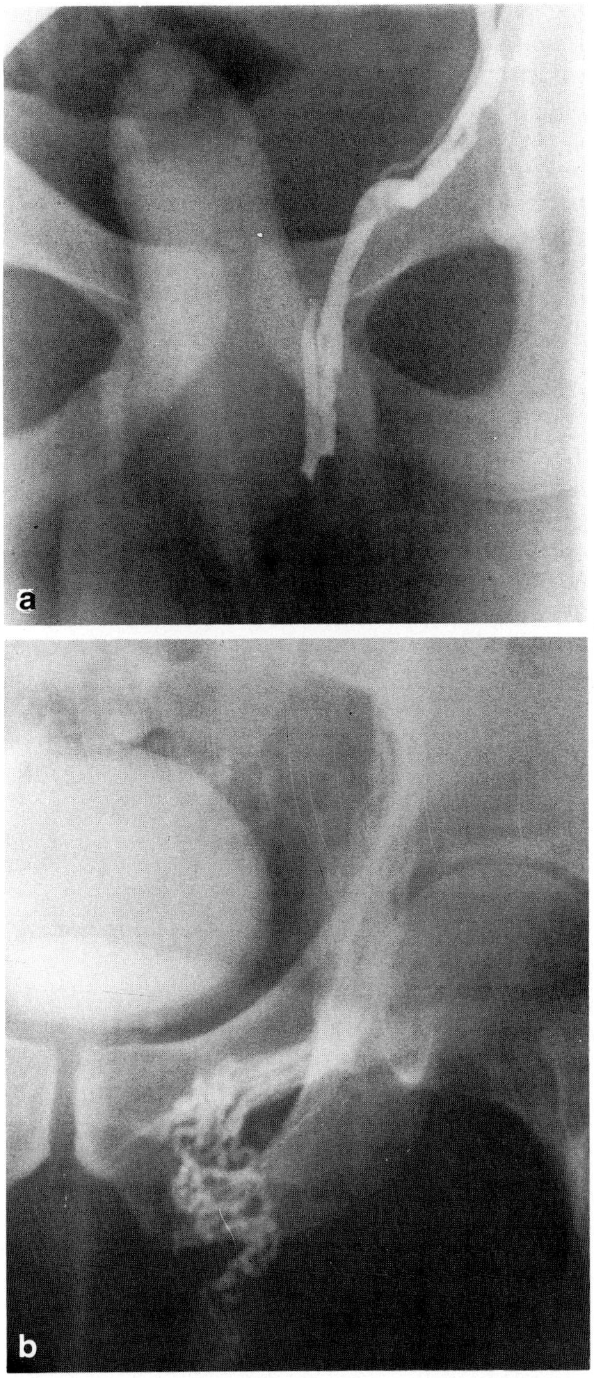

Fig. 17.4 a,b. A testicular venogram demonstrates well-opacified elements of the pampiniform plexus. On exploration the testis was found approximately 12 cm proximal to elements of the pampiniform plexus which led the testis along the gubernaculum testes

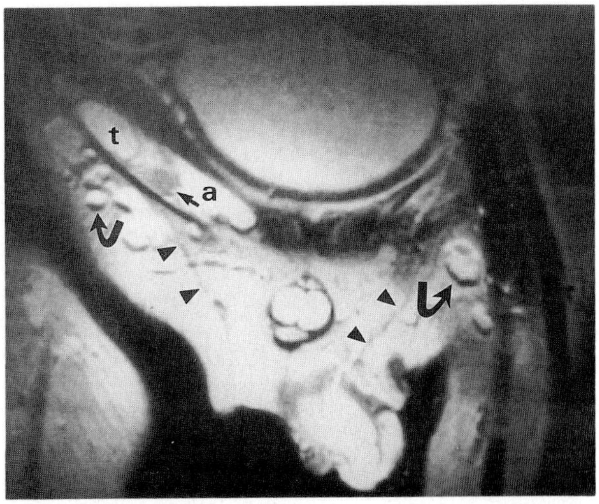

Fig. 17.5. Undescended impalpable right testis in a typical intracanalicular location. Note that the testis (*t*) has a normal bright signal on this T2-weighting image and has an associated normal epididymis (*arrow*) and ascites (*a*). In this location fluid is technically ascitic since the vaginal process is patent. Note that the gubernaculum is seen bilaterally, extending from the external inguinal ring to the base of the scrotum (*arrowheads*). Note also the presence of inguinal adenopathy (*curved arrows*) lateral to the right and left canals. (MATTREY and TRAMBERT 1990)

can be discerned, they are surrounded by fluid, and they are located in the path of the spermatic cord on axial scans. Lymph nodes, while of similar signal behavior, present different morphologies and are lateral to the spermatic canal.

Testicular atrophy, most likely related to missed extravaginal torsion, can be easily diagnosed. This noninvasive diagnosis, only possible with MRI, has far-reaching clinical implications. This diagnosis must be reserved for those cases with an atrophic cord that reaches the base of the empty scrotum (Fig. 17.6). This finding has been specific for testicular atrophy and proven surgically in nine of nine cases (MATTREY and TRAMBERT 1990). Given the reliability of the MRI diagnosis and given the proper clinical setting, the remaining cases with atrophy that were diagnosed by MRI in our series are being followed clinically (MATTREY and TRAMBERT 1990). Surgical resection to eliminate the potential for malignant degeneration is not required in these cases since viable testicular tissue is no longer present. If further clinical experience shows that MRI can indeed diagnose this entity with no false-positive diagnoses, surgical exploration in this group of patients could be eliminated.

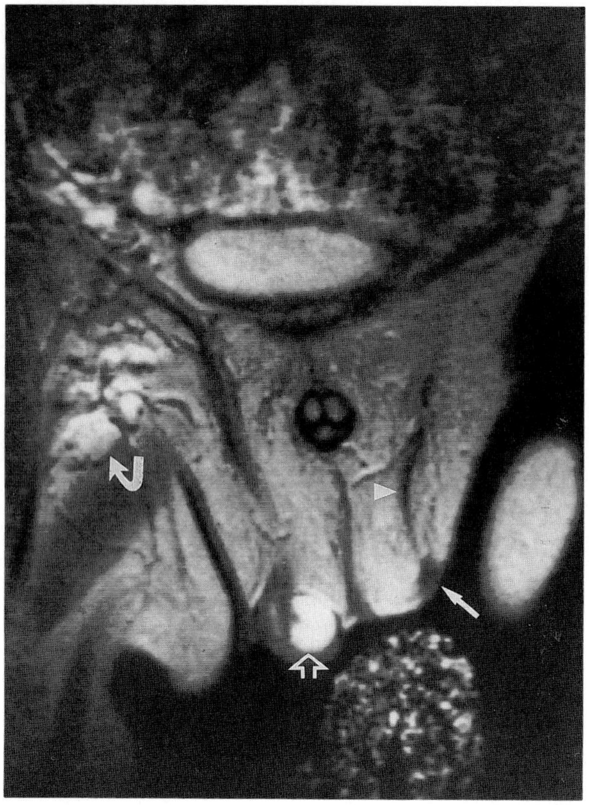

Fig. 17.6. Atrophic left testis seen on a T2-weighted image (*arrow*). Note the presence of an atrophic cord that is thinner than the normal contralateral cord (*arrowhead*) and thicker than the gubernaculum seen in Fig. 17.14. Also note that the atrophic cord reaches the base of the scrotum, and the presence of inguinal adenopathy lateral to the right cord (*curved arrow*). The normal right testis and its mediastinum are seen in the right hemiscrotum (*open arrow*). The heterogeneous signal seen below the scrotum is urine in a diaper. (MATTREY and TRAMBERT 1990)

17.6.1.2 Polyorchidism

Polyorchidism, defined as the presence of more than two histologically proven testes, is a rare congenital anomaly (HANCOCK and HODGINS 1984; SINGER et al. 1992). Occasionally it may be diagnosed as a scrotal mass palpated on physical examination in the older child or adult that does not transilluminate, but frequently it is not discovered until autopsy. The etiology of polyorchidism is uncertain, but several hypotheses have been proposed: (a) duplication of the urogenital ridge, (b) faulty disappearance or division of the mesonephric tubules during descent, (c) incmplete degeneration of a portion of the mesonephros, and (d) separation of the mesonephric tubules by the peritoneal bands (SINGER et al. 1992). The supernumerary testis may be located in the scrotum (most commonly found on the left side), in the inguinal canal , or in the retroperitoneum. It is usually asymptomatic, but has been occasionally encountered with testicular torsion, inguinal hernia, or neoplasms (GRECHI et al. 1980; SHAH et al. 1992). Of 47 cases with polyorchidism, torsion was encountered in 13%, indirect inguinal hernia in 30%, and neoplasm in 7.1% (SHAH et al. 1992). The histologic diagnoses of associated malignant lesions have been seminoma and teratocarcinoma (GRECHI et al. 1980).

Ultrasonography easily detects this anomaly. The echogenicity of the supernumerary testis is homogeneous but may be slightly different from the adjacent testis (RIFKIN et al. 1983; GOLDBERG et al. 1987; CARDIGAN 1989). MRI can demonstrate both the duplication and its associated anomalies. The normal polyorchid testis assumes a homogeneous signal that is similar to the ipsilateral testis on all pulsing sequences (BAKER et al. 1987c). Surgical intervention is not necessary when no complications are encountered. However, if clinical and ultrasonographic examinations present any doubt in the diagnosis or normal status of the supernumerary testis, MRI should be done. If MRI does not resolve the question, surgical exploration would be required (THUM 1991).

17.6.2 Neoplasms

Masses palpated clinically can be intra- and/or extratesticular. Ability of the imaging technique to distinguish these two locations is of great importance since most intratesticular lesions are malignant and most extratesticular lesions are benign (KRONE and CARROLL 1985; O'MARA and RIFKIN 1991). Ultrasonography can provide this distinction with an accuracy approaching 90%–95% (KRONE and CARROLL 1985).

Testicular neoplasms can be primary or metastatic. Primary cancers can take origin from any of the cell types of testicular tissue and account for 5500 new cases and 1000 deaths per year in the United States (RICHIE 1992). Testicular neoplasms are most frequently detected in males below 10 years of age, between 20 and 40 years of age, and then over 60. They have peak incidence and are the most common solid tumors detected between the ages of 20 and 34. Primary testicular neoplasms are grouped into germ cell and stromal tumors.

Germ cell tumors account for 90%–95% of all primary testicular malignancies, while stromal tumors account for 5%–10%. Germ cell lesions are in turn grouped into seminomatous cancers which account for 40% of all testicular neoplasms, and nonseminomatous cancers, responsible for 55%. Tumors of mixed cellularity, seminomatous and nonseminomatous elements, occur in 10%–15% of cases and are regarded and treated as nonseminomatous tumors. Germ cell tumors of yolk sac origin are the predominant lesions of infancy and lymphoma the predominant lesion of older men.

Testicular tumors are bilateral, either at the time of diagnosis or on follow-up, in 1%–3% of cases (Aristizabal et al. 1978; Sokal et al. 1980), mandating the careful examination of the contralateral testis at the time of diagnosis and close follow-up of the contralateral testis.

The differentiation of seminomatous from nonseminomatous lesions has remained important, in that patients with pure seminoma are irradiated and those with nonseminoma undergo retroperitoneal dissection and chemotherapy. While these modes of therapy have become controversial (Richie 1992), they remain standard practice at this time. Since seminomatous lesions may harbor small islands of nonseminomatous histology in 10%–15% of cases (Richie 1992), treatment is planned following detailed histologic analysis of the resected specimen. This is particularly true when there is elevation of β-human chorionic gonadotropin (HCG) or α-fetoprotein, findings suggesting the presence of nonseminomatous elements. From our data (Johnson et al. 1990) and those presented in the literature to date (Rholl et al. 1987; Seidenwurm et al. 1987; Thurner et al. 1988), it appears that MRI may offer such differentiation, although one group reported an inability to consistently distinguish these two cell types (Schultz Lampel et al. 1991).

Ultrasonographically, testicular neoplasms produce focal alterations in testicular homogeneity (see Fig. 17.7). They are usually well-defined hypoechoic focal lesions, but when hemorrhagic, fibrotic, or calcific, they may become hyperechoic (Vick et al. 1982; Krone and Carroll 1985; Grantham et al. 1985). When a focal echogenic focus is seen in a hypoechoic lesion, it may represent focal scarring due to infarction, granuloma, or "burned-out" neoplasm. A focus of calcification without mass may represent an inactive or treated germ cell tumor (Shawker et al. 1983; Krone and Carroll 1985). Diffuse bilateral calcifications, "microlithiasis," are a benign process that will be discussed later (Janzen et al. 1992). Calcifications in testicular tumors are uncommon, but may exist (Grantham et al. 1985). Some neoplasms, particularly lymphoma and leukemia, are diffusely infiltrative and can resemble inflammation, infarction, or hemorrhage. It can be difficult to differentiate benign from malignant infiltrative disease. However, some criteria may help in this differentiation (Rifkin et al. 1984): (a) residual normal testicular tissue can be visualized in neoplastic disease; (b) the epididymis is usually affected by infectious processes or spermatic cord torsion but is typically spared from neoplasia; (c) thickening of the scrotal wall may be observed with inflammation but is normal with neoplastic disorders; and (d) a diffusely homogeneous and hyperechoic testis is nearly always benign (Rifkin et al. 1984).

It is difficult to render a specific diagnosis of neoplasia or to classify a neoplasm as being of seminomatous or nonseminomatous histology by ultrasonography alone. The diagnosis of malignancy is suggested when typical ultrasonographic findings are encountered in the proper clinical setting. Although the sensitivity and negative predictive value of a technically adequate sonogram in testicular neoplasia have been reported to be as high as 100% (Schwerk et al. 1983), ultrasonography has missed 4 of 14 lesions which were either infiltrative or had totally replaced the testis (Thurner et al. 1988). Ultrasonography can also be useful in the detection of retroperitoneal adenopathy, with an accuracy ranging from 77% to 82% (Burney and Klatte 1979; Hutschenreiter et al. 1979; William et al. 1980). Although ultrasonography remains the primary imaging modality when malignancy is suspected (Glazer et al. 1982; Kirschling et al. 1983; Emory et al. 1984; Krone and Carroll 1985; Scott et al. 1986), computed tomography or MRI should be used for staging testicular tumors (Pillari et al. 1980; Baker et al. 1987b; Mattrey and Trambert 1990). In a recent study where 377 subjects underwent retroperitoneal lymph node dissection, preoperative staging agreed with pathologic staging in 75% and the addition of bipedal lymphography did not improve the accuracy over CT alone (Klepp et al. 1991). In the setting of neoplasm, ultrasonography can (a) aid in differentiating intratesticular from extratesticular masses; (b) exclude impalpable lesions in males with unexplained gynecomastia;

(c) detect occult testicular tumors in males with extratesticular germ cell tumors; and (d) monitor the contralateral testis of patients with prior testicular malignancy.

Color Doppler of testicular tumors has not been fully evaluated in that only a few studies have been published. Preliminary data suggest that degree of vascularity tends to be related to tumor size where tumors larger than 1.5 cm were hypervascular and those smaller than 1.5 cm were hypovascular compared to normal parenchyma (HORSTMAN et al. 1991a). Tumors may or may not cause distortion of normal vasculature. Infiltrative-type tumors such as lymphoma and leukemia can be hypervascular and therefore indistinguishable from orchitis (HORSTMAN et al. 1991a). The exact role of color Doppler imaging in the assessment of neoplasia is as yet unknown.

The overall MR appearance of testicular tumors is dependent upon tumor histology. Tumor margination as well as its influence on testicular size and shape are well depicted. Although invasion into peritesticular tissues such as the epididymis or cord is clearly seen (BAKER et al. 1987b), the accuracy of detecting extension may be limited (THURNER et al. 1988). However, this apparent handicap is irrelevant, since testicular cancer, regardless of the stage of disease, requires orchiectomy for pathologic staging. When comparing their ability to detect tumors, MRI detected 14 of 14 tumors and ultrasonography detected only ten (THURNER et al. 1988). In a study reviewing the MRI experience in 205 patients with scrotal disease, there were 88 patients studied for suspicion of cancer, all of whom underwent surgical exploration and 67 of whom had cancer. No false-positive or -negative studies were reported (100% sensitivity and specificity) (SCHULTZ LAMPEL et al. 1991). Although MRI is highly sensitive and likely more so than ultrasonography (THURNER et al. 1988), it is not clear what would be the minimum consistently detectable lesion size. It is possible, given the relatively long imaging time (minutes) and the continuous contraction of the dartos muscle producing wormian motion of the scrotal wall and testes, that small lesions may lose contrast as their dark signal will be averaged with the bright signal of the testis. The smallest lesion detected by MRI prospectively and proven surgically was a 3-mm germ cell tumor. Imaging time has been decreased by the availability of FSE, whcih we have now adopted as the standard technique. Given the limitation due to motion, any study compromised by motion aimed at detecting occult testicular neoplasm should be repeated in another plane if no lesions are found. On the other hand, when clear depiction of the interlobular septa or intratesticular morphology is achieved, it should be regarded as evidence of minimal partial volume and therefore negating the presence of disease.

17.6.2.1 Seminomatous Tumors

Seminomatous elements are present in nearly 60% of germ cell malignancies and pure seminomas account for 40%–45% of all testicular neoplasms. Seminoma is rare below the age of 10 and above 60 years and has a peak incidence in the late 30s; they are the most common cell type in cryptorchid testes (O'MARA and RIFKIN 1991). Spermatocystic seminoma, a subtype accounting for 10% of all detected seminomas, occurs most frequently in men over the age of 50 years. Nearly 10%–15% of seminomatous lesions are not pure seminomas. They contain scattered islands of nonseminomatous elements which change the classification to a nonseminomatous lesion and thus require careful pathologic evaluation for proper treatment planning. Elevation of β-HCG or α-fetoprotein suggests mixed cellularity. Seminomatous lesions are sheets of cells intermixed with fibrous strands presenting a homogeneous histologic pattern. They rarely bleed or necrose centrally. Seminoma is less aggressive, but 25% of cases are metastatic on initial manifestation. This tumor is radiosensitive and has a relatively good prognosis. The survival rate of stage 1 seminoma is better than 95% (CALDWELL et al. 1980).

Ultrasonographic findings of seminoma consist of a relatively well-defined, homogeneous, hypoechoic focal testicular lesion (Fig. 17.7). Echogenicity of the tumors are dependent upon tumor size and the presence of cystic degeneration (KRONE and CARROLL 1985). At times, echogenic foci can be seen in the tumor due to fibrosis, "burned-out" tumor lesion, or rarely calcifications. However, it should be noted that there is significant overlap between the ultrasonographic appearance of seminomatous and nonseminomatous tumors.

The MRI appearance of seminoma reflects the histologic pattern of the lesion. Like its histology, the mass is relatively homogeneous in signal intensity, is well marginated from normal testicular tissue, and lacks a fibrous tumor capsule (Fig. 17.8) (BAKER et al. 1987b; RHOLL et al. 1987; SEIDENWURM et al. 1987; JOHNSON et al. 1990). At times, dark bands can be seen within it that correlate with fibrous bands histologically (JOHNSON et al. 1990). The intensity of the tumor is constantly lower than that of normal testicular tissue or hydrocele fluid on T2-weighted images (Fig. 17.8). The tumors may contain well-defined regions of lower signal that have correlated with regions of increased fibrosis and cellular condensation (JOHNSON et al. 1990). While it is atypical, some seminomatous lesions may bleed internally, resulting in a focus of different signal dependent on the age of the bleed. Metastases to the epididymis and cord were well demonstrated in one case (BAKER et al. 1987b). The signal intensity of the metastatic lesion was similar to that of the intratesticular mass (BAKER et al. 1987b). While seminomatous lesions present darker signal than testis, similar to that of infection or infarction, some characteristic features may allow their distinction. Seminomatous mass is generally well defined while orchitis is poorly marginated, patchy in appearance, and does not produce a mass effect (MATTREY and TRAMBERT 1990). Seminoma usually spares the epididymis while orchitis is typically secondary to epididymitis (MATTREY and TRAMBERT 1990). Further, infection is associated with swelling of the peritesticular tissues and hypervascularity of these tissues and cord, two unusual associations with testicular malignancy.

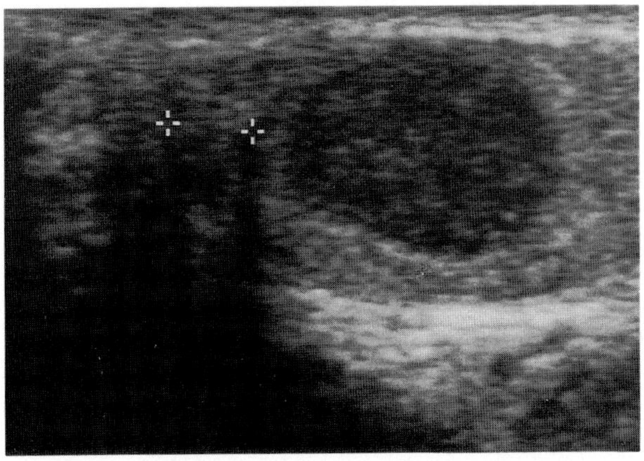

Fig. 17.7. A typical intratesticular seminoma (*arrow*) is shown on a longitudinal sonogram. Note that the lesion is homogeneous, hypoechoic relative to the normal testis, and well marginated. The cursors superior to the testis are marking the normal epididymal head. (Courtesy of JOHN GORMAN, M.D., Dept. of Radiology, Naval Medical Center, San Diego, CA, USA)

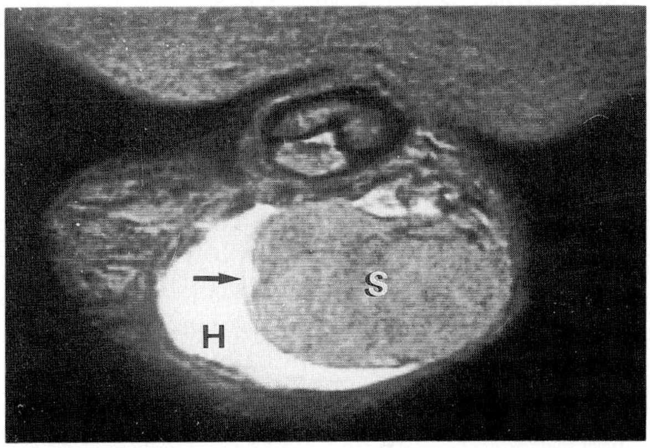

Fig. 17.8. Left testicular seminoma (*S*) is mildly inhomogeneous on a T2-weighted coronal image and is markedly lower in signal than the small amount of remaining normal testicular tissue (*arrow*) and hydrocele (*H*). (BAKER et al. 1987b)

17.6.2.2 Nonseminomatous Tumors

These tumors are typically of mixed histology where one cell type may predominate over the others. In order of frequency are teratocarcinoma, embryonal cell carcinoma, teratoma, and choriocarcinoma. Nearly 40% of nonseminomatous lesions are a mixture of two or three of these elements. They all carry a similar prognosis and are treated in a similar fashion. Therefore, preoperative distinction of the cell type is not necessary. These lesions account for nearly 50% of all primary testicular neoplasms and peak in incidence in the 20s and early 30s. They afflict slightly younger males than seminomatous lesions. These lesions present heterogeneous histology owing to their mixed cellularity, their attempt at tubular formation, and their high propensity to invade vessels, causing internal hemorrhage and necrosis. Choriocarcinoma is more aggressive than the other cell types, resulting in metastatic manifestation while the testicular mass is still small and clinically impalpable (KRONE and CARROLL 1985; O'MARA and RIFKIN 1991).

Their classic ultrasonographic appearance is that of a hypoechoic mass with heterogeneous echotexture that is not as well marginated from normal testicular tissue (KRONE and CARROLL 1985; O'MARA and RIFKIN 1991). The heterogeneous signal results from the frequent hemorrhage and necrosis and, particularly with teratoma and teratocarcinoma, from the multiple tissue

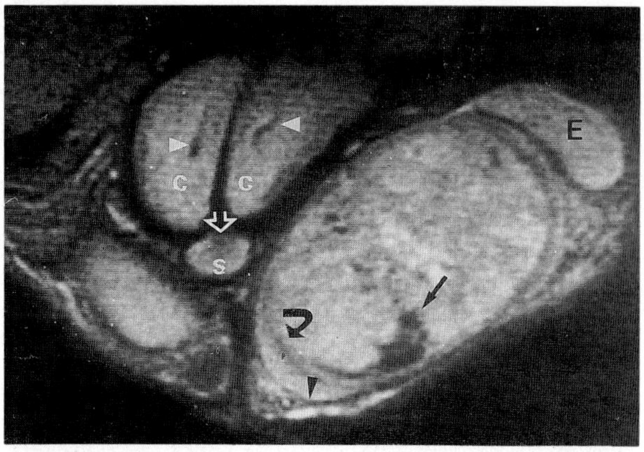

Fig. 17.9. T2-weighted image of a left testicular embryonal cell carcinoma, which is markedly heterogeneous in signal. The dark area was intermediate in signal on proton density (not shown), consistent with hemorrhage as was seen histologically. The intact tunica albuginea was demonstrated (*black arrowhead*) as a dark bank spearate from the fibrous tumor capsule which was seen as a dark band (*curved arrow*) separating the tumor from normal testicular tissue. An epididymal cyst (*E*) filled with fluid characteristic of water can be seen. Interestingly, the urethra (*open arrow*) can be seen in the corpora spongiosa (*S*) and the penile arteries (*white arrowheads*) can be seen in the right and left corpora cavernosa (*C*). (Baker et al. 1987b)

components such as bone, cartilage, muscle, mucus, and keratinaceous materials as well as the frequent occurrence of calcifications (Krone and Carroll 1985; O'Mara and Rifkin 1991).

The MRI appearance of nonseminomatous tumors is markedly different from that of seminomatous tumors owing to their heterogeneous histologic pattern, hemorrhage, and calcification (Mattrey and Trambert 1990; Johnson et al. 1990). The background of most nonseminomatous lesions is isointense or slightly brighter than normal testis on T2-weighted images (Fig. 17.9). Typically there are multiple areas of high and low signal intensities on both T1- and T2-weighted images representing hemorrhage of various ages within the mass. The degree of heterogeneity and the overall signal intensity are much greater than with seminoma. Unlike seminoma, which is typically isointense with testis on T1- and intermediately weighted images, nonseminomatous lesions are frequently heterogeneous and visible on these sequences. A band of low signal intensity is visible circumscribing the mass in most cases (Fig. 17.9). This has been shown histologically to represent the fibrous tumor capsule, also typical for these lesions (Johnson et al. 1990). Although some nonseminomas may be dark in signal and may lack the fibrous capsule, it is their heterogeneity on T2- and frequently on T1-weighted images that allows their differentiation from seminoma (Johnson et al. 1990). In fact, the degree of heterogeneity of signal was the most discriminating factor in our study (Johnson et al. 1990). It should be noted that another group with a larger experience than ours in imaging cancer patients was not able to distinguish one cell type from another (Schultz Lampel et al. 1991). It is not clear whether their criterion was similar to ours or whether their patient population had more advanced disease. Since our description of the MRI appearance of testicular tumors, our error rate in distinguishing seminoma from nonseminoma has decreased from 1 in 13 to 1 in 20 cancers (Johnson et al. 1990).

17.6.2.3 Stromal Tumors

Stromal tumors account for nearly 5% of all primary testicular tumors. They usually occur between the ages of 20 and 60 years. They are typically well circumscribed and rarely exhibit hemorrhage or necrosis. Since these lesions generally produce hormones, prepubertal boys can present with precocious puberty and adults with gynecomastia and even galactorrhea. The cell types include Leydig and Sertoli cells. These lesions are malignant in 10% of cases. Malignancy is suspected histologically when the lesions are large, necrotic, infiltrative, or have invaded blood vessels. Malignancy is clearly established when metastases are detected.

The ultrasonographic appearance of stromal cell tumors is the same as that of other solid testicular tumors. They cannot be differentiated from other testicular lesions, especially seminomatous tumors. They appear as well-defined homogeneous hypoechoic focal masses occasionally with a cystic component (Krone and Carroll 1985).

The MRI appearances of these lesions are not established yet, although published reports of Leydig cell tumors show them to be of moderately darker signal intensity than normal testis on T2-weighted images (Baker et al. 1987b; Thurner et al. 1988). One could hypothesize that, given their homogeneous histology and lack of hemorrhage and necrosis, their appearance on MRI would mimic seminomatous tumors (Baker et al. 1987b; Thurner et al. 1988). However, when malignant, the hemorrhage and necrosis would change their appearance to mimic nonseminomatous lesions. The experience with these lesions is limited, and this hypothesis needs to be tested.

17.6.2.4 Lymphoma and Leukemia

Lymphomatous or leukemic infiltration of the testis is common. Lymphoma accounts for nearly 5% of all testicular neoplasms (RICHIE 1992). It may be primary in the testis, the manifestation of occult disease seated elsewhere, or the late manifestation of disseminated lymphoma. Lymphomatous lesions are the most common testicular neoplasm over the age of 50 (RICHIE 1992). The majority of these lesions are infiltrative and may extend into or originate in the epididymis. The major cell type is histiocytic lymphoma.

The testis is the principal site of relapse of leukemia in children. A blood–testis barrier exists, similar to the blood–brain barrier; this barrier prevents chemotherapeutics from eradicating disease in the testes. Testicular evaluation and biopsy are commonly performed at the end of chemotherapy treatment to exclude testicular involvement.

Lymphomatous and leukemic infiltration of the testis has been accurately demonstrated on ultrasonographic examination, but the sensitivity of ultrasonography is limited (THURNER et al. 1988). There are two ultrasonographic patterns observed with tumor infiltration. The most common is an irregular hypoechoic lesion involving a part of or the entire testis. The second pattern is a well-defined intratesticular anechoic or hypoechoic focal lesion surrounded by normal parenchyma (O'MARA and RIFKIN 1991). The latter lesion is indistinguishable ultrasonographically from primary testicular tumors. The diagnosis can be suggested when the disease is bilateral or in the proper clinical setting (PHILLIPS et al. 1983; LUPETIN et al. 1983a).

The exact sensitivity of MRI in detecting leukemic or lymphomatous infiltration is not yet established. There were, however, four cases detected on MRI that were missed on ultrasonography (THURNER et al. 1988). In these cases, tumors affected the entire testis diffusely and decreased its signal relative to the contralateral normal testis (Fig. 17.10).

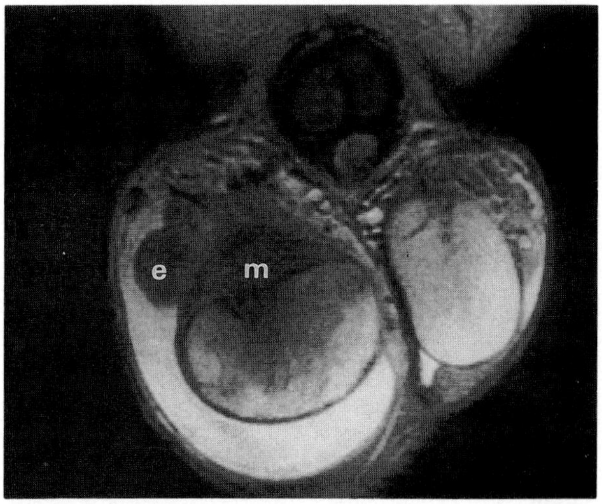

Fig. 17.10. Scrotal lymphoma involving the right epididymis and testis is shown on a T2-weighted image. Note that the center of the mass (*m*) is in the epididymis (*e*) and infiltrates the testis from the hilum. The mass, located along the "bare area" of the testis, rotated the testis into a horizontal position. Note that the mass within the testis is patchy and its margins with normal testicular tissue are generally poorly defined. There is mild hypervascularity and moderate ipsilateral hydrocele. (MATTREY and TRAMBERT 1990)

17.6.2.5 Benign Testicular Lesions

Benign testicular tumors are relatively uncommon. The most common of these is benign intratesticular teratoma (KRONE and CARROLL 1985; O'MARA and RIFKIN 1991). The ultrasonographic and possibly the MRI appearance of teratoma would be similar to teratocarcinoma, from which differentiation may be difficult.

Epidermoid inclusion cysts are benign solitary tumors accounting for approximately 1% of all testicular tumors (SHAH et al. 1981; BERGER et al. 1985). They are well defined and homogeneous on ultrasonography. They may be hyperreflective due to calcifications in the wall. Only a few internal echoes are noted throughout the tumor (MAXWELL and MAMTORA 1990; MEICHES and NURENBERG 1991). One reported case imaged by MRI showed a bull's-eye appearance in the testis (BRENNER et al. 1989). We have reported on four cases imaged by MRI, all of which displayed similar findings. The epidermoid cysts were nearly isointense with testis on all pulsing sequences with a tendency to be slightly darker on T1- and slightly brighter on T2-weighted images. A low signal intensity wall was observed on the T2-weighted image in all four cases owing to the fibrous capsule

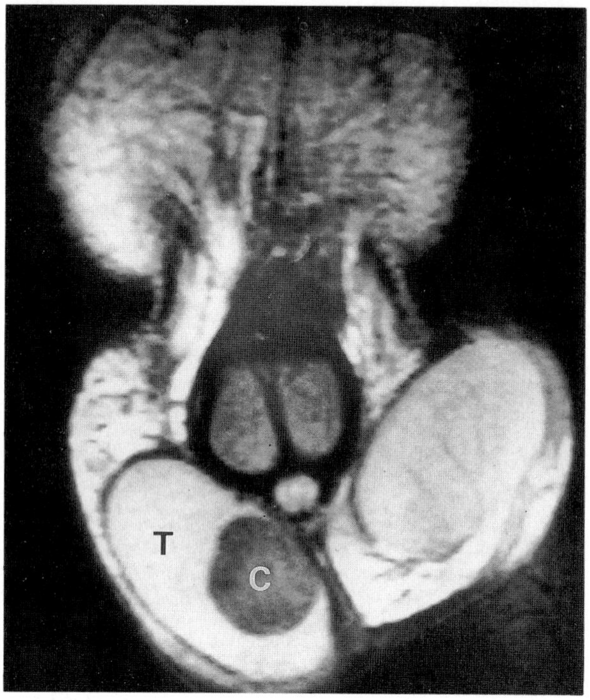

Fig. 17.11. Right intratesticular epidermoid cyst is shown on a T1-weighted scan acquired following the administration of Gd-DTPA. Note that the cyst (*C*) is well defined, round, and does not enhance relative to the normal testis (*T*), which enhances homogeneously. (CHO et al. 1993)

and epithelial lining. The lesions failed to enhance following the infusion of Gd-DTPA, confirming their avascular core (Fig. 17.11). Since normal testicular tissue enhances significantly, the postcontrast images increase their conspicuity.

Adenomatoid tumors are benign lesions characteristic of the genital tract that consist of fibrous stroma and epithelial cells. These lesions are benign and usually occur in the epididymis but may rarely occur in the testis or near the mediastinum testis. On MRI, their signal varies from being similar to testis to being darker than testis, dependent upon the degree of fibrosis (MATTREY and TRAMBERT 1990).

Prior to the use of high-resolution ultrasonography, simple intratesticular cysts were considered a rare condition; however, 8%–10% of sonograms demonstrate typical testicular cysts (LEUNG et al. 1984; GOODING et al. 1987; HAMM et al. 1988). Most are solitary, range in size from 2 to 18 mm, and are either intratesticular or tunical. Intratesticular cysts are impalpable and are incidental (KRONE and CARROLL 1985; O'MARA and RIFKIN 1991). They can occur anywhere within the testis and likely take origin from the rete testis in that their histology is similar to that of the rete testes (TRAINER 1987). Other hypotheses include degeneration following trauma or inflammation (HAMM et al. 1988). Tunical cysts are palpable, small, and usually detected in middle-aged men. The etiology of these lesions was considered to be posttraumatic or inflammatory degeneration (ARCADIA 1952); however, recent evidence suggests that they may derive from an embryologic remnant of mesothelial rest or from efferent ductules (MENNEMEYER and MASON 1979). MRI also displays characteristic findings for cysts. Although they are well depicted when they assume water signal (darker on T1- and brighter on T2-weighted than testis), they can be isointense with testis, requiring Gd-DTPA to increase their conspicuity (TARTAR et al. 1993).

The appearance of dilated intratesticular seminiferous tubules has been recently recognized and described on both ultrasonography and MRI (BROWN et al. 1992; WEINGARTEN et al. 1992; TARTAR et al. 1993). The findings are somewhat characteristic on ultrasonography, potentially allowing a specific diagnosis to be made, thereby obviating the need for surgery. In the three publications a total of 48 patients were reported, most of whom were over the age of 50. All had similar ultrasonographic appearances. The intratesticular process was associated with large ipsilateral spermatoceles, was centered at the mediastinum testis, and was contiguous with the body of the epididymis. The mass appeared hypoechoic with a coarse echotexture due to multitudes of small reflectors caused by the dilated tubules. It may also be associated with mediastinal cysts (Fig. 17.12). It was frequently bilateral and impalpable, although the testicular examination was compromised by the associated large spermatoceles. When this constellation of findings is encountered ultrasonographically, there is no need for further work up; however, short of that, Tartar et al. recommended the use of MRI to confirm the diagnosis. On MRI the findings may also be specific for this entity and distinguishable from those of neoplastic lesions. The mass of ectatic tubules at the mediastinum was homogeneous and of lower signal on T1- and intermediately weighted images and isointense with testis on T2-weighted images; it was identical to that of the ipsilateral spermatoceles on all sequences (Fig. 17.12). The MRI appearance of dilated tubules is different from that of seminomatous tumors in that the latter are typically isointense with testis

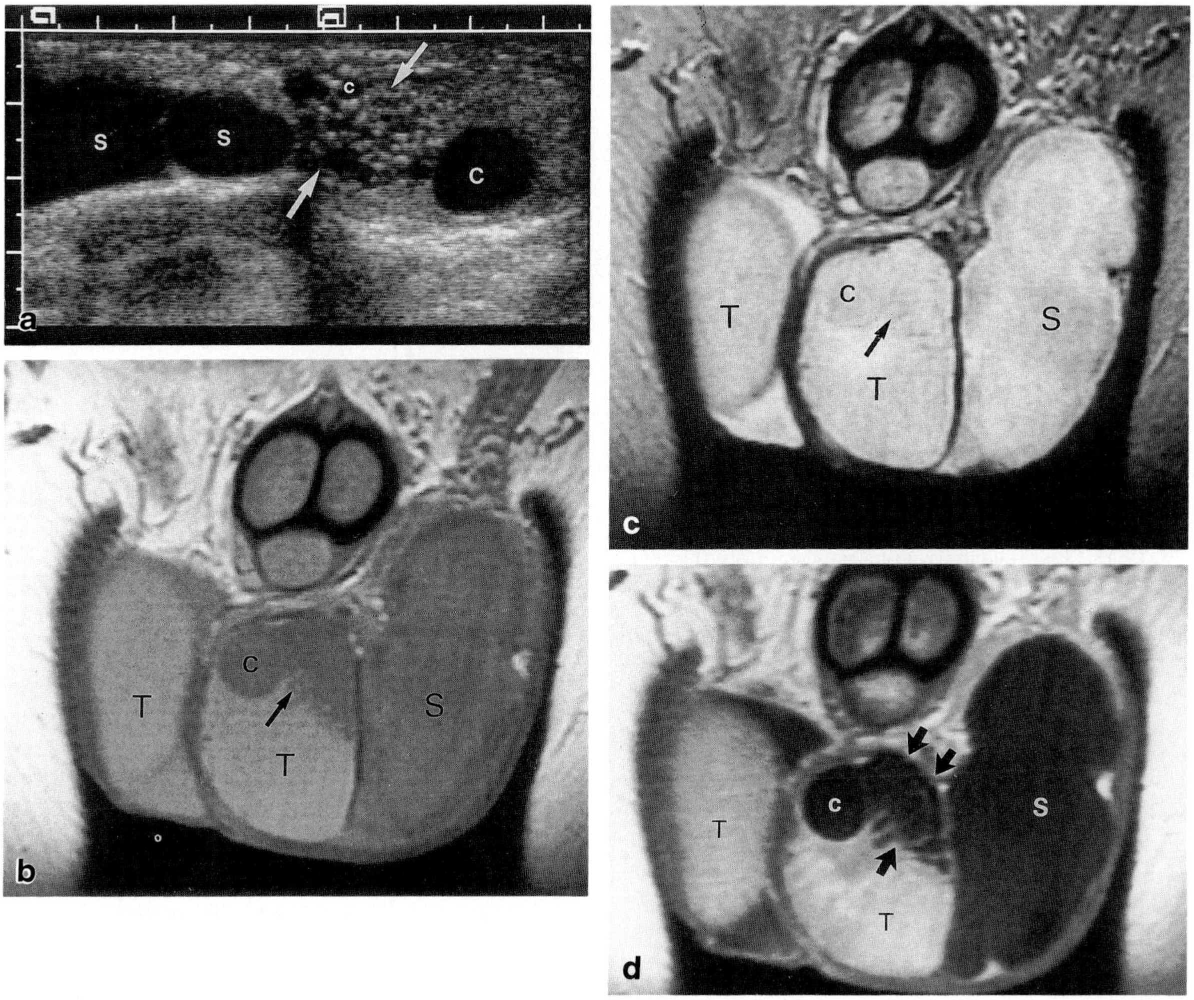

Fig. 17.12. **a** Longitudinal sonogram through left hemiscrotum shows several locules of a large multilocular spermatocele (*S*). A mediastinal lesion (*arrows*) has a coarse echotexture, with multiple contiguous tiny cysts (*c*) and a 1.5-cm-diameter intratesticular cyst (*C*). This lesion displayed no increased flow on color Doppler ultrasonography (not shown). **b** Proton density-weighted and **c** T2-weighted coronal MR images show the large spermatocele (*S*), intratesticular cyst (*C*), and mediastinal lesion (*arrow*) to be homogeneous and hypointense to testicular parenchyma (*T*) on proton density-weighted images, becoming isointense with and difficult to distinguish from testis on T2-weighted images. **d** Contrast-enhanced T1-weighted coronal MR image shows normal intense enhancement of testicular parenchyma. Contrast between testis (*T*) and spermatocele (*S*), intratesticular cyst (*C*), and mediastinal seminiferous tubule ectasia (*arrows*) is markedly increased, allowing recognition of tubular structures at the margin between the abnormal mediastinum and the testis. (Tartar et al. 1993)

on T1- and darker than testis on T2-weighted images (Baker et al. 1987b; Johnson et al. 1990). Nonseminomatous lesions are also different because they are heterogeneous in signal with all pulse sequences, especially on T2-weighted images (Baker et al. 1987b; Johnson et al. 1990). Because the tubules do not enhance with Gd, their conspicuity and tubular pattern become apparent following contrast administration.

Intratesticular varicocele, which also occurs in the mediastinum testis, may be indistinguishable ultrasonographically from the dilated seminiferous tubule on gray scale (Weiss et al. 1992). However, in the two cases reported, the hypoechoic spaces filled with color on Doppler ultrasonography, indicating flow (Weiss et al. 1992). The intratesticular varicoceles were associated with ipsilateral varicoceles in both patients. MRI should also allow this distinction (although no such cases

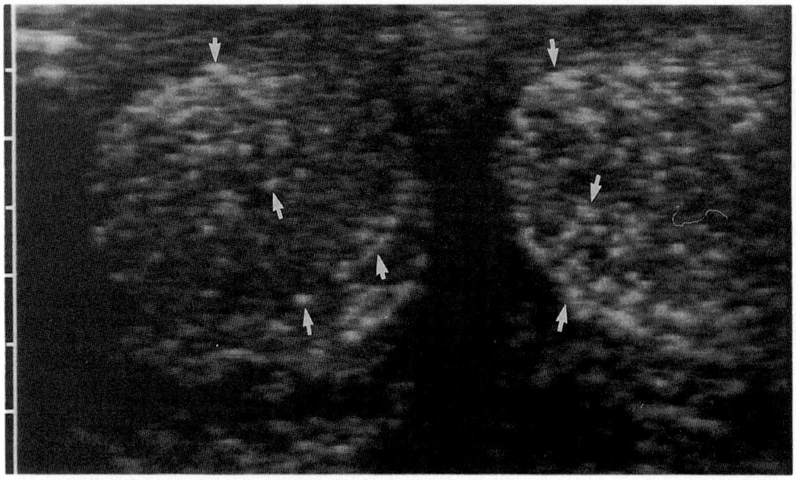

Fig. 17.13. Testicular microlithiasis is an entity that consistently involves both testes, as shown in this example. The multiple small echogenic foci (*arrows*) are caused by concretions within the seminiferous tubules. (Courtesy of John Gorman, M.D., Dept. of Radiology, Naval Medical Center, San Diego, CA, USA)

have been reported) because of the characteristic MRI appearance of flowing blood and because slowly flowing or static blood enhances markedly with IV contrast agents, unlike seminiferous tubules.

Testicular microlithiasis is caused by tiny (<2 mm) concentric calcifications within the seminiferous tubules throughout both testes (Fig. 17.13). It is typically incidental to the primary cause that brought the patient to medical attention. It is believed that these concretions form from degenerated tubular epithelial cells. Collagenous lamellae form and offer a nidus for dystrophic calcification. Although an exact etiology is not known, diffuse microlithiasis is more frequent in cryptorchidism or delayed testicular descent and a variety of genetic conditions, as well as with pulmonary alveolar microlithiasis. Although cancer and infertility have been associated with this condition, it is believed that the relationship with diffuse bilateral microlithiasis is incidental or may be related to the fact that these conditions also occur in association with cryptorchidism (Smith et al. 1991; Janzen et al. 1992).

17.6.3 Inflammation

17.6.3.1 Epididymitis

Epididymitis is the most common intrascrotal infection usually manifested by acute scrotal pain. It is seen in adolescent and middle-aged men, but it may be found in infants and young children (Mittemeyer et al. 1966; Gialason et al. 1980). Clinical manifestations of epididymitis include scrotal swelling, erythema, and tenderness. Most infections are unilateral and are associated with pain that increases over 1–2 days. Although on rare occasions epididymitis is secondary to vasculitis (Hayward et al. 1990), it is typically infectious. The common causative organisms include *Neisseria gonorrheae*, *Chlamydia trachomatis*, *Escherichia coli*, *Pseudomonas*, and *Aerobacter*. Less common causative organisms include *Schistosoma haematobium* and *Mycobacterium tuberculosis* (O'Mara and Rifkin 1991). The infection may be diffuse or focal and is frequently secondary to prostatitis. Most cases of epididymitis are treated conservatively. Surgery is reserved for complications such as abscess formation. Prolonged chemotherapy is required when orchitis complicates epididymitis, which can occur in as many as 20% of cases (Krone and Carroll 1985) and, when focal, is typically located near the epididymis (O'Mara and Rifkin 1991). Therefore imaging follow-up is warranted when symptoms do not resolve.

The ultrasonographic appearance includes enlargement of the epididymis (particularly the head) and a decrease in echogenicity due to edema (O'Mara and Rifkin 1991). Scrotal wall thickening

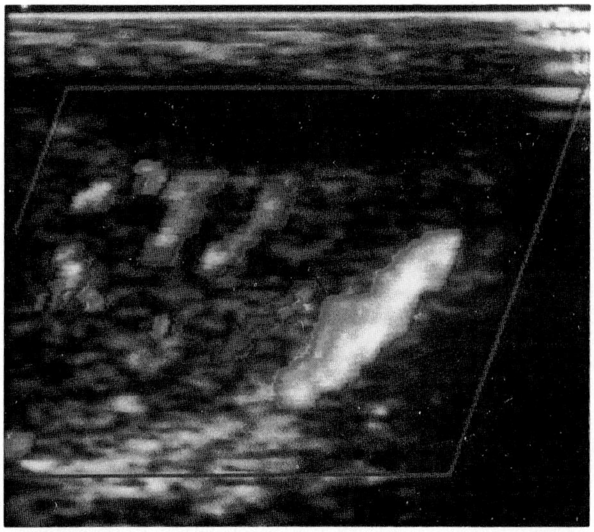

Fig. 17.14. Doppler image of the testis in a patient with acute epididymo-orchitis. Note the marked hypervascularity of the testis, demonstrating both the centripetal and the centrifugal arteries

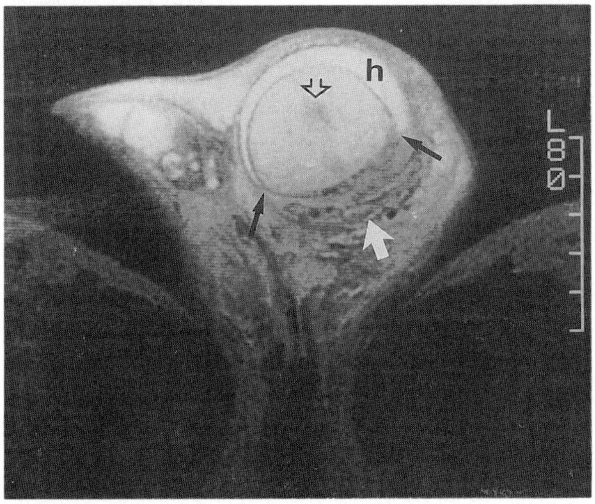

Fig. 17.15. Coronal T2-weighted image in a patient with acute scrotal pain due to epididymitis with associated orchitis shows prominence of the epididymal body (*white arrow*) and a mild hydrocele (*h*) that outlines the "bare area" of the testis (the edges of which are marked by *black arrows*), excluding torsion. Note the small, poorly defined focus of low signal in the testis (*open arrow*), which is compatible with infection. (TRAMBERT et al. 1990)

may be observed as well as a sympathetic hydrocele (MARTIN and CONTE 1987). At times, the hydrocele may become complex in appearance, suggesting a pyocele. When severe changes such as adhesions or septations become apparent, tuberculosis should be considered. Tuberculous epididymitis of the head likely results from hematogenous spread, while vas deferens and epididymal tail infections suggest retrograde spread from the prostate or bladder (WECHSLER et al. 1960). Chronic epididymitis typically causes enlargement and hyperechoic epididymis.

The main differential diagnoses of acute scrotal pain include epididymitis, spermatic cord torsion, or torsion of the testis or epididymal appendices. Color Doppler has added specificity. While a normal epididymis has no or scant flow, epididymitis causes significant hypervascularity of the affected side (Fig. 17.14) (LERNER et al. 1990; HORSTMAN et al. 1991a,b). Therefore, detecting any epididymal vascularity is abnormal and may be indicative of inflammation. When the testis is hypervascular, it may be secondary to orchitis or hyperemia. The diagnosis of orchitis should be reserved to those cases with focal abnormality on gray scale (LERNER et al. 1990; HORSTMAN et al. 1991a,b).

Acute epididymitis causes enlargement and an increase in signal of the epididymis, which is typically darker than testis on T2-weighted images (Fig. 17.15) (BAKER et al. 1987b; TRAMBERT et al. 1990). In chronic epididymitis, the epididymis is enlarged in a focal or diffuse manner and assumes a darker signal than normal on T2 weighting, becoming moderately darker than testis (BAKER et al. 1987b). In the setting of chronic epididymis, acute exacerbation may not be detectable. Severe acute epididymitis may be associated with hemorrhage within the epididymis. If hemorrhage is present, the MRI signal follows its resorptive stages. The most common appearance of hemorrhage has been signals associated with subacute bleeding (intermediate signal relative to fat and water on long TR, short TE sequences and dark on T2-weighted images). In acute epididymitis, hypervascularity and thickening and swelling of the spermatic cord, which increase its signal on T2-weighted images, are observed (Fig. 17.16) (TRAMBERT et al. 1990). While the degree of hypervascularity has been variable, it has been consistently present in all patients. Hypervascularity is seen as multiple serpiginous vessels with signal void due to high flow. This is in contradistinction to normal vessels, which are usually thinner and lack the very dark signal due to their slow flow. Hypervascularity of the testis associated with epididymitis has also been observed in some cases (TRAMBERT et al. 1990). Although scrotal thickening and swelling have been seen, they are

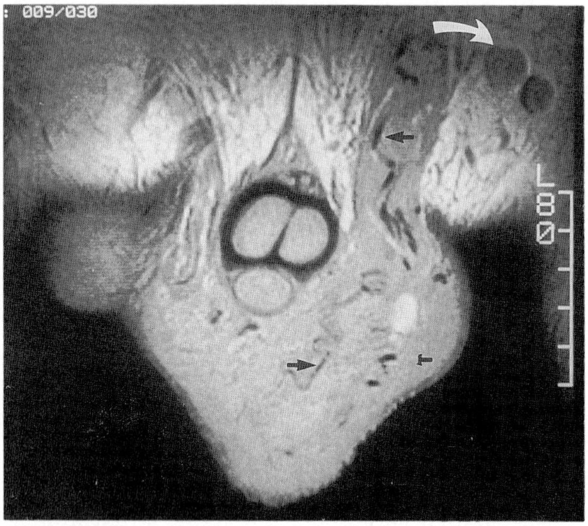

Fig. 17.16. Acute epididymitis shown on a coronal hydrogen density-weighted image demonstrating hypervascularity (*arrows*) and thickening of the extra- and intrascrotal spermatic cord. It also shows inguinal adenopathy (*curved arrow*). (TRAMBERT et al. 1990)

not specific to infection. Sympathetic hydrocele is present in most patients and yields a signal identical to those of water. Extensive inguinal adenopathy is also apparent but this finding is also not specific. Abscess formation has also been demonstrated (BAKER et al. 1987b) where it assumes a similar signal intensity to that of water and increases in conspicuity following IV contrast administration.

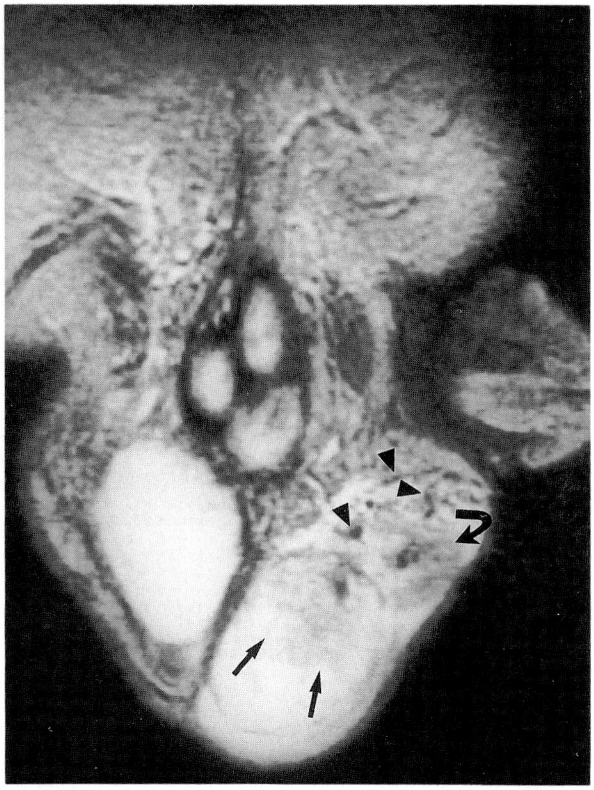

Fig. 17.17. Acute tuberculous epididymo-orchitis involving the upper pole of the left testis (*arrows*) and epididymal head (*curved arrow*) shown in the coronal plane on a T2-weighted image. Note patchy involvement of the testis and the enlarged epididymis that fails to darken on this T2-weighted image. Note the mild degree of hypervascularity (*arrowheads*) suggesting subacute inflammation. (MATTREY and TRAMBERT 1990)

17.6.3.2 Orchitis

Orchitis is often a sequela of epididymitis. Pure orchitis without epididymitis suggests a viral etiology. When orchitis accompanies epididymitis, treatment is extended over a longer period. Even when appropriately treated, orchitis may develop into an abscess requiring surgical intervention. Therefore, when a focus of orchitis is found and symptoms do not resolve appropriately, imaging follow-up is necessary. Testicular inflammation causes testicular enlargement, hypervascularity (HORSTMAN et al. 1991a), and loss in echogenicity resulting in diffuse or focal hypoechoic changes (GRANTHAM et al. 1985). At times, the testis may maintain normal echogenicity but assumes a heterogeneous echotexture.

Orchitis has caused loss of testicular signal on T2-weighted images as well as intratesticular, tunical, and cord hypervascularity. The areas of more severe changes have caused signal loss in patchy and poorly defined regions. Chronic orchitis, as in tuberculosis, has produced diffuse heterogeneous signal loss (BAKER et al. 1987b). Comparison between the affected and the contralateral testis or surrounding fat while taking into consideration coil shading can aid in the assessment of a diffusely abnormal testis. In a case of vasculitis from polyarteritis nodosa, patchy areas of inflammation, scarring, and infarction were apparent (HAYWARD et al. 1990).

Tuberculous orchitis is usually associated with tuberculous epididymitis. On ultrasonography, focal hypoechoic lesions in the testis associated with previously mentioned epididymal changes may suggest tuberculous epididymo-orchitis. On MRI, testicular lesions were patchy and poorly marginated and of slightly lower signal intensity than that of the normal testis (Fig. 17.17). Epididymal changes are less severe than the other bacterial epididymides and hypervascularity is also less prominent (Mattrey and Trambert 1990).

In some patients with fulminating epididymitis, epididymal swelling may compromise the blood supply to the testis, resulting in infarction (Bird and Rosenfield 1984). On ultrasonography, the infarcted testis may demonstrate areas of markedly decreased echogenicity. Color Doppler may demonstrate decreased or absent blood flow in the infarcted testis compared to the contralateral normal side (O'Mara and Rifkin 1991). There are no published reports describing the MRI findings in fulminating epididymitis and resultant testicular ischemia. However, it would be expected that such ischemia would be on the basis of venous occlusion, followed by arterial occlusion mimicking torsion. This type of infarction has resulted in hemorrhagic changes rather than patchy ill-defined areas of diminished signal. This hypothesis requires further clinical testing (Mattrey and Trambert 1990).

17.6.4 Trauma

The testis is easily movable and is naturally protected from injury (Finkelstein et al. 1986). However, forceful blunt trauma to the scrotum may induce testicular contusion, rupture, peritesticular hematoma, or hematocele (Rao 1980; Baker et al. 1987b). The severe pain can compromise the clinical assessment of the testis as well as ultrasonography. Surgical intervention is generally reserved for patients with testicular rupture or when the intratesticular hematoma is extensive. Since the latter can increase intracapsular pressure and cause ischemia and necrosis (McConnell et al. 1982).

Ultrasonography can adequately assess the traumatized scrotum (Lupetin et al. 1983b). Scanning should, however, be performed from the anterior and posterior aspect of the testicle since a large intrascrotal hematoma may displace the testis posteriorly (O'Mara and Rifkin 1991). The loss of a smooth tunica albuginea and a nonlinear mediastinum testis indicates rupture of the testis. Heterogeneous signal is indicative of an intratesticular hematoma (Hricak and Filly 1983; Krone and Carroll 1985), while linear abnormalities suggest a fracture plane. Hematocele suggests testicular rupture (Krone and Carroll 1985; O'Mara and Rifkin 1991) and appears hypoechoic with coarse internal echoes (Fig. 17.18) (Lupetin et al. 1983b). If the hematocele is longstanding, the fluid appears complex with septa, debris, or thick-walled fluid collection. Commplex hydrocele is nonspecific and is indistinguishable from pyocele but is suggested in the proper clinical setting. Injury of supporting structures such as epididymis, scrotal wall, and septum can also be recognized (Hricak and Filly 1983; O'Mara and Rifkin 1991). Color Doppler has not been fully evaluated in the setting of trauma;

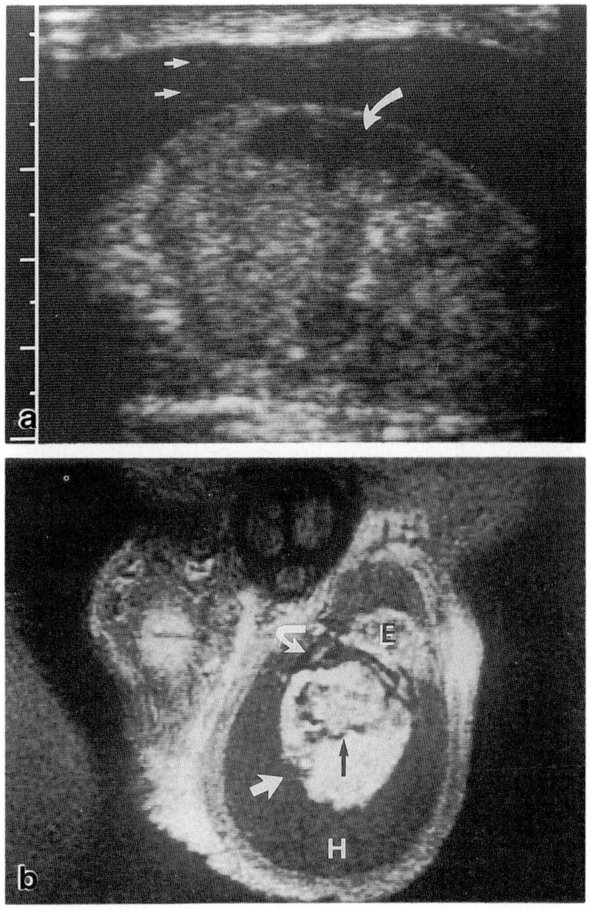

Fig. 17.18. a Subacute testicular trauma is shown on a longitudinal sonogram. Anechoic fluid with scattered internal echoes (*arrows*) is noted in the left scrotal sac surrounding the testis, indicating hematocele. Heterogeneous internal architecture and a subtunical anechoic space (*curved arrow*) confirm intratesticular hematoma. **b** A T2-weighted coronal scan of the scrotum depicts the intratesticular hematoma (*black arrow*), a tunical defect (*thick white arrow*) that was not suspected on the sonogram, subtunical hemorrhage (*curved arrow*), enlarged swollen epididymis (*E*), and a hematocele (*H*). (Baker et al. 1987)

however, it can exclude testicular ischemia caused by trauma as well as possibly aid in the differential diagnosis between hematoma (avascular) and tumor (vascular) (HORSTMAN et al. 1991a).

Magnetic resonance imaging is well suited to assess both the integrity of the tunica albuginea and the degree of intratesticular hematoma. Because the normal tunica is well visualized as a band of low signal intensity surrounding the testes on both intermediately and T2-weighted images, clear assessment of its integrity is possible (Fig. 17.18). In this setting multiple imaging planes may be required to ensure that all surfaces are optimally imaged without partial volume effect. Because all three imaging planes may be required with T2 weighting, gradient echo images with small flip angles or FSE techniques may be used to shorten the imaging time (BAKER et al. 1987b; MATTREY and TRAMBERT 1990). The appearance of the traumatized testis is highly inhomogeneous, with regions of high and low signal intensity compared with normal testicular tissue on both intermediately and T2-weighted images due to hemorrhage. Hematocele frequently accompanies trauma and yields a signal commensurate with the age of hemorrhage. Intratesticular trauma causes more linear than spherical changes, decreasing its confusion with mass lesions. Furthermore, associated clinical and scrotal changes with trauma differ from those of tumors. However, if a discrepancy exists between the severity of trauma and the degree of abnormality observed, the possibility of an underlying malignancy, such as a nonseminoma, should be raised and imaging follow-up is warranted.

17.6.5 Torsion

17.6.5.1 Intravaginal Spermatic Cord Torsion

The testis develops in a retroperitoneal location and as it descends into the scrotum it carries a layer of peritoneum called the vaginal process. This covering fuses to the scrotal wall and a significant portion of the tunica albuginea. The tunica vaginalis invests the entire contour of the testis except for a stripe that extends from the upper to the lower pole, leaving the region of the mediastinum testis uncovered. The transverse dimension of the bare area is variable but typically extends for at least one-third of the perimeter of the testis. The bare area serves as a passage for support structures into the testis and as an anchor fixing the testis to the posteromedial scrotal wall. This broad attachment prevents the testis from twisting. The surface area of this bare region can, however, be small, leaving a thin stalk for the passage of vessels and other support structures. This anomalous condition, called the "bell-clapper" deformity, predisposes the affected testis to twist and strangulate (Fig. 17.19). When the testis rotates upon its stalk, the veins become occluded, increasing intratesticular pressure. When arterial pressure is exceeded, blood flow ceases and the testis undergoes hemorrhagic necrosis. The bell-clapper deformity is thought to occur bilaterally in a large percentage of patients who present with torsion since subsequent contralateral torsion, if the unaffected testis was not fixed, has been observed in as many as 40% in one series (GULLENWATER et al. 1987).

Spermatic cord torsion typically occurs in the teens and 20 s, when the incidence is three times greater than in older men (O'MARA and RIFKIN 1991). This condition affects 1 in 4000 males younger than 25 years (GULLENWATER et al. 1987). The classic presentation is waking up with severe testicular pain radiating to the lower abdomen and/or groin that gradually worsens. Nausea and vomiting may occur (FINKELSTEIN et al. 1986). The affected hemiscrotum becomes indurated, enlarged, and tender, mimicking acute epididymitis and leading to clinical misdiagnosis in a large percentage of cases. If torsion is suspected, immediate surgery is required, since the likelihood of salvage of testicular function decreases with time. While nearly all testes can be salvaged if ischemic for 5 h or less, the salvage rate decreases to 20% if surgery is done at or beyond 12 h (HRICAK and JEFFREY 1983). When patients present in the subacute phase (24 h or later), surgery is still required to fix the contralateral testis to the scrotum to prevent subsequent torsion of the unaffected testis (GULLENWATER et al. 1987) and to remove the necrotic testis. The testis should be removed to establish the diagnosis, to stop the pain, which could last 3–4 weeks, and to prevent the development of infertility in the contralateral testis due to the possible development of antisperm antibodies, although the latter is controversial (WILLIAMSON and ANDERSON 1986; RYAN et al. 1988).

Color Doppler has successfully replaced radionuclide scanning for the diagnosis testicular torsion. The classic finding in nuclear scanning is a defect in the affected hemiscrotum (Holder et al. 1981; Chen et al. 1983a,b). Within 7 h from torsion, there is decreased flow on the affected side relative to the normal side and a photon defect is observed on the delayed images. One to 10 days after torsion, flow may be symmetric because of the hyperemia in the scrotal skin. A "halo" sign develops on delayed images caused by the hyperemic peritesticular tissue which surrounds the photon defect of necrotic testis (Holder et al. 1981; Chen et al. 1983a,b).

The findings on gray-scale ultrasound are not specific for torsion (Bird et al. 1979; Vordermark and Favila 1982). Within 7 h after torsion there is enlargement of the testis which becomes diffusely or focally inhomogeneous and hypoechoic (O'Mara and Rifkin 1991). The epididymis may or may not be enlarged. These findings are analogous to those of epididymo-orchitis. Scrotal skin thickening and reactive hydrocele may be presented. In the subacute stage, over 24 h, anechoic areas may be noted in the testis representing hemorrhage or infarction (Hricak and Jeffrey 1983; O'Mara and Rifkin 1991). At times a large echogenic or complex extratesticular mass may be present secondary to hemorrhage (Vick et al. 1986). Over time the necrotic testicle loses volume and its echogenicity may become variable. The combination of nuclear scanning and gray-scale ultrasonography is required to render a diagnosis because one study decreases the false-positive and false-negative diagnoses of the other.

Gray-scale and color Doppler ultrasonography have essentially replaced nuclear scanning since the combination can recognize each of the causes of an acute scrotum, spermatic cord torsion,

▷

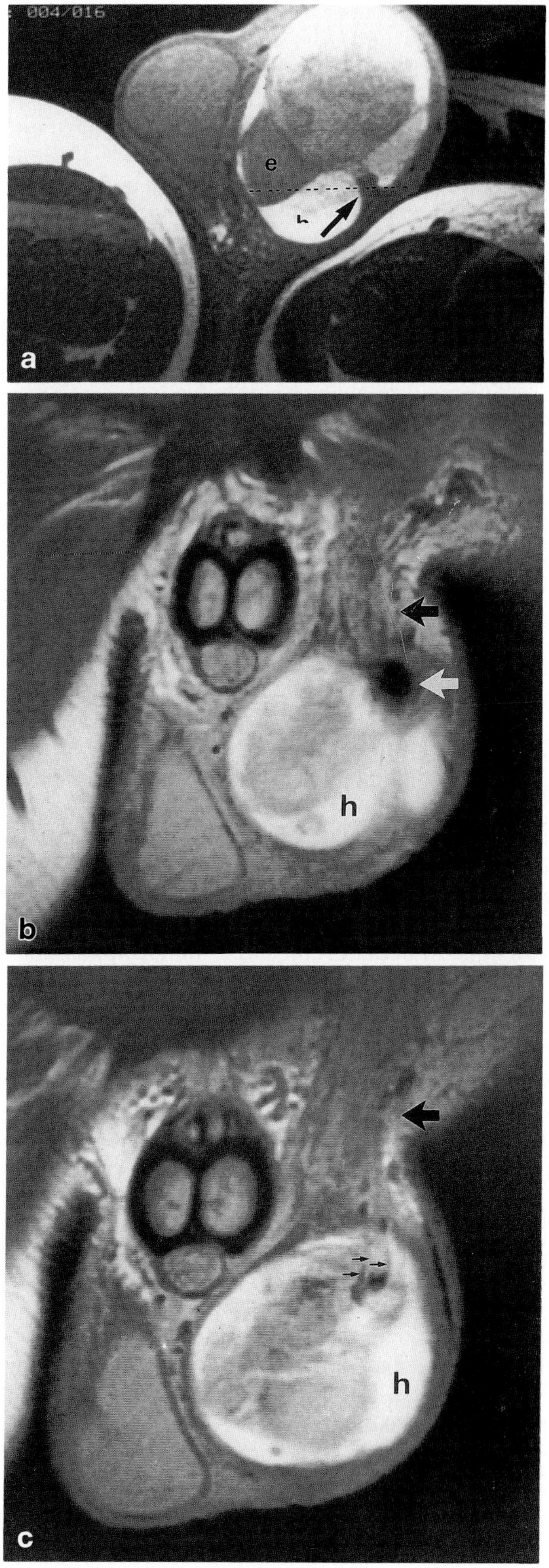

Fig. 17.19 a–c. Five-day-old torsion. **a,b** Hydrogen density-weighted coronal images and **c** a T1-weighted axial image demonstrating most of the constellation of findings seen in torsion: (1) Torsion knot (*white arrow* in **b**) is a dark region that represents the point of twist. It is thought to be due to the wringing out of water from the cord at the point of twist. (2) The "whirlpool" pattern (*small arrows* in **c**) represents the twisted facial planes of the cord emanating from the point of twist seen just anterior to image **b**. (3) The swollen hypovascular cord is seen in **b** and **c** (*thick black arrow*). (4) The "bell clapper" deformity is seen because of the hematocele (*h*) highlighting the stalk (*arrow* in **a**), proven surgically, perpendicular to which images **b** and **c** were obtained (*dashed line* in **a** is level of image **b**). (5) The hematocele (*h*) is seen as bright fluid within the scrotum (all three images). (6) The enlarged epididymis was partly edematous and partly hemorrhagic (*e* in **a**) (areas of hemorrhage not shown). (Trambert et al. 1990)

epididymo-orchitis, tumor, and trauma (Middleton and Melson 1989; Burks et al. 1990; Lerner et al. 1990; Middleton et al. 1990; Krieger et al. 1990). When testicular flow is absent in the affected testis and the instrumentation is sensitive to slow flow, torsion is identified in nearly all subjects (Lerner et al. 1990; Middleton et al. 1990; Burks et al. 1990; Feld and Middleton 1992; Dewire et al. 1992; Atkinson et al. 1992). When flow is present and symmetric with the contralateral side, torsion is effectively excluded. There are certain limitations that should be highlighted: (a) spontaneous detorsion may occur which may not only demonstrate flow but in fact hypervascularity due to postischemic hyperemia which may delay appropriate treatment (Horstman et al. 1991a); (b) although duplex ultrasonography can exclude torsion in the adult, it is more difficult in children. When testes were smaller than 1 cc, flow was not detected or was scant in 9 of 13 boys, leading the authors to recommend the use of scintigraphy to exclude torsion (Atkinson et al. 1992).

There are two specific findings of torsion on MRI: absent or diminished vascularity in a swollen spermatic cord on the affected side, and the presence of anatomic changes produced by the twisted stalk (Trambert et al. 1990). The findings of a twisted stalk were described in a rat study where torsion was produced by a 720° twist of one spermatic cord (Landa et al. 1988). The twisted cord produced a whirlpool pattern characteristic of torsion. In human subjects, a similar appearance was seen (Trambert et al. 1990). The twisted stalk was very dark at the point of twist (Fig. 17.19). From this dark point emanated several curvilinear dark lines resembling a whirlpool, presumably representing the spiraling facial planes. To best demonstrate the whirlpool pattern, the stalk must be imaged perpendicular to its axis (Fig. 17.19) (Mattrey and Trambert 1990). Other anatomic findings on MRI relate to changes in the epididymis and testis. The epididymis is markedly thickened with areas of swelling and hemorrhage. In the acute phase, the testis may be swollen and may have increased signal intensity on the T1-weighted images due to hemorrhage and clotting (Fig. 17.19). In the subacute phase the testis becomes smaller, loses signal, and becomes inhomogeneous on T2-weighted images. The inhomogeneity appears as linear bands of slightly diminished signal separated by thin lines of increased signal emanating from the mediastinum testis. When the episode is remote in time, the testis becomes small and diffusely dark on T2-weighted images, and the tunica becomes thickened and dark. The exact role of MRI in the setting of torsion is not clear but it could certainly serve to confirm the suspicion of torsion raised on ultrasonography when the ultrasonographic findings are equivocal.

17.6.5.2 Extravaginal Torsion

Extravaginal torsion occurs in the perinatal period and involves the testis, its support structures, and the vaginal process (Gullenwater et al. 1987). The clinical presentation of this condition may mimic a strangulated inguinal hernia because of the involvement of the vaginal process. Imaging is helpful when the diagnosis cannot be made clinically with certainty. In general, this condition does not need surgical intervention because it is detected too late to preserve testicular function and is not associated with any developmental anomalies such as bell-clapper deformity to warrant contralateral orchiopexy (Gullenwater et al. 1987).

Ultrasonographically the torsed testis is hypoechoic and inhomogeneous. Fluid may be present around the testis and around the not yet fused tunica vaginalis. The rim of the testis may appear echogenic due to edema or fibrous change of the tunica albuginea (Hubbard et al. 1984; Zafaranloo et al. 1986; Zerin et al. 1990). When subacute, the testis appears small, diffusely dark, and surrounded by a thickened tunica albuginea on MRI, similar to the appearance of chronic torsion in adults (Mattrey and Trambert 1990). No data are available in the acute phase to assess whether MRI could distinguish a torsed from an untorsed testis. However, IV contrast combined with fat suppression technique should produce significant enhancement differences between the normal and abnormal testes. This hypothesis requires clinical investigation.

17.6.5.3 Torsion of the Testicular Appendage

Testicular appendages are common and represent vestigial remnants of the degenerating embryologic müllerian and wolffian ducts. There are four types of testicular appendage (Rolnick et al. 1968): the appendix testis, appendix epididymis, paradidymis, and superior and inferior vas aberrans. The appendix testis is located near the upper pole of the testis, outside the tunica albuginea of the normal testis, and has its own tunical covering. The appendix epididymis is attached along the cranial aspect of the epididymis. An autopsy series demonstrated that the appendix testis and appendix epididymis were present in 92% and 34% of men (ROLNICK et al. 1968).

Torsion of the testicular appendage, a common cause of acute painful scrotal swelling in pubescent and adolescent boys, often presents with clinical features similar to those of acute spermatic cord torsion and epididymitis. The early detection of a torsed appendage is crucial since its management is conservative and differs from the other two commonly encountered acute conditions. Imaging diagnosis is very helpful in the detection and differentiation of these conditions. In a review of 171 patients who presented with an acute scrotum in whom scrotal exploration was performed, spermatic cord torsion and torsion of an appendage accounted for 89% of cases. Appendix torsion was more frequent than spermatic cord torsion in children under 12 years of age, accounting for unnecessary explorations of the scrotum twice as often in children as in adolescents or adults. Because unnecessary surgery was done in 66% of children, the authors feel that the delay associated with obtaining an imaging study is warranted (BEN CHAIM et al. 1992).

Ultrasonography of the torsed testicular appendage demonstrates a circular mass of increased echogenicity of variable size with a central hypoechoic region representing hemorrhage (COHEN et al. 1992). These findings are, however, nonspecific and may even be seen in normal testicular appendages. Color Doppler ultrasonography may show hypervascularity due to an inflammatory reaction adjacent to torsed testicular appendage, which may be difficult to differentiate from epididymo-orchitis (ATKINSON et al. 1992).

In three cases with testicular appendage torsion, MRI showed masses of variable size containing blood of variable degrees of degradation (CHO et al. 1993). The nodules were along the testis or epididymis and were associated with a hydrocele in two of the three cases (Fig. 17.20). In this setting, MRI can exclude with confidence testicular torsion, infection, or hemorrhage within a tumor, the three clinical conditions that can present with similar signs and symptoms.

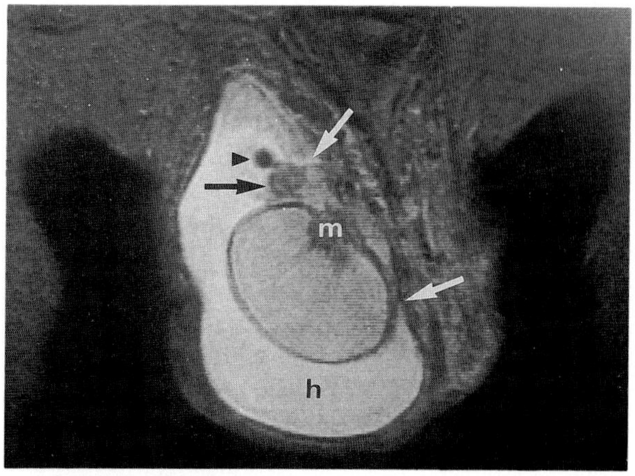

Fig. 17.20. Torsion of the epididymal appendix is shown on a T2-weighted coronal scan obtained in a patient with acute scrotal pain. Note the "bare area" of the testis (*distance between white arrows*), made visible by the hydrocele (*h*) excluding testicular torsion. The torsed appendix is full of blood that appears dark on T2-weighting (*arrowhead*) (it was bright on a hydrogen density weighted image not shown here), and is attached to a normal epididymal head (*black arrow*). Also note the normal testis and its mediastinum (*m*). (BAKER et al. 1987b)

17.6.6 Extratesticular Lesions

17.6.6.1 Spermatocele

Spermatoceles are retention cysts arising from the rete testis. They are usually located in the epididymal head. The fluid within them is thick and yellowish white and is composed of dead spermatozoa, fat, cellular debris, and sediment of lymphocytes. The cysts have a variable appearance and may be quite large. They are easily differentiated from hydrocele fluid because of their location and mass effect (O'MARA and RIFKIN 1991). Ultrasonographically, the spermatocele appears as a simple cyst but may at times be multiseptated (KRONE and CARROLL 1985; O'MARA and RIFKIN 1991). On MRI spermatoceles are round, well circumscribed, and of variable signal intensity. They may be dark or bright on T1-weighted images and are typically bright on T2-weighted images. At times, their signal is identical to the testis on all pulsing sequences (MATTREY and TRAMBERT 1990; TARTAR et al. 1993).

17.6.6.2 Hydrocele

Unless loculated, hydrocele fluid fills the vaginal space and surrounds the entire testis except for the bare area as well as the epididymal head and at times the tail and is the most common cause of scrotal swellings (Krone and Carroll 1985; O'Mara and Rifkin 1991). It accumulates because of congenital, idiopathic (primary), and local irritation (secondary) such as trauma, infarction, infection (epididymo-orchitis), or neoplasm (Hricak and Filly 1983). Reactive causes are more common than the primary or congenital causes. Although both hydrocele and hernia will transilluminate, a hydrocele with thickened tunica vaginalis might not (O'Mara and Rifkin 1991). The diagnosis of hydrocele and its distinction from hernia is easily made by imaging techniques. Simple hydroceles are anechoic and complex hydroceles (pyocele or hematocele) are multiseptated, contain debris, and may be associated with thickened scrotal wall. Analogous findings are observed on MRI except that the signal intensity of the fluid will reflect its composition.

17.6.6.3 Varicocele

Varicoceles are present in 8%–15% of adult men (Clarke 1966) and may or may not be associated with infertility. However, 21%–39% of infertile men may have varicoceles (Amelar and Dubin 1973; Hamm et al. 1986). Multiple etiologic factors have been proposed, including the obstruction of venous drainage from the testis and incompetent valves in the testicular vein allowing retrograde venous flow and increased venous pressure at the level of the pampiniform plexus (Belker 1981). More than 85% of unilateral varicoceles are left sided owing to the longer and more tortuous left testicular vein, which drains into the left renal vein before reaching the inferior vena cava (Greenberg 1977). Unilateral right-sided varicoceles suggest the presence of venous obstruction from pelvic disease (Rogers et al. 1980) and an acute left varicocele suggests obstruction of the left renal vein as in adenopathy at the left renal hilum.

Duplex ultrasonography is the primary modality for the diagnosis of varicoceles (Gonda et al. 1986; Petros et al. 1991). Examinations are usually performed in both supine and erect positions, before and after the Valsalva maneuver. The normal appearance of the spermatic cord includes the presence of veins less than 1.5 mm in diameter. Varicoceles are suspected when the diameter is increased, possibly reaching 5–6 mm. The major criterion on color Doppler imaging is the detection of dilated peritesticular vascular structures that demonstrate prolonged augmentation of venous flow during the Valsalva maneuver. However, it should be noted that mild transient flow augmentation may occur with the Valsalva maneuver in normal males (Horstman et al. 1991a).

Data are still lacking to assess the sensitivity and specificity of MRI in the diagnosis of varicoceles. However, men with known varicoceles have shown prominence of the pampiniform plexus and at times widening of the spermatic canal with a heterogeneous cord that contained a greater number of serpiginous vessels with slow flow. Abdominal compression over the sacral promontory may exaggerate the appearance of vessels in the cord in patients with varicoceles (Ziffer et al. 1989). While clinically palpable varicoceles are easily depicted on MRI, it is not clear at this time whether MRI will be able to diagnose subclinical varicoceles with sufficient accuracy.

17.7 Conclusion

Ultrasonography remains the primary imaging modality in scrotal disease but suffers from lack of specificity which may have improved with the advent of color Doppler imaging. Ultrasonography provides excellent depiction of scrotal anatomy and can distinguish with high accuracy intra- from extratesticular disease. Because of its wider field of view and higher tissue contrast and tissue characterization, MRI provides a greater constellation of findings, allowing for a more specific diagnosis (Semba et al. 1990). However, MRI is three to four times more expensive and as yet has limited patient access, thus serving as a secondary tool to ultrasonography. Because of its higher specificity, MRI should be performed when the ultrasonographic findings are equivocal, confusing, or do not explain the clinical picture.

References

Amelar RD, Dubin L (1973) Male infertility: current diagnosis and treatment. Urology 1:1–31

Arcadia JA (1952) Cysts of the tunica albuginea testis. J Urol 68:631–635

Aristizabal S, Davis JR, Miller RC et al. (1978) Bilateral primary germ cell testicular tumors: report of four cases and review of the literature. Cancer 42:591

Atkinson GO Jr, Patrick LE, Ball TI Jr, Stephenson CA, Broecker BH, Woodard JR (1992) The normal and

abnormal scrotum in children: evaluation with color Doppler sonography. AJR 158:613–617
Baker LL, Hajek PC, Burkhard TK, et al. (1987a) Magnetic resonance imaging of the scrotum: normal anatomy. Radiology 163:89–92
Baker LL, Hajek PC, Burkhard TK et al. (1987b) Magnetic resonance imaging of the scrotum: pathologic conditions. Radiology 163:93–98
Baker LL, Hajek PC, Burkhard TK, Mattrey RF (1987c) Polyorchidism: evaluation by MR. AJR 148:305–306
Batata MA, Whitmore WF Jr, Hilaris BS et al. (1980) Cryptorchidism and testicular cancer. J Urol 124:382
Belker AM (1981) The varicocele and male infertility. Urol Clin North Am 8:41–51
Ben Chaim J, Leibovitch I, Ramon J, Winberg D, Goldwasser B (1992) Etiology of acute scrotum at surgical exploration in children, adolescents and adults. Eur Urol 21:45–47
Benson CB, Doubilet PM, Richie JP (1989) Sonography of the male genital tract. AJR 153:705–713
Berger Y, Srinivas V, Hajdu SI, Herr HW (1985) Epidermoid cysts of the testis: role of conservative surgery. J Urol 134:962–963
Bird K, Rosenfield AT (1984) Testicular infarction secondary to acute inflammatory disease: demonstration by B-scan ultrasound. Radiology 152:785–788
Bird K, Rosenfield AT, Taylor KJW (1979) Ultrasonography in testicular torsion. Radiology 147:527–543
Brenner JS, Cumming WA, Ros PR (1989) Testicular epidermoid cyst: sonographic and MR findings. AJR 152:1344
Brown DL, Benson CB, Doherty FJ et al. (1992) Cystic testicular mass caused by dilated rete testis: sonographic findings in 31 cases. AJR 158:1257–1259
Burks DD, Markey BJ, Burkhard TK, Balsara ZN, Haluszka HM, Canning DA (1990) Suspected testicular torsion and ischemia: evaluation with color Doppler sonography. Radiology 175:815–821
Burney B, Klatte E (1979) Ultrasound and computed tomography of the abdomen in the staging and management of testicular carcinoma. Radiology 132: 415–419
Caldwell WL, Kudemian MT, Frias Z et al. (1980) The management of testicular seminomas. Cancer 45 [Suppl]:1768–1774
Cardigan P (1989) Polyorchidism diagnosed by ultrasound. Br J Radiol 62:82–83
Carroll BA, Gross DM (1983) High frequency scrotal sonography. AJR 140:511–515
Chen DCP, Holder L, Melloul M (1983a) Radionuclide scrotal imaging: further experience with 210 patients. Part I. Anatomy, pathology and methods. J Nucl Med 24:735–742
Chen DCP, Holder L, Melloul M (1983b) Radionuclide scrotal imaging: further experience with 210 patients. Part II. Results and discussion. J Nucl Med 24:841–853
Cho KS, Auh YH, Lee MG, Choi HY, Lee SG, Ahn HJ (1991) Testicular tumor: conventional MR imaging and Gd-DTPA enhancement. In: Book of abstracts, 77th scientific assembly and annual meeting. Radiology 181 [Suppl]:115
Cho KS, Semba CP, Trambert MA, Mattrey RF (1993) Torsion of the testicular appendages assessed with magnetic resonance imaging. JMRI
Clarke BG (1966) Incidence of varicocele in normal men and among men of different age. JAMA 198:1121–1122
Cohen HL, Shapiro MA, Haller JO, Glassberg K (1992) Torsion of the testicular appendage sonographic diagnosis. J Ultrasound Med 11:81–83
Cour-Palar IJ (1966) Spontaneous descent of the testicle. Lancet I:430
Dewire DM, Begun FP, Lawson RK, Fitzgerald S, Foley WD (1992) Color Doppler ultrasonography in the evaluation of the acute scrotum. J Urol 147:89–91
Emory TH, Charboneau JW, Randall RV, Scheithauer BW, Grantham JG (1984) Occult testicular interstitial-cell tumor in patients with gynecomastia: ultrasonic detection. Radiology 151:474
Fakhry J, Khoury A, Barakat K (1989) The hypoechoic band: a normal finding on testicular sonography. AJR 153:321–323
Feld R, Middleton WD (1992) Recent advances in sonography of the testis and scrotum. Radiol Clin North Am 30:1033–1051
Finkelstein MS, Rosenberg HK, Snyder HM, Duckett JW (1986) Ultrasound evaluation of the scrotum in pediatrics. Urology 27:1–9
Fornage BD, Touche DH, Rifkin MD (1984) Small parts real-time sonography: a new "waterpath." J Ultrasound Med 3:355–357
Friedland GW, Chang P (1988) The role of imaging in the management of impalpable undescended testis. AJR 151:1107–1111
Fritzsche PJ, Hricak H, Kogan BA et al. (1987) Undescended testis: value of MRI. Radiology 164:169–173
Fritzsche PJ, Rifkin M, Hopkins CR, Piccoli CW (1992) Scrotum and testis. In: Stark DD, Bradley WG (eds) Magnetic resonance imaging, 2nd edn. Mosby Year Book, St. Louis, pp 2058–2079
Gialason T, Noronha RFX, Gregory JG (1980) Acute epididymitis in boys: a 5 year retrospective study. J Urol 124:533–534
Glazer HS, Lee JKT, Melson GL, McClennan BL (1982) Sonographic detection of occult testicular neoplasms. AJR 138:673–675
Glickman MF, Weiss RM, Itzchak Y (1977) Testicular venography for undescended testes. AJR 129:67–70
Goldberg RM, Chilcote W, Kay R, Bodie B (1987) Sonographic findings in polyorchidism. J Clin Ultrasound 15:412–415
Gonda RL, Karo JJ, Forte RA, O'Donell KT (1986) Diagnosis of subclinical varicocele in infertility. AJR 184:71–75
Gooding GAW, Leonhardt W, Stein R (1987) Testicular cysts: US findings. Radiology 163:537–538
Grantham JG, Charboneau JW, Janes EM et al. (1985) Testicular neoplasm: 29 tumors studied by high-resolution US. Radiology 157:775–780
Grechi G, Zampi GC, Selli C, Carini M, Ucci M (1980) Polyorchidism and seminoma in a child. J Urol 123: 291–292
Green JR (1985) Computerized axial tomography vs spermatic venography in localization of the cryptorchid testis. Urology 26:513–517
Greenberg SH (1977) Varicocele and male fertility. Fertil Steril 28:699–706
Gullenwater JY, Grayhack JT, Howards SS, Duckett JW (1987) Adult and pediatric urology. Year Book Medical, Chicago, pp 1955–1962
Hadziselimovic F (1983) Cryptorchidism. Springer, Berlin Heidelberg New York
Hamm B, Fobbe F, Sorensen R, Felsenberg D (1986) Varicoceles: combined sonography and thermography

in diagnosis and post therapeutic evaluation. Radiology 160:419–424
Hamm B, Frobbe F, Loy V (1988) Testicular cysts: differentiation with US and clinical findings. Radiology 168:19–23
Hancock RA, Hodgins TE (1984) Polyorchidism. Urology 24:303–307
Harrison RG, Barkeley AT (1948) The distribution of the testicular artery (internal spermatic artery) to the human testis. Br J Urol 2:57–66
Hayward I, Trambert MA, Mattrey RF, Saltzstein SL, Demby AM (1990) Case report: MR imaging of vasculitis of the testis. J Comput Assist Tomogr 15:502–504
Holder L, Melloul M, Chen DCP (1981) Current status of radionuclide scrotal imaging. Semin Nucl Med 11: 232–249
Horstman WG, Middleton WD, Melson GL, Siegel BA (1991a) Color Doppler US of the scrotum. Radiographics 11:941–957
Horstman WG, Middleton WD, Melson GL et al. (1991b) Scrotal inflammatory disease: color Doppler US findings. Radiology 179:55–59
Hricak H, Filly RA (1983) Sonography of the scrotum. Invest Radiol 18:112–121
Hricak H, Jeffrey RB (1983) Sonography of acute scrotal abnormalities. Radiol Clin North Am 21:595–603
Hubbard AE, Ayers AB, MacDonald LM, James CE (1984) In utero torsion of the testis: antenatal and postnatal ultrasonic appearance. Br J Radiol 57:644–646
Hutschenreiter G, Alken P, Schneider H (1979) The value of sonography and lymphography in the detection of retroperitoneal metastases in testicular tumor. J Urol 122:766–769
Janzen DL, Mathieson JR, Marsh JI, Cooperberg PL, del Rio P, Golding RH, Rifkin MD (1992) Testicular microlithiasis: sonographic and clinical features. AJR 158:1057–1060
Johnson JO, Mattrey RF, Philpson J (1990) Differentiation of seminomatous from nonseminomatous testicular tumors with MR imaging. AJR 154:539–543
Just M, Melchior S, Grebe P, Kreitner KF, Burger RA, Hohenfellner R, Thelen M (1992) MR tomography in testicular processes. The significance of Gd-DTPA enhanced sequence in comparison with plain T2-weighted sequences. ROFO 166:527–531
Kier R, McCarthy S, Rosenfield AT et al. (1988) Nonpalpable testes in young boys: evaluation with MR imaging. Radiology 169:429–433
Kirschling RJ, Kvols LK, Charboneau JW, Grantham JG, Zincke H (1983) High-resolution ultrasonographic and pathologic abnormalities of germ cell tumors in patients with clinically normal testes. Mayo Clin Proc 58: 648–653
Klepp O, Olsson AM, Ous S, Nilsson S, Hoisaether PA, Tveter K (1991) Early clinical stages of nonseminomatous testis cancer. Evaluation of the primary treatment and follow-up procedures of the SWENOTECA project. Scand J Urol Nephrol 25:179–190
Krieger JN, Wang K, Mack L (1990) Preliminary evaluation of color Doppler imaging for investigation of intrascrotal pathology. J Urol 144:904–907
Krone KD, Carroll BA (1985) Scrotal ultrasound. Radiol Clin North Am 23:121–139
Landa HM, Gylys-Morin V, Mattrey RF et al. (1987) MRI of the cryptorchid testis. Eur J Pediatr 146 [Suppl]: S16–S17
Landa HM, Gylys-Morin V, Mattrey RF et al. (1988) Detection of testicular torsion by magnetic resonance imaging in a rat model. J Urol 140:1178–1180
Lee JKT, Glazer HS (1982) Computed tomography in the localization of the nonpalpable testis. Urol Clin North Am 9:397–404
Leopold GR, Woo VL, Scheible FW et al. (1979) High resolution ultrasonography of scrotal pathology. Radiology 131:719–722
Lerner RM, Mevorach RA, Hulbert WC, Rabinowitz R (1990) Color Doppler US in the evaluation of acute scrotal disease. Radiology 176:355–358
Leung ML, Gooding GAW, Williams RD (1984) High-resolution sonography of scrotal contents in asymptomatic subjects. AJR 143:161–164
Lupetin AR, King W, Rich P, Lederman RB (1983a) Ultrasound diagnosis of testicular leukemia. Radiology 146:171–172
Lupetin AR, King W, Rich PJ, Lederman RB (1983b) The traumatized scrotum. Radiology 148:203–207
Martin B, Conte J (1987) Ultrasonography of the acute scrotum. J Clin Ultrasound 15:37–44
Mattrey RF (1991) Magnetic resonance imaging of the scrotum. Semin Ultrasound CT MR 12:95–108
Mattrey R, Trambert M (1990) MR imaging of the scrotum and testis. In: Edelman RR, Hesselink JR, Newhouse J, Sartoris DJ (eds) Clinical magnetic resonance imaging. W.B. Saunders, Philadelphia, pp 952–979
Maxwell AJ, Mamtora H (1990) Sonographic appearance of epidermoid cyst of the testis. J Clin Ultrasound 18:188–190
McConnell JD, Peters PC, Lewis SE (1982) Testicular rupture in blunt scrotal trauma: review of 15 cases with recent application of testicular scanning. J Urol 128: 309–311
Meiches MD, Nurenberg P (1991) Sonographic appearance of a calcified simple epidermoid cyst of the testis. J Clin Ultrasound 19:498–500
Mennemeyer RP, Mason JT (1979) Non-neoplastic cystic lesions of the tunica albuginea: an electron microscopic and clinical study of 2 cases. J Urol 121:373–375
Middleton WD, Melson GL (1989) Testicular ischemia: color Doppler sonographic findings in five patients. AJR 152:1237–1239
Middleton WD, Siegel BA, Melson GL, Yates CK, Andriole GL (1990) Acute scrotal disorders: prospective comparison of color Doppler US and testicular scintigraphy. Radiology 177:177–181
Mittemeyer BT, Lennox KW, Borski AA (1966) Epididymitis: a review of 10 cases. J Urol 95:390–392
Moore KL (1988) The urogenital system. In: The developing human. Clinical oriented embryology, 4th edn. W.B. Saunders, Philadelphia, pp 246–285
O'mara EM, Rifkin MD (1991) Scrotum and contents. In: Resnick MI, Rifkin MD (eds) Ultrasonography of the urinary tract, 3rd edn. William and Wilkins, Baltimore, pp 386–435
Petros JA, Andriole GL, Middleton WD, Picus DD (1991) Correlation of testicular color Doppler ultrasound, physical examination, and venography in the detection of left varicocele in men with infertility. J Urol 145: 785–788
Phillips G, Kumari-Subaiya S, Swaitsky A (1983) Ultrasonic evaluation of the scrotum in lymphoproliferative disease. J Ultrasound 6:169–175

Pillari G, Rubenstein WA, Siess J (1980) Seminoma: improved imaging and tumor characterization with computed tomography. J Urol 123:41–43
Pinch L, Aceto T Jr, Myer-Bahlburg HFL (1974) Cryptorchidism. A pediatric review. Urol Clin North Am 1:573–592
Rajfer J (1992) Congenital anomalies of the testis. In: Walsh PC, Retik AB, Stamey TA, Vaughan ED Jr (eds) Campbell's urology, 6th edn. W.B. Saunders, Philadelphia, pp 1543–1562
Ralls PW, Larsen D, Johnson MB, Lee KP (1991) Color Doppler sonography of the scrotum Semin Ultrasound CT MR 12:109–114
Rao KG (1980) Traumatic rupture of the testis. Urology 20:624–625
Rholl KS, Lee JKT, Ling D et al. (1987) MR imaging of the scrotum with a high resolution surface coil. Radiology 163:99–103
Richie JP (1992) Neoplasms of the testis. In: Walsh PC, Retik AB, Stamey TA, Vaughan ED Jr (eds) Campbell's urology. W.B. Saunders, Philadelphia, pp 1222–1263
Rifkin MD, Kurtz AB, Pasto ME, Goldberg BB (1983) Polyorchidism diagnosed preoperatively by ultrasonography. J Ultrasound Med 2:93–94
Rifkin MD, Kurtz AB, Pasto ME et al. (1984) The sonographic diagnosis of focal and diffuse infiltrative intracostal lesions. Urol Radiol 6:20–26
Rogers WF, Ralls PW, Boswell WD (1980) Obstruction of the inferior vena cava by seminoma. J Urol 124:613–614
Rolnick D, Kowanous S, Szanto P, Bush IM (1968) Anatomical incidence of testicular appendages. J Urol 100:775–766
Ryan PC, Whelan CA, Gaffney EF, Fitzpatrick JM (1988) The effect of unilateral experimental testicular torsion on spermatogenesis and fertility. Br J Urol 62:359–366
Sadler TW (1990) Urogenital system. In: Langman's medical embryology, 6th edn. William and Wilkins, Baltimore, pp 260–296
Schultz Lampel D, Bogaert G, Thuroff JW, Schlegel E, Cramer B (1991) MRI for evaluation of scrotal pathology. Urol Res 19:289–292
Schwerk WB, Schwerk WN, Rodeck G (1983) Testicular tumors: prospective analysis of real-time US patterns and abdominal staging. Radiology 151:369–374
Scorer CG, Farrington GH (1972) Congenital deformities of the testis and epididymis Appleton-Century-Crofts, New York
Scott RF, Bayliss AP, Calder JF, Gravie WH (1986) Indications for ultrasound in the evaluation of the pathological scrotum. Br J Urol 58:178–182
Seidenwurm D, Smathers RL, Lo RK et al. (1987) Testes and scrotum: MR imaging at 1.5T. Radiology 164: 393–398
Semba CP, Trambert MA, Mattrey RF (1990) Specificity of MRI in scrotal disease versus sonography. RSNA, Chicago, IL, 1990 Radiology 177(P) [Suppl]:129
Shah KH, Maxted WC, Chun B (1981) Epidermoid cysts of the testis: a report of three cases and an analysis of 141 cases from the world literature. Cancer 47:577–582
Shah SN, Miller BM, Geisler E (1992) Polyorchidism discovered as testicular torsion. Urology 39:543–544
Shawker TH, Nasser J, O'leary T et al. (1983) Ultrasonographic detection of "burned-out" primary testicular germ cell tumors in clinically normal testes. J Ultrasound Med 2:477–479
Singer BR, Donaldson JG, Jackson DS (1992) Polyorchidism: functional classification and management strategy. Urology 39:384–388
Smith WS, Brammer HM, Henry M, Frazier H (1991) Testicular microlithiasis: sonographic features with pathologic correlation. AJR 157:1003–1004
Sokal M, Peckham MJ, Hendry WF (1980) Bilateral germ cell tumours of the testis. Br J Urol 53:158
Tanagho EA (1992) Anatomy of the lower urinary tract. In: Walsh PC, Retik AB, Stamey TA, Vaughan ED Jr (eds) Campbell's urology, 6th edn. W.B. Saunders, Philadelphia, pp 40–69
Tartar VM, Trambert MA, Balsara ZN, Mattrey RF (1993) Tubular ectasia of the testicle: sonographic and MR imaging appearance. AJR 160:539–542
Thum G (1991) Polyorchidism: case report and review of literature. J Urol 145:370–372
Thurner S, Hricak H, Carroll PR et al. (1988) Imaging the testis: comparison between MR imaging and US. Radiology 167:631–636
Trainer TD (1987) Histology of the normal testis. Am J Surg Pathol 11:797–809
Trambert MA, Mattrey RF, Levine D, Berthoty D (1990) Subacute scrotal pain: evaluation of torsion versus epididymitis with MR imaging. Radiology 175:53–56
Vick CW, Bird KI Jr, Rosenfield AT et al. (1982) Ultrasound of the scrotal contents. Radiology 144:147–153
Vick CW, Bird K, Rosenfield A et al. (1986) Extratesticular hemorrhage associated with torsion of the spermatic cord: sonographic demonstration. Radiology 158: 401–404
Vordermark JS II, Favila MO (1982) Testicular necrosis: a preventable complication of epididymitis. J Urol 128: 1322–1324
Wechsler H, Westfall M, Lattimer JK (1960) The earliest signs and symptoms in 127 male patients with genitourinary tuberculosis. J Urol 83:801–803
Weingarten BJ, Kellman GM, Middleton WD, Gross ML (1992) Tubular ectasia within the mediastinum testis. J Ultrasound Med 11:349–353
Weiss RM, Carter AR, Rosenfield AT (1986) High resolution real-time ultrasonography in the localization of the undescended testis. J Urol 135:936–938
Weiss AJ, Kellman GM, Middleton WD, Kirkemo A (1992) Intratesticular varicocele: sonographic findings in two patients. AJR 158:1061–1063
William R, Feiberg S, Kneight L, Traley E (1980) Abdominal staging of testicular tumors using ultrasonography and computed tomography. J Urol 123:872–875
Williamson RCN, Anderson JB (1986) The fate of the human testes following unilateral torsion. Br J Urol 58:698–704
Wolveson MK, Houttin E, Heiberh E et al. (1983) Comparison of CT with high resolution ultrasound in the localization of the undescended testis. Radiology 146:133–136
Zafaranloo S, Gerard PS, Wise G (1986) Bilateral neonatal testicular torsion: ultrasonographic evaluation. J Urol 135:589–590
Zerin JM, DiPietro MA, Grignon A, Shea D (1990) Testicular infarction in the newborn: ultrasound findings. Pediatr Radiol 20:329–300
Ziffer JA, Nelson RC, Chezmar JL et al. (1989) Subclinical varicoceles: detection with MRI (abstract). Presented at SMRI Los Angeles. Magn Reson Imaging 7 [Suppl]: 78
Zoeller G, Ringert RH (1991) Color-coded duplex sonography for diagnosis of testicular torsion. J Urol 146: 1288–1290

18 The Urethra: Normal Anatomy, Radiology, Disease, and Injury

Ronald W. McCallum

CONTENTS

18.1 Normal Anatomy and Physiology

The male urethra is divided anatomically and radiologically into the anterior and posterior urethra. The anterior urethra extends from the inferior fascia of the urogenital diaphragm to the external meatus. The anterior urethra consists of the penile urethra, from the external meatus to the penoscrotal junction below and the suspensory ligament above, and the bulbous urethra, from the penoscrotal junction to the inferior aspect of the urogenital diaphragm. The posterior urethra consists of the membranous urethra within the urogenital diaphragm and is approximately 1–1.5 cm long. It extends from the inferior fascia of the urogenital diaphragm to the inferior aspect of the verumontanum. The prostatic urethra extends from the inferior aspect of the verumontanum to the bladder neck and passes through the prostate gland a little anterior to the middle of the prostate. The urogenital diaphragm, which divides the urethra into the anterior and posterior urethra, is a triangular ligament extending horizontally from the inferior rami of the pubic arch, posteriorly attaching to the tendinous plate of the perineum and continuous with the anal fascia.

18.1.1 The Anterior Urethra

The anterior urethra is surrounded by the cavernous tissue of the corpus spongiosum, which dilates proximally and inferiorly to form the bulbous spongiosum and distally and superiorly to form the glans penis. Within the glans penis the urethra dilates to form the fossa navicularis proximal to the external meatus. The corpora cavernosa are two cavernous bodies which lie parallel and superiorly on the corpus spongiosum. Proximally, each corpus cavernosum forms a crus which is firmly attached to the rami of the pubic arch. Scarpa's and Colles' fasciae extend distally to form an envelope of fascia around the corpora cavernosa and corpus spongiosum. Proximally the bulbous spongiosum is enveloped posteriorly by the bulbocavernosus muscle, which also provides a small tendinous sling anteriorly, the musculus compressor nuda (Morales and Romanus 1955; McCallum and Colapinto 1976). This extends

Ronald W. McCallum, M.B., F.R.C.P. (C), F.A.C.R., Professor of Radiology, Radiologist-in-Chief, Department of Diagnostic Imaging, St. Michael's Hospital, University of Toronto, 30 Bond Street, Toronto, Ontario M5B 1W8, Canada

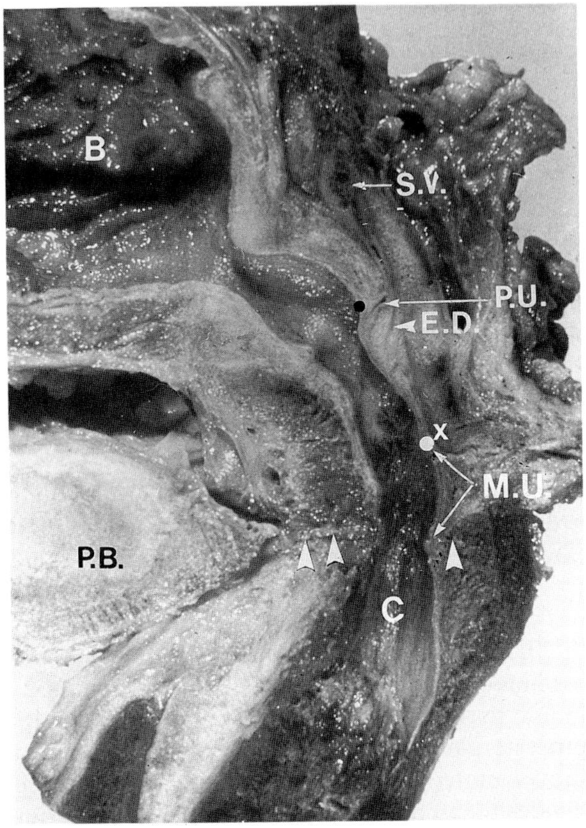

Fig. 18.1. Sagittal section through en bloc autopsy specimen includes bladder (*B*), prostatic utricle (*P.U.*), ejaculatory duct (*E.D.*), pubic bone (*P.B.*), cone of proximal bulbous urethra (*C*), membranous urethra (*M.U.*) and seminal vesicles (S.V.). *White vertical arrows* indicate fascia at inferior aspect of urogenital diaphragm. *Black dot*, superior edge of verumontanum; *X*, inferior edge of verumontanum; *white dot*, urethral crest. (Modified from McCallum 1979)

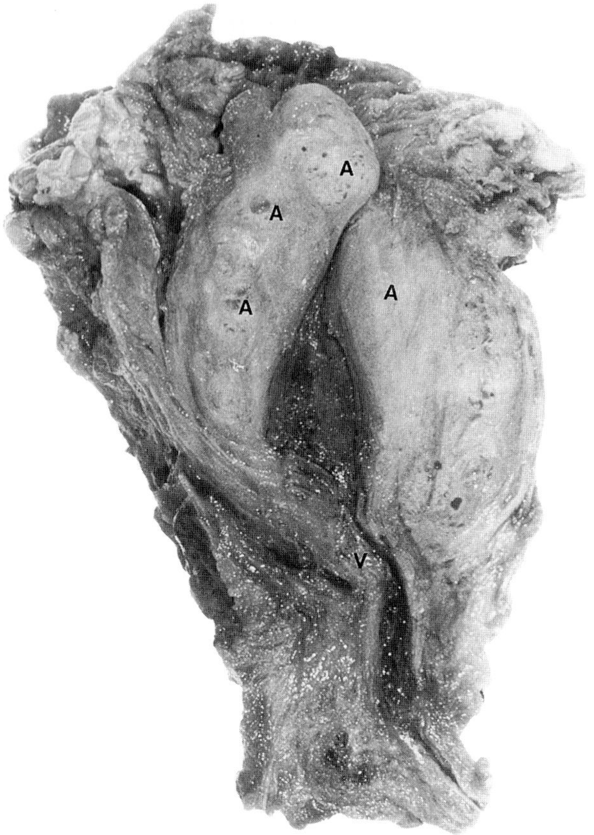

Fig. 18.2. Sagittal section through en bloc autopsy specimen showing multiple adenomas (*A*) arising from inner periurethral glands only present above the verumontanum (*V*)

anteriorly around the bare area of the proximal bulbous urethra. Contraction of the bulbocavernosus muscle indents the posterior urethra and musculus compressor nuda contraction produces a slight indentation in the anterior aspect of the proximal bulbous urethra. Numerous mucous and submucous glands, the glands of Littre, extend along the length of the anterior urethra, and the ducts of Cowper's glands empty into the mid bulbous urethra. Cowper's glands are contained within the urogenital diaphragm. The anterior urethra is emptied of urine at the end of micturition by contraction of the bulbocavernosus muscle and pelvic floor muscles.

18.1.2 The Posterior Urethra

The posterior urethra consisting of the membranous and prostatic urethra (Fig. 18.1) is more complex than the anterior urethra since it is the site of the verumontanum, is surrounded by prostatic tissue, and also is the location of the urinary sphincters.

The verumontanum is a mound of smooth muscle on the posterior wall of the prostatic urethra. The verumontanum rises abruptly, superiorly, slightly above the middle of the prostatic urethra and extends distally to the distal third of the prostatic urethra where it tapers inferiorly, forming the urethral crest, which extends as far as the membranous urethra. The ejaculatory ducts empty into the verumontanum through two small orifices close to the midline of the verumontanum. A little above the orifices of the ejaculatory ducts a third orifice represents the opening of the prostatic utricle which is a vestigial remnant of the müllerian duct. The prostatic utricle is homologous with the uterus and vagina of the female. On each side of the verumontanum are the prostatic sinuses into which the true prostatic ducts empty.

The ejaculatory ducts, formed by the junction of the ampulla of the vas deferens and the ducts of the seminal vesicles, separate the median lobe of the prostate above and the posterior lobe of prostate below. A true anterior lobe is said to atrophy at birth. A transverse section through the prostate above the verumontanum shows the true prostatic lobes peripherally (Franks 1954). Centrally, mucosal and submucosal glands lie adjacent to the urethra. These are the inner prostatic glands, only present above the verumontanum, which are subject to hypertrophy (Franks 1954) (Fig. 18.2). The true prostatic lobes or outer prostatic glands are subject to infection and malignancy but do not undergo hypertrophy. The inner prostatic (periurethral) glands correspond to the transitional zone of McNeal's (1972) anatomic description of the prostate. The true prostatic lobes correspond to McNeal's peripheral zone.

The posterior urethra is the site of influence of the urinary sphincters which govern passive and active continence (Fig. 18.3).

Muscles of Retention	
Primary Passive Continence	Internal Sphincter (Smooth muscle) Intrinsic Sphincter (Smooth muscle)
Secondary Active Continence	External Sphincter (Striated muscle) Pelvic Floor Muscles

Fig. 18.3. Primary and secondary muscles of continence

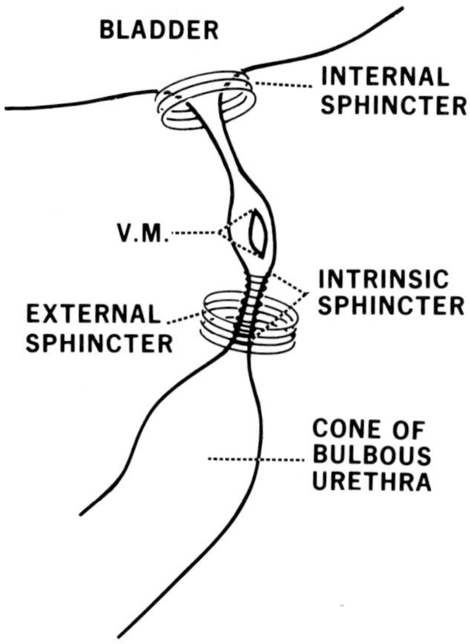

Fig. 18.4. Diagrammatic representation of the three urinary sphincters. The internal and intrinsic sphincters are smooth muscle. The external sphincter is striated muscle (verumontanum (V.M.)). (McCallum 1979)

18.1.3 The Urinary Sphincters

There are three urinary sphincters (McCallum and Colapinto 1976; Turner-Warwick and Whiteside 1970) (Fig. 18.4). Two are smooth muscle and the third is striated muscle. The smooth muscle sphincters circle the urethra. Proximally at the bladder neck the *internal sphincter* (smooth muscle) surrounds the proximal prostatic urethra adjacent to the bladder orifice. Distally around the distal prostatic and membranous urethra, closely applied to urethral mucosa, is the *intrinsic sphincter* (smooth muscle). Peripheral to the intrinsic sphincter, the *external sphincter* (striated muscle) surrounds the intrinsic sphincter and in addition passes arcuate fibers proximally within the prostatic capsule almost to the bladder neck. The internal sphincter at the bladder neck is the first line of defence against passive urinary incontinence. The internal sphincter may be damaged or obliterated, as may occur in urethral injury in pelvic fractures or in prostatectomy. However, this does not necessarily lead to urinary incontinence, since the intrinsic sphincter around the distal prostatic and membranous urethra is the second line of defence against passive incontinence. Consequently, passive continence is governed mainly by the two smooth muscle sphincters.

The external sphincter is striated muscle and has been shown histochemically to consist of specialized type I (slow twitch) fibers capable of maintaining tone for a considerable period of time without fatigue (Gosling 1981). It has also been shown that EMG activity is continuous while the patient is at rest, and only ceases when the patient voids. Whether the continuous tone of the type I fibers of the external sphincter is sufficient to maintain passive continence is questionable, since nerve block of the pudendal nerves (RAZ 1978) which innervate the external sphincter (TANAGHO et al. 1982) does not cause urinary incontinence. In addition, ELBADAWI and SCHENK (1974) have shown that part of the external sphincter area contains adrenergic and cholinergic fibers, which would support the concept that the smooth muscle sphincters are responsible for passive continence and that the external sphincter plays little part in maintaining passive continence. Active continence in response to stress is maintained by the external sphincter and pelvic floor muscles. The internal sphincter at the bladder neck has been shown to be rich in α-adrenergic receptors (ELBADAWI and SCHENK 1974) and has been made to contract and close the bladder neck under the action of sympathomimetic drugs even while the detrusor muscle is contracting (KLEEMAN 1970). In addition, the circular smooth muscle sphincters surround longitudinal bundles of smooth muscle which extend from the bladder neck to the urethral crest at the membranous urethra. These longitudinal bundles of smooth muscle relax during micturition so that the urethra lengthens and there is a descent of 1–1.5 cm of the posterior urethra during micturition. At the end of micturition the longitudinal smooth muscle contracts, shortening the urethra. In conjunction with this action of longitudinal smooth muscle at the end of micturition, the intrinsic sphincter performs its second function, which is, by contraction, to produce a milk-back action to empty the posterior urethra of urine, milking back the 1 or 2 cc of urine in the prostatic urethra into the bladder at the end of micturition. Consequently the whole urethra is empty of urine at the end of micturition. Finally, anatomic dissections of the urethra show that the proximal bulbous urethra forms a symmetric cone shape immediately adjacent to the inferior edge of the urogenital diaphragm (Fig. 18.1). The tip of this symmetric cone therefore represents the inferior edge of the membranous urethra, which extends to the inferior edge of the verumontanum and is approximately 1–1.5 cm in length.

18.1.4 Neurophysiology of the Lower Urinary Tract

In normal man, three separate coordinated nerve supplies are involved in micturition and sphincter function. There are:

The parasympathetic (pelvic nerves), S2–4
The sympathetic (hypogastric nerves), T11–L2
The somatic (pudendal nerves), S2–4

The parasympathetic nerve is motor and sensory to the bladder detrusor muscle. The pelvic nerves supply stretch receptors to the detrusor muscle. Bladder filling stimulates multiple superimposed stretch reflexes which are conveyed along the afferent fibers to the sacral segments S2–4 and which are conveyed back to the bladder via efferent parasympathetic fibers. This is the micturition reflex arc. As the bladder fills these impulses result in the final production of a strong bladder contraction. In infants the bladder is uninhibited and therefore micturition is more frequent. The inhibition of micturition occurs when micturition centers in the pons, hypothalamus, midbrain, and cortex develop. These centers are mainly inhibitory but occasionally may be excitatory during stress. Detrusor contraction resulting in micturition is coordinated with reciprocal sympathetic activity on the urinary sphincter mechanism causing the sphincters to relax. Parasympathetic activity also involves a response to hot and cold. Consequently the instillation of cold water into the bladder causes early bladder contraction.

The sympathetic hypogastric nerves supply adrenergic receptors to the bladder and to the urinary sphincters. Adrenergic mapping has shown the bladder to be rich in β-receptors and the smooth muscle sphincters to be rich in α-Receptors. β-Receptor stimulation causes smooth muscle relaxation. α-Receptor stimulation causes smooth muscle contraction. Consequently as the bladder fills the sphincters remain contracted and the detrusor relaxed. As the intravesical pressure increases above 20 cm water, the bladder is stretched enough to stimulate the micturition reflex arc and the detrusor contracts. Reciprocal relaxation of the sphincters which contain β-receptors allows urine to flow through the urethra and the bladder to empty.

The somatic pudendal nerves similarly reflexly relax the striated external sphincter and pelvic floor muscles to allow micturition. The distal sphincter mechanism consists of both the striated muscle external sphincter and the smooth muscle intrinsic sphincter.

The external sphincter contains fast and slow twitch fibers. The slow twitch fibers maintain tone in the external sphincters. The fast twitch fiber activity results when micturition is interrupted or reflexly to stop stress incontinence when the intra-abdominal pressure is increased. However, it has been shown that local pudendal block does not result in passive incontinence. Spinal cord lesions which interfere with normal autonomic activity may result in incoordination of sympathetic parasympathetic activity. Lesions below L2 (LMNLs) result in an aflexic bladder by interrupting the parasympathetic reflex arc. When the cord lesion is above L2 (UMNLs) the micturition reflex arc is intact and the detrusor muscle can contract, but the normal sphincter function is usually uncoordinated.

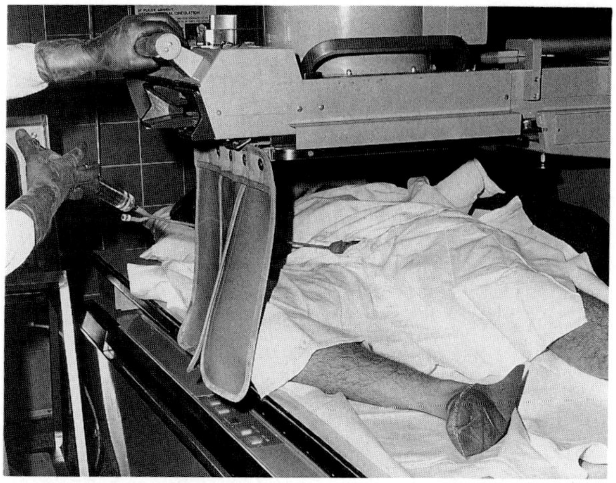

Fig. 18.5. The Foley catheter method. The patient is obliqued 30–40°. Tension is applied to the syringe and catheter to straighten the penis at the penoscrotal junction

18.2 Methods of Urethrography

18.2.1 Method in Urethral Stricture

Dynamic retrograde and voiding urethrography (McCallum and Colapinto 1976) are done as a single procedure. Dynamic retrograde urethrography requires motion of contrast medium through the urethra *during* exposure of the film. Exposure of the film during injection is the only way to consistently visualize the posterior urethra and verumontanum, which is an essential landmark for localization of the membranous urethra. The posterior urethra is rarely visualized in static retrograde urethrography (exposure of the film after the contrast medium has been injected into the urethra) because of the milk-back action of the intrinsic sphincter which will milk-back into the bladder the few cubic centimeters of contrast medium lying in the posterior urethra. Dynamic retrograde urethrography may be performed using a Brodny clamp, but this author prefers the Foley catheter method (Fig. 18.5).

A Foley catheter (size 14) is inserted 2–3 cm into the penis and 1 or 2 cc of saline is inserted into the balloon of the catheter. The balloon of the catheter is fixed in the fossa navicularis. No lubricant is used. To the catheter is attached an adaptor and 50 cc syringe containing 30% contrast medium. Mild traction is applied to the catheter and syringe during the retrograde injection in order to straighten the penis at the penoscrotal junction. Two or three films are obtained during the dynamic retrograde study, which is preferably done with fluoroscopy. Through the same catheter the bladder is filled and the voiding study obtained. The catheter is usually removed before the voiding study but the catheter may be left in place to obtain a choke voiding urethrogram with the patient voiding into the catheter and syringe. The whole procedure, dynamic retrograde and voiding urethrography, takes about 15–20 min. Occasionally, additional catheters are required when the patient presents with perineal fistulae. Additional catheters are inserted into the perineal fistulous tracts and two or three catheters injected simultaneously in order to visualize the whole urethra.

18.2.2 Method in Urethral Trauma

In acute urethral trauma usually only the dynamic retrograde urethrogram is obtained (McCallum and Colapinto 1976). This is sufficient to elucidate the site and degree of injury. As in urethral stricture, the examination is best performed under fluoroscopy but fluoroscopy may not be practical. The examination may be done successfully using an overhead beam or, as is occasionally necessary, portable equipment. The same Foley catheter method is used but modified so that the urethral injury may be assessed with the minimum amount of contrast medium injected. Too much contrast

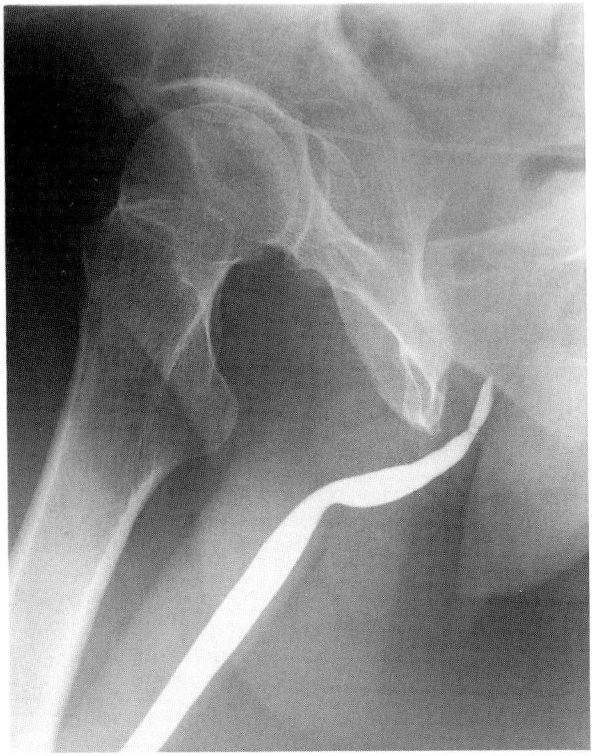

Fig. 18.6. Static retrograde urethrogram. Contrast medium lies static in the urethra during film exposure. The posterior urethra is not visualized. A stricture is seen in the proximal bulbous urethra. Extension of scarring from the proximal bulb stricture into the membranous urethra cannot be assessed

medium is likely to obliterate urethral landmarks and may produce a confusing film. Consequently it is recommended that the first film is exposed during the injection of the first 10 cc of contrast medium. This is sufficient to indicate whether the urethra is intact or whether there is extravasation due to either tear in the urethra or urethral separation.

In patients in whom urethrography demonstrates a urethral tear or urethral separation, the management may require primary urethral repair or delayed repair. In delayed repair a suprapubic catheter is inserted for temporary urinary diversion. In these cases follow-up urethrography requires both dynamic retrograde urethrography and attempted voiding urethrography. The bladder is filled via the suprapubic catheter. Dynamic retrograde and attempted voiding urethrography are performed simultaneously in order to visualize the extent of the urethral defect requiring repair by one- or two-stage urethroplasty via the perineal approach.

18.2.3 Method in Neurogenic Bladder

Patients with neurogenic bladder may have an unacceptable level of residual urine due to some degree of outlet obstruction. Consequently dynamic retrograde and voiding cystourethrography are required to elucidate the degree and site of outlet obstruction (McCallum 1974). Obstruction may occur at the bladder neck, which may not open on attempted voiding, or at the distal sphincter, due to sphincter dyssynergia. Prostatic hypertrophy or prostatitis may also contribute to outlet obstruction in patients with neurogenic bladder.

The method used to examine the bladder neck and urethra is identical to that used in urethral stricture. In neurogenic bladder patients the voiding study is essential. The method is slightly modified in that the catheter is not removed from the fossa navicularis when the patient voids. Voiding occurs into the catheter and syringe in the operator's hand. The site of outlet obstruction can be readily demonstrated by this method.

18.2.4 Other Methods of Urethrography

While the author has used the Foley catheter method successfully without significant complications in over 3000 patients, other methods are described in the literature.

1. *Static retrograde urethrography*. This procedure is performed by injecting contrast medium into the urethra, applying a clamp to the end of the penis, and exposing a film while the contrast medium lies static in the urethra. The examination may give information on the anterior urethra; however, it cannot assess the cone of the proximal bulbous urethra, and the posterior urethra is rarely visualized by this method (Fig. 18.6).

   Autourethrography, i.e., retrograde urethrography with the injection performed and controlled by the patient, has been lauded for excellent demonstration of the prostatic urethra in over 90% of the examinations performed (Kirshy et al. 1991).
2. *Excretory voiding urethrography* has recently been described in the literature (Fitts et al. 1977). This study includes a voiding cystourethrogram at the end of intravenous urography. The method has certain merit and may show

filling defects in the urethra, fistula, diverticulum, and stricture. However, the voiding study alone may give misleading information and soft or secondary scarring in the urethra may not be obvious. In addition, the author has found this procedure to be time consuming, and the fluoroscope and the radiologist must be available when the patient decides to void – not always a convenient situation.

18.3 Normal Radiologic Landmarks of the Urethra with Anatomic Correlation

18.3.1 Dynamic Retrograde Urethrography

The normal dynamic retrograde urethrogram (Fig. 18.7) correlates well with the normal anatomy described above. The balloon of the catheter in the fossa navicularis is well visualized. The penoscrotal junction dividing the anterior urethra into the penile and bulbous urethra is readily identified. The symmetric cone of the proximal bulbous urethra is visualized in all normal males. The tip of the cone represents the inferior aspect of the membranous urethra. Also well visualized is the verumontanum, the inferior aspect of which represents the proximal boundary of the membranous urethra. Therefore the membranous urethra is readily localized between the inferior edge of the verumontanum and the tip of the cone of the proximal bulbous urethra (McCallum and Colapinto 1976, 1979). Radiologic localization of the membranous urethra is of prime importance to the urologist, since disease or scar tissue within the membranous urethra necessitates an incision that involves the distal sphincters which surround the membranous urethra. Such an incision is not taken lightly by the urologist because of the possibility of producing urinary incontinence. On dynamic retrograde urethrography the membranous urethra is recognized as a thin wisp of contrast medium about 2 mm in width and 1–1.5 cm in length. The thin width of the membranous urethra on dynamic retrograde urethrography is due to the normal tone of contraction of the distal sphincters. The width of the membranous urethra can only be assessed on the voiding study. Proximal to the verumontanum the dynamic retrograde urethrogram shows the supracollicular prostatic urethra, and the bladder neck is shown by a jet of contrast medium flowing into the bladder. The jet of contrast medium

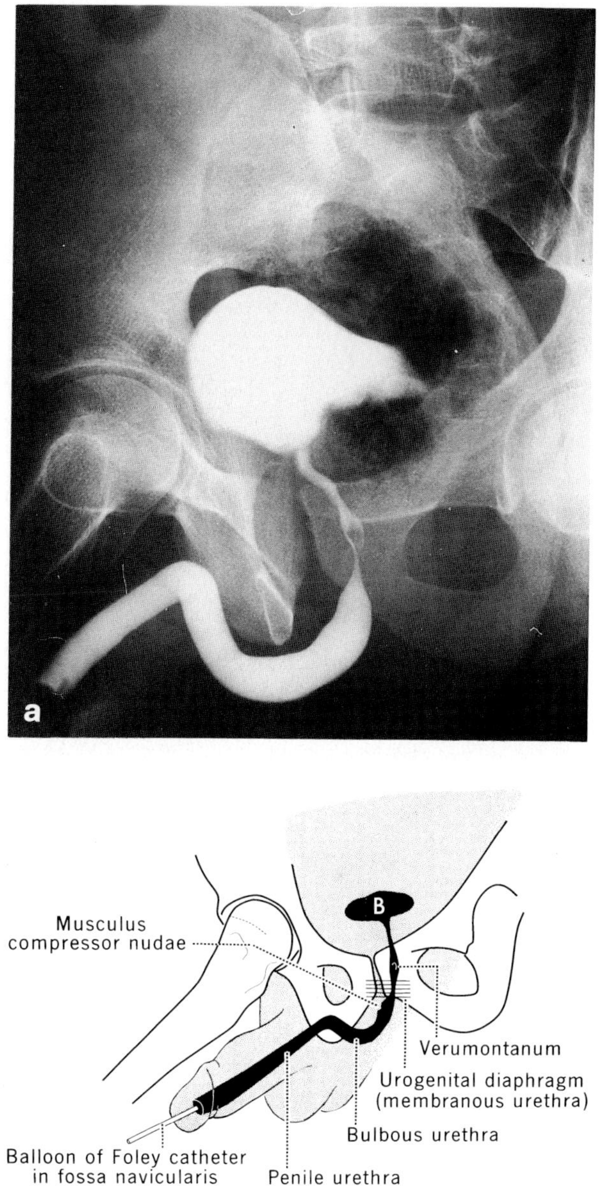

b

Fig. 18.7a,b. Normal dynamic retrograde urethrogram with tracing showing important radiologic landmarks. *B*, bladder

passing into the bladder is due to the resistance of the tone of the internal sphincter to the force of the injection applied by the operator's thumb on the barrel of the syringe. After bladder filling and removal of the catheter the patient voids (Fig. 18.8).

Occasionally, an anxious patient will contract the distal sphincters and pelvic floor muscles during injection. This may result in alterations in

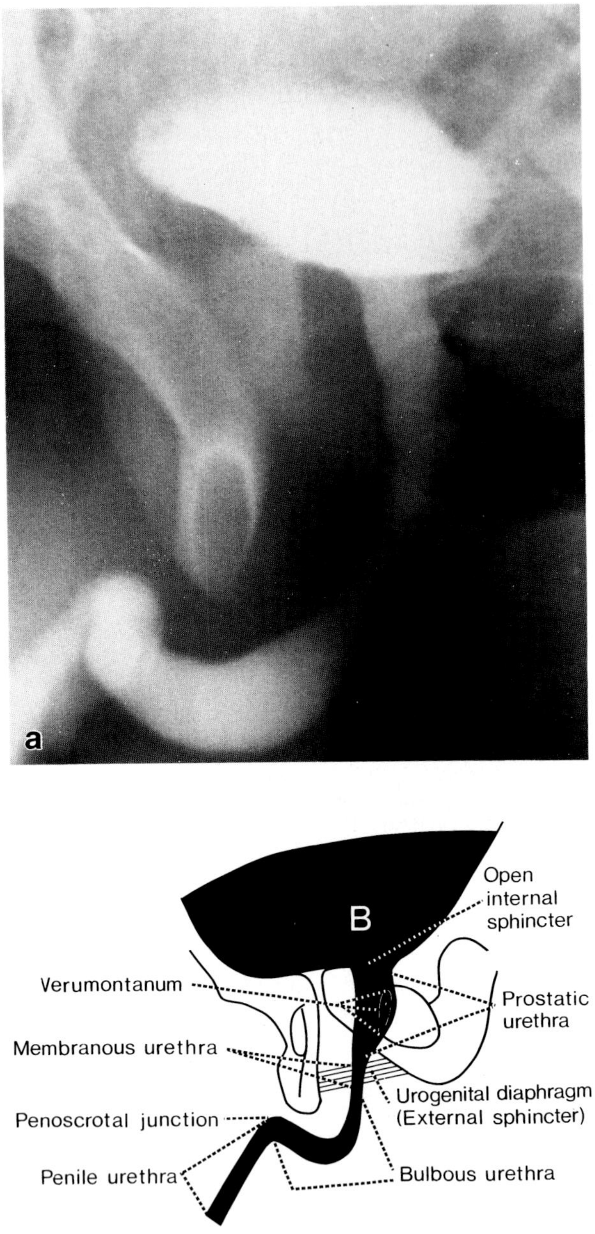

b

Fig. 18.8 a,b. Normal voiding urethrogram with tracing showing normal radiologic landmarks. *B*, bladder. (McCallum and Colapinto 1976)

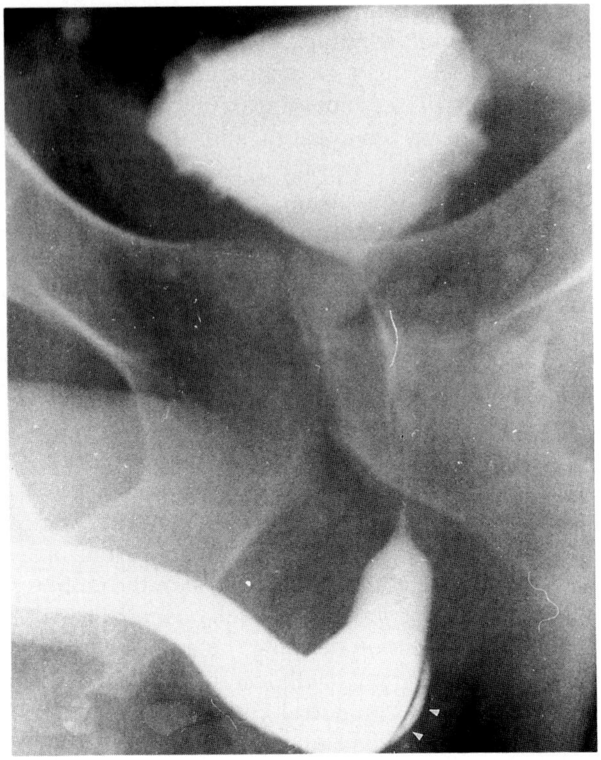

Fig. 18.9. The duct of the gland of Cowper is visualized (*arrows*) due to spasm of the distal sphincters during dynamic retrograde injection. No urethral pathology is demonstrated. Note that spasm of the distal sphincters produces a concave symmetric cone shape

the normal appearance of the dynamic retrograde urethrogram. A little contrast medium may be forced into the duct of the gland of Cowper. Visualization of the duct of the gland of Cowper does not necessarily mean an abnormality and in the absence of urethral pathology can be ignored (Fig. 18.9). Occasionally, the musculus compressor nuda may contract, producing an anterolateral indentation in the proximal bulbous urethra (see Fig. 18.7b). The appearance is characteristic and commonly seen in patients with neurogenic bladder. The radiologist should be aware of this possibility in order that it is not confused with urethral stricture. The complications of the procedure are few. Extravasation of contrast medium into penile and perineal veins may occur either by overenthusiastic dilatation of the catheter balloon causing a mucosal tear, or at the site of a severe stricture if too much pressure is applied during the retrograde injection. Although extravasation is rare if the examination is carefully performed under fluoroscopy, the possibility of extravasation into penile and perineal veins raises the same risk of reactions to contrast medium associated with any intravenous injection of contrast medium.

18.3.2 Voiding Cystourethrography

The bladder is filled through the dynamic retrograde catheter (Yoder and Papanicolaou 1992). When the patient is ready to void the catheter is removed from the fossa navicularis. When voiding occurs under fluoroscopy the bladder neck is seen to open to 1–2 cm in diameter and the posterior and anterior urethra fills with contrast medium under the parasympathetic activity of detrusor contraction and reciprocal sympathetic and pudendal relaxation of the sphincters. The verumontanum is well visualized and is seen to elongate due to relaxation of the longitudinal smooth muscle. The posterior urethra descends approximately 1.5 cm during voiding due to relaxation of the longitudinal smooth muscle, the urogenital diaphragm, and the pelvic floor muscles. The cone of the proximal bulbous urethra disappears on voiding and the membranous urethra is localized immediately adjacent to the inferior edge of the verumontanum for a distance of 1–1.5 cm. The bulbous urethra dilates slightly at its most inferior aspect (the sump of the bulbous urethra) and commonly is at a lower level than the penoscrotal junction. The penoscrotal junction is readily visualized on voiding. Because of the suspension of the penis at this point, the flow of contrast medium distal to the penoscrotal junction may be of smaller caliber than seen on the dynamic retrograde urethrogram. This is a normal finding and does not indicate any urethral abnormality.

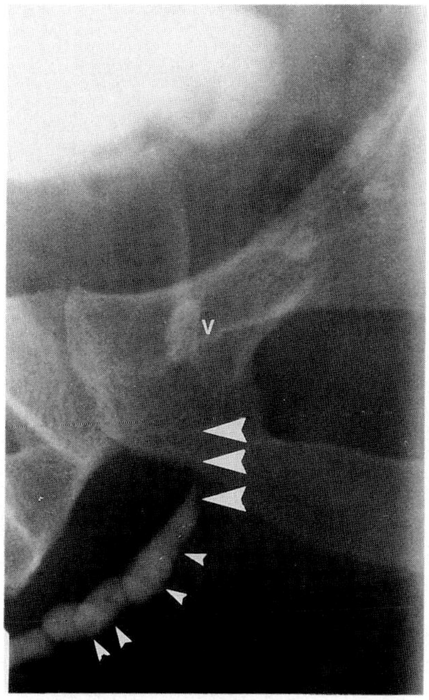

Fig. 18.10. A patient with gonococcal scarring in the mid-proximal bulbous urethral (*small arrows*). The cone of the proximal bulbous urethra is abnormal, being narrowed, elongated, and asymmetric (*large arrows*), indicating scarring extending into the membranous urethra (confirmed at operation)

18.4 Abnormal Urethrography

18.4.1 Urethral Infections

Infections affecting the urethra are the gonorrhea, tuberculosis, schistosomiasis (bilharziasis), viral, and mixed infections associated with catheterization.

18.4.1.1 Gonorrhea

Gonorrhea is the major cause of urethral stricture in undeveloped countries, since the majority of patients are untreated or inadequately treated. If adequate early antibiotic therapy is applied, urethral scarring is avoided. Only 40% of urethral strictures are due to the gonococcus in North America. Gonococcal infection ascends the urethra, causing a mucosal and submucosal inflammatory reaction in the anterior urethra, and involves the glands of Littre. Spread of the infection into the glands of Littre and corpus spongiosum causes venous thrombosis and eventual scarring. The preponderance of glands of Littre in the bulbous urethral sump make this the most common site of gonococcal scarring. The urethrographic study usually shows a long irregular area of scarring in the bulbous urethral sump, frequently with visualization of the glands of Littre. Of prime importance in the assessment of mid or proximal bulbous urethral stricture is an evaluation of the cone of the proximal bulbous urethra, which in normal patients is symmetric, smooth, and convex (Fig. 20.7a) on dynamic retrograde urethrography. If the cone of the proximal bulbous urethra is not symmetric, smooth, and convex but narrowed, elongated, irregular, or asymmetric (Fig. 18.10), the radiologist and urologists have a strong radiologic indication that the proximal bulbous urethral disease extends into the membranous urethra (McCallum and Colapinto 1979) and that transsphincter urethroplasty will be required for complete eradication (Colapinto and McCallum 1979) of the scarring. This finding is not uncommon in gonococcal urethral scarring.

The normal convex cone shape of the proximal bulbous urethra may be completely obliterated

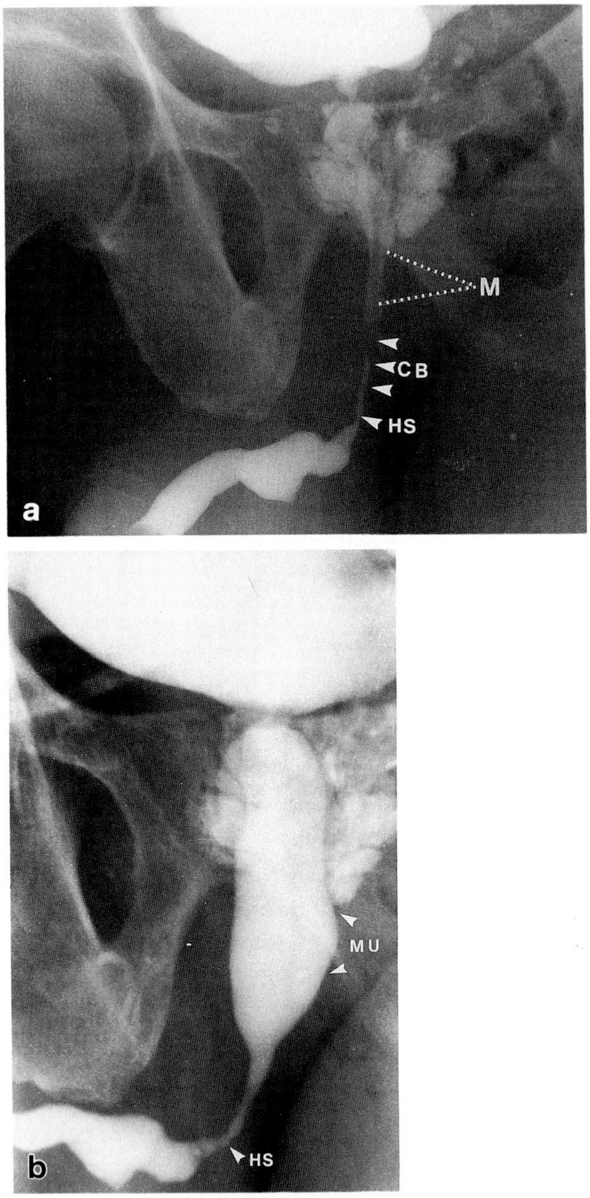

Fig. 18.11. **a** Dynamic retrograde urethrogram in a patient who has had several failed anterior urethroplasties. Hard scarring is present in the proximal bulbous urethra (*HS*). The normal cone of the proximal bulbous urethra is obliterated (*three arrows, CB*). *M*, membranous urethra. Reflux into prostatic ducts is demonstrated. The patient has outlet obstruction requiring suprapubic cystostomy. **b** Attempted voiding. The hard scar (*HS*) causes severe narrowing and obstruction. The scarred membranous urethra (*MU*) is paradoxically dilated. (McCallum 1979)

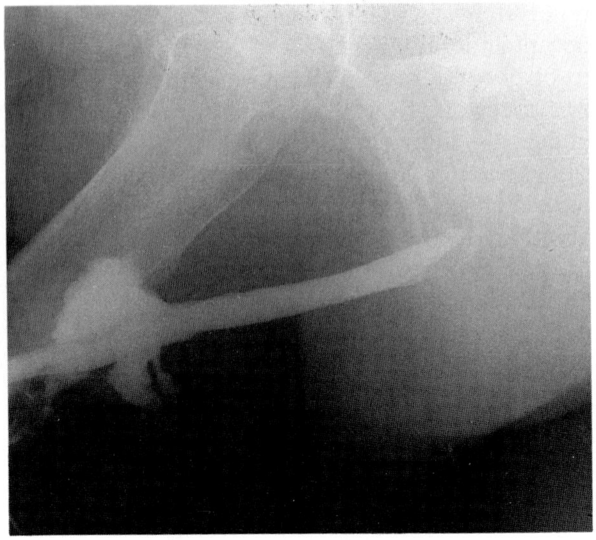

Fig. 18.12. Dynamic retrograde urethrogram in a patient with known active pulmonary tuberculosis. Periurethral abscess and small penile fistulous tracts are demonstrated

and unrecognizable due to gonococcal scarring in the bulbous urethra extending into the membranous urethra (Fig. 18.11a). Hard scarring in the bulbous urethra may produce sufficiently high proximal hydrostatic pressure to dilate softer scarring proximally in the membranous urethra. This results in dilatation of the scarred membranous urethra and has been described as paradoxical dilatation (Colapinto and McCallum 1979) (Fig. 18.11b).

18.4.1.2 Tuberculosis

Tuberculosis rarely affects the lower urinary tract. When present, it is a descending infection, most patients having concurrent manifestations of renal tuberculosis. Tuberculous prostatitis and granulomatous prostatic abscess are the most common manifestations. Calcific epididymitis may also occur from tuberculosis. Rarely, periurethral abscess (Fig. 18.12) and perineal fistula result from urethral scarring. Antituberculous therapy promotes healing with calcification and fibrous tissue development and treatment of the disease may lead to urethral stricture.

18.4.1.3 Schistosomiasis (Bilharziasis)

Schistosoma haematobium is a parasitic infection prevalent in Africa and the Nile Valley. It is rare in Europe and there is no known geographic site in North America. Abscess formation, calcification, and scarring affect the ureters, bladder, seminal vesicles, prostate, and urethra. Unlike other urethral infections, urethral fistula develops before urethral scarring. Urethral fistulae invariably result in urethral stricture. Fistula between the bowel and urinary tract are common and carcinoma of the bladder is a frequent complication in untreated cases.

18.4.1.4 Viral Infection

Viral infection causing condyloma acuminatum is uncommon in the urethra. It is an ascending infection spreading from condyloma on the glans penis. Approximately 5% of patients with penile condyloma have intraurethral verrucae which rarely extend into the bladder (POLLACK et al. 1978). Multiple irregular frond-like filling defects are seen on urethrography.

18.4.1.5 Urethral Infection Associated with Catheterization

Bladder catheterization per urethra may result in urethral infection usually of mixed gram-negative organisms. In the author's experience in a series of 300 patients requiring transsphincter urethroplasty for bulbomembranous urethral stricture, 19% were due to indwelling catheters. The initial injury to the urethra produced by the catheter is pressure necrosis which occurs at the fixed points of the urethra, i.e., the penoscrotal junction and the membranous urethra. If the catheter is too large a caliber for the urethra, pressure necrosis may occur at the fixed points. In addition, if the penis is not strapped up the anterior abdominal wall but is left to hang loose or be strapped to the thigh, pressure necrosis may occur at the penoscrotal junction. This latter situation is the most common cause of catheter strictures. It is almost inevitable that the area of pressure necrosis becomes infected, resulting in further urethral damage. Strictures due to pressure necrosis alone are generally short. Strictures due to pressure necrosis and superimposed infection are generally long and irregular, and glands of Littre are commonly visualized. Consequently, 75% of catheter strictures occur at the penoscrotal junction and are long and irregular (McCALLUM et al. 1985) (Fig. 18.13). Occasionally a catheter stricture is due to pressure necrosis alone without superimposed infection and is short and well defined.

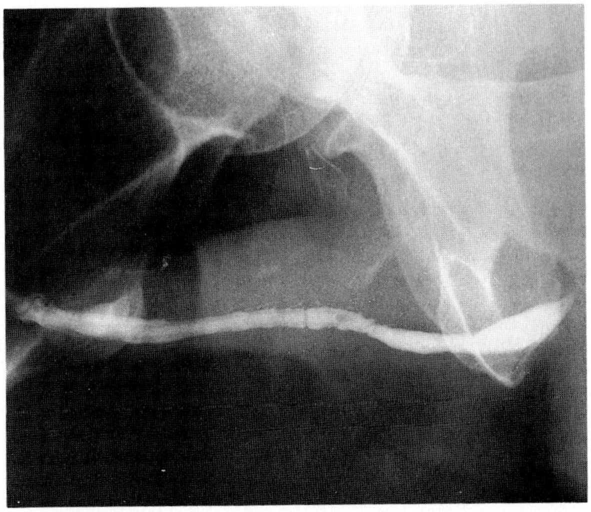

Fig. 18.13. Irregular urethral scarring extending distally and proximally from the penoscrotal junction due to 10 days with an indwelling catheter. Note: the glands of Littre are well visualized

18.4.2 Urethral Trauma

Urethral trauma results from urethral injury in pelvic fracture, straddle injury, iatrogenic trauma, and penetrating wounds.

18.4.2.1 Urethral Injury in Pelvic Fracture

Some degree of urethral injury occurs in 4%–17% (McCALLUM and COLAPINTO 1976; HILDSWORTH 1963; WILKINSON 1961; KISNER 1958; McCAGUE and SEMANS 1944) of male patients sustaining pelvic fracture. Urethral injury may be classified clinically as incomplete (urethral contusion), partial (a tear in the urethra), or complete (rupture of the urethra, usually with separation of the avulsed ends). Clinical criteria for the assessment of urethral injury in pelvic fracture include blood at the urethral meatus, inability to void, a high or hypermobile prostate on rectal examination, and inability to pass a catheter into the bladder. Radiologically, a high tear-drop bladder has been considered to be evidence of complete urethral rupture until recently. These criteria have led to wide discrepancies in literature reports regarding complete rupture at the time of injury (8%–100%) (MITCHELL 1968; PETROVIC 1956; GIBSON 1974) and resulting urethral stricture (14%–100%) (GIBSON 1974; MYERS and DEWEERD 1972; TRAFFORD 1955; MOREHOUSE et al. 1972).

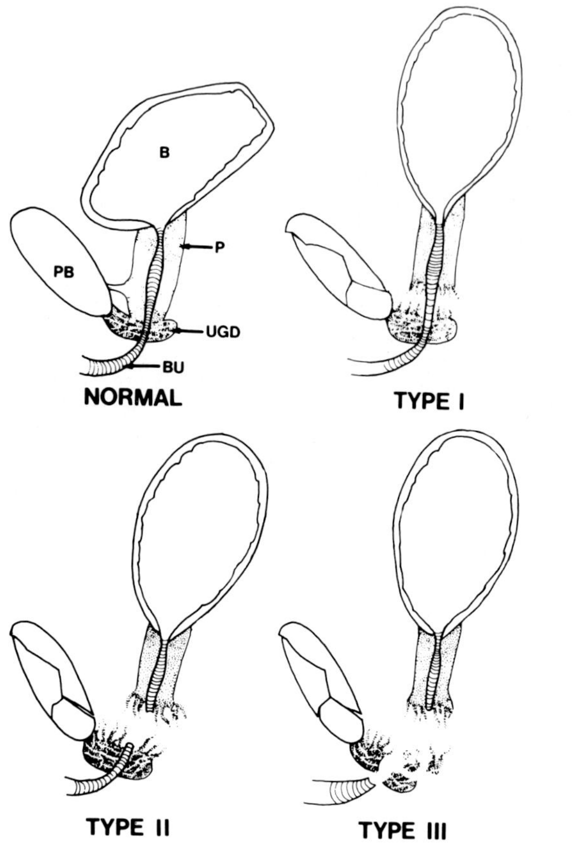

Fig. 18.14. Diagrammatic presentation of radiologic classification of acute urethral injury in pelvic fracture. *B*, bladder; *PB*, pubic bone; *UGD*, urogenital diaphragm; *P*, prostate; *BU*, bulbous urethra. (Modified from McCallum and Colapinto 1976)

Urethrography before catheterization is the best method of assessing urethral injury. This has resulted in an objective radiologic classification (Fig. 18.14) of urethral injury in pelvic fracture (McCallum and Colapinto 1976; Colapinto and McCallum 1977).

Using the previously described clinical criteria and surgical exploration, the classical urethral injury was thought to be complete separation of the urethra at the proximal end of the membranous urethra above the urogenital diaphragm due to a shearing separation at the superior aspect of the urogenital diaphragm. Recent literature indicates that when urethrography is done prior to attempting to pass a catheter, the so-called classical injury is rare, and that the most common injury occurs at the bare area of the proximal bulbous urethra below the urogenital diaphragm (McCallum and Colapinto 1976; Colapinto and McCallum 1977; McCallum 1979; Sandler et al. 1981). This would be in keeping with the anatomic findings since the membranous urethra and distal prostatic urethra are firmly supported by the distal sphincters and prostate, whereas the proximal bulbous urethra has only some fatty connective tissue anteriorly at the bare area where the crura of the corpora cavernosa separate for insertion into the inferior pubic rami.

Radiologic Classification. Retrograde urethrography provides an objective assessment of the degree and site of acute urethral injury. Three types of injury are recognized on urethrography:

- *Type I* is urethral contusion, compression, and stretching; the urethra, however, is intact.
- *Type II* is urethral "separation" above the urogenital diaphragm. This is the so-called classical injury and may be a partial tear or complete separation.
- *Type III* is urethral injury below the urogenital diaphragm. This may be a partial urethral tear or complete separation.

In the author's experience with 81 male patients with urethral injury in pelvic fracture, 30 cases occurred before urethrography was the initial assessment. All but two of these cases were assumed to be the classical injury (i.e., type II) and two were classified as incomplete (type I) because a catheter could be passed into the bladder. Following the advent of urethrography before catheterization 51 cases were initially assessed by urethrography. Seven patients had type I injury, two patients has type II injury, and 42 patients had type III injury, i.e., separation or partial tear below the urogenital diaphragm. Of the 42 type III injuries 32 were complete ruptures, while ten were partial.

The Foley catheter method is used in such patients. The examination can be done with fluoroscopy or overhead beam or, in an emergency, with a portable machine. As opposed to urethrography for urethral disease, in urethral injury the initial dynamic retrograde film is exposed during injection of a small quantity of contrast medium (8–10 cc). This film will show whether the urethra is intact, as in type I injury (Fig. 18.15), or whether a site of extravasation can be recognized, i.e., above or below the urogenital diaphragm. If the urethral tear is above the urogenital diaphragm, extravasation should extend into the pelvic cavity (Fig. 18.16). If extravasation occurs below the urogenital diaphragm,

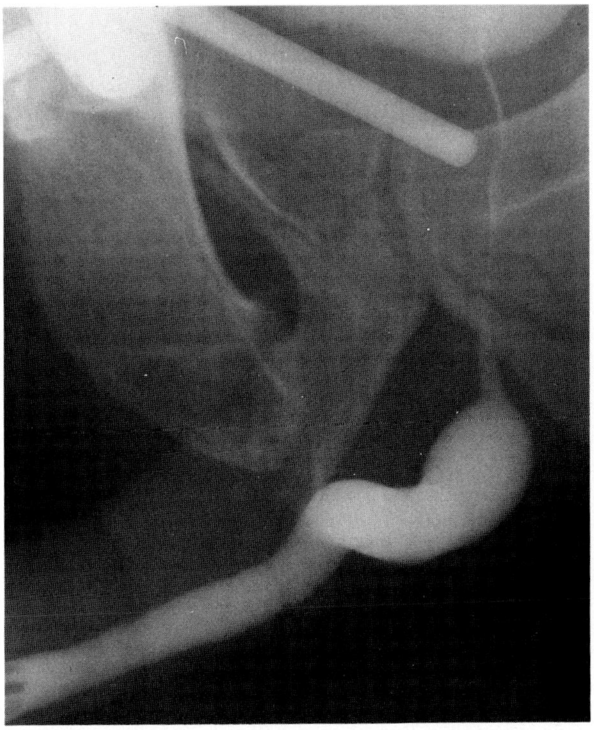

Fig. 18.15. Type I urethral injury in pelvic fracture. The proximal bulbous and posterior urethra are stretched and compressed but intact

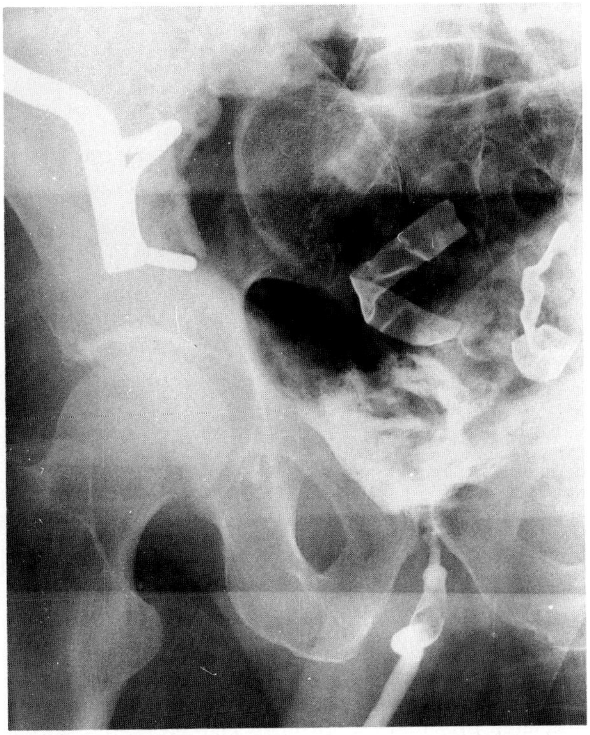

Fig. 18.16. Type II injury – complete urethral separation with extravasation of contrast medium above the urogenital diaphragm into the true pelvis. No contrast medium below urogenital diaphragm. The urethrogram was performed in the operating room

no contrast will be seen in the pelvis but contrast medium will be seen in the perineum and possibly the scrotum (Fig. 18.17). Urethrography and the radiologic classification are helpful to the urologist since they pinpoint the site of urethral injury. Complete and partial rupture of the urethra can commonly be distinguished, but occasionally a partial rupture may present on urethrography as a complete rupture. This problem can often be clarified by repeating the study in a few days if immediate primary urethral repair is not performed.

At the present time, there is a shift of emphasis away from primary repair of urethral injury to delayed repair. This change in policy has been initiated in order to preserve potency since most cases of urethral injury in pelvic fracture occur in young patients. The reported incidence of impotence following urethral injury in pelvic fracture ranges from 0% to 52% (MITCHELL 1968; PETROVIC 1956; GIBSON 1974; MYERS and DEWEERD 1972; TRAFFORD 1955; MOREHOUSE et al. 1972). In type II or type III injury, delayed repair involves the initial urethrographic assessment and insertion of a suprapubic catheter which is left in the

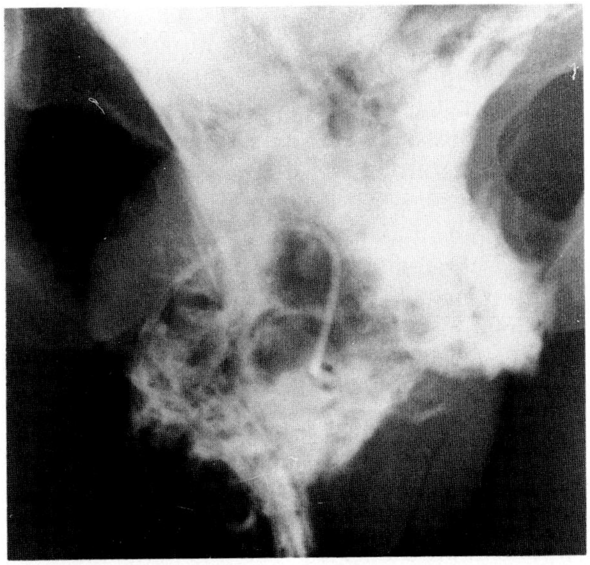

Fig. 18.17. Type III injury – urethral rupture below the urogenital diaphragm in the bulbous urethra showing extravasation into the perineum and scrotum. Some contrast medium has extravasated proximally into the anterior abdominal wall beneath Scarpa's fascia. (COLAPINTO and MCCALLUM 1977)

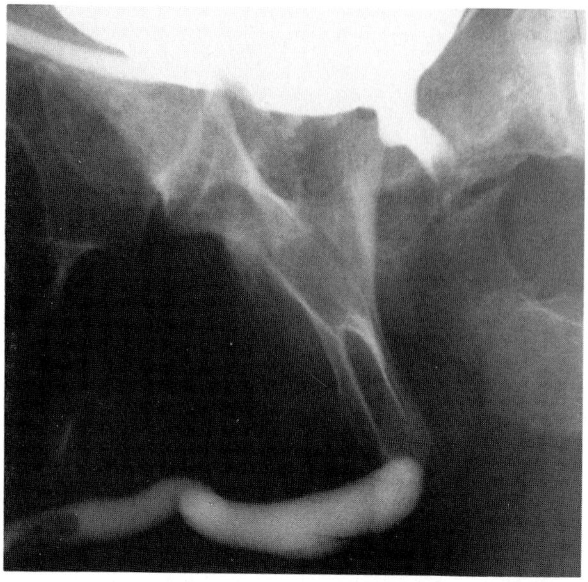

Fig. 18.18. Pelvic fracture with type III urethral rupture 1 month after the insertion of a suprapubic tube. The patient is having delayed repair. Dynamic retrograde injection into the urethra at the same time as the patient tries to void, after bladder filling via suprapubic catheter. Note the large gap from the proximal bulbous urethra to the verumontanum requiring repair. This study was performed immediately prior to delayed repair (two-stages transsphincter urethroplasty)

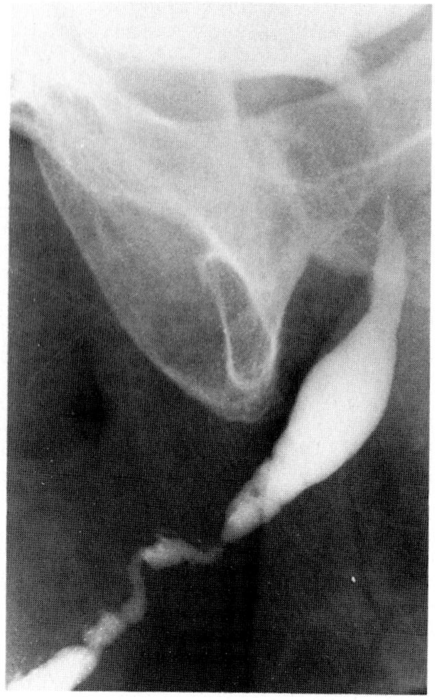

Fig. 18.19. Dynamic retrograde urethrogram 6 months after transurethral resection of the prostate and 10 days' postoperative catheterization. Note: well-defined stricture at the penoscrotal junction with glands of Littre due to pressure necrosis and superimposed infection

bladder for 1–3 months to allow time for the reduction of edema and resorption of blood clot. However, if the injury is shown to be a complete type III injury, the ensuing delay before perineal transsphincter urethroplasty produces considerable fibrous tissue in the region of the injury, making the urologist's delayed repair more difficult, since the area of fibrosis is usually long, (approximately 4–6 cm) (Fig. 18.18) and involves incision through the distal sphincters. Even with such a long 4–6 cm area of scarring, end-to-end anastomosis of the severed urethral ends is possible. Delayed repair of type II injury also involves the development of fibrous tissue but the defect in the urethra at the time of surgery is usually shorter and can be managed by the suprapubic approach or by the perineal approach to complete an end-to-end anastomosis. The demonstration of type I injury indicates that the patient can be catheterized, which should be done carefully with a well-lubricated catheter. Most patients who undergo primary urethral repair at the time of injury will develop urethral stricture months or years later at the site of injury.

18.4.2.2 Straddle Injury

Straddle injury is uncommon and is the result of falling astride a fixed object or sustaining a kick in the perineum. The bulbous urethra is compressed between the external object and the pubic arch and may be contused, partially ruptured, or completely ruptured. Urethrographic examination is essential before attempted catheterization. All degrees of this urethral injury will eventually result in urethral stricture.

18.4.2.3 Iatrogenic Urethral Injury

Iatrogenic urethral injury (McCallum et al. 1985) resulting in urethral stricture is the end result of pressure necrosis produced by the passage of a straight metallic instrument along the "S"-shaped urethra. Pressure necrosis occurs at the fixed points of the urethra, namely the penoscrotal junction (Fig. 18.19) and/or the membranous urethra (Fig. 18.20). This injury is therefore a complication of cystoscopy, transurethral resection of the prostate, transurethral resection of

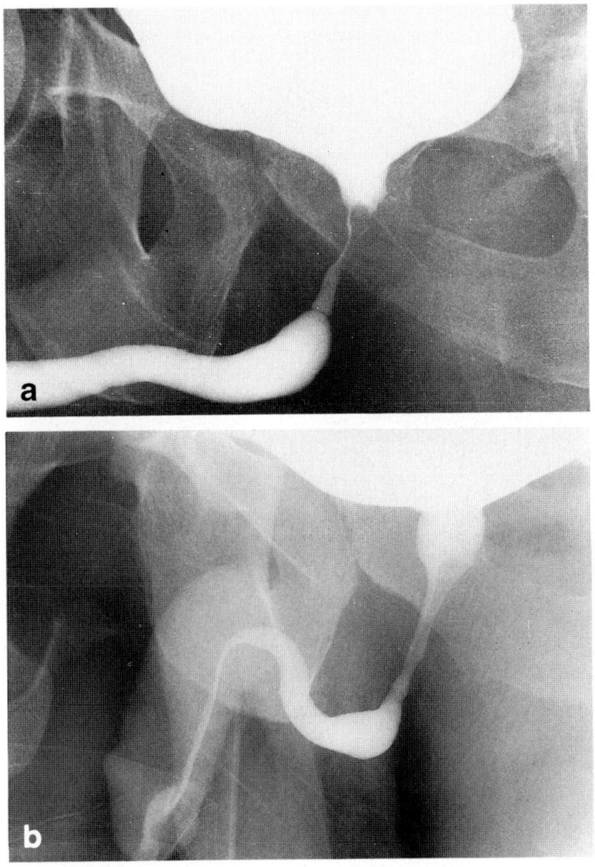

Fig. 18.20. a Dynamic retrograde urethrogram 1 year after transurethral resection of prostate. Note: resected prostate bed. Stricture in the proximal bulbous urethra with abnormal cone indicating scarring extends into the membranous urethra. **b** Same patient voiding. The membranous urethra and proximal bulbous urethra are narrowed

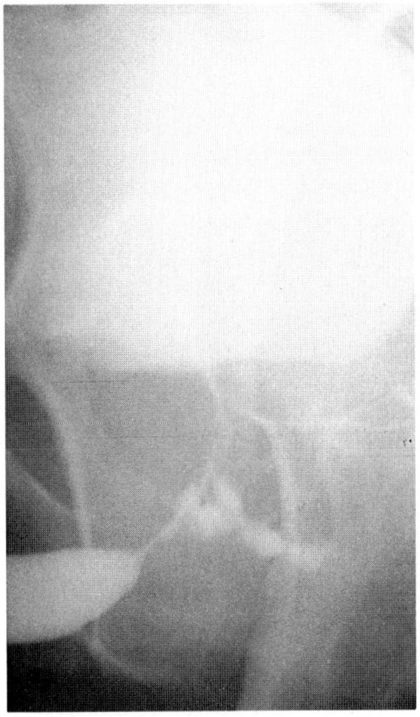

Fig. 18.21. Appearance following abdominoperineal resection for carcinoma of rectum. A fistulous tract has been produced due to a tear in the bulbomembranous urethra

bladder tumor, and transurethral removal of ureteric stone. If the cystoscope or resectoscope is too large for the urethra, or undue pressure is applied to straighten the urethra during the procedure, or the procedure takes a long time, pressure necrosis may occur at the fixed points, resulting in stricture. Strictures produced by pressure necrosis alone (without superimposed infection) are generally short and well defined (McCallum et al. 1985). Superimposed infection is uncommon after instrumentation. Following transurethral resection, a catheter is usually left in the bladder and urethra for a maximum of 3 days, which is usually not long enough for infection to supervene, provided the catheter has been placed with the normal aseptic technique. A catheter left in place for more that 3–4 days increases the possibility of superimposed infection in the area of pressure necrosis, resulting in long irregular strictures as previously discussed under urethral infection. In a series of 88 traumatic strictures, 37 (42%) were due to instrumentation. In a retrospective study of 300 patients requiring transsphincter urethroplasty 109 (36%) were due to instrumentation. Seventy-five percent of instrument strictures occur at the bulbomembranous urethra. The remaining 25% occur at the penoscrotal junction.

Rarely the urethra is iatrogenically traumatized during the pull-through portion of abdominoperineal resection for rectal carcinoma. This injury is usually a partial tear in the region of the bulbomembranous urethra and results in urethra-anal fistula (Fig. 18.21).

18.4.3 Urethral Stricture

Urethral stricture or scarring is classified as primary or secondary (Colapinto and McCallum 1979). The primary stricture is the cause of the patient's presenting symptoms and is usually a hard fibrous scar. There may also the areas of softer scarring in the urethra described as sec-

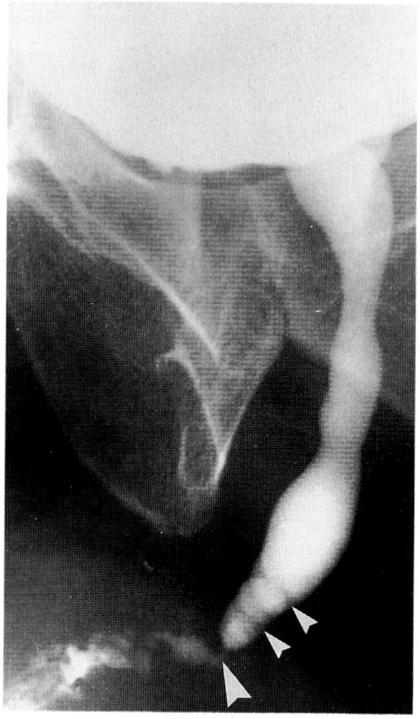

Fig. 18.22. The primary stricture (*big arrow*) is causing outlet obstruction. Secondary strictures (*small arrows*) proximal to the primary stricture are dilated

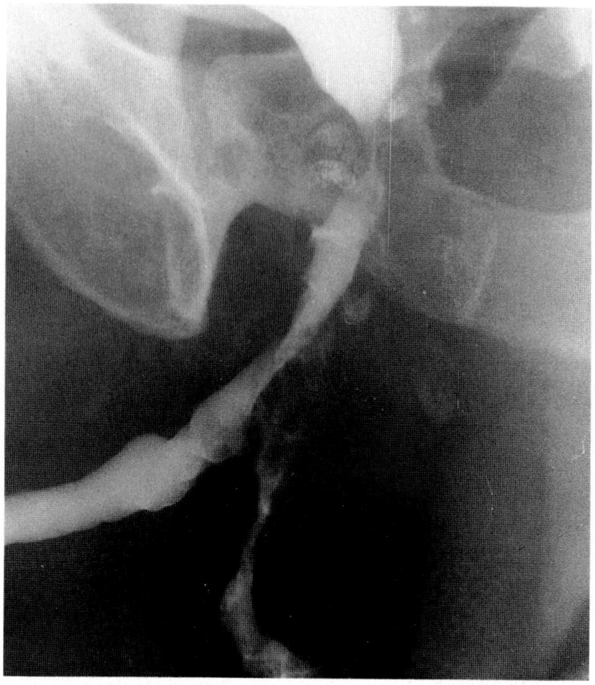

Fig. 18.24. Urethral carcinoma producing a malignant fistula to the perineum. The patient had bulbous urethral stricture repair 3 years previously. (McCallum and Colapinto 1976)

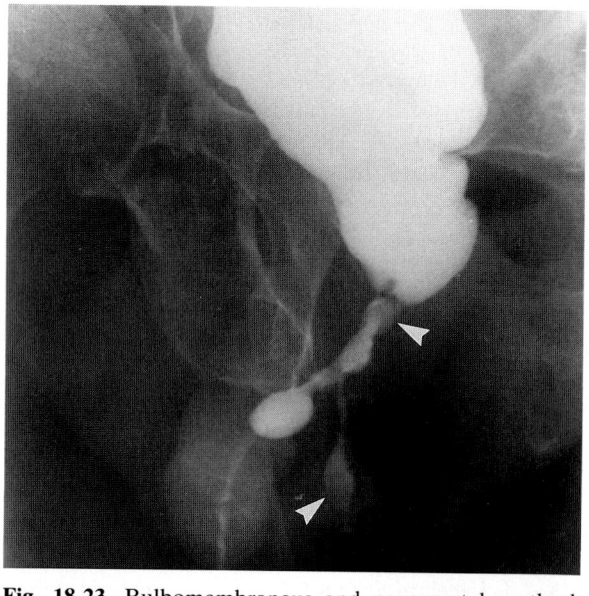

Fig. 18.23. Bulbomembranous and penoscrotal urethral scarring following transurethral prostatic resection. Severe obstruction at the penoscrotal junction. A perineal fistula is demonstrated originating from the mid bulbous urethra. Filling defects in the membranous urethra and fistulous tract represent urethral stones (*arrows*)

ondary stricture. Both the primary and secondary scarring must be identified by urethrography. If only the primary stricture is operated upon, the secondary scarring will eventually become hard and produce outlet obstruction. Retrospective and prospective urethrographic studies combined with urethroscopy indicate that an abnormal cone shape of the proximal bulbous urethra indicates scarring extending into the membranous urethra in over 90% of cases (McCallum and Colapinto 1979). In addition, such studies have shown that the scarred membranous urethra will be dilated on a voiding study in 60% of cases. This situation is called paradoxical dilatation (Colapinto and McCallum 1979) (Figs. 18.11, 18.22), and occurs when the high back pressure produced by a hard primary scar of fibrous tissue in the mid or proximal bulbous urethra causes dilatation of the softer scarring in the membranous urethra. Consequently, voiding urethrography alone without dynamic retrograde urethrography may give misleading information and should not be relied upon for complete assessment of urethral scarring (McCallum and Colapinto 1979).

Urethral trauma will generally result in urethral stricture, even after primary urethral repair.

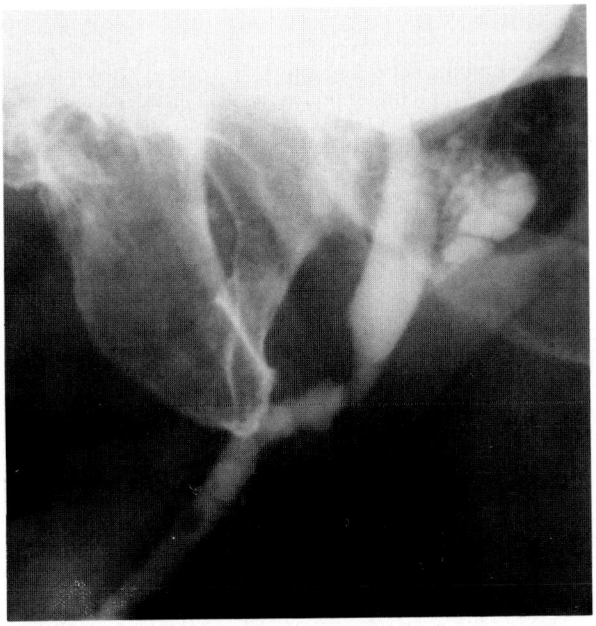

Fig. 18.25. Multiple urethral strictures in the anterior urethra. Reflux into dilated prostatic ducts is apparent on this voiding study

Urethral infection, if untreated, will also lead to urethral stricture. Dynamic retrograde urethrography and voiding cystourethrography combined with urethroscopy are the methods of choice for assessing the degree of scarring and the effects of scarring. Urethral scarring may result in proximal dilatation, either paradoxical or nonparadoxical, urethral fistula (Fig. 18.23), urethral diverticulum, urethral stone (Fig. 18.23), and urethral carcinoma (Fig. 18.24). The effect of urethral scarring on the prostate is frequently prostatitis with urethrographic visualization of dilated prostatic ducts (Fig. 18.25). The effects of urethral scarring on the bladder include trabeculation, diverticula, and vesicoureteral reflux. No longer is it sufficient for the radiologist to simply delineate the primary stricture and describe a tight stenosis in the anterior or membranous urethra. He must now identify secondary scarring and indicate the configuration of the cone of the proximal bulbous urethra. He must also pass an opinion on whether he thinks proximal dilatation is paradoxical or nonparadoxical. All of these radiologic findings are of significant help to the urologist, who will know what to expect to find on urethroscopy and at operation. Urethrography and urethroscopy combine to help the urologist decide which operation is best for the patient.

The following surgical procedures are employed for the repair of urethral stricture:

1. Anterior urethroplasty – urethral repair of urethral scarring which is more than 1.5 cm below the urogenital diaphragm.
2. Transsphincter urethroplasty – urethral repair of urethral scarring in the proximal bulbous urethra and membranous urethra; this operation involves incision through the membranous urethra and distal sphincters, raising the possibility of resulting urinary incontinence. It is not taken lightly and indications for this procedure are critical.

The surgical repair of urethral stricture from any cause is primarily an attempted end-to-end anastomosis, with removal of the scarred tissue. When end-to-end anastomosis is not practical, penile skin pedicle grafting or full thickness grafting is performed. Rarely full thickness grafts are obtained from a distant hairless site. Scrotal skin flaps have been used extensively in the past but are now in some disfavor because of the coarseness of scrotal skin and hair growth.

The operative repair of urethral stricture may be done as a one- or two-stage repair. End-to-end anastomosis is commonly a one-stage repair. Full thickness grafting and scrotal skin grafting are usually done as a two-stage operation.

18.5 Neurogenic Bladder and Urethral Sphincter Dysfunction

A classification of neurogenic bladder is given in Table 18.1; in this classification a distinction is drawn between upper (UMNLs) and lower motor neuron lesions (LMNLs). UMNLs are lesions to the brain or spinal cord above the level of L2. LMNLs are lesions below L2 resulting in interruption of the micturition reflex arc.

Upper motor neuron lesions therefore have an intact micturition reflex arc so that the detrusor muscle is capable of contraction. Micturition can be stimulated by bladder filling and suprapubic tapping. Bladder infection may produce irritability resulting in the irritable bladder with frequent contractions.

In LMNLs the micturition reflex arc is interrupted and therefore the bladder is unable to contract. In these cases outlet obstruction may result in the dilated flaccid or areflexic bladder with overflow incontinence and bladder infection

Table 18.1. McClellan's classification of neurogenic bladder (NGB)

Upper motor neuron lesion (contractile bladder lesion) Cord lesion above L2		Lower motor neuron lesion (poorly contractile or noncontractile bladder lesion) Cord lesion below L2	
Uninhibited NGB	Suprapontine lesions Cerebral atherosclerosis Multiple sclerosis Brain tumor Pernicious anemia Brain injury	Autonomous NGB	Vascular insufficiency Cauda equina lesions Abscess Disk protrusion Transverse myelitis Multiple sclerosis Chronic outlet obstruction
Reflex NGB	Subpontine lesions Cord trauma Cord tumor Disk protrusion Syringomyelia Extradural abscess Multiple sclerosis	Motor paralytic NGB	Poliomyelitis Anterior horn lesions Disk protrusion Pelvic surgery Vascular insufficiency
Uninhibited reflex	Subject to autonomic dysreflexia	Sensory paralytic NGB	Diabetes mellitus Tabes dorsalis Alcoholic neuropathy Disk protrusion Pelvic surgery
	Mixed NGB: features of both UMNL and LMNL	Thoracolumbar trauma Tabes dorsalis Multiple sclerosis Myelodysplasia Arachnoiditis	

leading to vesicoureteral reflux. Bladder emptying is accomplished only by suprapubic pressure or Credé's maneuver. Trauma to the spinal cord is the commonest cause of neurogenic bladder. Most trauma patients are young males whose injury to the cord most commonly results from motor vehicle accidents. Diving accidents and bullet wounds account for most of the remainder. In hospitals with recognized trauma units, most acute spinal cord injuries occur above the L2 level and are therefore UMNLs resulting in a neurogenic bladder in which the micturition reflex arc (S2–4) is intact and the bladder is capable of contraction. However, acute spinal cord injury above the L2 level initially presents in spinal shock which lasts for weeks or months. During the period of spinal shock, the micturition reflex arc is not functioning and therefore the initial presentation is that of an autonomous LMNL. These patients require intermittent clean catheterization to avoid bladder infection and vesicoureteral reflux. When spinal shock subsides the micturition arc function returns and bladder training can commence.

Lesions of the cervical and upper thoracic spine usually result in quadraplegia. Lesions of the mid and lower thoracic spine are usually paraplegic. Bladder training is successful in approximately 70% of paraplegic patients and acceptable residual urine is maintained. In the remainder the residual urine is increased and unacceptable and further investigation is required. This involves bladder and urethral pressure profiles and retrograde and voiding cystourethrography (McCallum 1974). To assess the cause of the unacceptable residual urine, voiding cystourethrography is necessary to elucidate the site of outlet obstruction. The method used is the Foley catheter method almost identical to that used in the assessment of urethral stricture. The dynamic retrograde study is necessary to exclude urethral stricture which may occur because of indwelling catheters. The bladder is filled via the catheter in the fossa navicularis. Persistence with bladder filling is usually sufficient to stimulate the intact micturition reflex arc, and the bladder is seen to contract and the bladder neck will open, usually to a diameter of 1–1.5 cm. The catheter is not removed from the fossa navicularis. If no outlet obstruction is demonstrated, voiding occurs into the catheter and syringe. When the syringe is filled, the catheter can be clamped and the syringe emptied. Reconnection usually shows continued voiding. When no outlet obstruction is present the UMNL patient will empty the bladder into the syringe. If outlet obstruction is present, the site of the obstruction is demonstrated.

In the author's experience, patients with UMNL and unacceptable residual urine commonly are obstructed at the level of the distal sphincter. This is sphincter dyssynergia. Voiding may occur spontaneously on bladder filling but suprapubic tapping may be required to initiate voiding. When voiding occurs, the bladder neck opens. The proximal prostatic urethra will fill with contrast medium. When sphincter dyssynergia is present, the distal sphincters do not relax, resulting in outlet obstruction (Fig. 18.26). Sphincter dyssynergia is commonly intermittent. The urine flow through the whole urethra may be normal initially, then distal sphincter spasm is seen and the flow of contrast medium is abruptly stopped below the verumontanum even when the bladder neck remains open. Continued suprapubic tapping may again produce a good flow of urine through the urethra. However, intermittent distal sphincter spasm usually results in significant residual urine. Distal sphincter dyssynergia is therefore a not uncommon cause of unacceptable residual urine in upper motor neuron quadraplegic and paraplegic patients. Patients with UMNLs whose cord lesion is above T7 are subject to autonomic dysreflexia. This applies to all quadraplegic patients and to those paraplegic patients whose lesion is above T7.

Autonomic dysreflexia is an unpredictable viscerovascular response resulting in vasodilation above the cord lesion and vasoconstriction below the cord lesion (McCallom 1974). The viscerovascular response results in the sudden and rapid rise in blood pressure, redness and sweating of the face, and pallor of the skin below the lesion. The viscerovascular response may produce a rapid (within 1 min) rise in blood pressure from normal to 260/150, resulting in severe headache. Aneurysmal rupture has been reported. Consequently, in any patient whose cord lesion is above T7, autonomic dysreflexia should be anticipated. Blood pressure monitoring after every 50 cc injection of contrast medium is mandatory. An α-adrenergic blocker such as rogitine should be readily available for intravenous administration. Blood pressure monitoring is a valuable indication of blood pressure increase. A small but rapid rise in pressure is an indication to pause in the injection of contrast medium. Slight elevation of the tabletop may be helpful and the blood pressure may stabilize a little above the patient's normal pressure. In this case, the procedure can continue. If the blood pressure continues to rise, the pocedure should be postponed and attempted at a later date. Although rogitine is readily available, the above routine has only required intravenous injection of rogitine in 2% of cases. Autonomic dysreflexia is unpredictable and may occur on one examination but not in a second examination on the same patient.

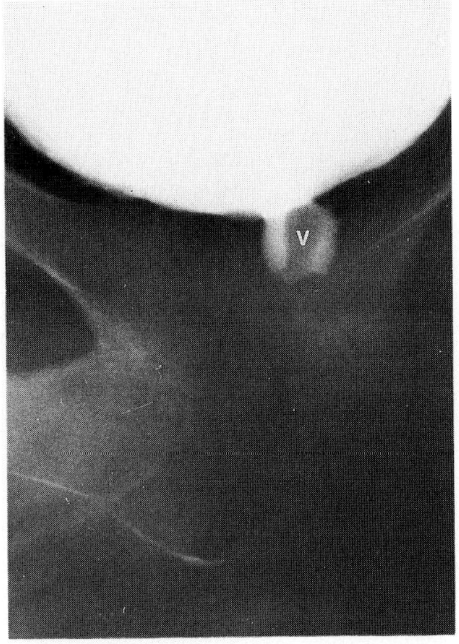

Fig. 18.26. Attempted voiding in a patient with a UMNL. The bladder neck is open. Voiding occurs as far as the distal sphincters. Complete obstruction is present due to sphincter dyssynergia. Note: verumontanum (*V*) which is high due to sphincter and pelvic floor muscle spasm

It is emphasized that when examining patients with neurogenic bladder, every attempt should be made to perform the examination without inserting a catheter into the bladder. Low and high pressure vesicoureteral reflux can be readily assessed by the described method.

Patients with LMNLs are assessed using the same method. However, since the micturition reflex arc is interrupted, bladder emptying is obtained by increased intra-abdominal pressure or by a Credé-type maneuver.

Patients with UMNLs and sphincter dyssynergia are usually managed by distal sphincterotomy (Fig. 18.27). Sphincter dyssynergia rarely is due to internal sphincter spasm, in which case wedge resection of the bladder neck is helpful.

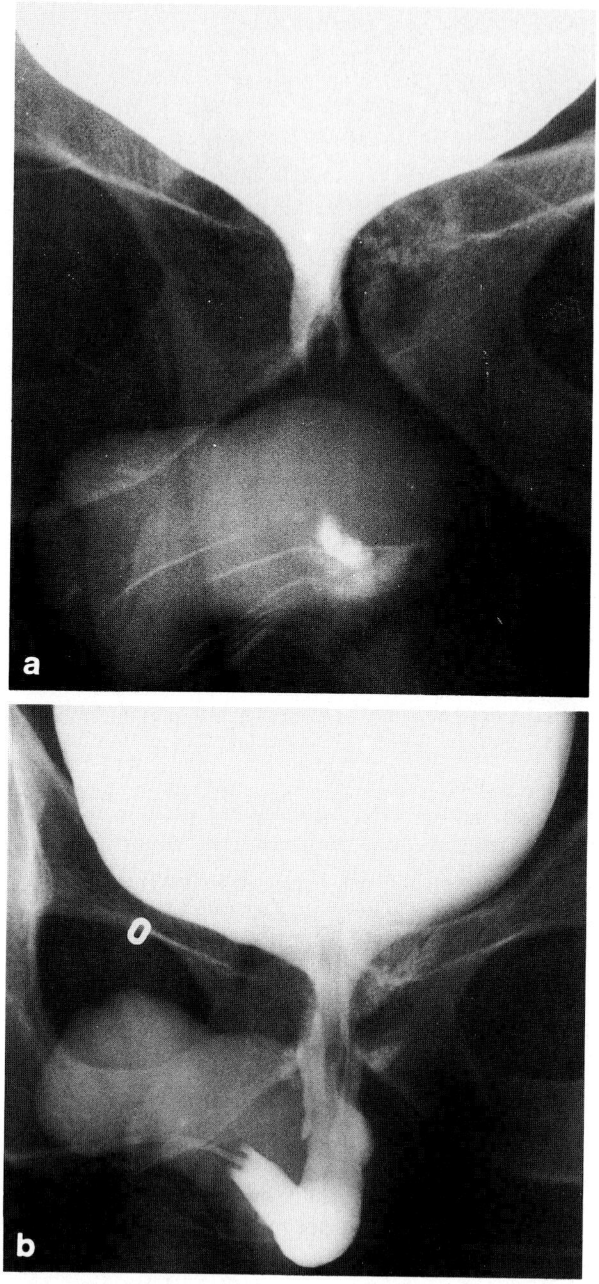

Fig. 18.27. **a** Voiding cystourethrogram in a patient with a UMNL. Complete obstruction is demonstrated due to sphincter dyssynergia. **b** Appearance following sphinctero-tomy. The distal sphincters have been incised. Voiding now occurs normally into the catheter and syringe. The distal sphincter region is now normally patent. (McCallum 1974)

The incidence of autonomic dysreflexia is said to be reduced by incision of the internal sphincter region. In some centers this is done routinely before radiologic and profile studies are attempted. Transrectal ultrasound has also been described as a method of assessing outlet obsturction in neurogenic bladder patients.

Radiologists and urologists involved in the investigation and management of patients with neurogenic bladder are aware that complete assessment requires insight into neurourology urodynamics and radiology (Camarr 1972). Good management depends on precise, detailed, and comprehensive information obtained from all of these investigations. The measurements of intravesical and rectal pressure during voiding cystourethrography are complementary. Urine flow rate measurement and cystometrography are essential initial parameters. Nonvoiding and voiding urethral pressure profiles are correlated with the radiography of voiding. Urethral pressures are obtained at the bladder neck and in the membranous urethra. Correlation of all of these investigations leads to good management; they provide an indication of the necessity for surgical intervention and, if surgical intervention is necessary, of the site and type of surgical procedure which would be most beneficial to the patient. These investigations include bladder training and the majority of patients with neurogenic bladder can be well managed without surgical intervention. Intermittent clean catheterization (Guttman and Frankel 1966) can maintain a neurogenic bladder free from infection. In those patients requiring surgical intervention the investigations lead to relatively minor operations and have markedly reduced the need for urinary diversion operations such as cutaneous vesicostomy (Lapides et al. 1971) and ileal conduit.

Recent literature advocates the use of transrectal ultrasound in the assessment of patients with neurogenic bladder (Shapeero et al. 1983). The transrectal ultrasound study is performed after natural bladder filling or bladder catheter filling. In UMNLs, suprapubic tapping is required to stimulate voiding. Voiding is assessed by real time ultrasound and the site of outlet obstruction can be visualized. Because of the possibility of autonomic dysreflexic stimulation produced by the insertion of the transrectal probe, the administration of an α-blocker or wedge resection of the bladder neck is required.

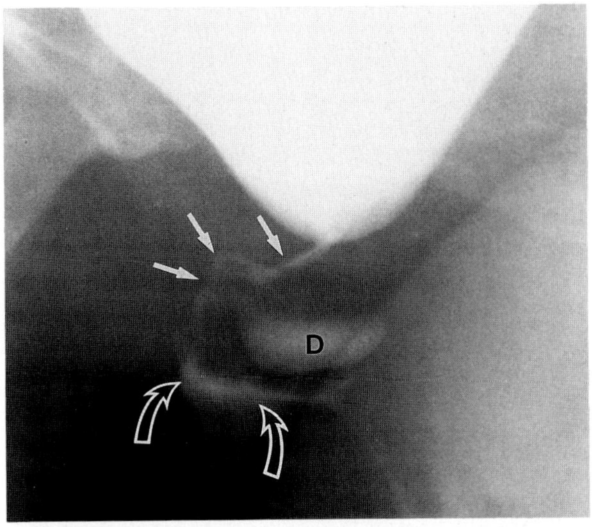

Fig. 18.28. Voiding cystourethrogram in a female with urethral symptoms. The upright voiding study shows a urethral diverticulum (*D*) containing a contrast medium fluid level. *Arrows*, urethra; *open arrows*, extraurethral contrast medium

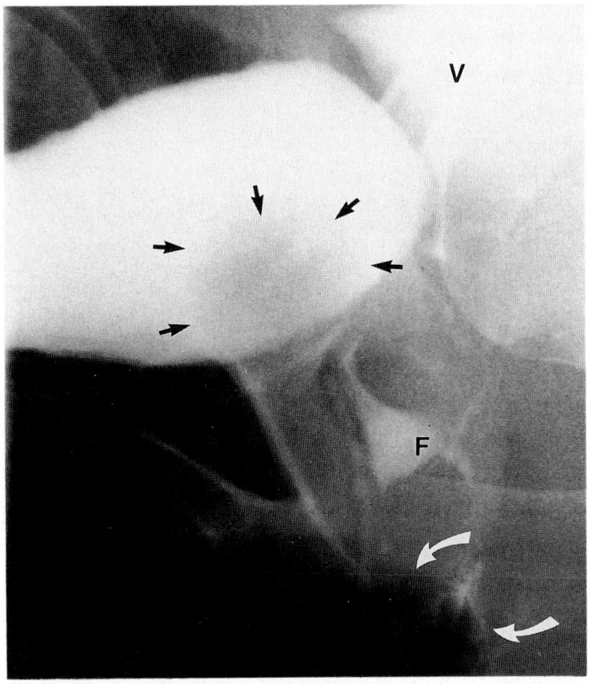

Fig. 18.29. The double balloon catheter method shows a urethrovaginal fistula (*F*) with contrast medium filling the vagina (*V*) following the urethral injection of contrast medium. *Black arrows*, internal balloon; *white arrows*, external balloon

18.6 Urethrography in the Female

Urethral stricture in females occurs at the urethral meatus and is managed by meatal urethrotomy. Urethrography in the female is indicated to demonstrate urethrovaginal fistula and urethral diverticulum. Both of these conditions may be urethrographically demonstrated by voiding cystourethrography (Fig. 18.28) or by using the double balloon catheter. This catheter has a balloon to block the bladder neck and a sliding balloon to block the urethral meatus. The only hole in the catheter is between both balloons, thus allowing contrast medium to fill the urethra. Although it is technically difficult to maintain traction on the bladder neck balloon so that contrast medium does not escape into the bladder, and to push the sliding balloon against the urethral meatus to stop contrast medium from leaking, it is possible to demonstrate both urethrovaginal fistula (Fig. 18.29) and urethral diverticulum (Fig. 18.30) by this method (Lang and Davis 1959).

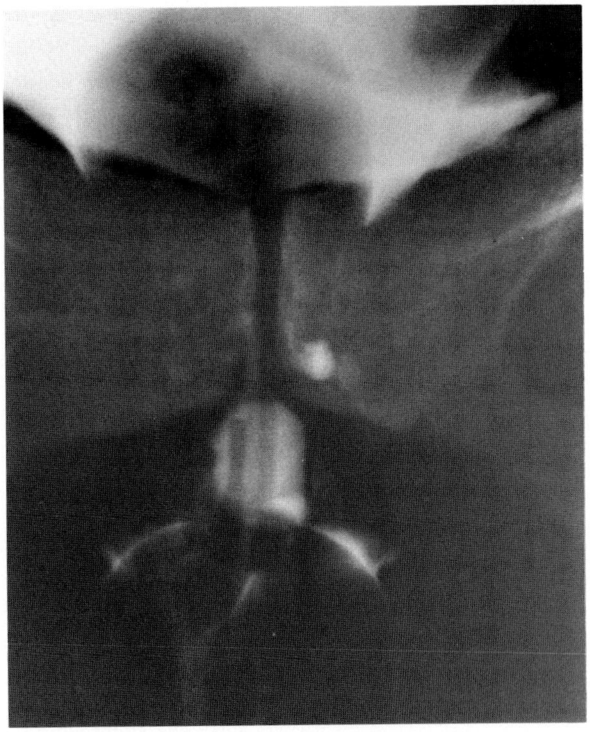

Fig. 18.30. Double balloon catheter method showing a small left diverticulum containing a small amount of contrast medium

18.7 Urethral Tumors

Urethral tumors are rare. The most common urethral tumors are malignant and are either squamous cell carcinoma or transitional cell carcinoma. Adenocarcinomas arising from the periu-

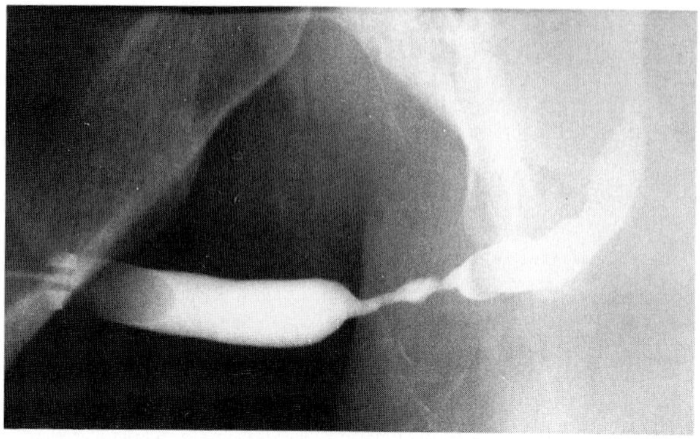

Fig. 18.31. Recurrent penoscrotal stricture with adjacent filling defect proximally. Biopsy-proven squamous cell carcinoma. (Courtesy of Dr. C. SANDLER)

rethral glands of Littre or Cowper's gland in the male or Skene's glands in the female may affect the urethra but are not true urethral tumors. In both males and females such adenocarcinomas typically present at an age above 50 years.

18.7.1 Squamous Cell Carcinoma

Squamous cell carcinoma accounts for almost 80% of urethral carcinomas in both males and females. The female to male ratio is 2:1. In the male, squamous cell carcinoma is a recognized complication of previous urethral stricture (BLANDY 1976), urethral infection, urethral instrumentation, and urethral trauma (RAY et al. 1977). Approximately 70% of male squamous cell carcinomas are associated with previous urethral stricture (BLANDY 1976). Recurrent stricture following urethroplasty should always raise the possibility of squamous cell carcinoma (WILLIAMS and ASHKEN 1980) and biopsy should be considered.

Squamous epithelium is only present in the urethra within the glans penis from the fossa navicularis to the external meatus and is continuous with the squamous epithelium of the glans penis. Small nests of squamous epithelium are randomly found within the stratified columnar epithelium of the bulbous and penile urethra. Consequently squamous cell carcinoma may occur spontaneously in the glans penis or anywhere in the anterior urethra at the site of squamous epithelial nests. However, in the presence of stricture or chronic inflammation, the normal pseudostratified columnar epithelium undergoes squamous metaplasia, resulting in the well-recognized association of stricture and squamous cell carcinoma

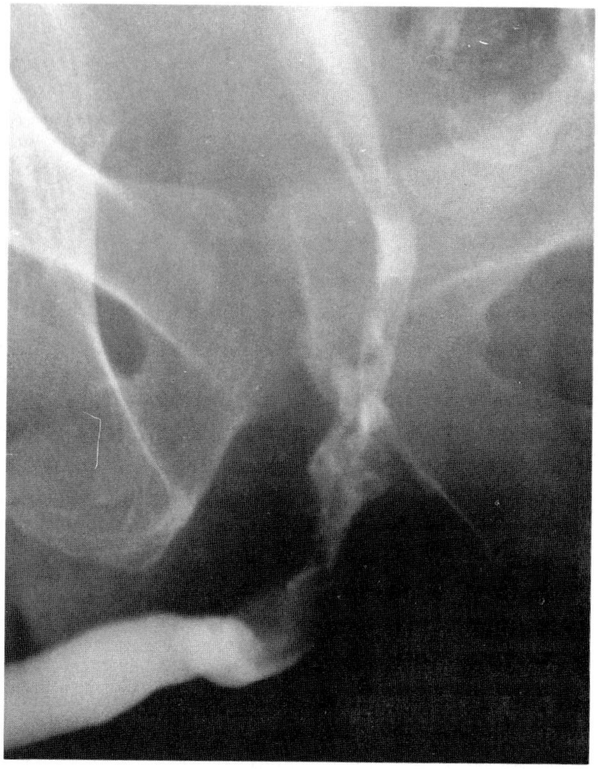

Fig. 18.32. Adenocarcinoma of the urethra probably arising from the duct of the gland of Cowper. A filling defect is seen in the proximal bulbous urethra extending into the membranous and prostatic urethra. (POLLACK 1990, p 1409)

(Fig. 18.31). The most common site of squamous cell carcinoma is in the proximal bulbous urethra: approximately 70% of cases occur at this site (Fig. 18.24).

In the female, squamous cell carcinoma accounts for 75% of urethral tumors (RAY and GUINAN 1979). Female urethral tumors are classified as anterior or entire. Anterior urethral tumors affect the distal third of the urethra and account for less than 50% of female carcinomas. These are usually low grade malignancies with a better prognosis than entire urethral carcinomas, which are commonly higher grade (GREBSTALD 1973).

18.7.2 Transitional Cell Carcinoma

Transitional cell epithelium continues from the bladder into the prostatic urethra in the male and into the proximal third of the female urethra. In males transitional cell carcinoma accounts for approximately 20% of all urethral carcinomas (RAY and GUINAN). Over 60% of transitional cell

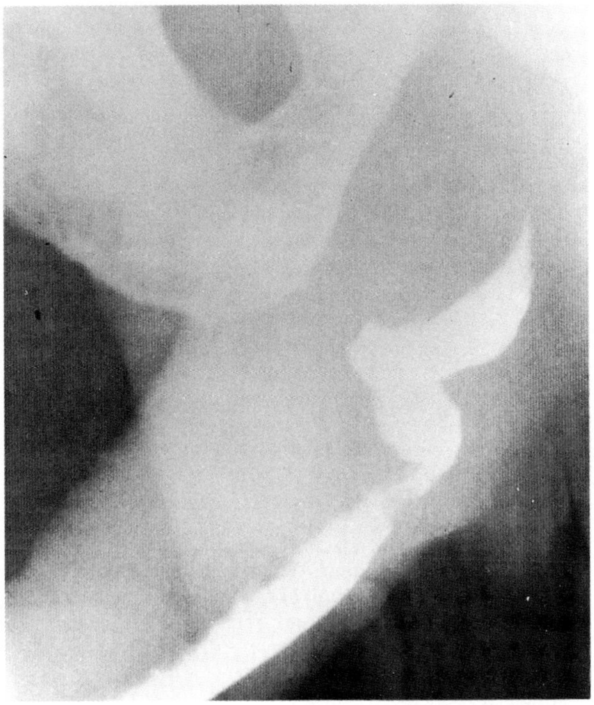

Fig. 18.33. Retrograde urethrogram in a patient with known carcinoma of the prostate. The study shows multiple extrinsic defects along the penile urethra and invasive carcinoma in the proximal penile urethra. (Courtesy of Dr. C. SANDLER)

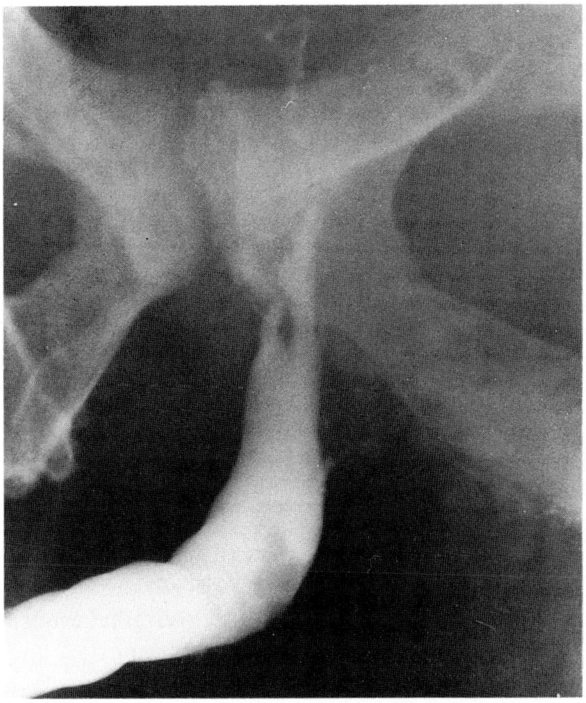

Fig. 18.34. Carcinoma of the prostate metastasizing to the corpus spongiosum, eroding into the bulbous urethra and producing filling defects. Note blastic metastasis in the visualized bones

carcinomas occur in the proximal urethra. The remainder occur in the anterior urethra and are thought to be the result of metaplasia or implantation of bladder transitional cell carcinoma. Up to 18% of male patients having cystectomy for bladder transitional cell carcinoma will later present with transitional cell carcinoma of the urethra (SCHELLHAMMER and WHITMORE 1976; FAYSAL 1980). This is thought to be due to implantation of malignant cells into the urethral mucosa but the possibility of multicentric tumor neogenesis has not been excluded. Many patients having total cystectomy for transitional cell carcinoma of the bladder have total urethrectomy as part of the operative procedure because of the incidence of transitional cell carcinoma of the urethra following cystectomy. Rarely spontaneous transitional cell carcinoma occurs in the prostatic urethra without evidence of transitional cell carcinoma elsewhere.

18.7.3 Adenocarcinoma

Adenocarcinoma of the urethra accounts for approximately 5% of all urethral carcinomas (Fig. 18.32). These tumors almost invariably arise in periurethral glands or in Cowper's gland in the male or Skene's glands in females. It has been reported in a female urethral diverticulum (TINES and BIGONGIARI 1982).

18.7.4 Other Urethral Malignancies

Primary melanoma, leiomyosarcoma, pigmented epidermoid carcinoma, and metastases have all been reported. All are extremely rare. Of these tumors, metastases are the most common. Contiguous spread of carcinoma of the prostate to the corpus spongiosum may indent or erode into the urethra (KOTECHA and GENTILE 1974) (Figs. 18.33, 18.34). Carcinoma of the bladder may result in implantation of malignant cells in urethral mucosa (or because of multicentric origin). Metastases from renal cell carcinoma and colon

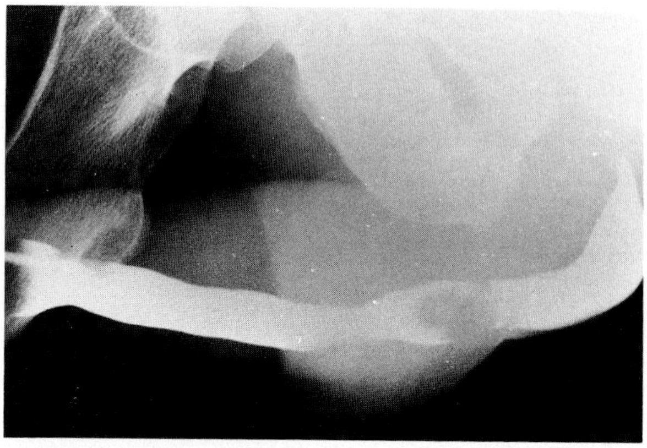

Fig. 18.35. Dynamic retrograde urethrogram in a 53-year-old patient who had colonic carcinoma resected 2 years previously. The filling defect in the distal bulbous urethra is metastasis to the corpus spongiosum eroding into the bulbous urethra. (POLLACK 1990, p 1411)

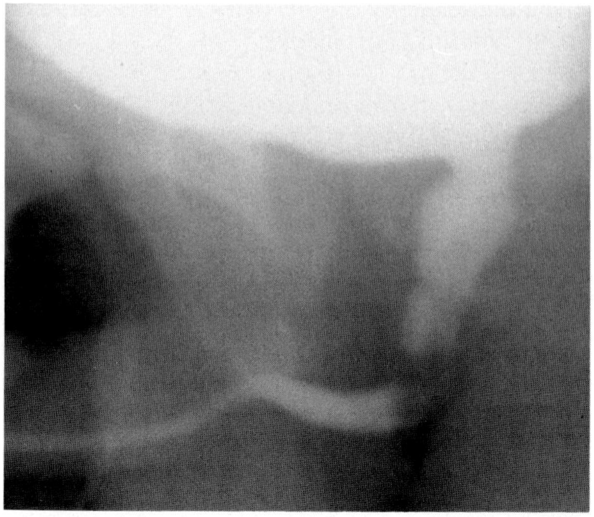

Fig. 18.36. Voiding cystourethrography in a male infant with obstructive symptoms. The filling defect in the bulbous urethra is a fibrous polyp, the stalk of which arises at the inferior aspect of the verumontanum. (POLLACK 1990, p 1404)

carcinoma (Fig. 18.35) to the corpora cavernosa and corpus spongiosum have been reported and are most likely blood borne.

18.7.5 Pseudotumors

Amyloidosis of the urethra is rare but simulates urethral carcinoma clinically (WALZER et al. 1983). Amyloidosis in the urethra is usually primary, there being no previous urethral disease. The presence of a hard ventral palpable mass and penile bleeding in a young male (usually below the age of 50 years) with no previous history of urethral disease should raise the possibility of amyloidosis. Biopsy is mandatory. The lesion may be short and well defined or long and irregular, producing narrowing of the urethra. The prognosis is excellent.

Sarcoidosis of the female urethra simulating urethral carcinoma has been reported (HO and HAYDEN 1979) but is exceedingly rare.

Urethral carcinoma is clinically insidious. Most patients have obstructive symptoms due to urethral stricture. The development of urethral carcinoma in these patients may result in serosanguineous urethral bleeding, palpable urethral mass, perineal abscess, or fistula; it may also be diagnosed by biopsy when suspected in cases of recurrent stricture. Carcinomas in the urethra not associated with previous stricture usually present with urethral bleeding and obstructive symptoms. Amyloidosis may clinically be impossible to differentiate from carcinoma.

Urethrography alone is not diagnostic for urethral carcinoma (OCCHIPINTI et al. 1992). Metastases and amyloidosis have a similar appearance, usually being seen as long irregular areas of narrowing. Unlike long urethral infectious stricture, the glands of Littre are not visualized. Urethral carcinoma may appear as a mass partially filling the urethra and there may be associated perirenal fistula. The same urethrographic appearance may be produced but abscess and partial filling defects may be due to stones or benign palpable lesions. However, the urethrographic appearance together with the clinical history may be diagnostic.

18.7.6 Benign Urethral Tumors

Benign tumors of the urethra are extremely rare. They may be of mesenchymal or epithelial origin.

Tumors of mesenchymal origin include fibrous polyp (congenital polyp), hemangioma, and myoblastoma. The most important of these is the fibrous polyp, which is congenital and most commonly found in children and young adults (ZULIAN et al. 1982). Fibrous polyps are usually pedunculated on a connective tissue stalk which is commonly long enough to produce a to-and-fro movement within the urethra. They originate in the posterior urethra and may produce obstructive frequency and dysuric symptoms. Elongation of the stalk allows the polyp to extend into the bulbous urethra on voiding (Fig. 18.36) and into the bladder at the end of voiding. On urethrography the mobility of the polyp is pathognomonic of congenital fibrous polyp. Resection of the polyp and stalk causes no risk of recurrence.

Benign tumors of epithelial origin include papillary adenoma, adenomatous polyp (Mostofi and Price 1973), adenomatoid metaplasia (Martin and Santa Cruz 1981), papillary urethritis (Schinella et al. 1974), inflammatory polyps, squamous cell papillomas, and transitional cell papillomas (Occhipinti et al. 1992). Papillary adenoma, adenomatous polyp, adenomatoid metaplasia, and papillary urethritis are all benign conditions which occur in the prostatic urethra. The clinical presentations of these lesions include hematuria, nocturia, and partial outlet obstruction. Papillary adenomas arise in the transitional cell epithelium in the prostatic urethra. These lesions usually present when small and are diagnosed on urethroscopy as a sessile polyp. They are most common in elderly men and are not associated with other urothelial tumors. There is no malignant potential.

Adenomatous polyps arise from prostatic epithelium and project into the prostatic urethra, commonly with a sessile base (Occhipinti et al. 1992). Immunohistologic techniques identify their prostatic origin by being positive for prostatic acid phosphatase and the identification of prostatic specific epithelial antigen. Resection usually results in a complete cure and recurrence is rare. Although generally considered benign and not premalignant, adenocarcinoma within a villous adenomatous polyp has been reported (Walker et al. 1982).

Adenomatoid metaplasia is extremely rare and is sufficiently confusing pathologically to command several names which include adenomatoid tumor, nephrogenic adenoma, and nephrogenic metaplasia. It is seen in elderly men who have had previous lower urinary tract surgery or trauma. It is more common in the bladder than in the prostatic urethra. These lesions are small and may be multiple. Diagnosis is by urethroscopy, the lesion being too small for detection by urethrography. Pathologically metaplasia tubules may be seen, resulting in the confusing array of names for the condition.

Papillary urethritis is the result of urothelial proliferation and adenoma due to an inflammatory reaction. Multiple edematous cystic filling defects are present in the prostatic urethra and may be diagnosed on urethroscopy and urethrography.

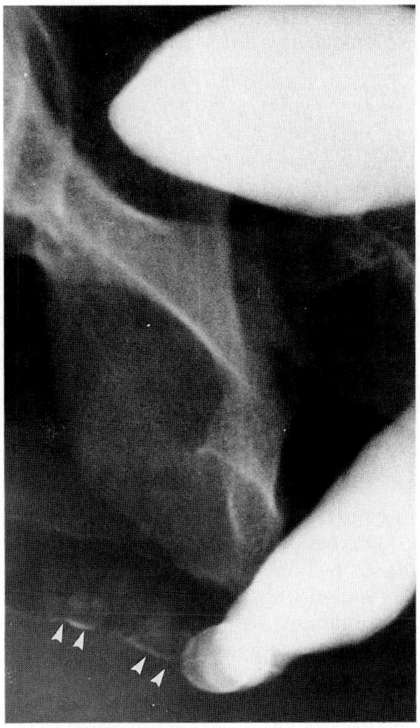

Fig. 18.37. Dynamic retrograde urethrogram following urethroplasty. After the injection of contrast medium, a small amount of air has been injected. Two inflammatory polyps are seen (*arrows*)

Inflammatory polyps and squamous and transitional cell polyps occur in the anterior urethra.

Inflammatory polyps are seen in the anterior urethra in patients with a previous history of urethral infections or stricture. They are more common in the bulbous urethra and may reach 1 cm in size and cause mild obstructive symptoms. Diagnosis is made by either urethoscopy or urethrography (Fig. 18.37). Squamous and transitional cell papillomas may occur anywhere in the anterior urethra. These lesions may occur spontaneously from squamous cell nests or transitional cell epithelium. They are found in younger men and are readily resectable. However, close follow-up is necessary since recurrence is not uncommon and malignant change within recurrent lesions has been reported.

Though rare, diverticulum of the male urethra can he highly symptomatic and must therefore be diagnosed and eradicated (Rimon et al. 1992).

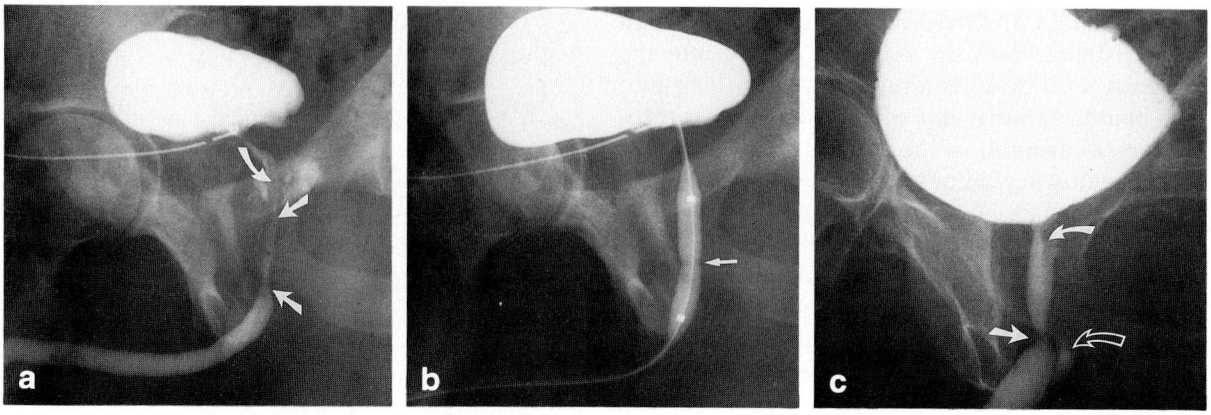

Fig. 18.38. **a** Dynamic retrograde urethrogram in a patient with complete outlet obstruction and suprapubic drainage. Severe hard scarring is present involving the proximal bulbous and membranous urethra (*between arrows*). *Curved arrows*, verumontanum. Reflux has occurred into prostatic ducts. **b** A balloon catheter has been inserted over a guidewire and the balloon placed in the strictured region. Dilatation of the balloon with contrast medium shows a waist defect (*arrow*) which persisted throughout the procedure. **c** Dynamic retrograde urethrogram immediately after dilatation. Most of the strictured area has been dilated. Some narrowing persists in the proximal bulbous urethra (*arrow*). Mild extravasation is present at the narrowed area (*open arrow*). *Curved closed arrow*, verumontanum. The patient spontaneously passed urine per urethra following the procedure and the suprapubic tube was removed 2 days later

18.8 Interventional Urethrography

Most urethral strictures are managed by urethrotomy or urethroplasty. Recent literature discusses the innovation of balloon dilatation of urethral strictures under fluoroscopy (Pinot et al. 1983; Russinovich et al. 1980; Scales et al. 1985; Wasserman et al. 1990; Castaneda et al. 1990). Pre- and postdilatation urethrography films are obtained. Three methods of balloon dilatation are described.

Following urethrography, delineating the site and extent of the urethral stricture, 5–10 cc of 2% xylocaine is introduced into the urethra. Attempted passage of a balloon catheter into the stricture area may be achieved without the use of a guidewire (Russinovich et al. 1980), if the stricture can accommodate the balloon catheter. The balloon of the catheter is dilated within the strictured area, and maintained dilated for 2–5 min. Fluoroscopic observation while the balloon is dilated may show a waist defect in the balloon which represents hard fibrous tissue poorly dilated. The balloon of the catheter is emptied and the dilatation of the balloon repeated after several minutes. This process is repeated until the waist defect in the balloon disappears. The balloon catheter is then removed and dynamic retrograde and voiding urethrography repeated. If extravasation occurs at the stricture site on the dynamic retrograde study, the urethrography is terminated and repeated after 5–6 days for assessment of the dilatation.

More commonly the balloon catheter cannot be passed into the stricture area. In this case an attempt is made to pass a guidewire through the strictured area. Usually a 0.038 guidewire is successful. When the guidewire is through the stricture and into the bladder, the balloon catheter is inserted over the guidewire into the stricture area under fluoroscopy. The balloon is then dilated as previously described (Fig. 18.38). Strictures which are impassable with a guidewire from below should be approached from above (Scales et al. 1985). These patients are usually completely obstructed and have a suprapublic catheter in place. This transvesical approach employs the passage of a guidewire through the cystostomy to the bladder neck. A steerable BF cathether then guides the wire through the urethral orifice and the guidewire is passed through the strictured area. This approach from above allows easier passage of the wire through the stricture since voiding pressure produces a funneled proximal end to a urethral stricture. The distal end of a severe stricture is usually a pinhole opening. The guidewire is then pushed through the stricture and exits the external meatus. The steerable catheter is then removed and the balloon catheter is inserted antegradely over the wire through the cystostomy into the strictured area. The balloon is then dilated as described until the waist defect in the balloon disappears.

The transvesical approach may initially involve use of a Cobra 3 shaped angiographic catheter to locate the urethral orifice. When the Cobra 3 catheter is through the urethral orifice, a 0.035 guidewire is passed through the catheter into the stricture area and passed through the urethra to exit the external meatus. Removal of the Cobra 3 catheter is followed by fixation of the guidewire at both ends. The stricture may then be approached by the catheter balloon over the wire retrogradely from the external meatus. The balloon may then enter the stricture site and the balloon dilated as described. Failure of passage of the balloon into the stricture site from the retrograde approach necessitates use of the above-described antegrade approach. Balloon dilatation of urethral stricture has achieved some success in relieving obstructive symptoms but repeat dilatation may be necessary any time between a few months to 2 years after the initial dilatation.

Care must be taken in the choice of balloon length and size (McCallum 1986). Many of the patients referred for balloon dilatation are post-prostatectomy patients with bulbomembranous urethral stricture. Surgical correction of such strictures entails the incision of the distal sphincters with the possibility of producing urinary incontinence since the internal sphincter at the bladder neck is already ablated by the transurethral prostatectomy. Balloon dilatation of bulbomembranous strictures may also interfere with distal sphincter function. However, damage to the distal sphincter mechanism is less likely than damage produced by metallic sound dilatation or surgical incision. Balloon dilatation is likely to stretch the distal sphincter but unlikely to produce muscle tearing and pressure necrosis. The fibrotic scar may be dilated without damaging the sphincter. Consequently in patients with stricture involving the membranous urethra the balloon diameter of choice should not be more than 5–6 mm, which is the normal voiding diameter of the membranous urethra. Stricture in the bulbous urethral sump may require a 9–10 mm balloon diameter since the normal bulbous urethral diameter is approximately 1 cm. In such a case the length of the balloon catheter is important. When dilating a balloon catheter within a stricture, it is usual to place the middle of the balloon at the tightest part of the stricture. Placing a 6-cm balloon in proper position to dilate a proximal bulbous urethral stricture may cause the distal end of the balloon to reach the distal sphincter and membranous urethra. Therefore it is advisable to use a shorter length of balloon (2–4 cm) to dilate proximal bulbous urethral strictures.

Complications of balloon dilatation of urethral stricture include urethral bleeding, which is usually slight and temporary. Redilatation is required within 1 year in approximately 10% of cases.

Coaxial balloon dilators especially designed for urethral stricture are now available. Coaxial balloon dilators used in males have a collapsed outer diameter of 9F and an inflated diameter of 24F. Using these balloon dilators, mild to moderate resistance of soft strictures was experienced in approximately 90% of cases, as evidenced by balloon pressure monitoring. Hard scars produced severe resistance to dilatation but are dilatable since these coaxial balloon dilators can be dilated to a maximum of 120 lb/in.^{2}.

18.9 Balloon Dilatation and Urethral Stent Insertion

Balloon dilatation of urethral stricture has recently been complemented by the insertion of a wire mesh urethral stent (Milroy et al. 1988; Donald et al. 1991; McInerney et al. 1991). Recurrent strictures following urethrotomy and urethroplasty are major problems for the patient and urologist. Such strictures may be balloon dilated and a stent inserted into the stricture area. The stent is collapsed and inserted over a balloon catheter. When the stent is in place in the stricture area, the balloon is dilated, which expands the stent, thus preventing stricture recurrence. The balloon catheter is then deflated and the catheter removed. It has been demonstrated that urethral stents become covered by a layer of stratified columnar epithelium within a few weeks. These stents are visible on plain radiography. Follow-up retrograde and voiding urethrography commonly shows the stent maintaining good urethral caliber (Fig. 18.39). Occasionally urethral narrowing is seen at the distal or proximal end of the stent. This usually results because the initial balloon dilatation has not adequately dilated all of the hard scarring, but may be due to secondary softer scarring progressing to the development of hard fibrous tissue.

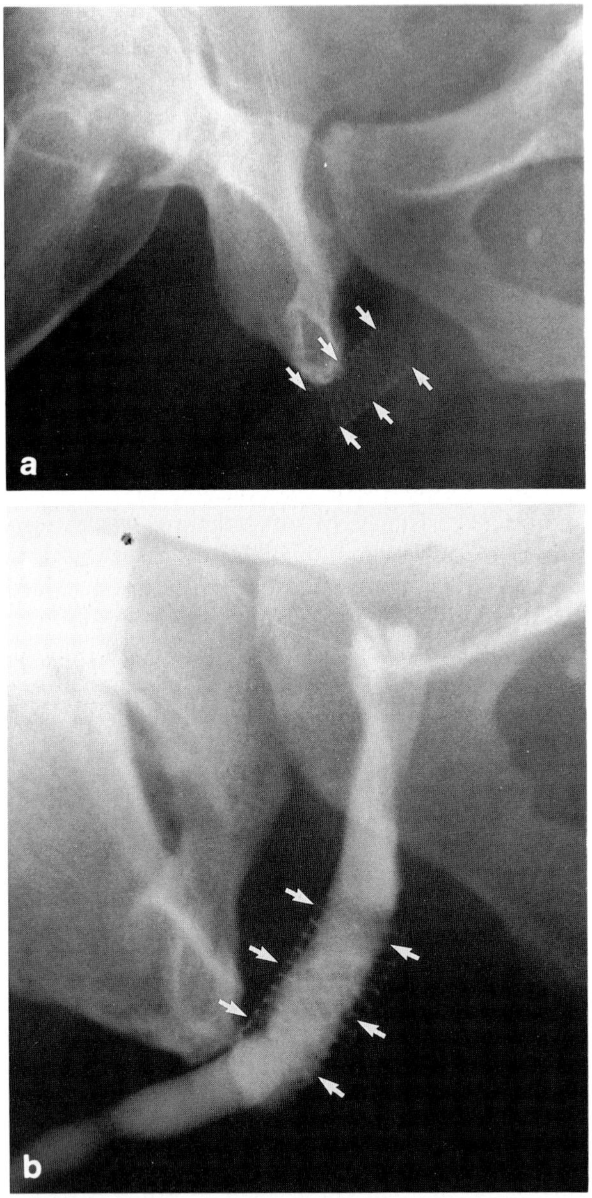

Fig. 18.39. **a** A plain film showing an expandable stent (*arrows*) in the region of the proximal bulbous urethra. **b** Dynamic retrograde urethrogram showing good caliber urethra maintained by the stent

Balloon dilatation and urethral stent insertion is still in its infancy. Hopefully, further improvement in stent design and length will obviate the above complications.

18.10 Balloon Dilatation of Prostatic Hypertrophy

Prostatic hypertrophy initially results in reduction of urinary stream, hesitancy in initiating micturition, and occasional urgency. Progressive hypertrophy leads to outlet obstruction and usually requires surgical intervention. This sequence of events is due to prostatic adenomas arising in the transitional zone of the prostate (inner periurethral glands) above the verumontanum. Therefore the site of obstruction is at the bladder neck and proximal prostatic urethra. Transurethral prostatectomy involves resection of these obstructing adenomas.

Balloon dilatation of the prostatic urethra involves applying high pressure balloon dilatation with compression of the adenomas. When first attempted by Burhenne and colleagues (1984) in the cadaver, eight out of ten cadaveric prostatic urethral dilatations were successful. Quinn and colleagues (1985) performed balloon dilatation of the proximal prostatic urethra in eight dogs (in six in vivo and in two in vitro) and one human (in vitro) (Quinn et al. 1985). The dilatation of the prostatic urethra was significant in all cases. This required three 5-min periods of balloon dilatation to 20 mm. Microscopic dissections of these prostates showed initial periurethral hemorrhage and chronic inflammatory change later. The prostatic glandular tissue elastic and collagen fibers and the lamina propria remained intact. All cases demonstrated successful persistent prostatic urethral widening. One human then performed self prostatic urethral dilatation resulting in an improved urinary stream. The procedure has required repetition almost on a yearly basis.

Since these first experiments, transrectal ultrasound has been incorporated as part of prostatic dilatation, and the dilatation maintained in real time as the dilatation proceeds. The method involves the passage of a guidewire per urethra into the bladder. The balloon catheter is passed over the guidewire with the balloon in the prostatic urethra. Care must be taken in positioning the balloon so that when dilated it is not in the region of the distal sphincter. Usually the balloon extends through the bladder neck. When the balloon is being dilated, traction must be applied to the catheter since there is a tendency for the dilated balloon to slip through the bladder neck into the bladder. Balloon catheters are now available up to 27 mm in dilated diameter. Transrectal ultrasound monitoring of the dilatation (Castaneda et al. 1987) is helpful and is also a method of assessing the widening of the prostatic urethra and bladder neck at the end of the procedure. If transrectal ultrasound is not used pre- and postdilatation, retrograde and voiding cystourethrography are necessary for the assessment of the degree of dilatation. The innovative use of balloon catheters in the dilatation of urethral strictures and in prostatic hypertrophy is likely to reduce the number of failed urethroplasties and transurethral resections of the prostate. In particular, the introduction of a urethral stent implant with associated balloon dilatation may indeed be the eventual method of management of failed urethroplasty and may even replace urethroplasty. However, it is to be emphasized that it is not sufficient to deal with a hard primary stricture alone since it is recognized that secondary softer scarring may progress to hard scarring. This is the common cause of failed urethroplasty and also applies to balloon dilatation. It is also necessary to emphasize that balloon dilatation of a bulbomembranous urethral stricture in a patient who has previously undergone transurethral prostatic resection carries the risk of urinary incontinence, although the risk of producing pressure necrosis into the membranous urethra and therefore the intrinsic sphincter is less with balloon dilatation than with metallic sound dilatation. The former provides a multidirectional force on the membranous urethra, providing compression and stretching of fibrous tissue. Metallic sound dilatation provides a shearing force to the strictured area, resulting in tearing of fibrous tissue and trauma which is more likely to produce more fibrous tissue, leading to recurrence of the stricture. Excess force applied with a metallic sound may indeed damage the intrinsic sphincter, resulting in some degree of urinary incontinence.

References

Bejany DE, Lockhart LL, Politano BA (1991) Ilial segment for ureteral substitution or for improvement of ureteral function. J Urol 46:302–305

Blandy JP (1976) Urethroplasty in males. In: Hendry WF (ed) Recent advances in urology, no. 2, sect. 10. Churchill Livinstone, New York, p 208

Burhenne HJ, Chisholm RJ, Quenville NF (1984) Prostatic hyperplasia: radiological intervention. Radiology 152: 655–657

Camarr AE (1972) Traumatic cord bladder treatment without diversion. In: Scott R (ed) Current controversies in urologic management. W.B. Saunders, Philadelphia, p 179

Carter HB, Brem RF, Tempany CM, Yang A, Epstein JI, Walsh PJ, Zerhounie A (1991) None papable prostate cancer: detection with MR imaging. Radiology 178: 523–526

Castaneda F, Reddy PK, Wasserman N et al. (1987) Benign prostatic hypertrophy: retrograde transurethral dilation of the prostatic urethra in humans. Radiology 163:649

Castaneda F, Hulbert JC, Letourneau JG, Hunter DW, Castaneda-Zuniga WR, Amplatz K (1990) Perineal abscess after prostatic urethroplasty with balloon catheter: report of a case. Radiology 174:49–50

Colapinto V, McCallum RW (1977) Injury to the male posterior urethra in fractured pelvis: a new classification. J Urol 118:575

Colapinto V, McCallum RW (1979) The role of urethrography in urethral disease, part II: Indication for transsphincter urethroplasty in patients with primary bulb strictures. J Urol 122:612

Dixon FJ, Moore RW (1953) In: Atlas of tumour pathology, fasc. 32. Armed Forces Institute of Pathology, Washington, DC, p 143

Donald JJ, Rickards D, Milroy EJG (1991) Stricture disease: radiology of urethral stents. Radiology 180: 447–450

Elbadawi A, Schenk EA (1974) A new theory of the innervation of bladder incontinence, part 4. Innervation of the vesicourethral junction and external urethral sphincter. J Urol 111:613

Faysal MH (1980) Urethrectomy in men with transitional cell carcinoma of bladder. Urology 16:23–26

Fisk NM, Dhillon HK, Ellis CE, Nicolini U, Tannirandorn Y, Rodeck CH (1990) Antenatal diagnosis of megalourethra in a fetus with prune belly syndrome. JCU 18:124–128

Fitts FB Jr, Herbert SG, Mellins HZ (1977) Criteria for examination of the urethra during excretory urology. Radiology 125:47

Fornage BD, Toubas O (1989) Transrectal sonographic monitoring of balloon dilatation of the prostatic urethra. J Ultrasound Med 8:53–55

Franks LM (1954) Benign nodular hyperplasia of the prostate: review. Ann R Coll Surg Engl 14:92

Gibson GR (1974) Urological management and complications of fractured pelvis and ruptured urethra. J Urol 111:353

Gosling JA, Dixon JS, Crutchley HOD, Thompson SA (1981) A comparative study of the human external sphincter and periurethral levator ani muscle. Br J Urol 53:35

Grebstald H (1973) Tumors of the urethra in men and women. Cancer 32:1236

Guttman L, Frankel H (1966) The value of intermittent catheterisation in the early management of traumatic paraplegia and tetraplegia. Paraplegia 4:63

Hildsworth FW (1963) Injury to the genito-urinary tract associated with fractures of the pelvis. Proc R Soc Med 56:1044

Ho KL, Hayden MT (1979) Sarcoidosis of urethra simulating carcinoma. Urology 13:197–199

Hricak H, Secaf E, Buckley DW, Brown JJ, Tanagho EA, McAninch JW (1991) Female urethra: MR imaging. Radiology 178:527–536

Jaramillo D, Lebowitz RL, Hendren WH (1990) Cloacal malformation: radiologic findings and imaging recommendations. Radiology 177:441–448

Kirshy DM, Pollack AH, Becker JA, Horowitz M (1991) Autourethrography. Radiology 180:443–445

Kisner CD (1958) Injuries of the urethra with special reference to those occurring in fractures of the pelvis. S Afr Med J 32:1105

Kleeman FJ (1970) The physiology of the internal urinary sphincter. J Urol 104:549
Kotecha N, Gentile RL (1974) Carcinoma of prostate with urethral metastasis. Urology 3:85–86
Lang EK, Davis JJ (1959) Positive pressure urethrography: a roentgenographic diagnostic method for urethral diverticula in the female. Radiology 72: 401–405
Lapides J, Koyanagi T, Diokno AC (1971) Cutaneous vesicotomy: 10 year survey. J Urol 105:76
Martin SA, Santa Cruz DJ (1981) Adenomatoid metaplasia of prostatic urethra. Am J Clin Pathol 75:185–189
McCague EJ, Semans JH (1944) The management of traumatic rupture of the urethra and bladder complicating fracture of the pelvis. J Urol 52:36
McCallum RW (1974) The radiologic assessment of the lower urinary tract in paraplegics – a new method. J Can Assoc Radiol 25:34
McCallum RW (1979) The adult male urethra: normal anatomy, pathology and method of urethrography. Radiol Clin North Am 17:227
McCallum RW (1986) Urethral disease and interventional cystourethrography. Radiol Clin North Am 24, no. 4
McCallum RW, Colapinto V (1976) Urological radiology of the adult male lower urinary tract. Charles C. Thomas, Springfield, Ill.
McCallum RW, Colapinto V (1979) The role of urethrography in urethral disease, part I: Accurate radiological localization of the membranous urethra and distal sphincter in normal males. J Urol 122:607
McCallum RW, Rogers J, Alexander M (1985) Iatrogenic urethral injury. J Can Assoc Radiol 36:122
McInerney PD, Banner TF, Harris SAB, Stephenson TB (1991) Permanent urethral stents for detrusor sphincter dyssynergia. Br J Urol 67:291–294
McNeal JE (1972) The prostate and prostatic urethra: a morphological synthesis. J Urol 107:1008
Milroy EJG, Cooper JE, Wallsten H et al. (1988) A new treatment for urethral strictures. Lancet I:1424–1427
Mitchell JP (1968) Injuries to the urethra. Br J Urol 40:649
Morales O, Romanus R (1955) Urethrography in the Male. J Urol 73:162
Morehouse DD, Belitsky P, MacKinnon K (1972) Rupture of the posterior urethra. J Urol 107:255
Mostofi FK, Price EB (1973) Tumors of the male genital system. Armed Forces Institute of Pathology, Washington, DC, p 195
Myers RP, DeWeerd JH (1972) Incidence of stricture following primary realignment of the disrupted proximal urethra. J Urol 107:765
Occhipinti K, Kutcher R, Gentile RL (1992) Prolapsing inverted papilloma of the prostatic urethra: diagnosis by transrectal sonography. AJR 159:93–94
Petrovic SD (1956) A clinical study of urethral injuries. J Urol 75:81
Pinot JJ, Hermanowicz M, Bonnet JL et al. (1983) Dilatation of the urethra by inflatable balloon catheter. Presse Med 12:163–164
Pollack HM (ed) (1990) Clinical urography. W.B. Saunders, Philadelphia
Pollack HM, DeBenedictis TJ, Marmar JL et al. (1978) Urethrographic manifestations of veneral warts (condyloma acuminata). Radiology 126:643
Quinn SF, Dyer R, Smathers R et al. (1985) Balloon dilatation of the prostatic urethra. Radiology 157:57–58
Ray B, Guinan PD (1979) Primary carcinoma of the urethra. In: Jawadpour N (ed) Principles and management of urologic cancer. Williams & Wilkins, Baltimore, p 461
Ray B, Canto AR, Whitmore WF (1977) Experience with primary carcinoma of the male urethra. J Urol 117: 591–594
Raz S (1978) Pathophysiology of male incontinence. Urol Clinic North Am 5:295
Rimon U, Hertz M, Jonas P (1992) Diverticular of the male urethra: a review of 61 cases. Urol Radiol 14: 49–55
Russinovich NAE, Lloyd LK, Griggs WP et al. (1980) Balloon dilatation of urethra strictures. Urol Radiol 2:33–37
Sandler CM, Phillips TM, Harris JD, Toombs BD (1981) Radiology of the bladder and urethra in blunt pelvic trauma. Radiol Clin North Am 19:195
Scales FE, Katzen BT, van Breden A et al. (1985) Impassable urethral strictures: percutaneous transvesical catheterization and balloon dilatation. Radiology 157: 59–61
Schellhammer PF, Whitmore WF (1976) Transitional cell carcinoma of the urethra in men having cystectomy for bladder cancer. J Urol 115:56–60
Schinella R, Thurm J, Feiner H (1974) Papillary pseudotumor of the prostatic urethra: proliferative papillary urethritis. J Urol 111:38–40
Shapeero LG, Friedland GW, Perkash I (1983) Transrectal sonographic voiding cystourethrography: studies in neuromuscular bladder dysfunction. AJR 141:83
Shokeir AA, Gaballah MA, Ashamallah AA, Ghoneim MA (1991) Optimisation of replacement of ureter by ilium. J Urol 146:306–310
Tanagho EA, Schmidt RA, Gomes de Araujo C (1982) The urinary striated sphincter: what is its nerve supply? Invest Urol 20:415
Tines SC, Bigongiari LR (1982) Carcinoma in diverticulum of the female urethra. AJR 138:582
Trafford HS (1955) Traumatic rupture of the posterior urethra with review of 32 civilian cases. Br J Urol 27:165
Turner-Warwick RT, Whiteside CG (1970) Investigation and management of bladder neck dysfunction. Mod Trends Urol 3:295
Walker AN, Mills SE, Fechner RE, Perry JM (1982) "Endometrial" adenocarcinoma of the prostatic urethra arising in a villous polyp. Arch Pathol Lab Med 106:624–627
Walzer Y, Bear RA, Colapinto V, McCallum RW, Lang A (1983) Localized amyloidosis of the urethra. Urology 21:406–407
Wasserman NF, Reddy PK, Zhang G, Berg BA (1990) Experimental treatment of benign prostatic hyperplasia with transurethral balloon dilatation of the prostate: preliminary study in 73 humans. Radiology 177: 485–494
Wilkinson FOW (1961) Rupture of the posterior urethra with a review of 12 cases. Lancet I:1125
Williams G, Ashken MH (1980) Urethral carcinoma following urethroplasty. J R Soc Med 73:370–371
Yoder RC, Papanicolaou N (1992) Imaging of the urethra in men and women. Urol Radiol 14:24–28
Zulian RAS, Brito RR, Broges GJ (1982) Transurethral resection of pedunculated congenital polyps of the posterior urethra. Br J Urol 54:45–48

19 Seminal Vesicles

João Martins Pisco

CONTENTS

19.1 Normal Seminal Vesicles

19.1.1 Anatomy

Seminal vesicles are secretory glands that produce seminal fluid to support and maintain sperm. Seminal fluid constitutes the major volume of the ejaculate. The seminal vesicles are paired glands located within the perivesical space behind and anterior to the rectum. Pathologic processes from the prostate, bladder, or rectum can, therefore, involve the seminal vesicles. The rectovesical fascia is placed between the seminal vesicles and the rectum (Lierse 1984). The seminal vesicles are largely extraperitoneal and only the lateral parts are covered by the peritoneum. Normally there is a 50°–60° angle between the seminal vesicles and the horizontal plane, the angle varying with the degree of distention of the bladder and rectum (Secaf et al. 1991). Because of the angle of orientation of the seminal vesicles, their medial and lateral ends are not included in the same cut (Higgins et al. 1992). After an abdominal perineal resection, the position and orientation of the seminal vesicles change and they fill the empty space.

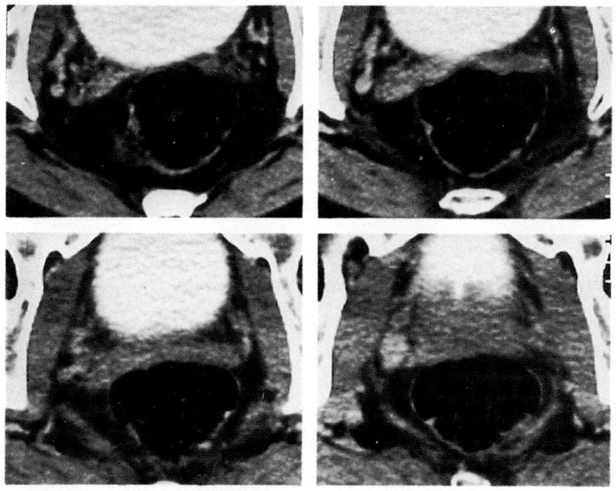

Fig. 19.1. CT of the pelvis. The enhanced venous plexus is shown posterior and lateral to the bladder

Between the bladder and the seminal vesicles there is a deep cleft that contains tributaries of prostatic venous plexus embedded in fat (Fig. 19.1).

The vas deferens becomes convoluted as it passes alongside the upper medial border of the seminal vesicle, where its diameter widens significantly as it forms the ampulla of the vas deferens. The seminal vesicle is highly convoluted, roughly ovoid, and lateral to the ampulla. There is constriction of the medial part of the seminal vesicle, which forms the seminal vesicle duct that joins with the vas deferens to form the ejaculatory duct (Lierse 1984). The paired ejaculatory ducts are placed within the posterior aspect of the prostate and reach the verumontanum.

Each gland measures 4.5–5.5 cm in length and 3–4 mm in diameter. There is great variation in the size of seminal vesicles of normal individuals. Seminal vesicles are dissimilar in size in nearly one-third of patients. The seminal vesicles are small in pediatric patients; they tend to be wider

João Martins Pisco, M.D., Ph.D., Director de Servico de Radiologia, Hospital de Santa Marta, Rua de Santa Marta, 1100 Lisboa, Portuga

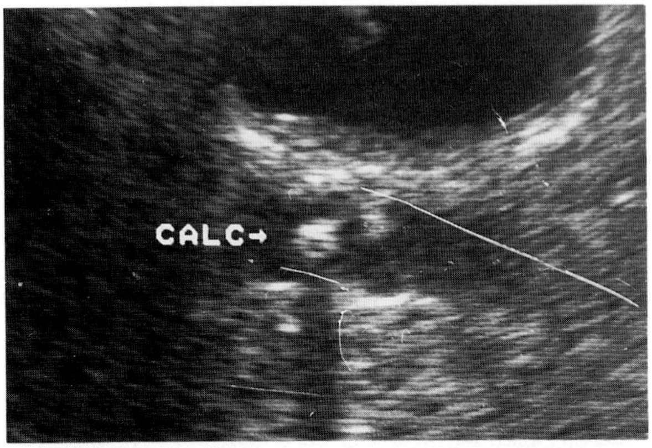

Fig. 19.2. Transabdominal pelvic ultrasonography. Transverse scan showing calcifications (*CALC*) of the seminal vesicle

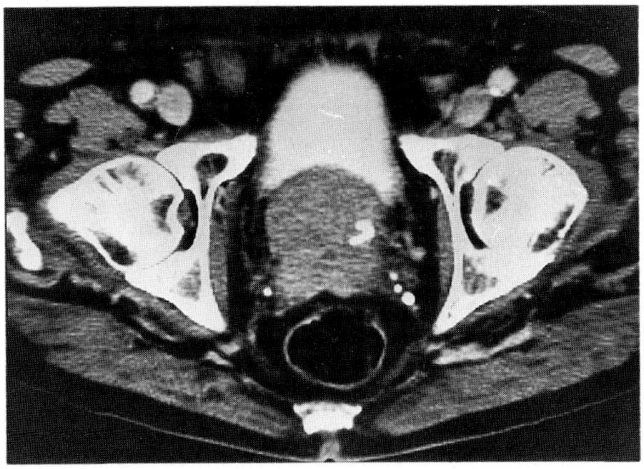
Fig. 19.3. CT of the pelvis. Calcifications of the seminal vesicles in a diabetic patient

in the fifth and sixth decades, probably owing to stasis and distention associated with benign prostatic hyperplasia and resultant ejaculatory duct compression (Secaf et al. 1991). The seminal vesicles decrease in size after the age of 70 years, probably owing to decreased androgen stimulation and, therefore, smaller volumes of seminal vesicle fluid production (Higgins et al. 1992).

Seminal vesicle calcifications are occasionally seen in diabetic patients (Figs. 19.2, 19.3).

19.1.2 Vesiculography

Initially, the seminal vesicles were shown as an impression on the opacified urethra, bladder, or rectum or by vesiculography.

Seminal vesiculography entails cannulation of the vas deferens. Vesiculography requires general anesthesia, opening of the scrotal sac, needle puncture of the vas deferens, and instillation of iodinated contrast medium (Dunnick et al. 1982). Although it is an invasive procedure, it is still used for detailed study of the morphology.

Belfield performed the first seminal vesiculography in 1913 (Witten et al. 1977). After surgical exposure of the vas deferens in the scrotum he injected 5% collargol into the vas deferens and demonstrated the abdominal portion of the vas, the seminal vesicles, and the ejaculatory ducts. Most of the early studies were performed to investigate chronic inflammatory disease of the seminal vesicles.

Vasography is used most frequently to define the level of a block within the vas in the investigation of azoospermia or extreme oligospermia and also in the investigation of patients with intractable chronic prostatitis and epididymitis.

With the development of ultrasonography (particularly transrectal ultrasonography) computed tomography (CT), and magnetic resonance imaging (MRI), the indications for seminal vesiculography have decreased. The development of urodynamic investigations has contributed a small number of patients who would benefit from seminal vesiculography. Nowadays, the most common indication for vasovesiculography is the evaluation of male infertility, particularly in patients suspected of having obstructive azoospermia. Obstruction of the ejaculatory ducts can be diagnosed definitively by vesiculography.

19.2 Imaging

In the past, evaluation of the seminal vesicles was attempted by means of intravenous urography, cystography, barium enema examination, and seminal vesiculography. Findings on the first three of these examinations were not specific, showing displacement of the bladder and sigmoid by an extrinsic mass.

Seminal vesicle lesions are uncommon but might be diagnosed more often with increased use of cross-sectional imaging for evaluation of pelvic masses in the male.

The most frequent indication for evaluation of the seminal vesicles is assessment of tumor extension from prostate, and occasionally from bladder or rectum. Other indications are cysts, absence of the seminal vesicles, postsurgical acquired disease, seminal vesicle or ejaculatory duct calculi, and primary neoplasms.

19.2.1 Ultrasonography

Transabdominal ultrasonography is noninvasive and more readily available and economical that CT or MRI. Ultrasound-guided needle biopsy is expeditious.

With transabdominal ultrasonography, the seminal vesicles can be examined through the acoustic window of the bladder (CARTER et al. 1989). The seminal vesicles are seen as paired structures placed behind the bladder. The seminal vesicles have medium echogenicity, slightly less than that of the prostate gland, with a typical bowtie appearance on transverse scans and an elongated elliptic appearance on oblique parasagittal scans. The center of the gland is hypoechoic, with areas of increased echogenicity due to the folds of the excretory epithelium. The junction of the seminal vesicle with the ejaculatory duct is usually within the prostate. The ejaculatory ducts can be followed to an area of slightly increased echogenicity – the verumontanum (CARTER et al. 1989).

Transrectal ultrasonography is indicated for seminal vesicle disease and for evaluation of male infertility. Among the many entities causing male infertility, some may be diagnosed by transrectal ultrasonography. These include absence of the seminal vesicles, ejaculatory duct dilatation, and unilateral obstruction of the ejaculatory duct (Fig. 19.4).

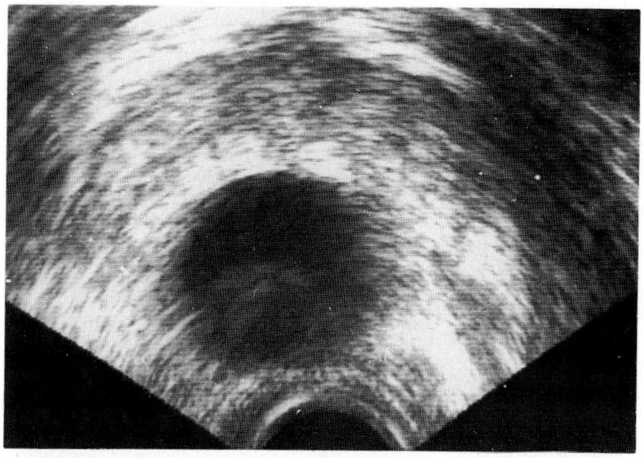

Fig. 19.4. Pelvic ultrasonography. Transrectal scan in a patient with an ejaculatory duct cyst

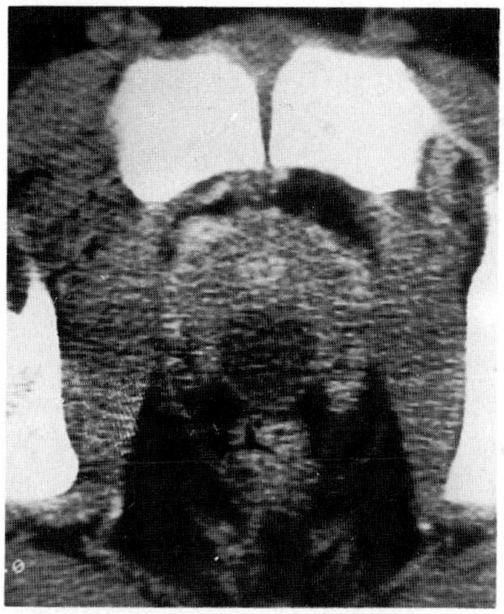

Fig. 19.5. Pelvic CT of the same patient as in Fig. 19.4

Absence of the seminal vesicles may be unilateral or bilateral and occasionally may be associated with mucoviscidosis.

Seminal vesicle cysts present as discrete anechoic areas. Ejaculatory duct cyst and müllerian duct remnants are present as discrete anechoic or hypoechoic areas in the posterior base of the prostate. Calculi within the seminal vesicle or ejaculatory ducts appear as well-circumscribed hyperechoic foci with or without acoustic shadowing (LITTRUP et al. 1988).

Seminal vesical cysts may be congenital or secondary to a congenital obstruction of the seminal vesicle and the ejaculatory duct. They may be seen on conventional sonograms, but small cysts will only be shown on transrectal sonograms. The differential diagnosis of seminal vesicle cyst includes wolffian duct cysts, müllerian duct remnant cysts, prostate cysts, diverticula of the ejaculatory duct, and seminal vesicle dilatation due to obstruction.

19.2.2 Computed Tomography

On CT, the paired seminal vesicles lie posterior to the bladder, extending cephalad and laterally from the prostate. On axial scans, the seminal vesicles and the vas deferens appear as bowtie-shaped structures, well delineated by low attenuation extraperitoneal fat, between the bladder and rectum.

One of the most frequent indications for CT for the seminal vesicles is determination of in-

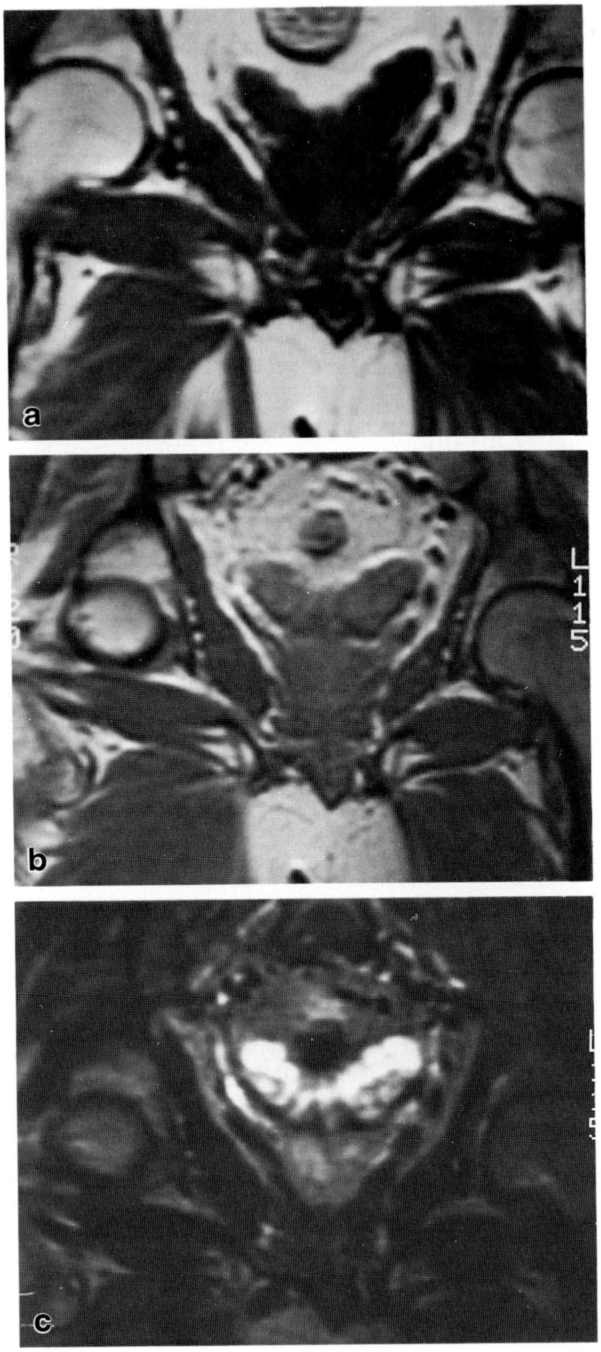

Fig. 19.6a–c. MRI of the pelvis. Coronal scan showing a normal seminal vesicle. **a** T1, TR 600, TE 12; **b** PD, TR 2000, TE 20; **c** T2, TR 2000, TE 80

vasion by prostatic carcinoma. CT may also be used in the evaluation of cysts either in the seminal vesicles or of the ejaculatory duct (Fig. 19.5).

19.2.3 Magnetic Resonance Imaging

Magnetic resonance imaging clearly displays the size and configuration of the seminal vesicles behind the bladder, embedded in retroperitoneal fat. On transaxial and sagittal scans, the angle between the seminal vesicles and the urinary bladder can be demonstrated.

Both T1- and T2-weighted images are used for evaluation of the seminal vesicles. T1-weighted scans are used for studying the anatomy of the seminal vesicles and for assessment of perivesical tumor invasion. T2-weighted images show the internal structure of the seminal vesicles, their fluid content, and tumor invasion (Gevenois et al. 1990).

There is asymmetry of seminal vesicle size in about one-third of normal subjects.

On coronal MR images, the seminal vesicles are seen as oval structures projecting obliquely from the posteromedial surface of the prostate. On a T1-weighted spin-echo pulse sequence, the seminal vesicles have a medium to low signal intensity. On a T2-weighted sequence, there is a relative increase in signal intensity due to the fluid within the seminal vesicles (Fig. 19.6).

On T2-weighted images, the glands' signal intensities vary according to age. In prepubertal patients, the signal intensity of seminal vesicles is lower than that of fat. In adult patients, the signal intensity of seminal vesicles is similar to or higher than that of fat. In patients older than 70 years, the signal intensity may decrease (Secaf et al. 1991).

On gadolinium-DTPA-enhanced T1-weighted images, the walls of the seminal vesicle enhance, but the fluid contents remain at the same low signal intensity.

Magnetic resonance imaging is ideal for evaluation of male infertility. The absence of ionizing radiation is an advantage in patients of reproductive age. Due to the very sensitive soft tissue contrast resolution, MRI displays clearly visible interfaces between pelvic fat and the genitourinary organs; therefore, the anatomy of the seminal vesicles, prostate, and urinary bladder is well shown. Moreover, it has the ability to yield multiplanar sections. MRI has provided more specific tissue characterization and is less operator dependent than ultrasonography (GEVENOIS et al. 1990). Moreover, MRI is not affected by the patient's body habitus or intestinal gas (HIGGINS et al. 1992).

19.3 Seminal Vesicle Cysts

Seminal vesicle cysts are usually unilocular, rarely multilocular. Usually they are unilateral, but they may be bilateral. They may involve one or more convolutions of the seminal vesicle or the entire vesicle.

Seminal vesicle cysts are more frequent between the ages of 20 and 30 years. If the cyst is large, it may obstruct the bladder, causing difficulty in voiding, or it may obstruct the vas, causing pain on ejaculation. Usually, they are asymptomatic and small cysts tend to be incidental findings.

The seminal vesicle cyst, although unusual, is the most frequent primary vesicle mass and the most frequent congenital abnormality of the seminal vesicles. It is often associated with ipsilateral anomalies of the ureter and kidney. ZINNER, in 1914, described the first case of seminal vesicle cyst associated with ipsilateral renal agenesis. Approximately two-thirds of seminal vesicle cysts are associated with ipsilateral renal agenesis (KING et al. 1989; HEANEY et al. 1987). Therefore, upper urinary tract imaging is indicated when a seminal vesicle cyst is encountered. Apart from ipsilateral renal agenesis, seminal vesicle cysts may be associated with an ectopic ureter draining into the seminal vesicle from a dysplastic kidney (ROCHOBORN et al. 1986). Ectopic ureteral insertion into the ejaculatory duct, vas deferens, or prostatic urethra can also be associated with seminal vesical cysts (KING et al. 1989).

Congenital cysts of the seminal vesicles probably result from congenital obstruction of the junction of the seminal vesicle and ejaculatory duct (ZINNER et al. 1914).

Transabdominal and transrectal ultrasonography and CT should be the initial diagnostic studies for seminal vesicle cysts; MRI is reserved for more complex situations. Transrectal ultrasonography has an advantage over the transabdominal approach in that it better delineates the configuration of the contralateral seminal vesicle and the cyst (CARTER et al. 1989). Sonographically, seminal vesicle cysts display typical cyst findings with no internal echoes unless complicated by hemorrhage or infection (Fig. 19.7). Under ultrasonographic guidance via the transabdominal or, better, the transrectal route, the cyst may be aspirated and injected with contrast medium (ABE et al. 1989; ASCH and TOI 1991).

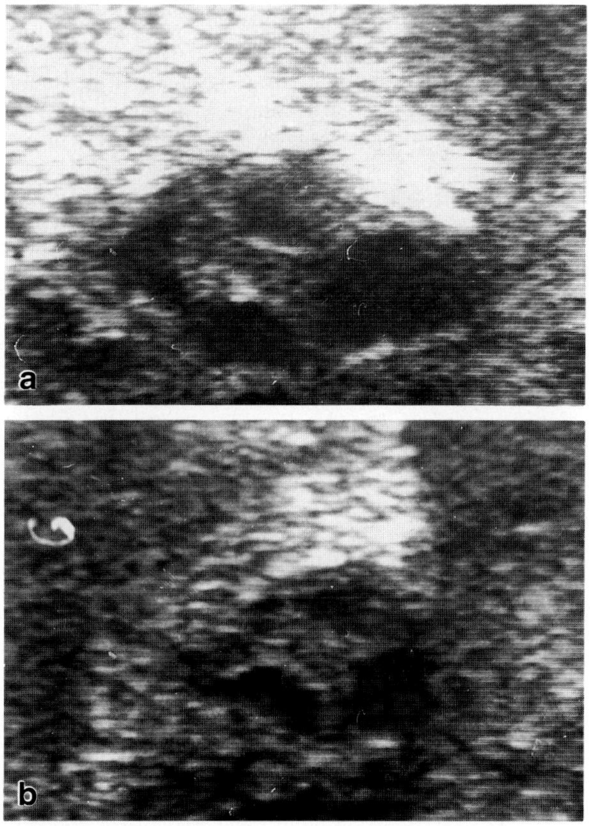

Fig. 19.7a,b. Ultrasonography of the seminal vesicles, in a patient with several cysts. **a** Right seminal vesicle; **b** left seminal vesicle

Computed tomography confirms the cystic nature of a mass; simple cysts present as a low density, nonenhancing, thin-walled mass and complicated cysts, such as hemorrhagic cysts, as a thick-walled mass of higher density (KNEELAND et al. 1985) (Fig. 19.8).

Uncomplicated cysts in most organs feature a low signal intensity on T1- and high a signal intensity on T2-weighted scans. If the cyst is complicated by hemorrhage, an increased signal intensity may be demonstrated on the T1-weighted sequence, depending on the time of imaging in relation to the hemorrhage.

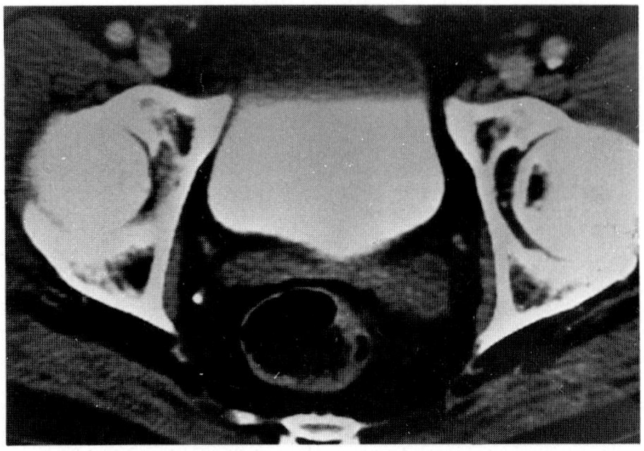

Fig. 19.8. CT of the pelvis. Enlarged left seminal vesicle with two small cysts

Seminal vesicle cysts are not simple cysts; rather they feature a brownish fluid containing spermatozoa and their precursors (KNEELAND et al. 1985). Therefore, the seminal vesicle cyst may display a high signal intensity on both T1- and T2-weighted images (due to a short T1 and a long T2). KING et al. established that such a finding indicates a hemorrhagic etiology and is often associated with hemospermia (WITTEN et al. 1977).

Acquired seminal vesicle cysts are usually associated with partial or complete obstruction of the ejaculatory ducts, which can be caused by urinary tract infection (generally ascending from the lumen of the prostatic urethra into the seminal vesicles), stones, or stenosis resulting from surgery (ROCHOBORN et al. 1986). They can be associated with benign prostatic hyperplasia due to compression of the ejaculatory ducts by prostatic nodules (KING et al. 1989). They should be suspected in the presence of any one of these predisposing factors and a normal ipsilateral kidney and vas deferens.

The differential diagnosis of seminal vesicle cyst includes the müllerian duct cyst that is located at the midline at the base of the prostate. This cyst tends to present in older men with normal genitalia and is due to incomplete resorption of the müllerian duct (RITCHEY et al. 1988). Seminal vesicle cysts, lateral in location, often cause obstruction of the ipsilateral seminal vesicle. Müllerian duct cysts are located at the midline and extend superiorly from the level of the verumontanum even beyond the prostate. The contents of müllerian duct cysts vary (mucoid, purulent, serous, or hemorrhagic). When blood is present, both T1- and T2-weighted scans show a high signal within the cyst (THURNER et al. 1988) (Fig. 19.9).

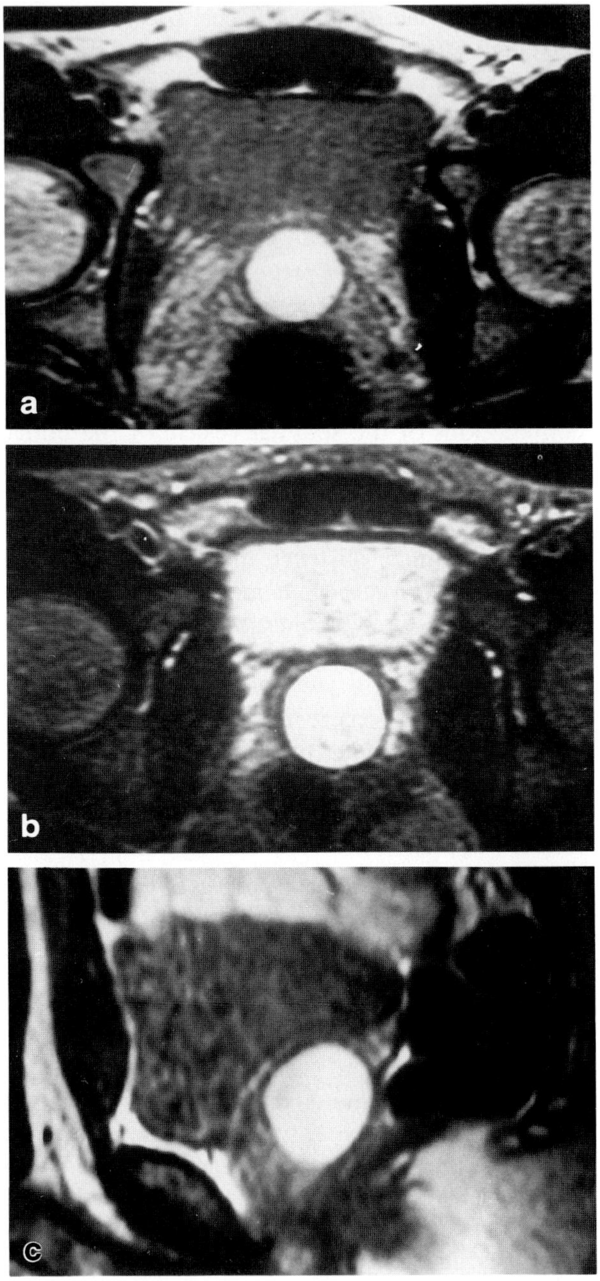

Fig. 19.9a-c. MRI of the pelvis in a patient with a hemorrhagic müllerian duct cyst. **a** Axial T1, TR 600, TE 12; **b** axial T2, TR 2200, TE 30; **c** sagittal T2, TR 2200, TE 30

19.4 Other Congenital Anomalies

Ectopic insertion of the ureter into the seminal vesicle is one congenital abnormality that is frequently associated with ipsilateral renal agenesis or dysgenesis and contralateral renal hypertrophy.

Bilateral or unilateral dilatation of the seminal vesicles may occur following transurethral resection. There is associated tubular dilatation of the ejaculatory duct that can be demonstrated by transrectal ultrasonography.

Other congenital anomalies are agenesis, hypoplasia, and ectopia. Any of the cross-sectional imaging modalities can be used in the evaluation of congenital anomalies of the seminal vesicles. However, for the diagnosis of ectopia, vesiculography is still the most accurate modality.

Unilateral or bilateral agenesis of the seminal vesicle is often an incidental finding on CT or transrectal ultrasonography. Low ejaculatory volume is almost invariably associated with congenital absence or hypoplasia of the seminal vesicles, often with vasal aplasia (CARTER et al. 1989). Another rare cause of low ejaculate volume is failure of the seminal vesicles and ejaculatory duct to empty (GOLDWASSER et al. 1985). The sonogram of such patients shows dilated seminal vesicles. Obstruction of the ejaculatory duct is another infrequent cause of male infertility, in which there is also dilatation of the seminal vesicle (COLFI et al. 1987).

When the vas is absent, the ejaculatory duct is absent. Bilateral congenital absence is associated with cystic fibrosis.

Diverticula can occur in the seminal vesicle.

Ectopia of the seminal vesicle may be associated with agenesis on the same side or with an ectopic ureter.

Arteriovenous malformation is a rare anomaly in which there are large vessels along the lateral aspect of the seminal vesicles (KING et al. 1989).

19.5 Inflammatory Disease

The signs and symptoms of seminal vesiculitis are nonspecific and include vague lower abdominal, pelvic, perineal, and scrotal pain and hematospermia.

Infection of the seminal vesicles usually arises from the prostate or the epididymis. Seminal vesiculitis can be a difficult clinical diagnosis due to complex symptoms (MEARS 1986; BAHN et al. 1990).

In acute inflammation, the seminal vesicles may be normal or one or both of the vesicles may be enlarged. Seminal vesiculitis is usually a secondary inflammatory process associated with prostatitis. Transrectal ultrasonography shows enlarged and hyperechoic seminal vesicles.

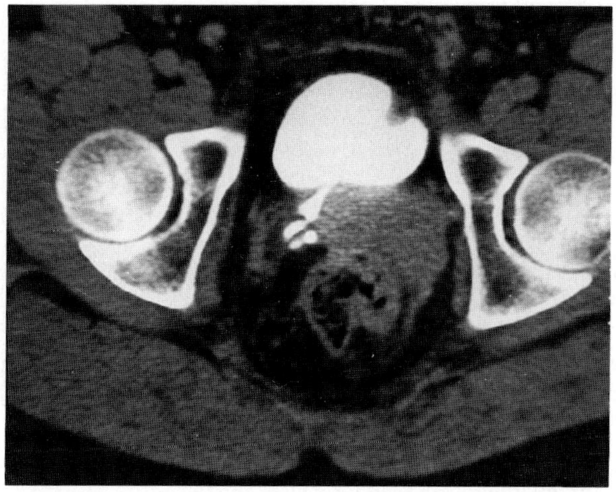

Fig. 19.10. CT of the pelvis. The left seminal vesicle is enlarged, and there is low attenuation in the posterior aspect due to a chronic abscess. This 28-year-old male had undergone an operation for an imperforate anus as a newborn. However, a fistula from the rectum to the seminal vesicle remained

In acute vesiculitis, the signal intensity on either the T1- or the T2-weighted images may be normal or the infected seminal vesicle may show a signal intensity lower than the normal contralateral seminal vesicle (BAHN et al. 1990). On T2-weighted images, the signal of the involved seminal vesicle is higher than that of fat and the contralateral noninvolved vesicle. If a hemorrhagic component is present, there will be increased signal on both the T1- and the T2-weighted sequences.

In subacute infection the seminal vesicles may show normal to high signal intensity depending on the age of the accumulated blood (HIGGINS et al. 1992; BAHN et al. 1990).

In chronic inflammation, the small fibrotic seminal vesicles show lower signal intensity on T2-weighted images.

Seminal vesiculitis may progress to abscess formation. Ectopic ureteral insertion into the seminal vesicles may also lead to abscess formation. Other predisposing factors are diabetes, urologic intervention, renal agenesis, seminal vesicle cysts, and recto-seminal vesicle fistula. Seminal vesicle abscess causes asymmetric enlargement of one seminal vesicle (Fig. 19.10).

Abdominal ultrasonography, transrectal ultrasonography, and CT are used for pelvic abscess

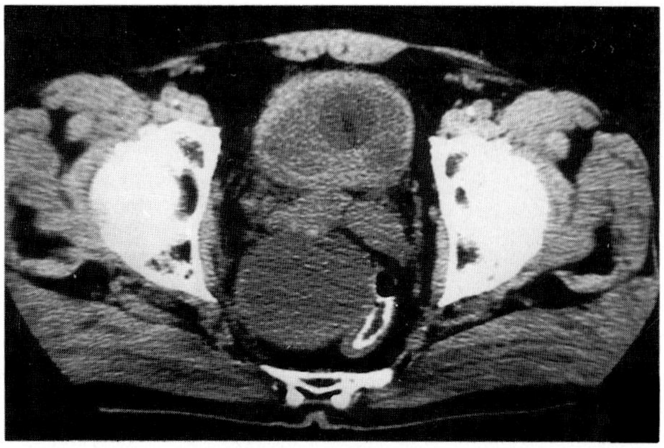

Fig. 19.11. CT of the pelvis. Perirectal abscess with invasion of the right seminal vesicle. Both seminal vesicle are enlarged. The bladder wall is thick

identification (Fig. 19.11). Transrectal ultrasonography is used for localization and guide needle aspiration of a seminal vesicle abscess. Ultrasonography shows an anechoic or hypoechoic fluid-filled mass.

Abscess of the seminal vesicle presents on T1-weighted images as an ill-defined mass of low signal intensity, and perivesicular adipose tissue shows low signal intensity.

19.6 Tumors

19.6.1 Secondary Tumors

The most frequent tumor of the seminal vesicle is invasive cancer from the prostate. The invasion of seminal vesicle by prostatic carcinoma may be by contiguous extension or from tumor infiltration along the course of the ejaculatory ducts (SECAF et al. 1991). Tumor permeation may be total or focal. Detection of seminal vesicle involvement by prostatic carcinoma is important for staging. Invasion of prostatic carcinoma into the seminal vesicles indicates a poor prognosis and at least a stage "C." Surgery is reserved only for stage A and B carcinoma of the prostate (JEWETT et al. 1972).

Prostatic carcinoma extends into the seminal vesicle by growing towards and through the prostate base within the muscular wall of the ejaculatory duct. Thus, the earliest and most extensive involvement by cancer is localized within the seminal vesicle wall near its point of junction with the vas deferens. VILLERS et al. (1990) showed that none of 38 transition zone carcinomas showed evidence of seminal vesicle invasion but that 47 nontransitional zone tumors displayed seminal vesicle invasion. The frequency and extent of seminal vesicle invasion are strongly related to cancer volume. Invasion of the seminal vesicles was observed in only 6% of VILLERS et al.'s patients.

Without invasion of the seminal vesicles, these organs will be symmetric with a recognizable fluid-filled lumen on sonograms. In the presence of invasion, the internal echo pattern is diffusely heterogeneous and irregular. Transrectal ultrasonography in combination with biopsy allows more precise preoperative staging and particularly differentiation of stage B from stage C cancer.

Ultrasonography is highly accurate (82%) in detecting extension of prostatic tumor into the seminal vesicles. Invasion of the seminal vesicles may produce abnormal ultrasonographic findings, the most consistent and reliable of which is asymmetry in size, shape, and internal echo pattern (SCARDINO et al. 1989). There are three patterns of invasion of the seminal vesicles. The most common is invasion along the ejaculatory ducts into the seminal vesicles (type I), usually shown as a posterior convexity. The second most common pattern is extension to the seminal vesicles from a tumor that penetrates the capsule and surrounds and subsequently invades the seminal vesicles from without (type II). In general, this type of invasion is shown as an "adhesion," the seminal vesicle appearing to be adherent to the prostate. The least common pattern is small isolated foci of tumor in the seminal vesicles representing micrometastases (type III) (SCARDINO et al. 1989).

The most common ultrasonographic finding in patients with seminal vesicle invasion is a hypoechoic lesion at the base of the prostate.

Invasion of the seminal vesicles is diagnosed on CT either by morphologic alteration or by obliteration of intervening fat planes. Therefore, one of the signs of tumor invasion is asymmetry of the seminal vesicles.

Enlargement of one or both seminal vesicles is a strong indicator of tumor invasion (Figs. 19.12, 19.13). Another finding is obliteration of the normal fat plane between the posterior wall of the bladder and seminal vesicles – the seminal vesicle angle sign. This sign can be simulated by a distended rectum if the CT scan is obtained in the prone position. Asymmetry of the seminal vesicle

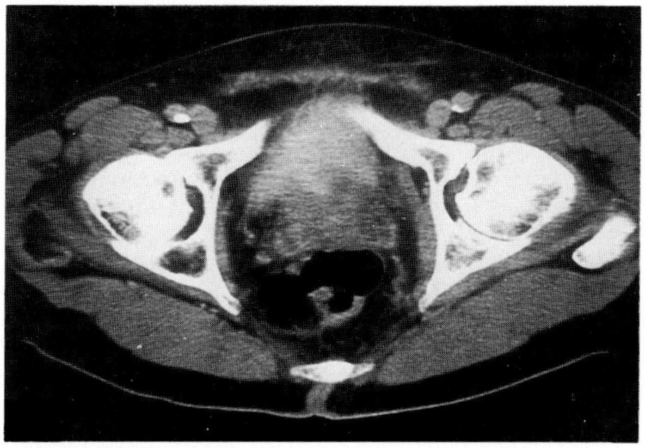

Fig. 19.12. CT of the pelvis. Carcinoma of the prostate invading both seminal vesicles, which are enlarged with low attenuation zones

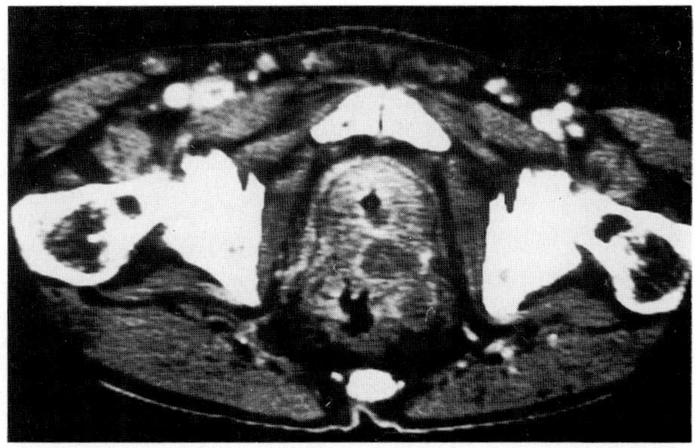

Fig. 19.13. Pelvic CT in a patient who had undergone prostatectomy. There is local recurrence of prostatic carcinoma with invasion of both seminal vesicles

angle may also occur with benign prostatic enlargement.

For evaluation of seminal vesicle extension of a tumor, the axial plane is the preferred plane with both CT and MR.

As prostatic carcinoma has a low signal intensity on T2-weighted images, and the seminal vesicles have a high signal intensity, early infiltration into the seminal vesicles can be diagnosed before the tumor changes their size and shape.

The signal intensity of normal seminal vesicles is similar to that of muscle on T1-weighted images and equal to or higher than that of fat on T2-weighted images.

In the evaluation of prostatic carcinoma the seminal vesicles are considered normal on MRI when they are symmetric in signal intensity, of intermediate signal intensity on T1-weighted images, and of high signal intensity on T2-weighted images. Seminal vesicles are considered abnormal if, on T2-weighted images, they are (a) asymmetric in signal intensity or (b) of low signal intensity or (c) of high signal intensity but with focal defects of low signal intensity or (d) grossly enlarged on the side where high intensity fat located in the seminal vesicular angle is disrupted (Fig. 19.14). BEZZI et al. (1988) found that in the evaluation of seminal vesicle invasion by prostatic carcinoma, MRI has a sensitivity of 83%, a specificity of 88%, and an accuracy of 86% (BEZZI et al. 1988). Similar data have been reported by BIONDETTI et al. (1987).

Tumors of the urinary bladder or rectum invade the seminal vesicles much less frequently (Fig. 19.15).

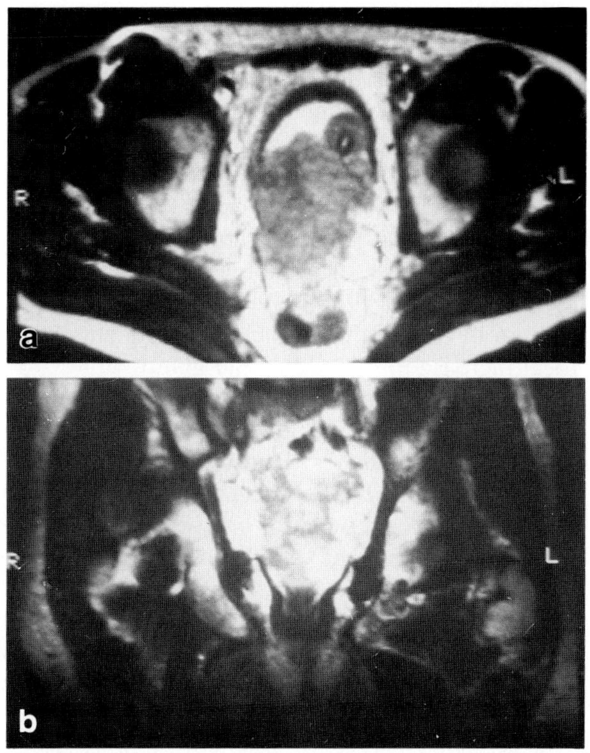

Fig. 19.14a,b. Pelvic MRI. Carcinoma of the prostate invading the seminal vesicles. **a** Axial T1, TR 600, TE 12; **b** coronal T2, TR 2000, TE 80

19.6.2 Primary Tumors

Primary tumors of the seminal vesicles are extremely rare and are either malignant or benign. The benign ones are shown as a sharply defined mass within the seminal vesicles, with a smooth outline.

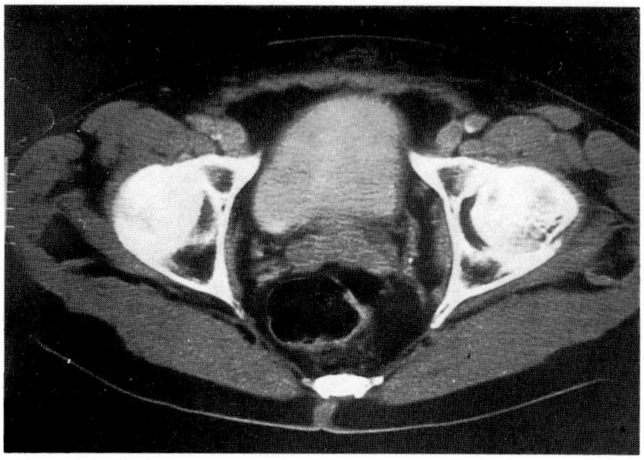

Fig. 19.15. CT of the pelvis. Bladder carcinoma invading the seminal vesicles, indicated by some low attenuation foci, particularly on the *left*

Carcinoma is the most common primary tumor; others include cystadenoma and benign and malignant mesenchymal tumors. It is usually difficult to establish the diagnosis of primary carcinoma of the seminal vesicle without surgery, and differential diagnosis includes invasion of the seminal vesicle by prostatic tumor (KAWAHARA et al. 1988). Primary tumor is considered when no associated bladder or prostatic mass is identified (SUSSMAN et al. 1986). On CT a primary carcinoma of the seminal vesicle shows a mass or a focal increase in the size of the gland.

Primary tumors show medium signal intensity on T1-weighted images and low signal intensity on T2-weighted images. This is because the tumor tissue that replaces the gland has a lower water content. The glands may be asymmetrically enlarged due to seminal vesicle obstruction.

Acknowledgments. The author is indebted to Drs. José Miguel Martins, Ma da Graça Correia, Nuno Jalles Tavares, and Joäo Franco for the loan of some of the case material.

References

Abbitt PL, Watson L, Howards S (1991) Abnormalities of the seminal tract causing infertility: diagnosis with endorectal sonography. AJR 157:337–340

Abe M, Watanabe H, Kojima M et al. (1989) Puncture of the seminal vesicles guided by transrectal real-time linear scanner. JCU 17:173–175

Alpern MB, Dorfman RE, Gross BH, Gottlieb CA, Sandler MA (1991) Seminal vesicle cysts: association with adult polycystic disease. Radiology 180:79–80

Asch MR, Toi A (1991) Seminal vesicles: imaging and intervention using transrectal ultrasound. J US Med 10:19–23

Bahn DK, Brown RKJ, Shei KY et al. (1990) Sonographic findings of leiomyoma in the seminal vesicle. JCU 18:517–520

Bezzi M, Kressel HY, Allen KS et al. (1988) Prostatic carcinoma staging with MR imaging at 1.5T. Radiology 169:339–346

Biondetti PR, Lee JKT, Ling D et al. (1987) Clinical stage B prostatic carcinoma: staging with MR imaging. Radiology 162:325–329

Carter SSC, Shinohara K, Lipshultz LI (1989) Transrectal ultrasonography in disorders of the seminal vesicles and ejaculatory ducts. Urol Clin North Am 16:773–789

Colfi GM, Zanollo CA, Ballerin G et al. (1987) Functional voiding disturbances of the ampullo-vesicular seminal tract: cause of male infertility. Acta Eur Fertil 18:165

Dunnick NR, Ford K, Osborne D et al. (1982) Seminal vesiculography: limited value in vesiculitis. Urology 20:454–457

Gevenois PA, Van Sinoy ML, Sintzoff SA Jr et al. (1990) Cyst of the prostate and seminal vesicles. AJR 155: 1021–1024

Goldwasser BZ, Weinerth JL, Carson CC III (1985) Ejaculatory duct obstruction: the case for aggressive diagnosis and treatment. J Urol 134:964

Heaney JA, Pfister RC, Meares EJ Jr (1987) Giant cyst of the seminal vesicle with renal agenesis. AJR 149:139

Higgins C, Hricak H, Helms C (1992) Magnetic resonance imaging of the body, 2nd edn. Raven, New York, pp 930–936

Jewett HJ, Eggleston JC, Yawn DH (1972) Radical prostatectomy in the management of carcinoma of the prostate: probable cause of some therapeutic failures. J Urol 107:1034

Kawahara M, Matsuhashi M, Tajima M et al. (1988) Primary carcinoma of seminal vesicle. Diagnosis assisted by sonography. Uroradiology 32:269–272

King BF, Hattery RR, Lieber MM et al. (1989) Seminal vesicle imaging. Radiographics 4:653–676

King BF, Hattery RR, Lieber MM, Berquist TO, Williamson B Jr, Hartman GW (1991) Congenital cystic disease of the seminal vesicle. Radiology 178:207–211

Kneeland BJ, Auh YH, MacCarron JP et al. (1985) Computed tomography, sonography, vesiculography and MR imaging of seminal vesicle cyst. JCAT 9:964–966

Lierse W (1984) Applied anatomy of the pelvis. Springer, Berlin Heidelberg New York, pp 169–170

Littrup PS, Lee F, MacLeary RD et al. (1988) Transrectal US of the seminal vesicles and ejaculatory ducts: clinical correlation. Radiology 168:625–628

Martin JF, Hajek P, Beker L et al. (1988) Inflatable surface coil for MR imaging of the prostate. Radiology 167:228–232

Mears EM (1986) Prostatitis and related disorders. In: Walsh PC, Gittes RF, Perlmutter AD et al. (1986) Campbell's urology. W.B. Saunders, Philadelphia, pp 868–885

Rholl SK, Lee JKT, Ling V et al. (1987) MR imaging of the scrotum with high resolution surface coil. Radiology 163:99–103

Ritchey MI, Benson RC, Kramer SA, Kelalis PP (1988) Management of muellerian duct remnants in the male patient. J Urol 140:795

Rochoborn CG, Scheineder HJ, Rugenderf EW et al. (1986) Embryological and diagnostic aspects of seminal vesicle tract malformations. J Urol 135:1029–1032

Scardino PT, Shinohara K, Wheeler TM et al. (1989) Staging of prostate cancer, value of ultrasonography. Urol Clin North Am 16:713–733

Secaf E, Nuruddin RN, Hricak H, MaClure RD, Demar B (1991) MR imaging of the seminal vesicles. AJR 156: 989–994

Sue DE, Chicola C, Brant-Zawadzki MN et al. (1989) MR imaging in seminal vesiculitis. JCAT 13:662–665

Sussman SK, Dunnick NR, Silverman PM et al. (1986) Carcinoma of the seminal vesicle: CT appearance. JCAT 10:519–520

Terris MK, McNeal JE, Stamey PA (1990) Invasion of the seminal vesicles by prostatic cancer: detection with transrectal sonography. AJR 155:811–815

Thurner S, Hricak H, Tanagho EA (1988) Muellerian duct cyst: diagnosis with MR imaging. Radiology 168:25–28

Villers AA, MacNeal JE, Redwine EA et al. (1990) Pathogenesis and biological significance of seminal vesicle invasion in prostatic adenocarcinoma. J Urol 143:1183–1187

Witten DM, Myers GH, Utz DC (1977) Clinical urography, 4th edn. W.B. Saunders, Philadelphia, p 76

Zinner A (1914) Ein Fall von intravesikaler Samenblasenzyste. Wien Med Wochenschr 64:605–676

Subject Index

List of Contributors

E. STEPHEN AMIS, Jr., M.D.
Professor and Chairman
Department of Radiology
Albert Einstein College of Medicine
and Montefiore Medical Center
111 East 210th Street
Bronx, NY 10467, USA

W. ANZBÖCK, M.D.
Institut für Röntgendiagnostik
Danubehospital, Sozialmedizinisches Zentrum Ost
Langobardenstraße 122
1220 Wien, Austria

LAWRENCE R. BIGONGIARI, M.D.
Clinical Associate Professor
1554 North Gatewood Court
Wichita, KS 67206, USA
formerly: Department of Radiology
St. Francis Regional Medical Center
University of Kansas
Medical School of Wichita
929 North Street Francis Street
Wichita, KS 67214, USA

KYOUNG-SIK CHO, M.D.
Associate Professor of Radiology
Asan Medical Center
University of Ulsan
388-1 Poongnap-Dong
Songpa-Ku
Seoul 138-040, Korea

ENRICO J. DOGANIERO, D.O.
Instructor of Radiology
Department Radiologic Sciences
PCOM, Graduate Health System
City Avenue Hospital
4150 City Avenue
Philadelphia, PA 19131, USA

GERALD W. FRIEDLAND, M.D.
Professor Emeritus of Radiology
790 Center Drive
Palo Alto, CA 94301-3009, USA
formerly: Chief, Radiology Service
Veterans Administration Medical Center
3801 Miranda Avenue
Palo Alto, CA 94304, USA

PEGGY F. FRITZSCHE, M.D.
Professor of Radiology
Loma Linda University, Medical Center
Schuman Pavilion, 11234 Anderson Street
Loma Linda, CA 92354, USA

WALTER HRUBY, M.D.
Professor and Chairman
Institut für Röntgendiagnostik
Danubehospital, Sozialmedizinisches Zentrum Ost
Langobardenstraße 122
1220 Wien, Austria

BARBARA HSU, M.D.
Sharp Rees-Stealy Medical
2001 Fourth Avenue
San Diego, CA 92101, USA

WOLFGANG KRAMPLA, M.D.
Institut für Röntgendiagnostik
Danubehospital, Sozialmedizinisches Zentrum Ost
Langobardenstraße 122
1220 Wien, Austria

ERICH K. LANG, M.D.
Professor and Chairman
Department of Radiology, School of Medicine
Louisiana State University, Medical Center
1542 Tulane Avenue
New Orleans, LA 70122-2822, USA

HOWARD M. LEVY, M.D.
Christina Hospital
Medical Center of Delaware
4755 Ogletown-Stanton Road
Newark, DE 19718, USA

ROBERT M. MATTREY, M.D.
Professor of Radiology
Magnetic Resonance Institute (8756)
UCSD Medical Center
410 West Arbor Drive
San Diego, CA 92103, USA

RONALD W. MCCALLUM, M.D., F.R.C.P. (C), F.A.C.R
Professor of Radiology, Radiologist-in-Chief
Department of Diagnostic Imaging
St. Michael's Hospital
University of Toronto
30 Bond Street
Toronto, Ontario M5B 1W8, Canada

REID M. MORSE, M. D.
Resident in Urology
Case Western Reserve University
School of Medicine
Cleveland, OH 44106, USA

DAVID S. MOSS, M. D.
Assistant Professor of Radiology
Department of Radiology
Columbia Presbyterian Medical Center
622 West 168th Street
New York, NY 10032, USA

H. MOSSER, M. D.
Institut für Röntgendiagnostik
Danubehospital, Sozialmedizinisches Zentrum Ost
Langobardenstraße 122
1220 Wien, Austria

JOSEPH ORTENBERG, M. D., F. A. A. P.
Associate Professor
Department of Urology and Pediatrics
LSU Medical Center, School of Medicine
Louisiana State University
1542 Tulane Avenue
New Orleans, LA 70112-2822, USA

JANET A. PARKER, M. D.
Professor of Radiology
Department Radiologic Sciences
PCOM, Graduate Health System
City Avenue Hospital
4150 City Avenue
Philadelphia, PA 19131, USA

INDER PERKASH, M. D.
Chief, Spinal Cord Injury Service
Veterans Administration, Medical Center
3801 Miranda Avenue
Palo Alto, CA 94304, USA

JOÃO MARTINS PISCO, M. D.
Professor da Faculdade de Ciência Médicas
Director de Servico de Radiologia
Hospital de Santa Marta
Rua de Santa Marta
1100 Lisboa, Portugal

GEORGE L. POPKY, M. D.
Professor and Chairman
Department Radiologic Sciences
PCOM, Graduate Health System
City Avenue Hospital
4150 City Avenue
Philadelphia, PA 19131, USA

MARTIN I. RESNICK, M. D.
Lester Persky Professor of Urology
Chairman, Department of Urology
University Hospitals of Cleveland
2074 Abington Road
Cleveland, OH 44106, USA

LINDA M. SANDERS, M. D.
Department of Radiology
Saint Barnabas Medical Center
Old Short Hill Road
Livingston, NJ 07039

GEORGE M. SEGALL, M. D.
Assistant Chief
Nuclear Medicine Service
Veterans Administration, Medical Center
3801 Miranda Avenue
Palo Alto, CA 94304, USA

DAVID B. SPRING, M. D.
Associate Professor
Department of Radiology
Kaiser Permanente Medical Center
The Permanente Medical Group, Inc.
280 West MacArthur Boulevard
Oakland, CA 94611-5693, USA

M. URBAN, M. D.
Institut für Röntgendiagnostik
Danubehospital, Sozialmedizinisches Zentrum Ost
Langobardenstraße 122
1220 Wien, Austria

J. CHRISTIAN WINTERS, M. D.
Resident in Urology
LSU/Ochsner Program, LSU Medical Center
School of Medicine, Louisiana State University
1542 Tulane Avenue
New Orleans, LA 70112-2822, USA

HILARY ZARNOW, M. D., M. S.
Clinical Associate Professor
Department of Urology
St. Francis Regional Medical Center
University of Kansas, Medical School at Wichita
929 North Street Francis Street
Wichita, KS 67214, USA

MEDICAL RADIOLOGY – Diagnostic Imaging and Radiation Oncology

Titles in the series already published

Lung Cancer
Edited by C. W. SCARANTINO

Innovations in Radiation Oncology
Edited by H. R. WITHERS and L. J. PETERS

Radiation Therapy of Head and Neck Cancer
Edited by G. E. LARAMORE

Gastrointestinal Cancer – Radiation Therapy
Edited by R. R. DOBELBOWER, Jr.

Radiation Exposure and Occupational Risks
Edited by E. SCHERER, C. STREFFER, and K.-R. TROTT

Radiation Therapy of Benign Diseases – A Clinical Guide
S. E. ORDER and S. S. DONALDSON

Innovations in Diagnostic Imaging
Edited by J. H. ANDERSON

Interventional Radiation Therapy Techniques – Brachytherapy
Edited by R. SAUER

Radiopathology of Organs and Tissues
Edited by E. SCHERER, C. STREFFER, and K.-R. TROTT

Concomitant Continuous Infusion Chemotherapy and Radiation
Edited by M. ROTMAN and C. J. ROSENTHAL

Radiology of the Upper Urinary Tract
Edited by E. K. LANG

Intraoperative Radiotherapy – Clinical Experiences and Results
Edited by F. A. CALVO, M. SANTOS, and L. W. BRADY

The Thymus – Diagnostic Imaging, Functions, and Pathologic Anatomy
Edited by E. WALTER, E. WILLICH, and W. R. WEBB

Radiotherapy of Intraocular and Orbital Tumors
Edited by W. E. ALBERTI and R. H. SAGERMAN

Interstitial and Intracavitary Thermoradiotherapy
Edited by M. H. SEEGENSCHMIEDT and R. SAUER

Interventional Neuroradiology
Edited by A. VALAVANIS

Non-Disseminated Breast Cancer Controversial Issues in Management
Edited by G. H. FLETCHER and S. H. LEVITT

Current Topics in Clinical Radiobiology of Tumors
Edited by H.-P. BECK-BORNHOLDT

Practical Approaches to Cancer Invasion and Metastases:
A Compendium of Radiation Oncologists' Responses to 40 Histories
Edited by A. R. KAGAN with the Assistance of R. J. STECKEL

Radiology of the Pancreas
Edited by A. L. BAERT, co-edited by G. DELORME

Radiation Therapy in Pediatric Oncology
Edited by J. R. CASSADY

Radiology of the Lower Urinary Tract
Edited by E. K. LANG

Radiation Therapy Physics
Edited by A. R. SMITH